Planning Your Career in Alternative Medicine

Planning Your Career in

In memory of
Gerard Boulrice
1925–1999

Acknowledgments

~~~~~~

It is very dangerous to go into eternity with possibilities which one has oneself prevented from becoming realities. A possibility is a hint from God. One must follow it.
—SØREN KIERKEGAARD

I THANK the Lord for giving me this mission—it's been a book well worth doing. I'm grateful to have had the opportunity to help prospective students find their calling, and help some struggling schools find their students. Though none of us is making a killing—or even a living!—on this project, it's been a valuable and rewarding experience just the same.

The letters I've received from readers have helped me realize just how important a resource this is. I thank all of you who took the time to write or e-mail; keep 'em coming.

A big thank-you to the good people at the schools and organizations who updated their listings (many of them twice) promptly, neatly, and without nagging—and a great big bear hug to those who made me laugh or were gushingly grateful. (Those of you who had to be nagged four or five times for information get a "Needs Improvement.")

Thanks to the husband and kids—Bub, Scotto, and Neen Bean—for ongoing support and remarkable tolerance for a steady diet of pizza and nachos. You guys are the best!

For keeping me sane, a warm fuzzy thanks to Liz Frenette; there is no better friend on the planet. You are what everyone ought to be: kind, compassionate, patient, thoughtful, tolerant, incredibly nice. Well—opposites attract.

Thanks to Ma, Krazy Karen, and Marloon—the family that never lets me forget that I'm a writer, not a housewife. (Though the melon-sized dustballs are also a reminder.)

To Kooie, Elmo, and Nikki—especially Nikki—thanks for keeping the lap warm while I write. And not biting. Much.

And a big thank-you to all the people at Avery—particularly Rudy Shur, who believed in this book wholeheartedly despite its limited profit potential. Some things are more important than making a buck; Rudy saw the significance of this project and made certain that it was not only the first, but the best of its kind. I wish you much success, Rudy, in your new ventures.

Contents

~~~~~~

Preface to the First Edition   ix

Preface to the Second Edition   xi

How to Use This Book   xiii

How Schools Are Selected   xvii

Introduction   xxi

PART ONE:
Understanding the Fields of Alternative Medicine   1

Acupuncture and Oriental Medicine   3

Aromatherapy   4

Ayurveda   5

Biofeedback   7

Chiropractic   8

Energetic Healing   9

Environmental Medicine   9

Guided Imagery   10

Herbal Medicine   11

Holistic Health Practitioner/
Holistic Health Education/Holistic Counseling   12

Holistic Nursing   13

Homeopathy   13

Hypnotherapy   14

Integrative Medicine   15

Iridology   15

Massage Therapy and Bodywork   16

Midwifery   22

Naprapathy   23

Naturopathy   23

Nutrition   24

Polarity Therapy   26

Reflexology   27

Vedic Psychology   27

Veterinary Massage   28

Yoga   28

PART TWO:
The Schools and Programs of Alternative Medicine   31

Choosing a School or Program   33

Listing of Programs by Field   34

Profiles of Schools and Programs   49

United States   49

  Arizona   49

  Arkansas   59

  California   59

  Colorado   129

  Connecticut   144

  District of Columbia   149

  Florida   150

  Georgia   168

  Hawaii   173

  Idaho   178

  Illinois   179

  Indiana   186

  Iowa   188

  Kansas   191

  Louisiana   191

Maine   191
Maryland   195
Massachusetts   198
Michigan   208
Minnesota   217
Mississippi   222
Missouri   222
Montana   226
Nebraska   227
Nevada   228
New Hampshire   229
New Jersey   230
New Mexico   242
New York   253
North Carolina   272
Ohio   276
Oklahoma   282
Oregon   283
Pennsylvania   295
Rhode Island   304
South Carolina   305
Tennessee   306
Texas   309
Utah   320
Vermont   322
Virginia   325
Washington   334
West Virginia   348
Wisconsin   349

Canada   353
Alberta   353
British Columbia   359
Ontario   366
Quebec   382
Saskatchewan   383

Multiple State Locations   383
United States   383
Canada   420

Appendices   425

**Accrediting Agencies and
Councils on Education   427**

Licensing and Certification   435

**Professional Associations and
Membership Organizations   445**

Self-Study Resources   462

**Conventional and Osteopathic Medical Schools
Offering Courses in Alternative Medicine   496**

Bibliography   503
Notes   511
Index   514

Preface to the First Edition

I find the medicine worse than the malady.
—JOHN FLETCHER, 1579-1625

OVER THE COURSE of my life, more often than not I have indeed found the medicine—allopathic medicine, that is—worse than the malady. As a child, a botched tonsillectomy left me with memories of terrifying, whirling sounds—an early part of the near-death experience, I'm told—not to mention another surgery six months later to finish the job. My adult medical experiences weren't much better—migraine medications that made me sicker than the migraine itself, and birth control pills that left me depressed.

What pushed me into alternative medicine, however, was my allergist. The doctor was concerned because I couldn't get past a particular vial in my immunotherapy; all her patients were supposed to go from vial one to vial three, and I couldn't get past vial two without massive welts. "But my dust mite allergies are controlled at this dose," I told her. "It doesn't matter," she said. "We need to push you up to the higher level." Five minutes after the shot, I had my first panic attack. Epinephrine stopped the reaction, but the "rain barrel" had already overflowed; from that point on, the bedroom carpet, grass, sulfites, dust mites, formaldehyde in stores, and almost anything else would cause extreme anxiety, shortness of breath, or swelling in my throat that made it nearly impossible to swallow. The turning point, though, was when the allergist declared that what I really needed was psychological help; I was producing these attacks myself, she said, from memories of the first one. At that point, I knew our association was over; as I left her office, my quest for health began.

Shortly after this, I read a newspaper article about Dr. Theron Randolph's clinic for the chemically sensitive. Dr. Randolph's pioneering work in clinical ecology, or environmental illness, seemed to be just what I was looking for. I went to the clinic, underwent weeks of testing, and found the correct doses of antigens for my specific allergies. I started a program of antigens, dietary changes, and vitamin and mineral supplements that had me feeling much better in a matter of weeks, and completely well in about a year.

Once I was well, I was so excited about what I had learned that I wanted to see what kinds of courses I could take in nutrition, herbology, and related alternative fields so that I might further help myself and others as well. I searched the library, *Books in Print,* anywhere I could think of, but I found no guide to educational programs in alternative medicine. Any writer, upon finding a gap, seeks immediately to fill it—and I'm doing just that with this book.

This is a book that is just as useful to serious students of alternative medicine—the would-be acupuncturists and naturopathic physicians—as it is to the individual who simply wants a better understanding of alternative therapies to treat family and friends. It is practical as a quick reference tool—for finding phone numbers, for example—and it is a good book to spend some time with, investigating schools within commuting distance or correspondence courses in various fields of interest. In fact, I couldn't wait to be finished writing it so that I might have time to take some classes myself! Like most of you,

I am a beginner, and very eager to learn; this book will help all of us to take more responsibility for our own health and to share our knowledge with others.

While I have tried hard to make this book as accurate and inclusive as possible, it does have its limitations (many of which are spelled out in the section "How Schools Are Selected"). As fast as we try to get this printed, area codes are changing, schools are moving, and programs are being restructured. I did the best I could to capture the alternative health education movement at a moment in time, but some changes will have occurred by the time this book reaches the stores. But while tuition has probably gone up a few dollars and a program may have been added, this book serves as a reliable, quick, and painless way to compare programs, tuition, accreditations, and so on, without ever leaving your home.

This is the first edition of a book that I plan to update and revise on a regular basis, and your input is an important part of making the next edition better. I want to know what you think. If I overlooked a program that you attended and found beneficial, send me the address. If I missed a professional organiza-

tion that has an informative newsletter, tell me about it. Likewise, if a school or program listed here was unsatisfactory to you, let me know that, too.

If you represent a school that should have been included (according to the criteria on page xvii) and wasn't, send a catalog and I may consider you for the next edition. Similarly, if you're a publisher who would like your books, catalogs, videos, or magazines mentioned next time, send them along for review.

I want this to be as complete and useful a guide as possible, and I sincerely welcome your input. Send inquiries, suggestions, catalogs, review copies, and other information to:

Dianne Lyons
c/o Avery
Penguin Putnam Inc.
375 Hudson Street
New York, NY 10014
dianneJBL@aol.com

Preface to the Second Edition

ONLY A COUPLE of years have passed since the first edition, and already so much has changed. Schools are growing like crazy; many more have moved to larger quarters than have closed their doors, and keeping up with all the change in this growing field is a bear. A few trends I've noticed:

- *The continued mainstreaming of alternative medicine.* Community colleges have programs in herbal medicine and massage therapy; greater numbers of conventional medical schools offer courses in alternative health care; you can go to the mall for a chair massage and the supplement of the month; and even my straightlaced gynecologist (Dr. Robert Olney—there's a plug) is pushing soy. It's everywhere!

- *The beefing up of educational standards.* As alternative therapies become more accepted, there are more unscrupulous people out to make a quick buck at the consumer's expense. Accrediting agencies and licensing bureaus are increasing the standards for schools and practitioners; even since the first edition, licensing laws in some states have gotten tougher, and agencies have formed to create laws in previously unregulated states. While some argue that this puts unnecessary restrictions on alternative therapists, I think it only adds to the professionalism of the field. Schools are adding hours, states are demanding testing—this is a good thing. I'm not getting naked for a guy with two weeks' training.

- *The competition!* When it came out, *Planning Your Career in Alternative Medicine* was the first and only guide of its kind;

now there are at least two others that offer essentially the same information (only now, mine is more current!). The solution to this is simple: buy mine! But, seriously—we're in this as a team, not as competitors. The more people we reach, the more people we can guide into alternative health care careers, the better our chances of coming up with natural solutions to everyday health problems, and the better our chances of leading full, productive, healthy lives. But . . . do buy mine.

So search through this book for the program that stirs your heart; I promise there'll be some very interesting people along your path. And keep in touch! Schools, students, prospective students, publishers, and people with large sums of money who'd like to reward me for my efforts can all reach me at this address:

Dianne J. B. Lyons
c/o Avery
Penguin Putnam Inc.
375 Hudson Street
New York, NY 10014
Email: dianneJBL@aol.com

Enjoy the journey.

How to Use This Book

THIS GUIDE is divided into two major sections. Part I contains short articles that briefly describe the history, philosophy, and treatments used in each field of study. Part II makes up the bulk of the book; it lists, alphabetically by state and within each state, schools that offer degree or certificate programs in various fields of alternative medicine. The key to finding the school you need is the Listing of Programs by Field, located on page 34.

THE LISTING OF PROGRAMS BY FIELD AND PROFILES OF SCHOOLS AND PROGRAMS

Many schools offer instruction in more than one subject area. Rather than listing schools by subjects offered—which would result in many duplications—we opted for the Listing of Programs by Field.

This section simplifies the task of finding programs of interest: just look under the desired field of study and you'll find an alphabetical, state-by-state listing of programs available. Scan the list for a state that you're interested in, check the name of the school, and locate its listing under that state in the Profiles of Schools and Programs. It's easy: to find schools of Ayurveda, look in the Listing of Programs by Field for "Ayurveda." The listing is reproduced below.

AYURVEDA

CALIFORNIA
California College of Ayurveda
Mount Madonna Center

COLORADO
Rocky Mountain Institute of Yoga and Ayurveda

MASSACHUSETTS
East West Institute of Alternative Medicine
International Ayurvedic Institute

NEW MEXICO
The Ayurvedic Institute

NEW YORK
Ayurveda Holistic Center

To read about The Ayurvedic Institute, find New Mexico in the Profiles section, then scan the alphabetical list of schools until you locate The Ayurvedic Institute.

There are several points to remember about the Listing of Programs by Field and the Profiles of Schools and Programs.

- The schools listed in this part of the book are all classroom-based programs; correspondence courses are listed in Self-Study Resources beginning on page 462.

- Entries are made under each specialty only for complete programs that result in a certificate, degree, or other credential relating to that specialty. Modalities that are taught as part of a larger specialty are not listed separately. For example, many schools of massage therapy offer instruction in polarity, reflexology, and aromatherapy, but they are listed only under Massage Therapy unless a separate, distinct certificate or program is also given in the subspecialty.

- Many of the terms used in the program descriptions are defined in the corresponding Part I chapter. For example, terms such as shiatsu, Rolfing, hydrotherapy, and Feldenkrais are defined in the Part I chapter on massage therapy.

- Canadian schools appear after the United States entries, alphabetized by province. Schools that offer instruction in many locations throughout the United States, Canada, and/or the world are listed in the section called "Multiple State Locations," which appears after the Canada section.

Reading the Listings

The listings for the various schools and programs are fairly self-explanatory. Each listing contains the school's name, address(es), phone number, fax number, e-mail address, and Internet address (URL) where applicable. Following this information is a general introduction to the school, including number of instructors and average or maximum class size, followed by as many of the following categories as apply: Accreditation, Program Description, Community and/or Continuing Education, Admission Requirements, Tuition and Fees, and Financial Assistance.

Each school or program was contacted at least twice: once to add or update its listing, and again to proofread it just prior to publication. We tried to keep some consistency between listings and worked to fit all sorts of programs into a single format; apologies to those schools that wrote lengthy listings that were subsequently hacked to pieces.

Accreditation

Prospective students should acquaint themselves with the principal accrediting agencies in their selected area of study. If the big-name accreditations are missing in a listing (i.e., COMTA, ACAOM, APTA), look carefully at what *is* included. Sometimes a school refuses to be locked in by the requirements of the accrediting agency; sometimes the program is too short or too new to meet the standards. A shorter program is virtu-

ally assured of being sufficient for licensing in the state in which it resides, but it may not be in yours; check first.

In general, if a school is accredited by one of the recognized agencies, the less important approvals are omitted; if a school is not accredited, it may list a lengthy series of lesser certifications or approvals. Don't assume that a longer list is better; in many cases, the reverse is true.

Other details that may be, but are not always, included in this section are facts about licensing, eligibility for certification exams and for membership in professional organizations, and other related information.

Program Description

Every listing, no matter how small, contains this section. Included here is a brief description of the programs offered: program name, the length of the programs (in hours and months wherever possible), course titles and/or details about the curriculum, and certain additional requirements for graduation (such as having five polarity sessions or receiving two massages per semester). Be sure to get the catalog for a more complete description of the program and individual courses.

Community and/or Continuing Education

Community education means classes or programs that are open to the public for entry-level instruction—for example, a weekend of massage or one-day herb seminars. *Continuing education* courses or programs offer advanced levels of training to practicing professionals or those who have completed a basic program.

Admission Requirements

Every applicant should expect to submit a completed application form, high school and/or college transcripts, and often a photo. What's listed in this section are additional requirements. Students should, of course, consult with an admissions representative if any of the requirements presents a problem.

Tuition and Fees

Schools were asked to supply 1999 or 2000 figures. As nothing changes more often than tuition and fees, these numbers should be viewed only as a basis for comparison between schools or for rough budgeting. Again, consult the school's current catalog or website or call the school directly for the most accurate figures.

Financial Assistance

Many, if not most, schools will take VISA or MasterCard—a simple, though usually high-interest, way to finance your education. All of them will take cash or checks. This section lists other forms of financial assistance for which you may qualify. Some of these—like payment plans—are usually open to everyone; others, like veterans benefits, are not. The underlying assumption for federal, provincial, and other forms of financial aid is "if eligible"; even though a school offers grants, that doesn't mean you'll qualify for one.

If you think you'll need assistance in paying for your education, you should speak directly with a financial aid representative at each school you're considering. Don't let a lack of funds keep you from a career; most schools will work very hard to find a way for qualified students to attend, even if they haven't listed financial aid of any kind.

MULTIPLE STATE LOCATIONS

This section lists schools that offer instruction in many locations throughout the United States, Canada, and/or the world. These schools are cross-referenced in the state-by-state listings based on their mailing addresses or the locations of their headquarters.

THE APPENDICES

Before spending thousands of dollars on a program, it's smart to learn as much as you can about both the field of study and the school. Naturally, you should contact potential schools for a catalog, but other organizations can provide important additional information about licensing requirements, accreditation standards, and career options. The appendices in this book show you where to go for more info.

Accrediting Agencies and Councils on Education lists the names and addresses of agencies that accredit, approve, or recommend schools or programs within schools. It gives a very brief description of the accrediting agency and some of the criteria they use to accredit or approve schools. You may want to contact these agencies about a particular program you have in mind.

Licensing and Certification gives only a general description of the types of laws and licensing requirements that are currently in place for a number of fields of alternative medicine.

New to this edition are suggested websites that provide licensing and regulatory information for the various fields. Even so, students are strongly urged to contact the appropriate boards or licensing agencies in the state and city in which they intend to practice prior to putting down a deposit on any educational program.

Professional Associations and Membership Organizations lists just some of the hundreds of organizations that cater to the needs of practicing professionals, students, and interested individuals. These organizations can be a valuable resource for newsletters, pamphlets, current research, referrals, and other information about the field.

Self-Study Resources provides a listing, arranged alphabetically by specialty, of catalogs, videos, correspondence courses, and other materials that offer basic instruction, serve as handy reference sources, offer a unique perspective, or provide ongoing education.

The correspondence programs listed should, in most cases, be considered an introduction to a field of study and not as preparation for a career. Programs that appeared suspect (i.e., those that offer Ph.D.s, N.D.s, or other advanced degrees through the mail) were not included in this guide. Even so, you need to closely scrutinize any home-study program and be honest about your ultimate goal. Correspondence courses can be valuable for learning how to treat oneself or one's family with nutrients or herbs, but those who are preparing for a career should really look into classroom training.

Think about this: would you rather be treated by a nutritionist who studied at an accredited and highly regarded school, or one who received a "degree" through the mail—and paid his sister to write his papers? Additionally, in most fields, licensing will be impossible with a correspondence-school education.

CONVENTIONAL MEDICAL SCHOOLS OFFERING COURSES IN ALTERNATIVE MEDICINE

As alternative (or complementary) medicine becomes more accepted, more and more conventional medical schools are including alternative medicine in their curriculums. In most cases, these schools offer only one or two courses, but some, such as the University of Arizona's Program in Integrative Medicine (see page 52), offer more complete programs.

THE SCHOOL AND ORGANIZATION INDEX

An alternative way to use this book, if you know a school's name but not its location, is to go directly to the School and Organization Index for a page number. This is also useful when you don't know whether a given institution is a school, an accrediting or certifying agency, or a membership organization.

LET THE BUYER BEWARE

In collecting information for this book, we tried to include only schools that are accredited, approved, or in some way recognized by an independent agency, but some fields of study are as yet so unregulated that this is simply impossible. You, the prospective student, are ultimately responsible for investigating the quality of the program you choose. What's beneficial to one person may be worthless to another, and inclusion in this book should not be construed as a personal recommendation.

Prospective students of alternative health care should be at least as careful in their selection of a school or training program as they would be in choosing a conventional college. But it's not a situation where you have to cross your fingers and hope for the best; there are guideposts along the way. The following are a few steps to getting a good return on your educational investment:

- Do some reading and educate yourself in the area in which you plan to specialize. Get a feel for the principles and philosophy, the diagnostic and treatment methods, and the job opportunities.

- Go for a treatment. There's no better way to find out what an acupuncturist, massage therapist, or naturopathic physician really does than to become a patient. Visit more than one practitioner for a broader view.

- Contact your local Board of Health or other agencies to determine the licensing requirements in your city. In many states, a specific number of hours of education are required to practice.

- Talk to practitioners in your area to see which schools they would recommend. Ask them about specific schools you have in mind.

- Send for catalogs from lots of schools. Compare programs between schools in your immediate area, and if circumstances permit, consider a longer commute or a relocation; convenience should not necessarily be your first criterion.

- Look at accreditations. In general, a school must be fairly well established, offer a quality program, and pass an on-site inspection to be approved by the major accrediting agencies.

- Compare program lengths. A 100-hour massage program will have you practicing before the month's out, but what will you learn? Be sure the training is sufficient to meet your future needs. That 100-hour program won't get you licensed in very many cities.

- Look at the course schedules and start dates. Some programs may be taken part-time and/or in the evenings; others are strictly full-time days. Some programs start four times per year, some just once a year or every two years.

- If finances are an issue, see what type of financial assistance the school offers. There is tremendous variation between schools in this area; one may offer scholarships, federal grants, and a variety of loans, while another may not have so much as a payment plan.

- Visit the school and get a feel for the place. Is it a warm, close-knit community or does it offer a cooler, more professional atmosphere? Which makes you more comfortable? Talk to the instructors and other students. If you can, speak with practitioners and ask how well their training prepared them for a career.

Please keep in mind that while all the information contained within this guide was accurate at press time—and that every school or program was given the opportunity to update their listing prior to publication—things change very quickly in this field. Schools outgrow their facilities, add or replace programs, become accredited, increase tuition; associations move, newsletters cease publication, telephone numbers and e-mail addresses change. This book is a general guide to what's out there and a basis for comparison between schools and programs—but always contact the schools directly before making any final decisions.

In work, do what you enjoy.
—LAO-TZU

How Schools Are Selected

A BOOK this size could not possibly contain every school or program offered in every form of alternative health care. Though alternative health care may seem like an emerging field, there are several hundreds of massage therapy schools alone; if all of these were listed in one volume, along with all the schools in other alternative fields, this would look less like a guide and more like a phone book, with room for little more than names and addresses.

But it's not just about space—it's about quality. Many schools were not included simply because, in the opinion of the author, they just don't offer sufficient training to produce a knowledgeable health care professional. It's legal in some cities to open a massage practice with two weeks' training, but would you want to be treated by that kind of practitioner?

The schools included in this book have been selected according to certain loosely applied criteria. You can count on finding schools accredited by the top agencies: COMTA, CNME, CCE, ACAOM. But some fields, such as herbal medicine or Ayurveda, as yet have no primary accrediting agency, or have several lesser ones, or have highly specific ones (i.e., the accreditation of Chinese herbology schools) that exclude almost everyone. In these cases, a school had only to offer an organized certification program of a healing nature that was at least several days in duration to qualify for inclusion.

The following are the criteria used to select the schools in each of the fields. Keep in mind that these criteria served as general guidelines during the selection process, not hard-and-fast rules.

Note: The selection criteria, loose as they may be, apply only to schools in the United States. Because Canada has fewer accrediting agencies in these fields, Canadian schools need only meet provincial licensing requirements to be included.

Acupuncture and Oriental Medicine

Programs that are accredited by, or are candidates for accreditation with, the Accreditation Commission for Acupuncture and Oriental Medicine (ACAOM) are included.

Ayurveda

There are no accredited programs of instruction in Ayurveda in the United States. A handful of schools offer programs in Ayurveda that may be taken by practitioners licensed in another field who would like to apply Ayurvedic principles to their practice, or as part of a Holistic Health Practitioner curriculum that may also include other modalities, or for treatment of self and family. Because there are so few, any school with an organized program of instruction in Ayurveda was included.

Biofeedback

Schools included here are accredited by the Biofeedback Certification Institute of America (BCIA) and/or offer instructional programs that prepare the student to become BCIA certified.

Chiropractic

All of the chiropractic schools included here are accredited by the Council on Chiropractic Education (CCE).

Herbology

Other than Chinese herbology taught as part of an Oriental medicine program, there is no accreditation in the field of herbal medicine. The programs in existence range from apprenticeships at family-run herb farms to extensive programs in Western, Chinese, and Ayurvedic herbology. Included are schools that offer a certificate program of at least several days' duration; those that offer individual courses not organized into a series or program were not included. It's up to the student to determine which type of program will meet his or her needs.

Homeopathy

Programs accredited by the Council on Homeopathic Education (CHE) or are candidates for accreditation are included. A handful of others are included as well: these are schools of homeopathy that have only recently opened their doors and are too new to be accredited, and/or those that appear to offer a comprehensive educational program. Students need to be clear about their goals and determine whether their expectations (and any legal requirements) will be satisfied by a given program.

Hypnotherapy

The schools listed here are endorsed by the International Medical and Dental Hypnotherapy Association or offer sufficient hours of training for graduates to pass certification exams, which generally require a minimum of 120 hours. There are several hypnotherapy associations that endorse or approve educational programs; none of these are recognized by the federal government as accrediting agencies.

Massage Therapy and Bodywork

With well over 600 massage and bodywork schools in existence, we couldn't include them all. Schools included here are either accredited by the Commission on Massage Training Accreditation (COMTA), the Integrative Massage and Somatic Therapies Accreditation Council (IMSTAC), or a regional or national accrediting agency; are approved by the American Oriental Bodywork Therapy Association (AOBTA) or other organization; or meet the requirements for state licensure *and* offer a program of at least 500 hours in length. Graduates of virtually all of the programs included here are eligible to take the National Certification Examination for Therapeutic Massage and Bodywork (NCETMB), which is used as the licensing exam in several states and is considered an indication of a highly trained massage professional. Be sure the program you select will prepare you to take this exam.

A couple of states still permit massage therapists to practice with only 100 or 300 hours of training, but most states now require at least 500 hours; some require 1,000 hours. We did lose a couple of schools by insisting on a 500-hour program, but by far the majority of schools who had previously offered shorter programs have upgraded them to 500 or more hours since the first edition. It's exciting to see schools staying ahead of licensing laws and most often offering the student even more than is legally required.

A few schools are included that don't meet these general criteria. Some offer continuing education for massage professionals or programs in specialized fields of bodywork, such as Equine Massage, Feldenkrais®, or Hellerwork, and are included regardless of hours because of the specialized nature of the course. Others have qualified for inclusion on other grounds—a polarity therapy or herbal medicine program, for example—and their massage program is described as well.

It is *imperative* that the student be familiar with the licensing laws of his state prior to enrolling in a massage therapy program.

Midwifery

Schools listed here are direct-entry midwifery schools accredited by the Midwifery Education Accreditation Council (MEAC). Certified Nurse-Midwifery programs are not included because there's really nothing alternative about them anymore; CNMs work in conventional settings and train in conventional colleges.

Naturopathy

All four of the schools that are accredited by, or are candidates for accreditation with, the Council on Naturopathic Medical Education (CNME) are included. Schools that offer ND degrees by mail are *not* included.

Polarity Therapy

The American Polarity Therapy Association (APTA) accredits polarity therapy schools and training programs—and there are quite a few. In keeping with the reasoning applied to massage therapy, included here are those schools that are accredited by APTA and that provide training leading to APTA registration as a Registered Polarity Practitioner (R.P.P.), rather than those that offer only Associate Polarity Practitioner (A.P.P.) training. However, an A.P.P.-only school may be included if it offers a program in another field that would qualify it.

Yoga

There is no agency that accredits schools of yoga. The schools included here offer vastly different instructor training programs with vastly different requirements—but all of them offer an organized program of teacher training.

Other

A handful of schools don't seem to fit the above criteria yet are included in this book. They may offer a hard-to-find program, such as iridology, or an independent degree program, in which students can major in virtually any aspect of holistic health. Though you may not see the inherent value of a given program, to someone immersed in the field, it may be filling a critical niche.

HEY, WHY ISN'T MY SCHOOL IN HERE?

If your school is accredited by one of the agencies mentioned above and is not listed in this book, it's likely because of human oversight—either yours or mine. Some schools have been nagged to death and still haven't delivered a catalog or website from which to write a listing, and it's certainly possible (though highly unlikely) that I failed to contact one or two along the line.

Some schools that were in the first edition are absent from this one; a few no longer qualified for inclusion because of a tightening of the criteria, and some never sent back corrections or catalogs despite four or five requests. Some moved and left no forwarding address; some changed names, were absorbed into other schools, or went belly-up.

If your school's not here and you think it should be included in the next edition, send a catalog to my attention. But do bear in mind that I was actively searching for you and didn't find you; how many potential students were also unable to find you and opted for the more visible school instead? Some schools

don't like to be harnessed by the restrictions of the accrediting agencies, but accredited schools get noticed; if you're not accredited, you've at least got to advertise. It seems obvious, but every school, no matter how small, should have a website.

Some schools aren't in here because we left them out on purpose. Schools deliberately excluded are those that:

- Offer advanced degrees (such as M.A., Ph.D., or N.D.) through correspondence. This is the one exclusion that makes people cranky, particularly in the case of N.D. degrees. Regardless of licensing requirements, I think it's important that a distinction be made between practitioners who've put in four years of postgraduate study in anatomy, biochemistry, microbiology, clinical diagnosis, cardiology, obstetrics, and the rest, and those who've taken correspondence courses and had little or, more often, no hands-on clinical training. Regarding master's and Ph.D. degrees through the mail, these are excluded to avoid including diploma mills. With the growing popularity of Internet-based distance learning courses offered by legitimate accredited colleges, we'll have to reassess this exclusion for the next edition; but for now, this is where we draw the line.

- offer only very short programs or single-day courses;

- offer only part of a recognized program (i.e., courses in polarity therapy that are not sufficient for R.P.P. or A.P.P. designation);

- offer training that is primarily of a spiritual nature;

- offer training that is of primary benefit to the individual, rather than training for a career in helping others;

- offer training in an area that is on the fringes of alternative medicine and for which the career prospects are questionable; or

- offer training in an area that is so mainstream that it can no longer be considered "alternative" at all (such as Osteopathy or Certified Nurse-Midwifery).

The most exciting part of the alternative medicine movement is that in time, *all* of the schools will be disqualified under that last provision! The ultimate goal of this book is to make itself obsolete.

Introduction

THE TERM "alternative medicine" is something of a misnomer, but it is one of a handful of terms used in the United States to identify various forms of healing that lie outside of mainstream (allopathic) medicine. Here in the United States, those who graduate from established medical schools and subscribe to conventional healing methods, including the prescribing of controlled medications and the use of surgery for the treatment of disease—the people we refer to as doctors, physicians, or M.D.s—are the norm. All other types of medicine are lumped under the terms "alternative" or "complementary."

What may seem odd to those just beginning to explore these alternative kinds of healing is that some of the philosophies and techniques dismissed by many physicians as quackery—including acupuncture, homeopathy, and herbal medicine—have been the standard way of treating illnesses in other parts of the world for thousands of years. Midwifery has got to be the oldest profession, practiced since Eve helped her daughter give birth, I imagine. The Bible is filled with references to medicinal herbs. Aromatherapy may have been embraced by at least one store in every mall, but it, too, has a long history—the Romans used scented oils in their baths, and Avicenna, a tenth-century Persian doctor, was the first to distill essential oils. Traditional Chinese medicine, including acupuncture, has been around for about 5,000 years. Homeopathy is an established practice in Great Britain today—Queen Elizabeth's medical staff includes a homeopathic physician—and may date back to 3,000 B.C. When compared to these time-honored traditions, our own allopathic medicine looks rather new and, some would argue, suspect.

Not even the most headstrong of alternative practitioners would deny that allopathic medicine has made important contributions to our national health and longevity. Even the most dedicated herbalist would welcome the sight of a skilled surgeon were his appendix to suddenly burst. But the emergence of deadly antibiotic-resistant germs, the lack of attention to disease prevention, and the many illnesses for which no cures have been found all point to a need for another kind of medicine. Alternative medicine seeks not to replace the allopathic tradition but to work alongside it, as partners in the healing process; hence, many now refer to "complementary" rather than "alternative" therapies.

A Chinese proverb nicely summarizes the relationship between alternative and allopathic medicine: "The superior doctor prevents sickness; the mediocre doctor attends to impending sickness; the inferior doctor treats actual sickness."[1] While allopathic medicine focuses on a malfunctioning heart or kidney, alternative approaches look at the whole person—his or her environment, diet, exercise and activities, stress level, and spiritual health. Most forms of alternative medicine focus on the reasons behind the illness; individualize treatment for each patient depending on other physical, mental, emotional, and/or spiritual considerations; and bolster the body that is trying to heal itself, rather than attacking the symptoms of that healing (for example, inflammation or fever). As one naturopathic physician says, "The first thing I tell people is, 'I will be your coach, not your doctor.' My role is to give patients the power of their own healing systems."[2]

Rather than replacing one healing system with another, it is the synthesis of these many fields that will bring American medicine into the twenty-first century. In the future, a trip to the doctor may mean seeing a physician, a naturopath, an herbalist, a homeopath, and/or an acupuncturist—all housed together in one office complex, consulting each other to determine the best course of treatment for the patient.

Actually, a few such holistic treatment centers already exist, but they are the exception rather than the rule. Generally, finding a reputable acupuncturist or herbalist can be a hit-or-miss proposition. Licensing laws vary from state to state, even from county to county; in some states, the acupuncture we feel may help us isn't even legally obtainable. The alternative practitioners we do find are often booked so far in advance that it's impossible to run in for a simple sinus infection with the same short notice we give our M.D.

While the current situation is frustrating for patients, it's a blessing for the student who plans to enter the field. Opportunities are everywhere, as alternative medicine is experiencing tremendous growth and ever-increasing legitimacy. A survey conducted by *The New England Journal of Medicine* in 1993 reported that 34 percent of Americans consulted alternative healers that year, spending nearly $14 billion for their largely uninsured services.[3] Even the United States government is beginning to see the light, as evidenced by the creation of the Office of Alternative Medicine, largely in response to pressure from Congress over the growing costs of health care and the frustrating lack of progress being made in the fight against the likes of AIDS, arthritis, and cancer.

This new way of thinking about age-old remedies presents tremendous opportunities for prospective students of naturopathy, homeopathy, massage therapy, herbal medicine, acupuncture, and other alternative therapies. Interest and acceptance by the public is growing daily, licensing laws are continually being reworked, and training programs are becoming more standardized and sophisticated. It's an exciting time to get involved in alternative medicine.

Let the healing begin.

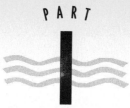

Understanding the Fields
of Alternative Medicine

THIS SECTION offers a brief introduction to some of the various fields of alternative or complementary medicine. The historical background, general philosophy, and treatments used in each field are explained, followed by a discussion of career opportunities as well as general licensing requirements.

While the legal status of a few fields, such as chiropractic, is pretty well established, many if not most of the fields included in this book are in the midst of a legal mess that gets progressively worse as more practitioners set up shop. For example, reflexologists and polarity therapists may practice without restriction in some states, while other states now require that they have a massage therapy license—even though polarity clients are fully clothed, and reflexologists never give a full-body massage. Naturopathy is another messy field, with correspondence-school graduates legally able to use the initials "N.D." after their names in the same way as graduates of a four-year hands-on naturopathic college do. Herbalists, like aromatherapists, iridologists, and lay homeopaths, can and do get into legal hot water for "practicing medicine without a license" by saying the right thing in the wrong way. And

all of it changes almost day to day. It can't be said enough: before enrolling in any school, a student needs to be intimately aware of the legal requirements and regulations in the city and state in which he or she intends to practice.

Accrediting agencies and professional organizations are a good first source for current licensure and regulatory information and are listed in the Appendices section; those whose websites discuss legislative issues are also mentioned here. A few sites discuss the legal status of many alternative fields; one such site is at www.healthy.net/public/legal-lg/regulations. Prospective students would do well to spend time on the Internet, investigating any and all websites pertaining to their field of interest; this will give the student a feel for the diversity of opinion out there and the legal battles that may lie ahead.

Keep in mind that what follows are general descriptions. Since you'll want to familiarize yourself as much as possible with a field of study before committing to it, take a look at the Bibliography on page 503; these recommended books discuss each topic in much greater depth.

ACUPUNCTURE AND ORIENTAL MEDICINE

Oriental medicine, or traditional Chinese medicine (TCM), has been in use for over 3,000 years and is still used by one-fourth of the earth's population.[1] Its emphasis is on prevention—correcting disharmonies and imbalances before they manifest themselves in the form of disease. As the legendary Yellow Emperor of China told doctors, treating a patient when disease had already taken hold is "like digging a well only when one feels thirsty. Is it not already too late?"[2] In traditional Chinese medicine, patients are partners in healing; educating the patient regarding diet, exercise, and relaxation is essential to the cure.

In TCM, the human body is seen as a microcosm of the natural world. The air, sea, and land of the earth correspond to the energy and fluids of the body. Just as the earth can be parched and dry, so can our skin; as rivers can swell and become bloated, so too can our feet or abdomen—hence the references to inner dampness, dryness, heat, or cold. Health is affected by both the internal and external climates, so to remain healthy, we must strive for the three harmonies: harmony with nature (being in tune with the seasons), internal harmony (among the five main organs), and mental and physical harmony (avoiding emotional and physical extremes).[3]

One concept essential to the understanding of traditional Chinese medicine is that of yin and yang. Every event or entity has both a yin and a yang aspect. Yin refers to more permanent states, such as solidity, concreteness, and completion; yang refers to the active component and to more transitional states such as being, moving, changing, and developing.[4] In TCM, yin and yang refer to opposing physical conditions of the body: yin refers to the tissue of an organ, yang to its activity.

Qi, or chi, is a critical concept that is completely absent from Western medicine. Qi is the life force that flows throughout the body along certain prescribed pathways, or meridians, on the skin and through the internal organs. A blockage in the flow of qi can result in illness.

The Five Phase Theory, another important concept in Chinese medicine, holds that each organ either aids or detracts from the functioning of another organ. Ten organs are assigned to the five elements of fire, earth, metal, water, and wood, and, as each element acts on another in particular ways on the earth, so too does each organ act on another organ in pre-

dictable ways. For example, water quenches fire, so the kidneys (a water organ) control the heart (a fire organ). Organs are also divided into yin and yang groupings. Yin organs are the more solid, substantive organs such as the heart, liver, lungs, spleen, and kidneys; yang organs are hollow areas through which materials pass, such as the small and large intestines, stomach, bladder, and gallbladder.

When a TCM practitioner examines a patient, he or she is likely to inspect the tongue, complexion, demeanor, and body language; take an extensive medical history and ask the patient about diet and lifestyle; listen to the sound of the voice; smell the patient's body, breath, and any excretions; and take the pulse at the wrists, abdomen, and meridians. The practitioner is looking for excesses of heat, cold, wind, dampness, and dryness, and deficiencies of blood, moisture, and qi. Herbs and acupuncture are the primary means of resolving imbalances and replenishing blood, moisture, and qi.

Western TCM doctors typically use no more than 200 different herbs, though some 50,000 are held at the Institute of Materia Medica in Beijing.[5] Herbs are classified according to the Four Natures (cold, cool, warm, and hot); the Five Flavors (bitter, sweet, pungent, sour, and salty); and the Four Directions (rising, sinking, floating, or descending), as well as by the organs and meridians affected.[6] Every herb is also either yin or yang; yin herbs act internally with a downward motion, whereas yang herbs rise upward and outward and act on the upper body, limbs, and skin. The actions of an herb are also affected by where it is grown and in what proportions it is used. Herbal remedies are used to treat a variety of symptoms, to regulate qi, to warm or cool, to expel dampness, and to otherwise regulate the internal environment.

Acupuncture, often thought to be synonymous with traditional Chinese medicine, originated some 5,000 years ago in China. It is an essentially painless procedure in which fine needles are inserted into several (usually just ten or twelve) of over 1,000 possible acupoints along the meridian system, helping to unblock the flow of qi, relieve pain, and restore health. Research conducted in the 1960s and 1970s has shown that radioactive isotopes and electrical currents did indeed flow along pathways that corresponded to the ancient Chinese meridians, and that 25 percent of acupuncture points lie along these proven meridians.[7] According to the World Health Organization, acupuncture has been successfully used to treat 104 conditions ranging from the common cold and tennis elbow to ulcers and paralysis.[8] It is particularly successful in pain relief and the treatment of addictions; this is no doubt due to the fact that acupuncture has been found to stimulate the release of endorphins, our body's natural painkillers. Proving that its success is not due to the placebo effect, veterinary acupuncture has been successful in relieving arthritic pain in 84 percent of animals.[9]

Acupuncture points are also used in other related therapies. Moxibustion, in which herbs are combusted on the skin above an acupoint, is often used in conjunction with acupuncture; the combination of these two techniques is referred to as acu-moxa-therapy. Laser acupuncture (which focuses a laser beam on acupoints), auriculotherapy (ear acupuncture that involves many more than the four classic acupoints of the ear), and acupressure or shiatsu (the application of pressure from a fingertip, pencil, or other blunt instrument to the acupoints) are other derivative therapies that have enjoyed varying degrees of success, but whose results are not thought to be as reliable as those of acupuncture itself.

A Career in Acupuncture and Oriental Medicine

Traditional Chinese medicine has become fairly well established in the United States. At the present time acupuncture licensing is required in thirty-two states and the District of Columbia. In almost all of these jurisdictions, NCCAOM certification is a requirement to fulfill some or all of the licensure requirements. Since giving its first examination in 1985, the NCCAOM has certified over 7,000 acupuncturists, over 2,000 Chinese herbologists, and over 200 Oriental bodywork therapists.

While the instruction itself is challenging, finding a school of acupuncture and Oriental medicine is not at all difficult. The Accreditation Commission for Acupuncture and Oriental Medicine (ACAOM) has accredited twenty-nine schools in the United States; an additional eleven programs are candidates for accreditation.[10] A master's degree program can generally be completed in three or four years of full-time study; applicants usually must have completed two years of college prior to enrollment.

Prospective students need to be aware that graduation from an ACAOM-accredited or candidate school is required for a large and increasing number of states for licensure eligibility. Students attending an unaccredited or noncandidate school may find upon graduation that they are unable to get a license in the state in which they'd hoped to practice.

For updated information on acupuncture laws by state, visit the website: www.acupuncture.com/StateLaws/statelaws.htm. For information on NCCAOM certification, visit www.nccaom.org.

AROMATHERAPY

Stopping to sniff the lavender, putting a pot of potpourri by the door, or using scented bath oils gives many of us a psychological lift, even if we've never heard of aromatherapy and aren't aware of the physiology involved.

But aromatherapy is not the same as flowers on the breakfast table. The inhalation or external application of essential oils—obtained by distilling or cold-pressing different parts of a plant—allows molecules to penetrate the tissues and create actual physiological changes within the body. In this way, aromatherapy has been found to have a healing effect on such diverse physical ailments as viral and bacterial infections, herpes simplex, shingles, arthritis, skin conditions, and muscular disorders—hence the use of essential oils in the practice of massage. Research conducted in 1973 showed that a blend of cloves, cinnamon, lavender, and melissa or lemon balm was as effective as prescription antibiotics in treating bronchial conditions—with none of the side effects.[1] Studies conducted in Munich, Germany, have demonstrated that essential oils of cloves, thyme, and cinnamon show anti-inflammatory effects in the treatment of arthritis.[2] And *The British Journal of Occupational Therapy* reported in 1992 that the potential uses of aromatherapy are vast, and include diminishing stress, relieving depression, promoting alertness, treating medical problems, and relieving pain.[3]

Aromatherapy is defined as the practice of using the naturally distilled essences, or essential oils, of plants to promote health and well-being.[4] These essential oils are extremely concentrated, with many pounds or even tons of plant material required to produce a small amount of oil. Though yield varies from plant to plant, on average the yield of essential oil from plant material is 1.5 percent; that is, seventy pounds of raw material produce just one pound of essential oil.[5]

Despite their name, essential oils are not greasy; they are

volatile oils that readily evaporate given the chance, and are closer in consistency to water than to oil. Some of our most fragrant flowers, such as lilac, gardenia, and lily of the valley, produce no essential oils whatsoever. Others yield oils that smell little or nothing like the original flower, and some of the most important essential oils, such as black pepper, ginger, fennel, and thyme, seem more at home in our spice rack.

Surprisingly, fewer than 300 essential oils can be produced from the hundreds of thousands of plants on earth using today's extraction methods. Essential oils are distilled by a variety of methods, including steam distillation, cold-pressing, solvent extraction, and carbon dioxide extraction. While extraction methods may vary, it's important to find reputable suppliers of pure essential oils rather than synthetic, laboratory-born scents. While there is no absolute way to be sure, the label should at least read "essential oil" or "pure essential oil," rather than "perfume oil" or "infused oil." Other indicators of a quality product include price (you get what you pay for, at least some of the time) and opaque glass bottles.

Undiluted essential oils can be so potent when used alone that they may actually burn the skin. For this reason, a few drops of an essential oil are often mixed with a much larger quantity of a carrier oil. Almond, grapeseed, canola, sunflower, sesame, and hazelnut are frequently used carrier oils; rose hip, evening primrose, borage, and other oils may also be added in small amounts. Any carrier oil should be cold-pressed, unscented, and organically grown.

Aromatherapy can be practiced in a number of ways. Essential oils can be used to treat specific mental or physical disorders, just as herbs and conventional Western medicines are used; added to a beauty routine; or used in the kitchen in the form of aromatic honeys or hydrosols. Some practitioners use aromatherapy as part of another modality; though many link aromatherapy with massage and, less often, with chiropractic, the energetics of particular oils are also recognized in Ayurvedic approaches. As such, aromatherapy can be seen as a complement to virtually any form of alternative or allopathic health care.

A Career in Aromatherapy

A handful of schools offer certificate programs in aromatherapy, either through classroom instruction or home study. Many more schools combine a study of essential oils with instruction in herbology, and a class in aromatherapy is frequently part of the curriculum at schools of massage therapy.

Most states require a license of some kind to practice massage, and, of course, all states require specific forms of medical training before permitting practitioners to diagnose and treat illnesses. Aside from these restrictions, the practice of aromatherapy is largely unregulated. That is, though aromatherapists can't legally diagnose and treat illnesses, they may teach others how to prepare blends, create aromatic bath oils, and use essential oils to treat themselves and their family members, and may produce and sell a variety of aromatic products.

There are as yet no legal standards for aromatherapy training or certification in the United States; however, the National Association for Holistic Aromatherapy (NAHA) is working to develop an Accreditation Committee and has developed guidelines for aromatherapy education and certification; see page 428. For a more complete description of the NAHA guidelines and additional information, visit the NAHA website at www.naha.org

AYURVEDA

Ayurveda is not only a healing science, but a philosophy and a religion as well, for it concerns itself with the whole journey of life, with love and truth, and with an open mind and heart; the word is Sanskrit for "science of life."[1] Ayurveda is indigenous to India, where it has been practiced for some 5,000 years. In contrast to Western allopathic medicine, Ayurveda teaches that each individual has the power to heal him- or herself.

Ayurveda teaches that man has four biological and spiritual instincts: religious, financial, procreative, and the instinct toward freedom. Good health is essential for the fulfillment of these instincts, and is the basis for happiness and growth. Consciousness is energy manifested into five basic principles or elements: Ether (space), Air, Fire, Water, and Earth. These five elements, the heart of Ayurvedic science, exist within each individual, as we are a microcosm of nature. For example, Ether exists in the mouth, respiratory tract, abdomen, and tissues; Air is in the movements of the lungs, stomach, and intestines, and in the larger movements of the muscles; Fire is present in our metabolism, in the digestive system, and in our intelligence; Water takes the form of digestive juices, mucous membranes, and plasma; and Earth is manifested in bones, cartilage, muscles, skin, and hair. The five senses of hearing, touch, vision, taste, and smell correspond to the five elements.

In Ayurveda, the human constitution manifests the five elements, combined in pairs, in one of three principles or humors known as doshas. The human constitution is determined at conception and is categorized as vata, pitta, or kapha. Within and between these types, there exist subtle variations depending on the predominance of one element over another. Ether and Air combine to produce vata; Fire and Water manifest as pitta; and Earth and Water produce kapha. Though one's constitution manifests a predominant dosha, all three doshas are present in every cell of the body.

Persons with a primarily vata constitution tend to be physically underdeveloped, with flat chests, thin frames, visible veins and tendons, and cold, rough, dry skin; either quite tall or quite short, with bent or turned-up noses, brittle nails, and cold hands and feet. Vata types are creative, active, and restless; talk and walk fast but tire easily; and tend to be nervous and fearful.

Those with a pitta constitution are of medium height, slender but not as flat-chested as vata types. The skin is soft and warm and not as wrinkled as that of vata persons; the nose is sharp; the hair is thin and may gray prematurely; and the body temperature is higher, with much perspiring. Pitta types are leaders, are generally very intelligent and ambitious, and tend toward anger and jealousy.

The kapha body is well-developed, often with excess weight, a broad chest, thick skin, and good muscle development. The skin of kapha people is fair and oily, and their hair is thick and wavy. They move and speak slowly, sleep soundly, and are generally happy, healthy, tolerant, and forgiving, though they may also be greedy and possessive.

The individual constitution comes with a corresponding susceptibility to disease. Vata types are prone to arthritis, lower back pain, paralysis, and gas; those with a pitta constitution suffer from skin disorders, gallbladder and liver disorders, ulcers, and gastritis; kapha types are more likely to suffer attacks of sinusitis, tonsillitis, bronchitis, and other types of lung congestion. Disease is caused by an imbalance of the humors, which may in turn be caused by repressed fear (excess vata), anger (pitta), or envy and greed (kapha). Food, lifestyle, and environment may also play a part in creating imbalance.

Ayurvedic diagnosis emphasizes day-to-day observation that detects an imbalance before any signs of disease are present. Observation of the pulse, tongue, face, eyes, nails, and lips yields important information regarding which organs are impaired and where toxins have accumulated.

Once there is an understanding of what has caused an illness, there are four main methods of treatment: cleansing and detoxifying, palliation, rejuvenation, and mental hygiene.[2] Cleansing and detoxification, or shodan, are used in cases where excess mucus, bile, or gas has accumulated. The pancha karma (five actions) of vomiting, purgatives or laxatives, enemas, the nasal administration of medication, and bloodletting are used to cleanse the body. Palliation, or shaman, uses herbs, fasting, yoga, breathing exercises, meditation, and exposure to sunlight to balance the doshas. Rejuvenation, or rasayana, uses herbs, mineral preparations, yoga, and breathing exercises to enhance the body's ability to function. Mental hygiene and spiritual healing, or satvajaya, uses sound therapy, meditation, crystals, and mental exercises to release stress and negative beliefs, and to direct energies through the body.

The three doshas exist in plants as they do in all forms of life. Their characteristics parallel those of the constitutional types: vata plants have rough, cracked bark and gnarled, spindly branches, and contain little sap; pitta plants are brightly colored and moderate in sap and strength; kapha plants are heavy, dense, and luxuriant, with abundant sap and leaves. In addition, herbs are classified according to which prana, or life force, they work on: prana (brain), vyana (heart), samana (small intestine), udana (throat), or apana (lower abdomen). Ayurveda also recognizes the energetic properties of herbs: taste, elements, heating or cooling effects, effect after digestion, and other properties.

A sound diet is essential to the maintenance of health. Foods should be selected in accordance with the constitution. For example, apples, melons, potatoes, tomatoes, ice cream, and beef aggravate vata; but brown rice, bananas, grapes, and oranges are beneficial. Spicy foods, peanut butter, tomatoes, and garlic aggravate pitta; pears, plums, oranges, green salads, and mushrooms inhibit it. Bananas, pineapples, melons, and dairy products increase kapha, while cranberries, basmati rice, chicken, and sprouts are beneficial for kapha types. General dietary recommendations include eating only when hungry and drinking only when thirsty; eating foods that work together and don't contradict one another's actions; chewing thoroughly; and eating only about two handfuls of food at one time. Fasting is sometimes recommended, but it should be done in accordance with the constitution. Supplementation of vitamins is normally not recommended.

A Career in Ayurvedic Medicine

In the United States, there are currently no legal licensing requirements for Ayurveda, nor are there any colleges offering the five years of training that is the educational standard in India, where some 108 colleges offer the degree.[3]

Some schools in the United States and Canada offer up to three years of training in Ayurveda. These programs may be taken by the public for their personal use, or by health care professionals who may want to incorporate principles of Ayurveda into their established practices, or by those who intend to practice as health care educators or consultants without diagnosing or prescribing.[4]

BIOFEEDBACK

The term "biofeedback" was coined in the late 1960s to describe a process used to develop control over certain biological responses. The process generally involves seeing and/or hearing an indicator of a biological state (for example, hearing a tone that indicates skin temperature) and learning to control the indicator, or feedback, by acquiring control over the physical response itself. Once the client can successfully control the indicator, the feedback is removed, leaving the client with control over the biological function whenever he or she feels the need to use it.

As odd as it may sound at first, we are in fact able to control a variety of physical states; in addition to skin temperature, subjects can learn to voluntarily influence brain waves, blood pressure, heart rate, and many other autonomic functions. The realization that we have such control has enabled individuals to make considerable progress in the self-treatment of a variety of ailments.

While the technology is relatively new, learning to control the autonomic functions is certainly not. Yogis in eighteenth-century colonial India astounded the British army physicians by exerting control over their breathing and heart rates, not to mention performing the bed-of-nails routine.[1] But it wasn't until the 1950s that Kamiya, Brown, and Green discovered that individuals could learn to control physiological processes when measuring instruments supplied them with information about these processes. It was Kamiya who first used EEG readings to teach subjects to produce alpha brain waves, which identify a very relaxed, waking state; he learned, too, that once subjects had learned how to produce the alpha state with biofeedback, they could do so when the machines were removed.

Later studies indicate that biofeedback, like hypnosis and guided imagery, works by altering the direction of blood flow, which is one of the most common factors in the resolution of mind-body problems. T. X. Barber and others have used this principle of redirected blood flow to control blushing, to cure dermatitis, to aid coagulation in hemophiliacs, and even, in a well-publicized study, to increase breast size.[2]

Today, psychologists, physicians, and other health professionals use biofeedback to treat migraines and tension headaches, high and low blood pressure, anxiety, insomnia, Raynaud's disease (characterized by cold extremities), epilepsy, paralysis, stomach and intestinal disorders, and a host of other ailments.

A Career in Biofeedback

The biofeedback training practitioner teaches the client how to use any of several types of biofeedback instruments available. Training programs certified by the Biofeedback Certification Institute of America (BCIA) typically include courses in introduction to biofeedback, preparing for clinical intervention, neuromuscular intervention, central nervous system interventions, autonomic nervous system interventions, biofeedback and distress, instrumentation, adjunctive techniques and cognitive interventions, and professional conduct.

Biofeedback practitioners are not required by law to be certified; in states that license psychologists, nurses, and other professionals, the state license is all that is required to practice biofeedback, and technicians may work under their employer's license.

Practitioners who wish to be certified by BCIA must have a bachelor's degree or higher in an approved health care field (licensed Registered Nurses are accepted with an associate's degree); must have completed 200 hours from the BCIA core curriculum, a course in human anatomy or physiology, and a course in counseling with practicum; and must pass a qualifying examination consisting of both a written and practical assessment.

CHIROPRACTIC

Of all the forms of alternative health care, chiropractic is perhaps the most mainstream. Many insurance companies pay for chiropractic care, and it's not hard to find someone you know who sees a chiropractor regularly: in 1993 over 30 million consumers received chiropractic care from some 60,000 Doctors of Chiropractic.[1] Chiropractic is no doubt so widely accepted because most Americans have some type of back trouble, and conventional medicine can do little to alleviate it. Allopathic physicians may recommend drugs or surgery, but those who have tried these methods will attest to their limited success and significant downsides. And yet patients who were told their only option was surgery frequently find that chiropractic relieves their chronic pain and restores freedom of movement in just a few sessions. As with many other alternative approaches, it's not only the positive results but the enthusiastic recommendations of chiropractic patients that have done the most to promote the practice.

Chiropractic (the word comes from the Greek *chiro* and *praktikos,* meaning "done by hand") was first developed by Daniel David Palmer, a self-taught healer who was informally educated under Paul Caster, a "magnetic healer," in the late nineteenth century. Palmer used a drug-free approach that involved the laying on of hands, and came to believe that most illnesses result from spinal misalignment. He based this belief on his experience with cases such as that of a janitor whose hearing was restored when Palmer slipped the man's protruding vertebra back into place, and another patient who reported relief from a persistent and painful heart condition after Palmer adjusted the misaligned spine.

Over the years, Palmer refined his system; he later recognized that it was the pressure of misaligned vertebrae on the nerves of the spinal column—what he termed "subluxation"—that interfered with nerve transmission and created disease. Palmer opened the first school of chiropractic in Davenport, Iowa, in 1897. Though he was fined and jailed for six months for practicing medicine without a license, at the time of his death in 1913, Kansas had passed the first state law licensing chiropractic. Today, every state and Canadian province licenses chiropractors, and millions of Americans are treated by them every year.

Just as Palmer did, today's chiropractors perform adjustments or manipulations, in which they ease the spinal vertebrae back into their normal positions. While innovative devices have been developed to aid in this process, most adjustments are still done by hand, usually on a specially designed table with separate sections that can move as the adjustment is being made. While the patient may hear some cracks or pops, the treatment is usually painless, though the patient may feel sore afterward. More interesting are the effects that sometimes show up after the third or fourth treatment—headaches, dizziness, digestive complaints, and a low-grade fever may accompany the muscle soreness and joint tenderness. These are called recovery symptoms, and are seen as an indication that the body is beginning to heal itself as it adapts to the new spinal alignment.

Today's chiropractor may use a number of other tools that Palmer had to do without. X-rays are a fairly standard part of the chiropractic exam, both for a determination of misalignment and to look for other pathologies, such as a fracture or growth. Activator instruments—small, pen-sized guns loaded with a powerful spring—may be used for applying thrust on a small area.

There are two schools of chiropractic practice. "Straight" chiropractic uses only the Palmer philosophy of adjustments—that is, locating and treating subluxations. "Mixed" chiropractic may involve nutritional counseling, heat, or hydrotherapy, as well as spinal adjustments.

While chiropractic may be an obvious choice for those with lower back or neck pain, it has also been successful in treating a host of seemingly unrelated problems. Although today's chiropractors have backed away from the idea that all disease is caused by spinal misalignment, according to Dr. Chester A. Wilk, disorders that have been successfully treated with chiropractic include arthritis, sciatica, bursitis, headache and migraine, nervous disorders and emotional problems, sinusitis, heart trouble, asthma, high blood pressure, respiratory conditions, and the common cold.[2] Anecdotal evidence points to the positive effects of chiropractic on patients with cancer and AIDS, not so much because chiropractic cures these diseases but because it aids in the restoration of the immune function, helping the body to better protect itself.[3]

A Career in Chiropractic

All fifty states plus the District of Columbia, the U.S. Virgin Islands, and Puerto Rico license chiropractors as health care providers. In general, students must have completed two years (in some states, four years) of a preprofessional, college-level education prior to attending a four-year (at least 4,200-hour) chiropractic college. For a graduate to be eligible for licensure, the chiropractic college must be accredited by the Council on Chiropractic Education (CCE) and/or approved by the state board; national exams and some state assessment are also required. Like other alternative health care fields, chiropractic is growing; between 1994 and 1995, the number of D.C. degrees bestowed by CCE-accredited institutions increased by 7 percent to nearly 2,900 degrees[4]; today, over 10,000 students are enrolled in CCE-accredited chiropractic schools.[5]

Legally, chiropractors are permitted to do much more than align a spine. Like any doctor, a chiropractor will take a medical history and conduct a physical exam, and may order lab tests or X-rays in order to arrive at a diagnosis. Most chiropractors will also work with their patients to develop a plan for a healthier lifestyle through better nutrition, exercise, improved posture, and other changes.

State statutes set boundaries for chiropractors that often fall far short of what is permissible for physicians, however: currently no state allows chiropractors to prescribe drugs or perform major surgery. Some states, like Michigan, prohibit venipuncture for lab diagnosis or the dispensing of vitamin supplements; others, like Oregon, are more liberal, allowing chiropractors to perform minor surgery and pelvic and rectal exams, and to collect blood specimens for diagnosis.

For specific information on licensure and legal scope of practice by state, visit the website www.ncschiropractic.com/ahcpr/part5.htm.[6]

ENERGETIC HEALING

Several schools offer certificate programs in what they call energetic healing or subtle energy therapies. These are hybrid programs that generally combine courses in color therapy, flower essence therapy, magnetic therapy, aromatherapy, hypnotherapy, the laying on of hands, meditation, sound healing, and other topics with a more mainstream base in massage, craniosacral therapy, polarity therapy, and/or reiki.

Practitioners of energetic healing can work as either unlicensed health care educators or consultants, or they may use their knowledge of these therapies to add another dimension of healing to a practice in such fields as massage, yoga, or polarity therapy.

ENVIRONMENTAL MEDICINE

In the 1940s, Theron G. Randolph, M.D., treated a woman named Sally who had been admitted to a mental hospital for psychosis. Dr. Randolph, convinced that food allergies could be contributing to her problem, put Sally in an allergen-free environment and started her on a water fast. By the fourth day, Sally had regained her sanity. Randolph reintroduced foods, one at a time, and found that beet sugar brought back her psychotic symptoms. Once the offending food was removed from her diet, Sally was no longer in need of hospitalization.[1]

In addition to food allergies, Randolph found that common environmental chemicals could also have profound effects on a patient's physical and emotional well-being. Every day, we encounter formaldehyde and toluene in our carpeting; artificial colorings, preservatives, and pesticides in our food; natural gas fumes and the toxic by-products of their combustion from our stoves and furnaces; and petroleum from our cars. All of these things can be the direct cause, depending on our susceptibility, of migraines, eczema, arthritis, anxiety, depression, gastrointestinal problems, attention deficit disorder, bed-wetting, lupus, and any number of other problems.[2] According to Sherry Rogers, M.D., a Fellow of the American Academy of Environmental Medicine, the most common symptoms of chemical sensitivity are feeling dopey, dizzy, "spacey," and unable to concentrate[3]—which should give pause to every parent of a "learning-disabled" child.

Of course, not everyone is sensitive to environmental chemicals. Those who are, according to the American Academy of Environmental Medicine, can blame a combination of genetics, poor nutrition, infection, stress, and excessive chemical exposure.[4] Exposure to formaldehyde, which is in our walls, cabinets, furniture, and carpeting, can cause an individual to become sensitive to a variety of other chemicals that previously had no effect.[5] Most of us are not born sensitive to new carpeting, but we are worn down by years of chemical attacks on our bodies, and one day, we fall apart. Many in the field speak of the "rain barrel effect," which is similar in concept to the straw that broke the camel's back. We begin with a fairly empty rain barrel. Over the years, our dust allergies develop; we get a pet and add dander allergies to the barrel. We eat too many colored and preserved snack foods, linger too long over the gas stove, and fill our barrel near to the brim. Then we get the new bedroom carpeting, and the barrel overflows. We suddenly develop breathing difficulties, panic attacks, scaly hands, or migraines—or all those and more. We can't understand why, all of a sudden, we're a physical wreck. But the rain barrel theory holds that it's not "all of a sudden" at all; we just overflowed our barrel's capacity.

Physicians trained in the treatment of environmental illness, or multiple chemical sensitivities (MCS), take an extensive medical history that helps both doctor and patient to see that it's not just the new carpeting—it's the accumulation of a lifetime of bad habits. The good news is that in many cases, the rain barrel can be effectively emptied, or at least decanted a little. Physicians accomplish this by identifying and treating the underlying allergies and sensitivities, and working to rebuild the immune system through diet, stress reduction, and other holistic means.

Environmental physicians may test for food and airborne allergies through blood tests, but some prefer the slower and, they believe, more accurate method of provocation/neutralization. In this form of testing, the patient is injected with a suspected allergen and waits a few minutes to see whether there is a reaction, either visible on the skin or felt by the patient as a change in mental state. The practitioner then finds a dose of the same substance that will turn off the reaction; this is the neutralizing dose. The patient is then able to self-administer the antigen on a regular basis for the control of symptoms.

Many practitioners and patients are reluctant to routinely inject possible carcinogens such as formaldehyde and natural gas. For these types of substances, education and avoidance are the key. Once a patient has identified the chemicals to which he or she is sensitive, they can be removed from the home. This is usually neither easy nor cheap; Dr. Randolph was responsible for the removal of many a natural gas furnace and hundreds of yards of wall-to-wall carpeting.

A Career in Environmental Medicine

Environmental physicians are generally just that—M.D.s or D.O.s who were trained by fellow physicians and/or have taken advanced courses in the treatment of environmental illness. However, a knowledge of the effects of food and chemical sensitivities can be beneficial in any area of alternative health care. Practitioners of any kind should be aware that a patient's headache could be caused not by overworked muscles, a spine out of adjustment, or blocked chi, but by the carpeting in the waiting room.

GUIDED IMAGERY

Goose bumps from a ghost story, salivating while reading a recipe, sweating when an actor teeters on a ledge—we've all experienced the physical effects of an image that existed only in our imagination. To our brains, real and imagined experiences look exactly alike; hence, our worrying about problems can cause as many—or more—hives and ulcers as the actual problems themselves. This powerful mind-body connection can be harnessed to work in our favor in a technique known as guided imagery, where we can learn to visualize positive outcomes and experiences rather than imagining the worst.

Belleruth Naparstek, author of *Staying Well with Guided Imagery*, enumerates several operating principles of imagery. These can be summarized as follows: first, our bodies can't tell the difference between sensory images in the mind and reality; second, in a relaxed state, we are capable of rapid healing, learning, and change; and third, we feel better when we have a sense of mastery over what happens to us.[1]

Therapists trained in guided imagery use these principles in developing techniques to help their clients cope with, and sometimes defeat, chronic diseases such as multiple sclerosis, cancer, AIDS, or back pain. Cases have been reported in which patients have visualized their tumors under attack by "bullets of energy" or Star Wars–type weapons, and their tumors have, in fact, disappeared.[2]

In its simplest form, a guided imagery session may go something like this: the client is asked to get comfortable, take some deep breaths, release all tension, and enter into a relaxed, peaceful state. The client is then asked to remember a specific instance in which he or she felt totally at peace—a special place, a particular time or event, in which all was well with the world. Depending on the client's needs, he or she may be asked to use a physical gesture, or anchoring device, that will become linked in his or her mind with the relaxed response—something as simple as touching two fingers together. After several weeks of practice evoking the peaceful scene and then making the gesture, the client will be able to make the gesture and then automatically feel the relaxed response, even in a time of stress, such as when giving a speech or boarding an airplane.

A Career In Guided Imagery

Workshops in helping others through guided imagery are generally open to professionals in the counseling field, including psychologists, certified counselors, social workers, and nurses. Many hospitals or health organizations offer self-help courses in guided imagery to patients or to the general public; several books and audiotapes are on the market that can teach an individual to use imagery to help solve specific problems.

HERBAL MEDICINE

Herbal medicine is a prime example of how what is considered alternative or unproven medicine in the United States is standard practice in most of the rest of the world. In 1985, the World Health Organization estimated that approximately 80 percent of the world's population relies primarily on herbs to meet their health care needs.[1] What Americans may find surprising is that it isn't only primitive cultures that rely on herbs; 30 to 40 percent of all medical doctors in Germany and France use herbs as their primary medicines.[2]

Despite its lack of acceptance in the United States, herbalism is by far the oldest form of medicine in the world, used by all cultures throughout every period of history. It remains an important part of traditional Chinese medicine, naturopathy, and Ayurvedic medicine. Indeed, plants are the source of many of the drugs sold by prescription in the United States; some 125 plant-derived drugs are in use here, and of these, three-fourths are used in similar ways in native cultures.[3] But despite the proliferation of news reports showing khaki-clad botanists roaming the rain forests in search of cancer cures, dozens of plants indigenous to North America are world-renowned for their healing powers. Not the least of these is the unassuming purple coneflower—better known in herbal circles as echinacea—which has been found to show anti-inflammatory, antiviral, antibacterial, and even anticancer properties.[4] Perhaps the answers to many of our health problems lie not in exotic jungle leaves, but in our own backyards.

Echinacea is just one of many substances derived from garden- (or roadside-) variety plants that can contribute to our collective wellness. The dandelions that our neighbors find so resistant to herbicides and uprooting are that hardy for a reason: this humble plant has been found to aid digestion, to improve liver conditions such as jaundice and hepatitis, and to act as a safe diuretic. It is also used by the Chinese to treat breast cancer. Peppermint has long been a treatment for indigestion and intestinal colic. And garlic has been in use for over 5,000 years in the treatment of a wide variety of conditions, including high blood pressure, diabetes, high cholesterol, and all sorts of infections. It is only we Americans who fail to fully recognize the herbal treasure trove under our feet; of the 232 monographs in the British Herbal Pharmacopoeia, seventy-three are about native North American plants that are exported to Britain for medicinal purposes.[5]

Though the vast majority of herbs are beneficial and well-tolerated, not all are harmless; some have the potential to be toxic when taken improperly. In 1994, a California woman died after trying to induce an abortion with pennyroyal; other herbs that have produced dangerous side effects include chaparral, comfrey (when taken internally), and ma huang, a stimulant sometimes used in weight-loss products.[6] Though extremely rare, stories of harmful side effects make headlines when they do occur, and are used as ammunition by those who would attempt to limit the public's access to herbs. However, the American Association of Poison Control Centers reported that in 1988 to 1989, pharmaceuticals caused a total of 809 deaths and 6,407 major nonfatal poisonings, while plants (most of which were houseplants, not herbs) caused two fatalities and fifty-three major poisonings.[7] Still, while herbs are considerably less toxic than what's in the medicine chest, it makes sense for anyone who wants to use medicinal herbs to become educated enough to do it safely and effectively.

Herbal Preparations

Courses offered at any of the classroom or correspondence schools will instruct the student in identifying, gathering, and growing herbs; Western and Eastern theories of healing; materia medica (healing properties and actions of specific herbs and conditions for their use); and creating a number of types of herbal preparations.

While herbal products may be purchased in a variety of forms, the simplest and often most effective herbal preparations are easily prepared at home with only a knife, strainer, and mortar and pestle. Can't tell an ointment from a salve? Here's a quick lesson:

- *Tinctures* are alcohol-based solutions of herbal extracts, and are among the more common formulations; they can be taken orally or used externally.

- *Infusions,* or teas, are made by pouring hot water or other liquid over fresh or powdered herbs, which are then allowed to steep for ten or twenty minutes. The infusion is then strained for drinking.

- A *decoction* is very similar to an infusion, but it is made from woody herbs that are not soluble in hot water; in this case, the herbs are simmered for up to twenty minutes and strained while hot.

- A *poultice* is a mashed or powdered herb applied directly to the skin to reduce inflammation or to draw out toxins.

- *Ointments* are prepared by boiling herbs together with a petroleum jellylike substance; these can be applied to the skin for long periods of time, such as in the treatment of injuries.

- *Compresses* involve soaking sterile gauze in a solution of boiled herbs, applying the warm pad to the affected area, and replacing it when cool.

- *Salves* are prepared by adding boiled herbs to a mixture of vegetable oil and beeswax.

A Career in Herbal Medicine

Naturopaths and practitioners of traditional Chinese and Ayurvedic medicine all use herbs as part of their arsenal of treatment options, though in somewhat different ways. In Western herbology, herbs are used to treat particular symptoms, in much the same way as Western medicines are used. In Chinese and Ayurvedic medicine, herbs are used energetically; that is, particular herbs are either "warm" or "cold," and the herb used would depend on an assessment of the individual's overall condition and constitution. Whatever the approach, a license to practice naturopathy or traditional Chinese medicine would permit a practitioner to prescribe herbal preparations.

In the United States, Native American reservations are the only places where a nonmedically trained herbalist can legally diagnose and prescribe.[8] The herbalist, then, takes on more of an advisory role, and is free to use his or her expertise in teaching, manufacturing, wildcrafting (harvesting native wild herbs), and growing herbs. Michael Tierra, a naturopath, certified acupuncturist, and developer of the home study East West Herb Course, notes that a properly trained herbalist may incorporate a practice as an herbal consultant because "the system of holistic analysis based upon principles of Oriental diagnosis has nothing to do with the Western concepts of pathological disease, and so can be used as a basis of practice without infringing on the law."[9]

Roger Wicke, Ph.D. and noted herbalist, discusses the legal ramifications of the practice of herbology in his web page, "The Right to Practice Herbology, Legal History and Basis." Wicke explains that while an herbalist can assist in building a client's general health, can recommend specific herbal preparations for a particular constitutional or body type, and may even show a client a page in a book that lists which diseases a particular herb will cure, he or she isn't legally allowed to say "This herb will cure your throat infection," or to diagnose illness or prescribe remedies. (Wicke's page is www.rmhiherbal.org/a/f.ahr3.rights.html).

The National Commission for the Certification of Acupuncturists has recently instituted an examination process for certification of practitioners as Diplomates of Chinese Herbology. But outside of accreditation in Chinese herbology, there is no association that regulates or accredits education in herbal medicine in this country.

HOLISTIC HEALTH PRACTITIONER/ HOLISTIC HEALTH EDUCATION/ HOLISTIC COUNSELING

Several schools offer programs, ranging from one month to as much as three years in length, in areas they call Holistic Health Practitioner, Holistic Health Education, or Holistic Counseling.

These programs typically combine a base program of massage, counseling, or yoga with offerings from many other fields of alternative health care, including nutrition, herbs, stress management, dreamwork, hypnotherapy, traditional Chinese medicine, acupressure, polarity, and others.

Such programs generally provide extra hours of education beyond licensing requirements in, for example, massage therapy, thereby allowing the therapist to incorporate an added dimension of healing into his or her practice. The shorter programs may not provide sufficient training for a career; like an herbologist, however, the Holistic Health Practitioner is free to work in a purely advisory role without diagnosing or prescribing.

Those schools that offer a degree in counseling with specialization in holistic health enable counselors to incorporate knowledge of nutrition and eating disorders, diet and disease, and the physiology and psychology of stress into their practices. While requirements vary by state, programs that offer a master's degree in counseling are generally sufficient for licensing as a counselor.

HOLISTIC NURSING

As alternative medicine becomes increasingly mainstream, there is more of an overlap between conventional, allopathic medicine and various alternative fields. Many professional Registered Nurses are seeking additional training in such areas as massage as a means of providing even better patient care.

Holistic nursing programs provide continuing education for licensed health care professionals, covering topics such as AMMA therapy, stress management, nutrition, herbology, Oriental diagnosis, tai chi, and others.

The American Holistic Nurses' Association website at www.ahna.org has information on holistic nursing certification.

HOMEOPATHY

Paracelsus said, "All things are poison, it is the dosage that makes a thing not poison."[1] This is as true in the various fields of alternative medicine, where treatments are generally viewed as wholesome and natural, as it is in the allopathic world of synthetic drugs with side effects that can be worse than the original affliction. Medicinal herbs may sometimes produce allergic or toxic reactions in some individuals, and certain vitamins and minerals can cause damage when taken in excess. But homeopathy uses remedies that not only can be toxic, but definitely *are* toxic, even in fairly small doses. Who wouldn't raise an eyebrow at the homeopath's remedies of petroleum, bee venom (*apis mellifica*), deadly nightshade (*belladonna*), mercury (*mercurius*), and snake venom (*lachesis*)?

The critical element in homeopathy, however, is the dose. Homeopathy is criticized on the basis that homeopathic remedies are so dilute that not a single molecule of the original substance is present. But homeopathy is an energetic system, much like Chinese medicine or Ayurveda; homeopathic remedies work because of the energy pattern, not the material content, of the substance used in its preparation. When a substance is shaken (known as succussion) and repeatedly diluted until no trace of the original substance is left, the resulting remedy is actually more potent than the tincture from which it was made.

It may sound like hocus-pocus, but it works: a survey of research published in the *British Medical Journal* shows that 81 out of 107 controlled clinical trials demonstrated that homeopathic remedies had beneficial results.[2] Critics have argued that any successes attributed to homeopathy were due to the placebo effect. This argument falls apart, however, when one looks at the numbers of successful homeopathic treatments on animals who were not, in all likelihood, staunch believers in the practice; and a 1997 review of research in *Lancet* showed that homeopathic medicines had an effect 2.45 times greater than placebo.[3]

The practice of homeopathy was founded by the German physician Samuel Hahnemann in 1790 (the word is derived from the Greek *homoios,* meaning "similar," and *pathos,* meaning "suffering"). Hahnemann believed that the symptoms produced by an illness are the body's attempt to heal itself. Therefore, he reasoned, a remedy that could mimic the symptoms of a particular illness would strengthen the healing response—a principle referred to as "like cures like" or the Law of Similars. In this regard, homeopathy differs only in potency from immunizations and allergy shots.

Hahnemann developed two other primary principles. One, the Law of the Infinitesimal Dose, states that the more dilute the remedy, the greater its potency. The other involves looking at each patient and his or her illness on an individual basis; no two cases will be manifested in exactly the same way, so the remedy given to one patient may be completely different from that given to the next.

To determine the proper remedy, the practitioner would need to look beyond the obvious stuffy nose and sore throat to find the more peculiar symptoms—a red face, waking in the night, bloating, twitching, or anxiety, for example. He or she would then select the proper potency. Potencies are expressed in centesimal (c) and decimal (x) scales. Commonly available potencies usually range from 6c (the lowest potency commonly available) to 30c (the highest potency normally obtained over the counter). In general, lower potencies are used for physical pathologies, while the highest potencies are used with diseases that are mental or emotional in nature.

Homeopathic remedies are derived not only from the poisonous substances mentioned earlier, but from a variety of plants (in whole or part), animals, reptiles, insects, and minerals. Potencies in the lower ranges are available in health food stores and through numerous mail-order companies. While a trained practitioner should be consulted for any serious illness, an individual can learn enough through courses or independent study to treat minor ailments in himself and in his family.

A Career in Homeopathy

In much of the world, homeopathy is not "alternative" at all; some 500 million people around the world receive homeopathic treatment, including Britain's royal family.[4] In Britain, homeopathic hospitals are part of the national health care system; in France, pharmacies are required to stock homeopathic remedies along with standard drugs. Even in the United States, an estimated 3,000 physicians and health care professionals practice homeopathy.[5] Because they are recognized by the FDA as over-the-counter drugs, anyone can buy homeopathic remedies to treat themselves or their families.

Training courses in homeopathy in the United States are typically three years in length, meeting perhaps one weekend per month during this time, and requiring a significant amount of home study. A number of certification programs are available.

The legal status of the practice of homeopathy is somewhat muddled. In most states, homeopathic remedies can legally be prescribed by M.D.s, D.O.s, N.D.s, dentists, and veterinarians;

in some states, chiropractors are also permitted to administer homeopathic remedies. The practice of homeopathy may also be legal if done under the supervision of a physician or other licensed practitioner.

Currently, eight states have laws protecting the physician's use of homeopathy and other alternative therapies; three states (Arizona, Connecticut, and Nevada) offer an additional homeopathic license to previously licensed physicians. Nevada also offers professional status for Advanced Practitioners of Homeopathy who work in collaboration with an M.D. or D.O. Homeopathy is currently unregulated in Canada.

Interested individuals should contact the National Center for Homeopathy or visit their website, www.homeopathic.org, for additional information on homeopathy and the law.

HYPNOTHERAPY

There's really nothing alternative about hypnotherapy; it's been approved by the American Medical Association as a valid medical treatment since 1958. It's also nothing new. Hypnotic trances have been in use for nearly all of recorded history; there are reports of hypnotic suggestion in the writings of ancient Egypt and Greece, and it is still observed in the ceremonies of primitive cultures. Franz Anton Mesmer, an eighteenth-century Austrian physician, is credited with the founding of modern hypnosis; he called it animal magnetism because he believed that the human body possessed a magnetic polarity. The term mesmerism, which is still used today, was derived from his name.

Despite its long history, the only hypnosis most of us have ever witnessed is the parlor-trick variety we see now and then on television. But hypnotherapy is actually quite effective in the treatment of a host of ailments, from migraines and ulcers to anxiety, phobias, and depression; over 15,000 doctors combine hypnosis with other forms of treatment.[1]

We have all experienced states of awareness that are very similar to the early stages of hypnosis. The feeling of drifting off, of being not quite asleep yet not awake, feels very much like the average hypnotic trance. In fact, the trancelike state in which we find ourselves when we drive past our exit ramp or get lost in a daydream at work is a common hypnotic experience that has been defined as "an altered state of consciousness, characterized by an inward focusing and temporary inattention to the ordinary environment."[2] Virtually everyone who is willing can be hypnotized; likewise, it is virtually impossible to hypnotize a subject against his or her will.[3] There is no difference in susceptibility to hypnosis between male and female or in correlation to body build, intelligence, or personality, though children and those with higher levels of anxiety are actually somewhat more susceptible than others.[4]

Inducing a trance is not complicated. The subject is usually asked to relax and to fix his or her gaze on an object; as the subject's eyes grow weary, the hypnotist suggests that they close. Subjects may also focus on a body part or on their breathing, a technique common to yoga, karate, and Lamaze.

There are several types or depths of trance. In a light trance, subjects feel calm and somewhat detached, muscles are relaxed, respiration slows, and the heart rate usually drops. In a medium trance, subjects may feel altered bodily perceptions (such as feeling smaller or larger, or floating in space), will lose their gag reflex, and may experience hallucinations. Surgery may be performed on people in a medium trance. In a deep trance, blood pressure may drop to very low levels and major surgery may be performed without pain.[5]

Hypnotherapy has been used to successfully treat a variety of disorders, including blindness, alcoholism, addictions, and phobias, and in such medical settings as anesthesiology, psychiatry, obstetrics, and dentistry.

A Career in Hypnotherapy

Just as nearly anyone can be hypnotized, nearly anyone can learn to perform hypnosis; several programs will teach just that in a weekend or less. There are many organizations that offer certification upon successful completion of a training program and an exam; usually these organizations require a minimum of 120 to 150 hours of classroom-based training. However, it's not difficult for a school to itself become a certifying agency, so beware: "certification" may only mean that you've completed their course.

Certification, whatever it means, has little to do with licensing. Indiana is the only state that licenses hypnotherapists and offers a State Certification for hypnotherapists; applicants must be graduates of state-licensed schools. Otherwise, hypnotherapists may work in any state with any amount of training.

INTEGRATIVE MEDICINE

The goal of integrative medicine is to combine the best of both conventional and alternative ideas and practices in an effort to produce an environment in which the body can heal itself. Neither standard medical practices nor alternative approaches are accepted blindly; both are subjected to laboratory research and testing in clinical settings in an attempt to sort the effective from the useless.

Practitioners of integrative medicine are encouraged to practice a healthy lifestyle themselves. In addition, they work from the assumption that prevention is medicine's primary responsibility, as many illnesses are entirely preventable; that the body has the ability to heal itself and that the best kind of medicine is that which stimulates and encourages this natural healing; and that simple, cost-effective treatments should be tried before invasive and costly procedures.

The University of Arizona's Program in Integrative Medicine is currently the only one of its kind. Physicians (licensed M.D.s and D.O.s) trained in this two-year program are educated in the use of botanical, nutritional, and energy medicine, as well as such modalities as homeopathy, acupuncture, guided imagery, osteopathic manipulation, and others.

IRIDOLOGY

Iridology had its beginnings, it is said, when a boy tried to capture an owl in his garden and inadvertently broke its leg in the struggle. As the boy looked into the owl's eye, he saw a black streak forming. After the owl's leg healed, the black line faded to white. That boy, Ignatz von Peczely, later became a physician and one of the fathers of iridology.[1]

In the practice of iridology, the eyes—or, more specifically, the irises—provide the knowledgeable practitioner with a map through which he or she can determine the health or weakness of the various systems of the body. Iridology is not designed to diagnosis specific diseases (and in fact, practitioners are not legally able to do so without a medical license); rather, the iridologist can discern the location of inherent weaknesses and various stages of inflammation. This can be done by using several tools.

The primary tool of the iridologist is the iris chart. Around

1880, Dr. Peczely and Swedish minister Nils Liljequist, working independently, developed iris charts that showed a striking similarity to one another. Such charts have been refined by various practitioners over the years. The charts created by Dr. Bernard Jensen, a twentieth-century chiropractor, nutritionist, and iridologist, contain some 166 named areas (86 in the left iris, 80 in the right) that correspond not only to the major organs like the liver, the kidneys, and the heart, but also to very specific regions, such as areas of the brain that control acquired mental speech, senses, and mental ability, the upper jaw, tonsils, scapula, or left foot.[2] These grids are superimposed over an enlarged photograph of the iris to help the iridologist identify areas more precisely than could be done with handheld magnifiers.

What does the iridologist look for? Fiber quality, or constitution, is rated from one to ten, and is determined by the graininess or weave of the iris fibers; a fine weave or tight grain would be a one, a very loose weave or grainy fibers would be a ten. An individual's constitutional pattern is inborn and cannot be changed. Beyond this, an iridologist might look for specific wreaths (rings around the pupil) that correspond to the autonomic nervous system, the stomach, or nutrient absorption; open or closed lesions or healing lines in specific areas; a string of puffs near the perimeter of the iris (indicating lymphatic system congestion); a dark rim (indicting a problem with the elimination of toxins) or a rim that is milky-white (indicating high sodium and high cholesterol levels); and other lines, rings, or lesions that appear in particular colors or patterns.

Dr. Jensen believes that iridology can reveal a host of conditions. He contends that, along with showing the inherent strength or weakness of organs, glands, and tissues, the iris reveals the nutritional needs of the body; which organs are in greatest need of rebuilding; where inflammation is located; sluggishness or spastic conditions of the bowel; pressure on the heart; nerve force and depletion; hyper- or hypoactivity of the organs, glands, and tissues; lymphatic system congestion; poor nutrient assimilation; the need for rest; high or low sex drive; allergy to wheat; potential for senility; and much more.[3]

A Career in Iridology

The National Iridology Research Association (NIRA) offers a certification program covering eye anatomy and physiology, topography and mapping of the iris, and case studies, as well as certification testing. In order to maintain certification, a certified iridologist is required to complete two NIRA-approved continuing education classes each year. The organization also maintains a referral listing of NIRA-certified iridologists.

As an iridologist does not attempt to diagnose or prescribe, no license is required. Iridology is often combined with other holistic approaches to health care.

MASSAGE THERAPY AND BODYWORK

Hippocrates taught his students, "The physician must be acquainted with many things and assuredly with rubbing," and used massage as a treatment for ailments from sprains to constipation. The ancient Japanese healing art of shiatsu, Ayurvedic massage from India, the massage techniques of Chinese Taoist priests, even texts found in Egyptian tombs all testify to the healing power of touch.

Some of the greatest physicians in history advocated the use of massage. Celsus (25 B.C.–A.D. 50), Galen (A.D. 131–A.D. 200), and Avicenna (A.D. 980–A.D. 1037), authors of the most authoritative medical texts of their times, all wrote about the techniques and indications for massage. But it wasn't until the 1850s that massage was introduced into the United States by New York physicians George and Charles Taylor, brothers who had studied massage in Sweden. Swedes opened the first massage therapy clinics in the United States just after the Civil War; Baron Nils Posse founded the Posse Institute in Boston and Hartwig Nissen opened the Swedish Health Institute in Washington, D.C., where several members of Congress and Presidents Benjamin Harrison and Ulysses S. Grant were clients.

By the early 1900s, massage was delegated to the nursing and physical therapy staff, and by the 1940s it had been all but abandoned by these health care workers as well. The resurgence of interest in massage in the 1970s occurred outside the medical establishment, in the gray area we call alternative health care.

Research conducted today is helping to bring massage therapy closer to the mainstream. Dr. Tiffany Field, director of the Touch Research Institute at the University of Miami, studied the effect of massage on premature babies and found that those who received massage gained 47 percent more weight and left the hospital six days earlier than those who did not.[1] Touching has also been found to reduce anxiety, high blood pressure, and a host of other ills—and it's not all in our heads. Research has shown that massage can increase levels of serotonin, a natural antidepressant, and encourages the release of endorphins—nature's painkillers. In a study of the effects of massage on cancer patients, subjects' perception of pain was reduced by 60 percent and anxiety by 24 percent; feelings of relaxation increased 58 percent, along with a measurable reduction in heart rate, blood pressure, and respiratory rate.[2]

Massage not only makes us feel better, it can make us smarter, too. Another study by the Touch Research Institute found that subjects were able to complete math problems in half the time with half as many errors following a twenty-minute chair massage.[3] Studies like this have helped fuel the boom in on-site massage at the workplace, with employers often picking up the tab.

According to the American Massage Therapy Association, the United States is the only developed country in which massage is not part of the official health care system. In Germany and the former Soviet Union, for example, every major hospital has a massage therapy department; China, Japan, and India also recognize massage as an important part of health care. But our society is coming to recognize the need for touch, and the field of massage therapy is growing at an astronomical rate. More than a million Americans get a massage each year, and over a recent ten-year period, membership in the American Massage Therapy Association increased tenfold. *The New England Journal of Medicine* reports that massage is the third most frequently used form of alternative health care.[4]

What Is Massage Therapy?

Massage therapy has been defined by the National Institutes of Health as "the scientific manipulation of the soft tissues of the body to normalize those tissues. It consists of a group of manual techniques that include applying fixed or movable pressure, holding, and/or causing movement of or to the body, using primarily the hands but sometimes other areas such as forearms, elbows, or feet."[5] The emphasis, in this and virtually all other forms of alternative medicine, is on assisting the body in healing itself.

Swedish massage started it all in the United States, but there are now some eighty different types of hands-on therapy. A massage therapist may incorporate one or several of these techniques into a given treatment, and schools of massage usually offer instruction in a number of them.

ACUPRESSURE

Acupressure is essentially acupuncture without needles. Finger pressure is applied to specific points along meridians, the highways of energy flow (chi or qi) that run through bones, muscles, organs, and the bloodstream. It is thought that the even distribution of chi along these meridians results in strength and health; when chi is unbalanced, physical or emotional problems may result. Acupressure seeks to restore the balance of chi. While most often used for relief of chronic pain, acupressure is also successful in treating hyperactivity, mood disorders, stress, asthma, and other physical or emotional problems. Individuals can learn to treat themselves with acupressure. In varying forms of acupressure, points are stimulated with heat, cold, electricity, ultrasound, or lasers. Burning herbs over the acupressure points is called moxibustion, a traditional Chinese method of stimulating the flow of chi.

ALEXANDER TECHNIQUE

F. Mathias Alexander, an Australian actor, suffered periodically from inexplicable voice loss; after nine years of study, he determined that the way he held his head contributed to the problem. He developed a philosophy founded on the principle that proper alignment of the spine was the key to good health, and that poor alignment was simply the result of habitual misuse of body motions. He taught students his techniques to free the neck, lengthen the spine, and reeducate patients though the use of massage and studied movements. Since exercises are developed for each individual, Alexander wrote no manual; techniques are passed down from teacher to teacher. The Alexander technique has been used to eliminate knee pain, tendinitis, chronic back pain, and a variety of other ills.

APPLIED KINESIOLOGY

In the 1960s, a chiropractor named Dr. George Goodheart introduced applied kinesiology in response to the connections he'd noticed between muscle weakness and dysfunctioning organs; for example, a weakness in a pectoral muscle might indicate gastric disease. Applied kinesiologists see health as a triangle—the chemical side takes into account nutrition and the effects of drugs; the structural side considers the interrelationship of muscles, bones, joints, and organs; and the mental side includes attitudes and expectations.

AROMATHERAPY

Aromatherapy may be used alone or in combination with some form of massage (see page 4).

CRANIOSACRAL THERAPY

Craniosacral therapists subtly manipulate bones in the face, head, and vertebral column, and the membranes beneath the skull in order to treat headache, TMJ-related jaw pain, ear infections, strokes, and other ailments. The therapist focuses on reducing tension and stress in the meningeal membrane and its fascial connections, allowing free movement by the cerebrospinal fluid and balancing energy fields.

DEEP MUSCLE THERAPY/ DEEP TISSUE MASSAGE

These therapies are corrective or therapeutic massages that use greater pressure to reach deeper layers of muscle, most often as a treatment for muscle spasms, scar tissue, or chronic patterns of muscular tension. In Pfrimmer deep muscle therapy, muscle fibers are worked back and forth in both directions. Cross-fiber friction works against the muscle grain to break up adhesions in the tendons and muscle fiber.

DO-IN

Do-in (pronounced dough-in) is a macrobiotic exercise program that was introduced into the United States in 1968. Do-in exercises resemble yoga postures and are thought to stimulate the same energy meridians as acupuncture or shiatsu. Foot massage, abdominal massage, neck extensions, nose squeezes, eye exercises, and ear stretches are all part of the do-in practice.

ESALEN MASSAGE

Esalen is a hybrid style of massage taught at the Esalen Institute in California that uses the techniques of Swedish massage, Rolfing, deep tissue massage, and others in long flowing stokes. The goal is to promote relaxation and healing.

FELDENKRAIS® METHOD

A series of exercises designed to release habitual patterns and introduce new ways of moving, the Feldenkrais method was developed by Moshe Feldenkrais in response to his own incapacitating injury. Feldenkrais used his knowledge of anatomy, physiology, physics, and the martial arts to produce a method of movement reeducation that can improve flexibility and coordination. As the client lies on a table, fully clothed, the practitioner guides the body in various movements and in essence reprograms the nervous system, resulting in more efficient body movement and relief of muscle tension.

HYDROTHERAPY

Usually used in conjunction with massage, hydrotherapy involves the use of water, heat, and ice in the form of hot and cold packs, saunas, whirlpools, and steam baths.

INFANT MASSAGE

Infant massage is common in many other countries, and is gaining a toehold in the United States and Europe, particularly in cases of drug-addicted babies. Massage is said to help the infants relax, move and react better, and bond more closely with their mothers.

JIN SHIN DO

This system employs sequences of meridian point pressure that are designed specifically for a particular illness or ailment. A product of the 1980s, Jin Shin Do was derived in part from Jin Shin Jyutsu, which was developed in Japan in the early 1900s and brought to the United States in the 1960s. Though similar to acupuncture and other meridian-based techniques, these systems differ in their use of specific patterns of pressure on particular points, depending on the ailment, in order to energize or enervate qi.

MANUAL LYMPH DRAINAGE

Edema, inflammation, and other conditions related to poor lymph drainage can be treated with manual lymph drainage, a system of light, rhythmic strokes. In a study conducted in 1984, it was found to be more effective than diuretic drugs in controlling lymphedema after radical mastectomy.[6] Used by European hospitals and clinics for decades, manual lymph drainage may be helpful for chronic infections, excess scar tissue, poor circulation, edema caused by surgery or other trauma, chronic pain, or stress.

MYOFASCIAL MASSAGE

This massage technique manipulates the connective tissue and fascia that surround the muscles for pain relief (as in the case of carpal tunnel syndrome) and structural integration (see page 20) of the entire body. Myofascial massage may incorporate light strokes or deep massage, depending on the muscle involved.

MYOTHERAPY

Similar to neuromuscular therapy (NMT) and using trigger points (see page 21), the aim of myotherapy is to eliminate pain and reeducate the muscles into healthy, pain-free patterns of movement. Myotherapy involves the use of knuckles, fingers, and elbows to press on trigger points, and stretching and exercises to unlearn painful habits.

NEUROMUSCULAR THERAPY (NMT)

A combination of myofascial, trigger point, and deep cross-fiber techniques, NMT is designed to relieve acute or chronic pain by balancing the muscular and neurological aspects of body alignment. Applied to individual muscles, it is used to increase blood flow, release trigger points (see page 21), release pressure on nerves, and relieve pain.

ON-SITE MASSAGE

In on-site massage, the therapist uses a specially designed chair to give employees a fifteen- to twenty-minute head, shoulder, and arm massage at the workplace, without disrobing or oils.

ORIENTAL MASSAGE/AMMA

Amma is the traditional Japanese massage, which is much more commonly taught in Japan than shiatsu. Prior to World War II, it was traditionally performed by the blind. Like shiatsu, amma focuses on energy meridians and points called tsubos (sue-boes). The thumbs are normally used for pressure, kneading, tapping, and rubbing. Unlike Swedish massage, Japanese massage doesn't use oils and may be performed through clothing, and whereas the strokes of Swedish massage move toward the heart, Japanese massage stresses movements away from the heart.

ORTHOBIONOMY

Gentle movements and comfortable positions, in harmony with the body's own preferred posture, are used in orthobionomy to relieve muscle tension and discomfort. Clients learn, under the guidance of a practitioner and through home exercises, to realign and reeducate nerves and muscles for the reduction of pain.

POLARITY THERAPY

Developed by Randolph Stone, an American osteopath, naturopath, and chiropractor, polarity therapy attempts to release obstructed energy flow and thereby reduce pain. (See page 26.)

PREGNANCY MASSAGE

Massage during pregnancy can help relieve fluid retention, improve muscle tone, and relieve the sore back, neck, and muscles that are often part of pregnancy. Shiatsu and massage of the abdomen are avoided, and large pillows are used for comfort.

QIGONG

Qigong exercises are somewhat similar to tai chi chuan, a nonaerobic, rhythmical series of exercises. Qigong differs in that the exercises do not flow from one to another and are done in shorter movement groups repeated a number of times. But it is the accompanying mental effort that is crucial; during the exercises, one must concentrate on moving qi along the meridian pathways, and in so doing, increase the amount of qi to aid in healing.

REFLEXOLOGY

In reflexology, deep pressure is applied to particular spots (or reflex points) on the hands or feet believed to correspond to particular organs and glands. One can visit a reflexologist for manipulation of only the feet and hands, or opt for the technique as part of a full-body massage (see page 16).

REIKI

One of the biofield therapies (see Therapeutic Touch, below), reiki (Japanese for "universal life force") was developed in Japan during the 1800s, but first appeared some 2,500 years ago in the Buddhist scriptures, the sutras. It was introduced into the United States in 1936. Using rituals, symbols, and spirit guides, the practitioner channels spiritual energy to heal the client's spiritual body, which in turn will heal the physical body. There is no massaging involved; practitioners simply hold or place their hands on the afflicted part and other key points for several minutes. One doesn't need a special spiritual gift to heal with reiki; anyone can learn to be a healer of others or of oneself.

ROLFING/STRUCTURAL INTEGRATION

Developed by Ida P. Rolf, Ph.D., during more than fifty years of study, Rolfing and structural therapy are systems of body manipulation and reeducation. The goal of the therapy is structural integration—that is, the balance and alignment of the body along a vertical axis. Withheld emotions, illness, surgery, and other actions can result in compression and distortion of the body; a properly aligned body can function more gracefully and effectively. The gospel of Rolfing, according to Ida Rolf herself, is that "when the body gets working appropriately, the force of gravity can flow through. Then, spontaneously, the body heals itself."[7]

The Rolfer or structural therapist uses thumbs, knuckles, and elbows in a deep, sometimes painful massage to manipu-late connective tissue and realign the body by altering the length and tone of these tissues. This method requires ten sessions to complete.

SHIATSU

Shiatsu, a Japanese method of activating the flow of chi, involves the firm and prolonged pressing of prescribed points that lie along meridians by the practitioner's fingers, thumbs, hands, elbows, feet, or knees in a rhythmic (often painful) pattern. This may be accompanied by stroking that resembles a traditional massage, and with rotating joints to increase range of motion. The client remains clothed and lies on a hard massage table, exercise mat, or floor. Benefits include increased mental alertness, deep relaxation, and relief from muscle soreness.

SPORTS MASSAGE

Techniques of Swedish massage, perhaps combined with other modalities, are used to relax an athlete before an event and to help speed recovery afterward. Sports massage focuses on the stresses, injuries, or sore muscles caused by exercise or vigorous athletic performances.

SWEDISH MASSAGE

The grandfather of the massage movement in this country, Swedish massage is what most of us think of when we hear "massage." Used to promote relaxation, improve circulation and range of motion, and relieve muscle tension, it was developed about 150 years ago by Peter Ling of Sweden, who combined ancient Oriental techniques and principles with modern physiology.

The five basic techniques used in Swedish massage are effleurage (long, soothing strokes), petrissage (squeezing and kneading the muscles), tapotement (a repetitive striking or drumming), vibration (a trembling movement of the hands and fingertips), and friction (a circular movement around joints and tendons). Oil is a must for a smooth, flowing massage. The client is generally undressed but draped with sheets for both warmth and modesty; only the part of the body being worked on is exposed.

THERAPEUTIC TOUCH

Therapeutic touch, SHEN therapy, healing science, healing touch, or the laying on of hands are all considered biofield therapies, a type of healing that dates back some 5,000 years. In these therapies, a practitioner places his or her hands directly on or just slightly above the client's (usually clothed) body and merges his or her biofield with that of the client to promote general well-being or to help heal a specific ailment. Both client and healer may detect subtle changes in temperature, tingles, pressure, or other sensations. Some practitioners attribute the healing power to an outside source—God, the cosmos, or a higher power; others believe that the manipulation of the biofield is itself the healing mechanism. Therapeutic touch is best used for stress-related illnesses, pain relief, and relaxation prior to dental or surgical procedures.

TRAGER® METHOD

Trager psychophysical integration was developed by a Hawaiian physician and former boxing trainer, Milton Trager. This method of movement reeducation employs light rocking, bouncing, and shaking movements to loosen joints and release chronic tension, as well as interrupting deep-seated psychophysiological patterns that project into body tissues. Another part of the method taught to clients, Trager Mentastics are mentally directed physical movements designed to enhance flexibility and a feeling of freedom. Improvement has been reported in patients suffering from multiple sclerosis, lung disease, cerebral palsy, TMJ, recovery from stroke, and a host of other ailments.[8]

TRIGGER POINT THERAPY

When compressed by tense muscles, particularly sensitive nerve bundles, known as trigger points, can send referred pain to areas of the body far removed from the source. Trigger point therapists use finger pressure to relax the spastic muscle and relieve pain.

A Career in Massage Therapy

It has been estimated that there are between 120,000 and 160,000 massage therapists practicing in the United States.[9]

Currently, twenty-nine states plus the District of Columbia regulate the massage and bodywork profession. Although twenty-one of those twenty-nine states utilize the National Certification Exam for Therapeutic Massage and Bodywork (NCETMB) either by statute or in rule, not all states regulate the profession by licensure. Whether or not a given state administers massage practice laws, local or county laws may still apply; large cities and counties often utilize the NCETMB in their local ordinances. In states that govern massage, the potential practitioner should contact the Board of Massage (generally a function of the Department of Health) for requirements. The American Massage Therapy Association (AMTA) chapter in any state will also be able to provide up-to-date information on massage laws; it might also be useful to contact a massage therapist currently practicing in the desired locality. Visit the AMTA website for more information: www.amtamassage.org/about/lawstate.htm.

The Commission on Massage Training Accreditation (COMTA) is the largest accrediting organization in the field of massage education. COMTA uses a minimum 500-hour, six-month curriculum as its standard for approval. Only about one-fourth of the massage schools in the United States are accredited or approved by COMTA.

In 1992, the National Certification Board for Therapeutic Massage and Bodywork (NCBTMB) began administering the only nationally accredited certification examination for the therapeutic massage and bodywork profession. In just seven years, more than 34,000 massage and bodywork practitioners have passed the NCETMB.[10] In order to become eligible to sit for the NCETMB, candidates must have graduated from a formal education training program of at least 500 hours, or its equivalent. This program must have included 100 hours of anatomy and physiology, 200 hours of massage/bodywork theory and application, and 200 hours of related education. For a copy of the current Candidate Handbook, contact the NCBTMB at (703) 610-0281, or visit their website at www.ncbtmb.com.

A massage therapist can work in a variety of settings: health clubs, spas and resorts, cruise ships, in medical offices with chiropractors or physical therapists, for an athletic team or department, or most commonly, as an entrepreneur. More than two-thirds of all massage therapists are self-employed.

MIDWIFERY

It's no contest: midwifery takes the prize as the oldest of the alternative therapies. Since the beginning of time, women have looked to older, more knowledgeable and experienced women to help them through childbirth. Though hospital births are viewed as the norm in much of the United States, midwives have delivered most of the world's babies.

Though midwifery continued to thrive around the world, in the United States the village midwife gave way to the male physician and virtually disappeared by the early 1900s; only those who couldn't afford a hospital stay continued to rely on a midwife's care. The field of nurse-midwifery was born in the 1920s, when Mary Breckenridge enlisted nurse-midwives who rode in on horseback to roadless areas of rural Appalachia. Her success in lowering infant mortality rates led to the founding of the Frontier School of Midwifery and Family Nursing in 1939. Home births experienced a resurgence in popularity in the 1970s and have since continued to account for a steady percentage of births.

Today in the United States, there are two primary types of midwifery, each requiring different training: the certified nurse midwife or the direct-entry midwife.

The Certified Nurse Midwife (C.N.M.) may work alongside a conventional obstetrician in a hospital or clinic, or have a private home-birth practice. C.N.M.s must have a bachelor of science in nursing, then pass board exams to become a Registered Nurse (R.N.). After completion of one to two years of obstetrical nursing or Labor and Delivery in a hospital setting, the R.N. would be a candidate for a master's degree or certificate program in Nurse-Midwifery. Upon completion of the Nurse-Midwifery program, the candidate must pass the American College of Nurse Midwifery (ACNM) board exam to achieve the title Certified Nurse Midwife.

Direct-entry midwifery is based on the European professional midwifery model, in which the midwife enters the field through study and experience, without having to become a nurse first (though nurses are not excluded from becoming direct-entry midwives). Licensed or certified (direct-entry) midwives may practice in a home or birth center, and may receive their training through formal schooling, correspondence courses, self-study, and apprenticeship with a senior midwife. These midwives are reimbursed by many insurance companies, and may sign birth certificates and order lab tests.

A Career in Direct-Entry Midwifery

Because Certified Nurse Midwives are accepted into mainstream medical practices and work in conventional medical settings, their training is not addressed in this book; any standard college guide will provide a listing of the numerous educational opportunities available.

Direct-entry midwives, who receive their training outside of medical schools, are the more "alternative" of the two types. These midwives are often graduates of a formal school of midwifery that, when coupled with hands-on experience, prepares the midwife for licensure and/or national certification.

There are eight schools in the United States that are accredited or in pre-accreditation status with the Midwifery Education Accreditation Council (MEAC). MEAC creates standards and criteria for the education of midwives that reflect the core competencies and principles developed by the Midwives Alliance of North America (MANA). Topics typically covered in MEAC-accredited programs include anatomy and physiology, physical assessment, labor and birth, prenatal and postpartum complications, newborn lab work, pharmacology, well woman care, counseling techniques, and others. Students may work at local hospitals as doulas or be paired with local midwives for apprenticeships.

To become licensed by the state or certified by the North American Registry of Midwives (NARM), a national certifying agency, a direct-entry midwife must demonstrate a certain level of skill and academic knowledge on the NARM or state exam, and must have participated as the primary midwife on a prescribed number of births and pre- and postnatal visits.

At this writing, direct-entry midwifery is legal and regulated, or legal and unregulated, in a total of twenty-nine states, including California, New York, and Texas; it is legally prohibited or effectively prohibited in a total of seventeen states, including Illinois, New Jersey, and Pennsylvania; and in five states, the legal status of direct-entry midwifery is unclear. Eleven states require national certification (NARM or ACNM) for direct-entry midwives.

For updated information on state midwifery laws, visit http://midwife.org/prof/direct.htm.

NAPRAPATHY

Naprapathy is the evaluation of persons with connective tissue disorders through the use of case history and palpation or treatment using connective tissue manipulation, postural and nutritional counseling, and assistive devices utilizing the properties of heat, cold, light, water, radiant energy, electricity, sound, and air. The practice includes the prevention and treatment of contractures, lesions, laxity, rigidity, structural imbalance, muscular atrophy, and other disorders.

Naprapathy was founded in 1905 by Oakley Smith, a graduate of the Palmer School of Chiropractic who was educated by D. D. Palmer, the founder of chiropractic. Dr. Smith conducted extensive research into the bony subluxation theory that was the heart of Palmer's philosophy, and through human dissection, histologic specimens, clinical observation, and patient record keeping, he found no scientific support for Palmer's theory. Rather, he found that the scarring and shortening of the soft connective tissue was the cause of many structural joint problems. Smith named his manipulative science "naprapathy," developed his own treatment system, wrote several books, and opened his own school in 1908.

Licensing generally requires that the applicant have graduated from a two-year, college-level program and be a graduate from a curriculum in naprapathy.

NATUROPATHY

Naturopathy, or naturopathic medicine, is based not on the treatment of specific symptoms or diseases but on achieving a state of optimal wellness in which the body can not only heal itself of any current afflictions but also prevent the occurrence of illness in the future. Though considered alternative in the United States, this approach, like most other forms of natural health care, is nothing new—Hippocrates, considered the first naturopathic doctor, looked for the causes of disease in the air, water, or food that the patient ingested.

Naturopathy took hold in Europe and the United States in the eighteenth and nineteenth centuries. The first school of naturopathic medicine in the United States, founded in New York by Dr. Benedict Lust, graduated its first class in 1902; by the 1920s, there were more than twenty naturopathic colleges in the country. Naturopathy fell out of favor around the 1940s, when allopathic medicine managed to eliminate virtually all conflicting modalities. However, in recent years, naturopathic medicine has staged a comeback, and there are now four colleges in North America devoted to increasing the number of naturopaths.

There are six philosophies that distinguish naturopathy from other forms of medical practice[1]:

1. The healing power of nature—that is, the body's natural ability to establish, maintain, and restore health. It is the physician's duty to assist in this natural, orderly healing process by removing obstacles to health.

2. Identify and treat the cause. An M.D. may have neither the time nor the interest to speculate as to why your hands break out in a scaly rash each October; it's quicker to prescribe a steroidal cream. An N.D., however, seeks out the causes underlying that nagging rash; perhaps it's that dye-filled Halloween candy or your mother-in-law's annual visit that triggers the flare-up. When the cause is known, the treatment can be much more effective.

3. First, do no harm. Symptoms are an expression of the body's efforts at healing; the suppression of symptoms without removing the underlying cause is considered harmful.

4. Treat the entire person. Physical, emotional, spiritual, mental, genetic, environmental, and social factors all contribute to a person's state of wellness and should all be taken into account by the physician.

5. The physician as teacher. The role of the physician is to educate the patient by showing him or her the relationships between actions and illnesses, thereby making the patient responsible for his or her own healing. The physician needs to inspire hope and be a catalyst for change.

6. Prevention. The ultimate goal of the naturopathic physician is to prevent disease through education and promotion of a healthy lifestyle.

In practice, naturopathic medicine is not so much a separate modality as a combination of many of the most widely used forms of alternative therapy. In this way, an N.D. is the general practitioner of complementary medicine—a one-stop shop for a host of natural alternatives. The following are some of the N.D.'s commonly used natural healing techniques.

Clinical nutrition, or diet therapy, is at the core of naturopathic medicine; even allopathic doctors recognize that a diet high in fats and sugars contributes to such illnesses as heart disease, diabetes, colitis, and premenstrual syndrome (PMS), among others. Naturopathy takes nutrition a step further by treating a wider variety of ailments—including eczema, depression, asthma, arthritis, and acne—with dietary changes and nutritional supplements.

Herbal remedies are also an important part of the naturopath's treatment plan. N.D.s are skilled herbologists familiar with the medicinal uses of plants, and they are likely to use herbs for illnesses from the common cold to AIDS.

Homeopathic medicine is another of the N.D.'s tools. Homeopathy uses extremely dilute formulations of substances that, were they given to the patient in a larger dose, would produce the same symptoms as the disease itself—the principle of "like cures like." Hippocrates noticed this effect in his studies of the actions of toxic herbs, and Hahnemann based homeopathy on this concept.

Acupuncture is used to stimulate the immune system through the insertion of fine needles into prescribed points along meridians, or energy pathways, in the body. In the West, acupuncture points may be stimulated with the traditional needles or with lasers, massage, or electrical pulses.

Physical medicine may include the therapeutic manipulation of bones and tissues, as well as hydrotherapy, ultrasound, massage, and exercise.

Psychological medicine such as hypnotherapy, counseling, stress management, and biofeedback may also be used or recommended by a naturopathic physician. As mental states can do much to produce either health or illness, these tools can be important in achieving a balanced emotional, and therefore physical, state.

Minor surgery can be performed by N.D.s in their offices. Such surgical procedures may include stitching a wound, lancing a boil, or removing a foreign object.

Naturopathic physicians can also rely on X-rays, ultrasound, and other forms of diagnostic testing, but they generally do not perform major surgery or prescribe synthetic drugs.

A Career in Naturopathic Medicine

There are currently only four naturopathic colleges in operation in the United States and Canada that are recognized by the Council on Naturopathic Medical Education (CNME), a nationally recognized accrediting agency. Admission to naturopathic colleges is competitive, and students are generally required to have completed all or the better part of a bachelor's degree with an emphasis on premed sciences.

Several correspondence schools (none included in this book) offer programs leading to an N.D. degree; it is not illegal for them to do so, nor for their graduates to use the initials "N.D." after their names. However, they may not legally represent themselves as physicians or engage in the practice of medicine unless they are otherwise licensed. The CNME does not consider graduates of such courses to be part of the naturopathic medical profession, and points out that the accrediting agencies listed by such schools are not recognized by the U.S. Secretary of Education or the Council for Higher Education Accreditation. For more information, visit the www.cnme.org.

Eleven states and four provinces have laws that specifically license or register naturopathic physicians, and N.D.s practice in virtually all of the remaining states and provinces under various legal provisions. Those states that license naturopathic physicians require graduation from an approved resident college program of 4,200 hours or more, and many require graduates to take the Naturopathic Physicians Licensing Exam (NPLEX), a national licensing examination, and/or another licensing exam.

For information on licensing legislation in the United States and Canada, visit www.naturopathic.org.

NUTRITION

There's nothing alternative about nutrition; we all were taught about the four basic food groups (children today learn the food pyramid) by the elementary school nurse or health teacher. Many of us watch our fat grams, calories, or sodium intake, depending on our own personal afflictions and dearly held beliefs. Everyone, from the medical establishment to the vegan, agrees that a bad diet leads to illness, and a good diet can prevent illness.

What we don't agree on, of course, is what constitutes a

"good diet." Therefore, before you embark on a career in nutrition, you must be aware of the many belief systems currently in existence.

Conventional approaches to nutrition include the aforementioned food pyramid school of thought—all foods are more or less good, but the foods near the bottom of the pyramid (grains, fruits, and vegetables) should be eaten in greater quantities than the fats, oils, and sweets at the top. Conventional nutrition is most of what we read in mainstream magazines, see on television, and get in menu form from our doctors in a usually belated attempt to stave off heart disease or diabetes. It's what most nutritional counselors are trained in; it's what most bachelor's or master's degree programs teach. And it's not at all alternative. In fairness, though, the world of nutrition is changing; vegetarianism is taught and practiced by many conventionally educated registered dietitians.

Alternative approaches to nutrition include many very different schools of thought, some of which are in direct opposition to one another. Vegetarianism, which eliminates the consumption of meat products, is probably the most widely known and accepted; in fact, the primarily vegetarian diet is the most common on the planet.[1] It can take the form of the lacto-ovo-vegetarian diet, which includes eggs and milk products, or the vegan diet, which includes no animal products of any kind. In either case, the diet consists primarily of fruits and vegetables, grains, legumes, nuts, and seeds. Through its elimination of meat, a vegetarian diet will reduce an individual's consumption of saturated fat and protein (unless excessive eggs and dairy products are consumed in its place), and increase fiber, vitamins, minerals, and other important nutrients, particularly if organically grown foods are chosen.

While there is not as much concern today about the combining of foods in order to obtain all the amino acids required to build proteins, there is still some concern that a strict vegetarian diet may result in deficiencies of particular vitamins and minerals, most notably vitamin B_{12}, iron, and zinc; for this reason some practitioners suggest a multivitamin and mineral supplement to their vegetarian clients. However, the health rewards of a vegetarian diet are great—lower blood pressure, lower weight, and a reduced risk of cancer, heart disease, diseases of the digestive tract, and osteoporosis[2]—and are usually even more pronounced in the vegan diet.

The macrobiotic diet was brought to the United States from Japan by George Ohsawa and expanded upon by Michio and Aveline Kushi, founders of the Kushi Institute. Ohsawa's beliefs, as presented in Essential Ohsawa, are based on the concept that good air, water, and sunshine are necessary for life, and therefore the most important foods; other necessary foods such as whole grains, vegetables, beans, sea vegetables, and fish are products of these three basic foods.[3] Furthermore, the proper foods are those that are traditionally eaten, grown locally and in season, and that provide a good balance of yin and yang. Whole grains provide the basis for each meal, and comprise 50 to 60 percent of the diet. Well-cooked vegetables and sea vegetables make up 20 to 25 percent of the diet; fresh fish is used in even smaller amounts, and dairy products, fruits, and nuts are used as pleasure foods. Drinks are to be used in the smallest quantity and only as dictated by thirst. Chewing should be thorough; each mouthful should be chewed at least fifty times, up to one hundred or 150 times. The macrobiotic diet contains adequate protein and nutrients, is low in fat and sugar, and would likely do much to improve the health of the average American.

Vitamin therapy is another approach to nutrition that is not exactly embraced by the American Medical Association but is slowly winning converts. While many physicians still tell patients they don't need supplements if they eat a healthy diet, most Americans simply won't eat a healthy diet. Deficiencies can and do develop in both children and adults because of poor eating habits, dependence on processed and fast foods, overworked soils, and poor absorption; simply cooking some foods diminishes or depletes essential nutrients. Physicians, naturopathic and otherwise, can order tests to determine a patient's vitamin and mineral levels and correct the identified deficiencies; or patients can educate themselves regarding the symptoms of deficiency (i.e., irregular heart rhythm as a symptom of magnesium deficiency,[4] Ménière's Syndrome as a symptom of a deficiency of the B vitamins[5]) and order tests only for the suspected deficiencies. Some physicians prefer to have their patients take the full range of vitamins, minerals, amino acids, and fatty acids instead of testing for individual deficiencies, which can be quite expensive. Consuming large quantities of particular nutrients in supplement form can, however, lead to an unbalanced, unhealthy nutritional state in which, for example, too much molybdenum causes a loss of copper, or too much manganese interferes with iron utilization.[6] For this reason, individuals should not take large quantities of individual supplements willy-nilly, but in a balanced fashion under the advice of a physician or other trained health care professional.

A Career in Nutrition

In contrast to conventional nutrition, there are very few schools that teach the alternative approaches. Many practitioners are licensed health care professionals who are self-taught in some aspect of nutrition or who have taken a course here or there; some may get a degree in conventional nutrition and swerve left after graduation, counseling clients in macrobiotics; and some learn the value of vitamin therapy in schools of naturopathy or the joys of macrobiotic cooking at a summer intensive.

The programs listed in this book offer several ways of beginning a career in alternative nutrition. Applicants should first be aware of the laws in their particular state regarding nutritional counseling and find a program that will meet their specific needs; in general, nutritional counselors are permitted to educate their clients about diet and nutrition but are not permitted to diagnose or prescribe.

POLARITY THERAPY

Polarity therapy is an energetic approach to healing that recognizes that energy flows through and around the body in bipolar currents, and that blockage or imbalance of this energy flow results in disease. The approach was developed in the mid–twentieth century by Dr. Randolph Stone, a chiropractor, naturopath, and osteopathic physician who believed, "Energy is the real substance behind the appearance of matter and forms."[1] Stone combined insights common to Eastern energy-based healing practices, such as Ayurveda and Chinese medicine, with his extensive knowledge of Western medicine and structural manipulation.

Polarity theory holds that the head is the source of a positive pole and the feet of a negative pole; the right side of the body is positive and the left side is negative; the joints are neutral, permitting a crossover of energy currents.[2] The pulsation between the two poles provides the basis for life; this is Stone's Polarity Principle.[3] Stone also borrowed the Ayurvedic concept of the Five Elements—ether, air, fire, water, and earth—that correlate to five of the seven chakras, or energy centers, that occur throughout the body. Energy enters through the forehead via the third eye, flows through the chakras, and is then directed by the nervous system to the various muscles and organs.

Polarity therapy in practice is vastly different from massage in that clients remain clothed and the focus is on energy systems rather than physical tissue; a massage education is not necessary for polarity work. In a typical polarity session, the practitioner uses touch (which may vary from light to firm), observation, and interview methods to assess energetic attributes. The practitioner helps the client to become aware of subtle energetic sensations, and may result in relaxation, new insights, and relief from pain or problematic situations. Polarity work does not involve manipulation of the soft tissues or muscles, and is not intended to affect the physical structures and tissues of the body.

Stone also taught that each person must take responsibility for his or her own health, and that wellness can be achieved through some simple steps. For that reason, the polarity practitioner counsels the client in regard to diet, emphasizing vegetarianism as a means of promoting internal cleansing and well-being; exercise, using self-help energy techniques known as polarity yoga; and self-awareness, so that a client might become aware of sources of tension.

Because polarity therapy rebalances the flow of energy so that the body may better heal itself, it can be of value in the treatment of almost any ailment. The deeply relaxed state it produces can be of particular value in the treatment of migraines, cramps, digestive disorders, and stress-related problems.

A Career in Polarity Therapy

The American Polarity Therapy Association (APTA) approves schools and training programs based on their Standards for Practice. A practitioner must complete 155 hours of accredited training for certification as an Associate Polarity Practitioner (A.P.P.), and 615 hours of training for certification as a Registered Polarity Practitioner (R.P.P.). Today there are more than 850 APTA-certified polarity practitioners.

The APTA is working to protect the right of its members to practice without the restrictions of laws pertaining to massage therapy. The APTA maintains that it is inappropriate to classify polarity therapy as massage therapy, bodywork, or somatic therapy, because it is a physically safe, clothes-on, noninvasive holistic system of health care involving energetic approaches to somatic contact, verbal facilitation, nutrition, exercise, and health education. Students interested in polarity therapy as a career should contact the APTA for specific information about licensing; the APTA website is www.PolarityTherapy.org.

REFLEXOLOGY

Far more than a foot massage, reflexology involves the application of pressure to areas of the feet and hands, called reflex areas, that are believed to correspond to specific organs, glands, and other parts of the body in an effort to relieve tension, improve blood flow, reduce pain, and unblock nerve impulses. The principles of reflexology are similar to those of acupuncture and acupressure in that the stimulation of specific points leads to an improvement in functioning in some distant area of the body.

Reflexology is the most popular form of alternative health care in Denmark, according to Dwight Byers, president of the International Institute of Reflexology.[1] While still relatively unknown here, the practice is catching on. Reflexology was first brought to the United States by William Fitzgerald, M.D., a laryngologist from Connecticut, who based the system on European zone therapy. Fitzgerald found he could induce numbness and relieve symptoms in various parts of the body by applying pressure to specific points on the hands and mouth. Physiotherapist Eunice Ingham expanded the system, creating maps of the reflex areas of the feet and developing techniques for stimulating them.

Some reflexologists believe that because of their position, the feet are the most likely site for accumulated toxins; as blood pools in the feet and is pushed back up the leg, these toxins, most often uric acid crystals, are deposited in the feet. Reflexologists break up these crystals so that they may be recirculated and cleansed from the body.[2]

Others see reflexology more as an energetic healing system. Reflex zones are akin to meridians, with life energy or qi flowing through them; a blockage of this energy results in illness. By reducing tension and breaking up deposits, a reflexologist can restore the flow of energy and rebalance the body.

In a typical foot reflexology session, the client either sits on a chair or lies on a massage table, fully clothed except for his or her socks and shoes. The reflexologist, using powder, lotion, or nothing at all, will stroke the foot with his or her thumbs and fingers for up to an hour. Hand reflexology may also be performed.

Research has demonstrated the effectiveness of such stimulation of the hands and feet. Bill Flocco, founder of the American Academy of Reflexology, found a 62 percent reduction in symptoms of premenstrual syndrome (PMS) in those receiving reflexology treatment.[3] Other problems that are relieved by reflexology include anxiety, hypertension, or painful conditions anywhere in the body.[4]

A Career in Reflexology

Reflexology is practiced worldwide by over 25,000 certified practitioners; while some practice only reflexology, it is also commonly used in conjunction with massage therapy, chiropractic, podiatry, and other alternative and conventional modalities. Many, if not most, massage schools include at least minimal instruction in reflexology in their curriculum, while a few schools devote their entire curriculum to the practice.

There is no national licensure for reflexologists, though practitioners may choose to be certified by the American Reflexology Certification Board (ARCB). In order to take the certification exam, applicants must have completed at least 110 hours of education and submit 90 documentations, along with other requirements.

In some states, reflexologists are categorized as massage therapists; nine states and six large cities require that reflexologists hold a massage therapy license.[5] In general, a reflexologist who is licensed for nursing, physical therapy, cosmetology, or barbering is probably not required to meet massage therapy standards. For detailed information on the increasingly mucky legal battle over the status of reflexology, visit the web pages prepared by Kevin and Barbara Kunz at www.footreflexologist.com.

VEDIC PSYCHOLOGY

The study of psychology at Maharishi International University, founded by Maharishi Mahesh Yogi, is based on a deep understanding of consciousness through both direct experience of the inner field of pure consciousness—through daily practice of transcendental meditation—and knowledge of the theoretical model of the Maharishi's Vedic psychology, which explores the full range of consciousness based on India's Vedic tradition. Students are taught to identify the deepest level of their own intelligence as the cosmic psyche, the fundamental intelligence underlying all of nature, and to recognize how it functions in their own psyche. Vocational psychology, psychophysiology, developmental psychology, and other fields are taught in terms of the Maharishi's theories.

Maharishi International University offers bachelor's-through doctorate-level programs in Vedic psychology; the faculty and students are currently developing a Vedic approach to counseling.

VETERINARY MASSAGE

Veterinary massage is just what you'd think: the application of therapeutic massage to animals, most commonly horses, dogs, and cats. Like its counterpart in the human population, veterinary massage has been shown to aid recovery from injury and increase performance and endurance. While cat and dog massage is typically performed by owners on their own pets, equine sports massage (ESM) has far greater career potential.

According to the Tufts University School of Veterinary Medicine, the most likely cause of a horse's poor performance is a musculoskeletal problem. By increasing circulation and relieving stress and muscular tension, equine sports massage can improve performance and reduce the likelihood of injury for racehorses, barrel racers, jumpers, or just about any horse.

In an article in *Practical Horseman,* Equissage originator Mary Schreiber gives a brief description of her equine sports massage technique.[1] Schreiber explains that the only tools required are your fingers, thumbs, and palms; the backs of your hands; and your elbows and fists, which at times will require the pressure of your full body weight. The therapist palpates the entire horse, one side at a time, gently at first to warm up the area and then applying more pressure to find the knotted muscles. These spots are marked with liniment for further work that may include percussion, compression, cross-fiber friction, and other strokes. Massage not only makes the animal more relaxed and cooperative, but can also create a special bond between a horse and its owner.

A Career in Equine Sports Massage

While equine sports massage is a relatively new field, the demand for ESM therapists is growing. As individuals seek out alternative therapies for themselves, they are increasingly interested in the same type of care for their animals.

Training programs in ESM are few in number. Programs run two weeks or less and, while no additional training in massage is required, it is usually recommended that those seeking a full-time career in ESM attend a professional massage therapy school either before or after ESM training in order to bring maximum knowledge of technique and theory to their work. Experience with horses is generally required.

A national ESM survey taken in 1995 by Equissage, operators of a training program in Virginia, indicates that of those who had taken the training with the intention of starting an income-producing business, about 84 percent were successful in starting either a full- or part-time business; about 16 percent were unsuccessful due to lack of persistent effort or perceived lack of acceptance of ESM in that area.[2] The same survey indicated that the mid-Atlantic region was the most receptive to equine sports massage.

Currently, no state recognizes certification in equine sports massage. As with any other career in alternative health care, prospective students should check with their own city and county for any applicable local regulations.

YOGA

Not long ago, many of us viewed yoga as a hippie, counterculture non-exercise, perhaps okay for those with lots of time to contemplate their navels but certainly not anything we could squeeze into our own frenetic schedules. Over the past couple of decades we've progressed from jogging to aerobics to power walking to spinning, and though our thighs may be a little firmer, we're still as stressed as ever. It's no surprise, then, that a quiet revolution is taking hold in the fitness world, as more and more of us are turning to yoga to quiet our minds and relax our muscles—not to mention help us get in touch with our spiritual selves.

It's been estimated that between three and five million Americans now practice some form of yoga.[1] Yoga's increasing popularity is evident in the increased circulation of *Yoga Jour-*

nal, up some 60 percent between 1988 and 1993.[2] And while traditional yoga exercises won't get your heart rate into your target zone, burn many calories, or get rid of the thirty pounds around your middle, the health benefits are very real. Not only have studies found that yoga can produce general health benefits, such as increased circulation, stronger immune systems, and reduced stress, but large percentages of individuals who have used yoga as a treatment for specific medical conditions have also reported positive effects. In a survey of 3,000 individuals conducted by the Yoga Biomedical Trust in the early 1980s, 98 percent of respondents with back pain claimed the practice of yoga was beneficial for them; the reported success rate was 94 percent for anxiety, 90 percent for arthritis, 84 percent for hypertension, 94 percent for heart disease, 90 percent for duodenal ulcers, 80 percent for diabetes, 90 percent for cancer, and 100 percent for alcoholism.[3]

While a few yoga schools are now teaching an aerobic style of power yoga and others don't hold to the traditional ideals of a vegetarian, substance-free lifestyle, by far the majority of schools are still teaching what we would consider classical yoga.

Classical yoga follows an eightfold path that combines postures, breathing, and meditation to produce harmony between the mind, body, and spirit. Purification is also an important aspect of yoga, and takes the form of a vegetarian diet and cleansing and detoxification routines.

Most people are familiar with yoga in the form of hatha yoga postures, or asanas ("ease" in Sanskrit). Meditative asanas align the head and spine, promote blood flow, and aid relaxation. Therapeutic asanas, such as the shoulder stand and cobra positions, are used today to benefit back or joint pain and other specific medical conditions, though originally they served as another way to produce a meditative state. Either type of asana requires little movement but a great deal of mental discipline, allowing an openness that permits the free flow of prana, or life energy.

Pranayama is the regulation of the breath, and hence, of the prana that flows throughout the body. A calm mind will produce regular, rhythmic breathing, and, as we are all aware in times of fright or flight, an anxious mind produces irregular, agitated breathing. The goal of pranayama is a smooth, deep breath from the diaphragm rather than the shallow chest breathing in which so many of us unconsciously engage. Pranayama, like the asanas, serve as preparation for meditation.

Meditation makes up four of the eight limbs of yoga. Meditation has been embraced for thousands of years as a path to spiritual enlightenment, and for the past decade or two as an effective means of treating stress-related illnesses. In fact, in 1984 the National Institutes of Health recommended meditation—rather than medication—as the first line of treatment for mild hypertension.[4]

Meditation is often thought to be a state of not thinking, but that description is not entirely accurate. Meditation is more the training of the mind to concentrate only on the breath or a particular sound or phrase; as other thoughts enter our consciousness—about breakfast, the ache in our knees, or how long this is taking—they are briefly noticed and released, and we resume our concentration on the breath or phrase. Nobody said it was easy: Buddhists say the untrained mind is like a drunken monkey stung by a bee, and once aware, we find it remarkable how much clamor goes on in there day after day. After much daily practice, meditation can calm the mind and put us in touch with our higher selves.

The spiritual culmination of a long, disciplined meditation practice is samadhi, or spiritual realization. At this stage we enter a fourth state of consciousness, neither awake nor asleep nor dreaming.

There are a number of different schools of yoga, including Ashtanga, Iyengar, Sivananda, Kundalini, Kriya, and others, and each has a different emphasis.

A Career in Yoga

For those interested in the classical approach to yoga, becoming a yoga instructor or yoga therapist involves much more personal dedication than many of the other fields of alternative health care. The prospective yoga instructor must not only attend a training program but must, on a daily basis, practice what he or she preaches. To be admitted to most teacher training programs, the student must have been practicing yoga—meaning asanas, pranayama, and meditation—daily for six months to a year or more; must abstain from drugs, alcohol, and tobacco; and must be committed to a vegetarian diet.

Even after completing the teacher training course, which

may take as little as a few weeks or as long as three years, the teacher is never finished learning; he or she must continue, even while teaching, to study under another and to continue his or her daily practice. At least in the case of traditional yoga, becoming an instructor is more a commitment to a lifestyle than just a career choice, and takes an extreme measure of dedication and perseverance.

There are alternatives to the classical approach, however. Many students are looking for less of a lifestyle change and more of an aerobic or fitness approach to yoga—the power-yoga type of workout. Prospective yoga teachers not wishing to commit to the lifestyle restrictions and/or spiritual emphasis of traditional yoga should investigate those schools that offer a more fitness-based approach.

PART

The Schools & Programs
of Alternative Medicine

THE FOLLOWING SECTION lists, alphabetically by state and within each state, schools that offer degree or certificate programs in various fields of alternative medicine. Classroom-based programs in the United States are listed first, followed by programs in Canada and a section called Multiple State Locations. These are schools that offer instruction in many different locations throughout the United States, Canada, and/or the world. The key to finding the school or program you need is the Listing of Programs by Field, located on page 34; just look under the desired field of study and you'll find an alphabetical, state-by-state listing of available programs. Scan the list for a state that you're interested in, check the name of the school, and locate its listing under that state in this section.

Following the state-by-state listing is the Self-Study Resources appendix. This appendix is arranged alphabetically by specialty and lists correspondence courses, periodicals, videos, and other materials that offer basic instruction, serve as handy reference sources, offer a unique perspective, provide ongoing education, or otherwise serve to familiarize you with a field of study. There is also a section on courses in alternative medicine that are now available at conventional medical schools.

Choosing a School or Program

Prospective students of alternative health care should be at least as careful in their selection of a school or training program as they would be in choosing a conventional college. But it's not a situation where you have to cross your fingers and hope for the best; there are guideposts along the way. The following are a few steps to getting a good return on your educational investment.

- Do some reading and educate yourself in the area in which you plan to specialize. Get a feel for the principles and philosophy, the diagnostic and treatment methods, and the job opportunities.

- Go for a treatment. There's no better way to find out what an acupuncturist, massage therapist, or naturopathic physician really does than to become a patient. Visit more than one practitioner for a broader view.

- Contact your local Board of Health or other agencies to determine the licensing requirements in your city. In many states, a specific number of hours of education are required to practice.

- Talk to practitioners in your area to see which schools they would recommend. Ask them about specific schools you have in mind.

- Send for catalogs from lots of schools. Compare programs between schools in your immediate area, and if circumstances permit, consider a longer commute or a relocation; convenience should not necessarily be your first criterion.

- Look at accreditations. In general, a school must be fairly well established, offer a quality program, and pass an on-site inspection to be approved by the major accrediting agencies.

- Compare program lengths. A 100-hour massage program will have you practicing before the month's out, but what will you learn? Be sure the training is sufficient to meet your future needs. That 100-hour program won't get you licensed in too many cities.

- Look at the course schedules and start dates. Some programs may be taken part-time and/or in the evenings; others are strictly full-time days. Some programs start four times per year, some just once a year or every two years.

- If finances are an issue, see what type of financial assistance the school offers. There is tremendous variation between schools in this area; one may offer scholarships, federal grants, and a variety of loans, while another may not have so much as a payment plan.

- Visit the school and get a feel for the place. Is it a warm, close-knit community or does it offer a cooler, more professional atmosphere? Which makes you more comfortable? Talk to the instructors and other students. If you can, speak with practitioners and ask how well their training prepared them for a career.

The best decisions are made with the heart *and* the mind. If your research tells you that a particular program will be sufficient to get you licensed, and if it feels like home—you're there!

Listing of Programs By Field

This section holds the key to finding the schools that interest you. Look under the desired field of study and you'll see an alphabetical, state-by-state listing of available programs. Scan the list for your home state (or one you'd like to visit for a while), check the name of the school, and locate its listing under that state in the Profiles of Schools and Programs.

Schools in the United States are listed first, followed by those in Canada, then schools that offer instruction in more than one state or province (Multiple State Locations). The schools listed here are all classroom-based programs; distance learning courses are listed in the Self-Study Resources appendix beginning on page 462.

NOTE: There are two headings for massage and bodywork schools: Massage and Bodywork and Massage and Bodywork Specialties and Advanced Training. The former lists schools that offer a program of instruction with few or no prerequisites which prepares the student for licensure; the latter are schools that specialize in a unique or narrowly defined field of bodywork whose courses are generally offered to licensed bodywork practitioners. Students looking for continuing education in massage or bodywork should assume that *all* of the schools in the Massage and Bodywork section also offer advanced courses; with the exception of one school (whose primary focus is on advanced training but which also offers a beginner-level program), they are not repeated in the Specialties section. Students seeking advanced training may find what they need under additional headings such as Shiatsu, Reflexology, Aromatherapy, Holistic Health Practitioner, and others.

ACUPRESSURE

CALIFORNIA
Acupressure Institute
Body Therapy Center
Jin Shin Do Foundation for Bodymind Acupressure
Mueller College of Holistic Studies
Taoist Sanctuary of San Diego

FLORIDA
Acupressure-Acupuncture Institute

NEW YORK
Academy of Natural Healing

Canada

ALBERTA
Mount Royal College

BRITISH COLUMBIA
Canadian Acupressure Institute

Multiple State Locations

Pacific College of Oriental Medicine

ACUPUNCTURE AND ORIENTAL MEDICINE

ARIZONA
Phoenix Institute of Herbal Medicine and Acupuncture
Southwest College of Naturopathic Medicine and Health Sciences

CALIFORNIA
Academy Chinese Culture and Health Sciences
American College of Traditional Chinese Medicine
Dongguk Royal University
Emperor's College of Traditional Oriental Medicine
Five Branches Institute
Five Element Training Program
Kyung San University

Meiji College of Oriental Medicine
Samra University of Oriental Medicine
Santa Barbara College of Oriental Medicine
South Baylo University
Yo San University

COLORADO
Colorado School of Traditional Chinese Medicine

FLORIDA
Academy for Five Element Acupuncture
Academy of Chinese Healing Arts
Acupressure-Acupuncture Institute
Atlantic Institute of Oriental Medicine
Florida Institute of Traditional Chinese Medicine
National College of Oriental Medicine

HAWAII
Hawai'i College of Traditional Oriental Medicine
Tai Hsuan Foundation College of Acupuncture and Herbal Medicine
Traditional Chinese Medical College of Hawaii

ILLINOIS
National College of Chiropractic

MARYLAND
Maryland Institute of Traditional Chinese Medicine
Traditional Acupuncture Institute

MASSACHUSETTS
New England School of Acupuncture

MINNESOTA
Minnesota Institute of Acupuncture and Herbal Studies

NEW MEXICO
International Institute of Chinese Medicine

NEW YORK
Mercy College
New York College for Wholistic Health Education and Research
Swedish Institute
Tri-State College of Acupuncture

OREGON
National College of Naturopathic Medicine
Oregon College of Oriental Medicine

TEXAS
Academy of Oriental Medicine—Austin
American College of Acupuncture and Oriental Medicine
Dallas Institute of Acupuncture and Oriental Medicine
Texas College of Traditional Chinese Medicine

WASHINGTON
Bastyr University
Northwest Institute of Acupuncture and Oriental Medicine
Seattle Institute of Oriental Medicine

WISCONSIN
Midwest College of Oriental Medicine

Canada

ALBERTA
University of Alberta

BRITISH COLUMBIA
Academy of Classical Oriental Sciences
Canadian College of Acupuncture and Oriental Medicine
International College of Traditional Chinese Medicine of Vancouver

ONTARIO
The Michener Institute for Applied Health Sciences
Toronto School of Traditional Chinese Medicine

Multiple State Locations

American Academy of Medical Acupuncture
Pacific College of Oriental Medicine
Southwest Acupuncture College

AROMATHERAPY AND FLOWER ESSENCE THERAPY

CALIFORNIA
Aromatherapy Institute and Research
College of the Botanical Healing Arts
Flower Essence Society
Twin Lakes College of the Healing Arts

COLORADO
Artemis Institute of Natural Therapies

CONNECTICUT
Connecticut Institute for Herbal Studies

FLORIDA
Atlantic Institute of Aromatherapy

MASSACHUSETTS
East West Institute of Alternative Medicine

NEW JERSEY
Institute of Aromatherapy
Our Lady of Lourdes Institute of Wholistic Studies

NEW YORK
Academy of Natural Healing
The American Institute for Aromatherapy and Herbal Studies
New York Open Center

OHIO
Ohio Academy of Holistic Health

OREGON
The Australasian College of Herbal Studies

VIRGINIA
Advanced Fuller School of Massage
Aromatherapy Center

WASHINGTON
The Institute of Dynamic Aromatherapy

Canada

ALBERTA
Mount Royal College

BRITISH COLUMBIA
Dominion Herbal College

ONTARIO
Aromaflex Centre of Healing Arts
The Institute of Aromatherapy

Multiple State Locations

Canadian Holistic Therapist Training School/Mississauga School of Aromatherapy
The Foundation for Aromatherapy Education and Research
Institute of Integrative Aromatherapy
The Michael Scholes School for Aromatic Studies

Pacific Institute of Aromatherapy
R.J. Buckle Associates, LLC

AYURVEDA

CALIFORNIA
California College of Ayurveda
Mount Madonna Center

COLORADO
Rocky Mountain Institute of Yoga and Ayurveda

MASSACHUSETTS
East West Institute of Alternative Medicine

NEW MEXICO
The Ayurvedic Institute

NEW YORK
Academy of Natural Healing
Ayurveda Holistic Center

Multiple State Locations

International Ayurvedic Institute

BIOFEEDBACK

CALIFORNIA
Biofeedback Institute of Los Angeles

Multiple State Locations

Biofeedback Instrument Corporation
Stens Corporation

CHIROPRACTIC

CALIFORNIA
Cleveland Chiropractic College of Los Angeles
Life Chiropractic College West
Los Angeles College of Chiropractic
Palmer College of Chiropractic West

CONNECTICUT
University of Bridgeport College of Chiropractic

GEORGIA
Life University School of Chiropractic

ILLINOIS
National College of Chiropractic

IOWA
Palmer College of Chiropractic

MINNESOTA
Northwestern College of Chiropractic

MISSOURI
Cleveland Chiropractic College
Logan College of Chiropractic

NEW YORK
New York Chiropractic College

OREGON
Western States Chiropractic College

SOUTH CAROLINA
Sherman College of Straight Chiropractic

TEXAS
Parker College of Chiropractic
Texas Chiropractic College

Canada

ONTARIO
Canadian Memorial Chiropractic College

CHIROPRACTIC ASSISTANT

GEORGIA
Life University

ENERGETIC HEALING

CALIFORNIA
Diamond Light School of Massage and Healing Arts

MICHIGAN
Health Enrichment Center

MISSOURI
Massage Therapy Training Institute LLC

NORTH CAROLINA
North Carolina School of Natural Healing

VERMONT
Wellness College of Vermont

Canada

ONTARIO
Spirit of the Earth Centre for Herbal Education and Earth Awareness

Multiple State Locations

Polarity Realization Institute

ENVIRONMENTAL MEDICINE

Multiple State Locations

American Academy of Environmental Medicine

GUIDED IMAGERY

CALIFORNIA
Academy for Guided Imagery

HERBOLOGY

ARIZONA
Phoenix Institute of Herbal Medicine and Acupuncture
Southwest Institute of Healing Arts
Southwest School of Botanical Medicine

CALIFORNIA
California School of Herbal Studies
California School of Traditional Hispanic Herbalism
Dandelion Herbal Center
Dry Creek Herb Farm and Learning Center
East West School of Herbology
EverGreen Herb Garden and School of Integrative Herbology
Natural Healing Institute of Naturopathy
Ohlone Center for Herbal Studies
Sierra Institute of Herbal Studies

COLORADO
Artemis Institute of Natural Therapies
Rocky Mountain Center for Botanical Studies

CONNECTICUT
Connecticut Institute for Herbal Studies
Northwestern Connecticut Community-Technical College

FLORIDA
Acupressure-Acupuncture Institute
Florida Health Academy

GEORGIA
Living With Herbs Institute

ILLINOIS
Northern Prairie Center for Education and Healing Arts

MAINE
Avena Botanicals

MASSACHUSETTS
Blazing Star Herbal School
Centre of the Web
Ellen Evert Hopman
Hands of Light

MONTANA
Rocky Mountain Herbal Institute

NEW JERSEY
The Chrysalis Center
Herbal Therapeutics School of Botanical Medicine

NEW MEXICO
National College of Phytotherapy
New Mexico College of Natural Healing
The New Mexico Herb Center

NEW YORK
Academy of Natural Healing
Flynn's School of Herbology
New York College for Wholistic Health Education and Research
New York Open Center
Northeast School of Botanical Medicine
Susun S. Weed / Wise Woman Center
Tri-State College of Acupuncture

NORTH CAROLINA
North Carolina School of Natural Healing

OHIO
Healing Heart Herbals
Ohio Academy of Holistic Health

OREGON
The American Herbal Institute
Brighid's Academy of Healing Arts
Center for Herbal Studies

PENNSYLVANIA
Mt. Nittany Institute of Natural Health

RHODE ISLAND
Apollo Herbs

VERMONT
Sage Mountain Herbal Retreat Center
Vermont School of Herbal Studies
Wellness College of Vermont

VIRGINIA
Dreamtime Center for Herbal Studies

WISCONSIN
Wisconsin Institute of Chinese Herbology

Canada

BRITISH COLUMBIA
Dominion Herbal College
International College of Traditional Chinese Medicine of Vancouver

ONTARIO
Spirit of the Earth Centre for Herbal Education and Earth Awareness
Toronto School of Traditional Chinese Medicine

HOLISTIC HEALTH EDUCATOR/ PRACTITIONER

ARIZONA
Southwest Institute of Healing Arts

CALIFORNIA
Academy of Professional Careers
American University of Complementary Medicine
California College of Physical Arts

California Institute of Integral Studies
Desert Resorts School of Somatherapy
Healing Hands School of Holistic Health
Heartwood Institute
John F. Kennedy University
Mendocino School of Holistic Massage and Advanced Healing
   Arts
Mueller College of Holistic Studies
National Holistic Institute
Natural Healing Institute of Naturopathy
School of Healing Arts

MISSOURI
Massage Therapy Training Institute LLC

NEW MEXICO
The Medicine Wheel—A School of Holistic Therapies

NEW YORK
Omega Institute

PENNSYLVANIA
Mt. Nittany Institute of Natural Health

Canada

ALBERTA
Grant MacEwan Community College
Centennial College

ONTARIO
The Institute of Aromatherapy

Multiple State Locations

DoveStar Institute
Pacific College of Oriental Medicine

HOLISTIC NURSING

NEW YORK
New York College for Wholistic Health Education and Research

HOMEOPATHY

CALIFORNIA
American University of Complementary Medicine

Hahnemann College of Homeopathy
Institute of Classical Homoeopathy
Pacific Academy of Homeopathy
Quantum-Veritas International University Systems
Valley Hypnosis Center

COLORADO
Colorado Institute for Classical Homeopathy

ILLINOIS
National College of Chiropractic

MICHIGAN
Institute of Natural Health Sciences

MINNESOTA
Northwestern School of Homeopathy

NEW JERSEY
Five Elements Center

NEW YORK
Atlantic Academy of Classical Homeopathy
The School of Homeopathy
Teleosis School of Homeopathy

VIRGINIA
National Center for Homeopathy

Canada

BRITISH COLUMBIA
Vancouver Homeopathic Academy

ONTARIO
Homeopathic College of Canada
Toronto School of Homeopathic Medicine Ltd.

Multiple State Locations

Canadian Academy of Homeopathy
New England School of Homeopathy

HYPNOTHERAPY

ARIZONA
Southwest Institute of Healing Arts
Wesland Institute

CALIFORNIA
Alchemy Institute of Healing Arts
Center for Hypnotherapy Certification
Diamond Light School of Massage and Healing Arts
Hypnosis Motivation Institute
Hypnotherapy Training Institute
Hypnotism Training Institute of Los Angeles
Natural Healing Institute of Naturopathy
School of Healing Arts
Twin Lakes College of the Healing Arts
Valley Hypnosis Center

CONNECTICUT
The Connecticut School for Hypnosis and NLP

ILLINOIS
Leidecker Institute

INDIANA
Midwest Training Institute of Hypnosis

MAINE
New England School of Clinical Hypnotherapy

MICHIGAN
Discovery Institute of Clinical Hypnotherapy
Infinity Institute International

NEW JERSEY
Light Lines Wholistic Center
Unlimited Potential Institute

NEW MEXICO
Hypnosis Career Institute

NORTH CAROLINA
The Wellness Training Center

OHIO
Ohio Academy of Holistic Health

VIRGINIA
Eastern Institute of Hypnotherapy

WASHINGTON
Institute for Therapeutic Learning

WISCONSIN
WMB Hypnosis Training Center

Multiple State Locations
Creativity Learning Institute
DoveStar Institute
The Wellness Institute (WA)

INDEPENDENT STUDY DEGREE PROGRAMS

VERMONT
Vermont College of Norwich University

INTEGRATIVE MEDICINE/THERAPIES

ARIZONA
Program in Integrative Medicine—University of Arizona

CALIFORNIA
Natural Healing Institute of Naturopathy

NEW YORK
Omega Institute

IRIDOLOGY

CALIFORNIA
Valley Hypnosis Center

OHIO
Ohio Academy of Holistic Health

Canada
ONTARIO
Spirit of the Earth Centre for Herbal Education and Earth Awareness

Multiple State Locations
Canadian Holistic Therapist Training School/Mississauga School of Aromatherapy

MASSAGE THERAPY AND BODYWORK

ARIZONA
Arizona School of Integrative Studies
Desert Institute of the Healing Arts

Phoenix Therapeutic Massage College
RainStar College
Southwest Institute of Healing Arts

ARKANSAS
White River School of Massage

CALIFORNIA
Academy of Professional Careers
Alive and Well! Institute of Conscious BodyWork
American Institute of Massage Therapy
Body Therapy Center
California College of Physical Arts
California Institute of Massage and Spa Services
Central California School of Body Therapy
Desert Resorts School of Somatherapy
Diamond Light School of Massage and Healing Arts
Esalen Institute
Healing Hands School of Holistic Health
Heartwood Institute
Institute of Psycho-Structural Balancing
International Professional School of Bodywork
Jin Shin Do Foundation for Bodymind Acupressure
McKinnon Institute
Mendocino School of Holistic Massage and Advanced Healing Arts
Monterey Institute of Touch
Mueller College of Holistic Studies
National Holistic Institute
Natural Healing Institute of Naturopathy
Phillips School of Massage
reSource
School of Healing Arts
School of Shiatsu and Massage at Harbin Hot Springs
Touching for Health Center
The Touch Therapy Institute
Trinity College
Twin Lakes College of the Healing Arts
Western Institute of Neuromuscular Therapy

COLORADO
Academy of Natural Therapy
Boulder College of Massage Therapy
Colorado Institute of Massage Therapy

Colorado School of Healing Arts
Cottonwood School of Massage Therapy
Crestone Healing Arts Center
Massage Therapy Institute of Colorado
MountainHeart School of Bodywork and Transformational Therapy
South West School of Massage

CONNECTICUT
Connecticut Center for Massage Therapy

DISTRICT OF COLUMBIA
Potomac Massage Training Institute

FLORIDA
Academy of Healing Arts
Acupressure-Acupuncture Institute
Boca Raton Institute
CORE Institute
Educating Hands School of Massage
Florida Academy of Massage
Florida College of Natural Health
Florida Health Academy
Florida School of Massage
Florida's Therapeutic Massage School
The Humanities Center Institute of Applied Health School of Massage
Loraine's Academy
Sarasota School of Massage Therapy
Seminar Network International

GEORGIA
Academy of Somatic Healing Arts
Atlanta School of Massage
Georgia Institute of Therapeutic Massage
Lake Lanier School of Massage

HAWAII
Hawaiian Islands School of Body Therapies
Honolulu School of Massage

IDAHO
Idaho Institute of Wholistic Studies

ILLINOIS
Chicago School of Massage Therapy

LifePath School of Massage Therapy
Northern Prairie Center for Education and Healing Arts
Redfern Training Systems School of Massage
Wellness and Massage Training Institute

INDIANA
Alexandria School of Scientific Therapeutics
Lewis School and Clinic of Massage Therapy

IOWA
Capri College
Carlson College of Massage Therapy

LOUISANA
Blue Cliff School of Therapeutic Massage

MAINE
Downeast School of Massage

MARYLAND
Baltimore School of Massage

MASSACHUSETTS
Bancroft School of Massage Therapy
Massage Institute of New England
Muscular Therapy Institute
The Stillpoint Program at Greenfield Community College

MICHIGAN
Ann Arbor Institute of Massage Therapy
Health Enrichment Center
Institute of Natural Therapies
Irene's Myomassology Institute
Kalamazoo Center for the Healing Arts
Kirtland Community College
Lansing Community College
Michigan School of Myomassology
Wellspring School of Therapeutic Bodywork

MINNESOTA
Center for a Balanced Life
Minneapolis School of Massage and Bodywork
Northern Lights School of Massage Therapy

MISSOURI
Massage Therapy Training Institute LLC
St. Charles School of Massage Therapy

NEBRASKA
Gateway College of Massage Therapy
Omaha School of Massage Therapy

NEW HAMPSHIRE
North Eastern Institute of Whole Health

NEW JERSEY
Academy of Massage Therapy
Garden State Center for Holistic Health Care
Healing Hands Institute for Massage Therapy
Healing Hands School of Massage
Health Choices
Helma Institute of Massage Therapy
Morris Institute of Natural Therapeutics
Our Lady of Lourdes Institute of Wholistic Studies
Somerset School of Massage Therapy

NEW MEXICO
Body Dynamics School of Massage Therapy
Crystal Mountain Apprenticeship in the Healing Arts
The Medicine Wheel—A School of Holistic Therapies
New Mexico Academy of Healing Arts
New Mexico College of Natural Healing
New Mexico School of Natural Therapeutics
Scherer Institute of Natural Healing
Taos School of Massage
Universal Therapeutic Massage Institute

NEW YORK
Finger Lakes School of Massage
New York College for Wholistic Health Education and Research
New York Institute of Massage
Swedish Institute

NORTH CAROLINA
Body Therapy Institute
Carolina School of Massage Therapy
North Carolina School of Natural Healing
Therapeutic Massage Training Institute
The Whole You School of Massage and Bodywork

OHIO
Central Ohio School of Massage
National Institute of Massotherapy
SHI Integrative Medical Massage School

OKLAHOMA
Oklahoma School of Natural Healing
Praxis College of Health Arts and Sciences

OREGON
Ashland Massage Institute
Cascade Institute of Massage and Body Therapies
East-West College of the Healing Arts
Oregon School of Massage

PENNSYLVANIA
The Alternative Conjunction Clinic and School of Massage
    Therapy
Career Training Academy
East-West School of Massage Therapy
Health Options Institute
Lancaster School of Massage
Lehigh Valley Healing Arts Academy
Mt. Nittany Institute of Natural Health
Pennsylvania Institute of Massage Therapy
Pennsylvania School of Muscle Therapy

SOUTH CAROLINA
Charleston School of Massage

TENNESSEE
Cumberland Institute for Wellness Education
The Massage Institute of Memphis
Middle Tennessee Institute of Therapeutic Massage
Tennessee Institute of Healing Arts
Tennessee School of Massage

TEXAS
Academy of Oriental Medicine—Austin
Austin School of Massage Therapy
Hands-On Therapy School of Massage
The Institute of Natural Healing Sciences
The Lauterstein-Conway Massage School
The Winters School

UTAH
Myotherapy College of Utah
Utah College of Massage Therapy

VERMONT
The Vermont School of Professional Massage
Wellness College of Vermont

VIRGINIA
Advanced Fuller School of Massage
Cayce/Reilly School of Massotherapy
Richmond Academy of Massage
The School of Applied Kinesthetic Studies
Virginia School of Massage

WASHINGTON
Alexandar School of Natural Therapeutics
Ashmead College School of Massage
Brenneke School of Massage
Brian Utting School of Massage
Cedar Mountain Center for Massage
Soma Institute
Spectrum Center School of Massage
Tri-City School of Massage

WEST VIRGINIA
Mountain State School of Massage

WISCONSIN
Blue Sky Educational Foundation
Lakeside School of Massage Therapy
Wisconsin Institute of Natural Wellness

Canada

ALBERTA
Alberta Institute of Massage
Edmonton School of Swedish Relaxation Massage
Foothills College of Massage Therapy
Grant MacEwan Community College
Mount Royal College
The Orthopaedic Massage Therapy Institute
Somatic Arts Institute

BRITISH COLUMBIA
Okanagan Valley College of Massage Therapy Ltd.

ONTARIO
Centennial College
D'Arcy Lane Institute School of Massage Therapy
ICT Kikkawa College / ICT Northumberland College
Sault College of Applied Arts and Technology
Sutherland-Chan School and Teaching Clinic

QUEBEC
Le Centre Psycho-Corporel

SASKATCHEWAN
McKay School of Massage and Hydrotherapy

Multiple State Locations

Asten Center of Natural Therapeutics
BioSomatics
Canadian College of Massage and Hydrotherapy/West Coast
   College of Massage Therapy
DoveStar Institute
New Hampshire Institute for Therapeutic Arts
Pacific College of Oriental Medicine
Polarity Realization Institute
Southeastern School of Neuromuscular and Massage Therapy

MASSAGE AND BODYWORK SPECIALTIES AND ADVANCED TRAINING

CALIFORNIA
The Breema Center
Polarity Healing Arts
Reese Movement Institute

COLORADO
Polarity Center of Colorado
Rolf Institute of Structural Integration

DISTRICT OF COLUMBIA
Institute for Integrated Therapies

FLORIDA
Florida Institute of Psychophysical Integration

MASSACHUSETTS
Kripalu Center for Yoga and Health

NEVADA
Aston-Patterning

PENNSYLVANIA
Academy for Myofascial Trigger Point Therapy

WASHINGTON
Soma Institute

Canada

QUEBEC
Feldenkrais Institute of Somatic Education

Multiple State Locations

BioSomatics
Day-Break Geriatric Massage Project
Feldenkrais Resources
Hellerwork International
Jin Shin Jyutsu
Myofascial Release Treatment Centers and Seminars
Nurturing the Mother
Ohashi Institute
The Rubenfeld Synergy Center
The School for Body-Mind Centering
School for Self-Healing
Touch for Health Kinesiology Association
The Trager Institute
Wellness Institute

Multiple State Locations—Canada

Dr. Vodder School—North America

MIDWIFERY

CALIFORNIA
Midwifery Institute of California

MAINE
Birthwise Midwifery School

OREGON
Birthingway Midwifery School
Oregon School of Midwifery

TEXAS
Maternidad La Luz

UTAH
Utah College of Midwifery

WASHINGTON
Seattle Midwifery School

Multiple State Locations

Sage Femme Midwifery School

NAPRAPATHY

ILLINOIS
Chicago National College of Naprapathy

NATUROPATHY

ARIZONA
Southwest College of Naturopathic Medicine and Health Sciences

CONNECTICUT
University of Bridgeport College of Naturopathic Medicine

OREGON
National College of Naturopathic Medicine

WASHINGTON
Bastyr University

Canada

ONTARIO
The Canadian College of Naturopathic Medicine

Multiple State Locations

Canadian College of Massage and Hydrotherapy/West Coast College of Massage Therapy

NUTRITION

ARIZONA
Southwest Institute of Healing Arts

CALIFORNIA
Heartwood Institute
Los Angeles East West Center Institute for Macrobiotic Studies
Natural Healing Institute of Naturopathy
School of Healing Arts
Vega Institute

GEORGIA
Life University

MASSACHUSETTS
Kushi Institute

NEW YORK
Gulliver's Institute
The Natural Gourmet Cookery School

OHIO
Ohio Academy of Holistic Health

WASHINGTON
Bastyr University

Canada

ONTARIO
Canadian College of Natural Nutrition

PERSONAL TRAINER/WELLNESS CONSULTANT

(See Holistic Health Educator / Practitioner)

POLARITY THERAPY

ARIZONA
Southwest Institute of Healing Arts

CALIFORNIA
Heartwood Institute
Polarity Healing Arts
Polarity Therapy Center of Marin

COLORADO
Polarity Center of Colorado

FLORIDA
Florida School of Massage

MASSACHUSETTS
American School for Energy Therapies

NEW MEXICO
New Mexico Academy of Healing Arts

NEW YORK
Academy of Natural Healing
International Woodstock Retreat Center

The Linden Tree Center for Wholistic Health
New York Open Center

VIRGINIA
The Polarity Center and Shamanic Studies

Canada

ONTARIO
Reaching Your Potential

Multiple State Locations

Polarity Realization Institute
Wellness Institute

QIGONG

ARIZONA
Southwest Institute of Healing Arts

FLORIDA
Seminar Network International

OHIO
The Qigong and Human Life Research Foundation

TEXAS
Academy of Oriental Medicine—Austin

Multiple State Locations

East West Academy of Healing Arts / Qigong Institute

REFLEXOLOGY

ARIZONA
Southwest Institute of Healing Arts

COLORADO
Colorado School of Healing Arts
MountainHeart School of Bodywork and Transformational Therapy

DISTRICT OF COLUMBIA
Institute for Integrated Therapies

FLORIDA
Florida School of Massage

ILLINOIS
Redfern Training Systems School of Massage

MAINE
Footloose

NEW JERSEY
Our Lady of Lourdes Institute of Wholistic Studies

NEW YORK
New York Open Center
Omega Institute

OHIO
Central Ohio School of Massage
International Academy for Reflexology Studies
Ohio Academy of Holistic Health

PENNSYLVANIA
Lehigh Valley Healing Arts Academy
Mt. Nittany Institute of Natural Health
Pennsylvania School of Muscle Therapy

VIRGINIA
Advanced Fuller School of Massage

Canada

ALBERTA
Mount Royal College

ONTARIO
Aromaflex Centre of Healing Arts
The Institute of Aromatherapy

Multiple State Locations

Canadian Holistic Therapist Training School/Mississauga School of Aromatherapy
International Institute of Reflexology

REIKI

CALIFORNIA
Valley Hypnosis Center

FLORIDA
Reiki Plus Institute

MICHIGAN
International Center for Reiki Training

NEW JERSEY
Unlimited Potential Institute

NEW YORK
The Linden Tree Center for Wholistic Health

OHIO
Ohio Academy of Holistic Health

Multiple State Locations
· DoveStar Institute

SHIATSU

ARIZONA
Desert Institute of the Healing Arts
Southwest Institute of Healing Arts

CALIFORNIA
Acupressure Institute
Body Therapy Center
California Institute of Massage and Spa Services
School of Shiatsu and Massage at Harbin Hot Springs
Shiatsu Massage School of California

COLORADO
Colorado School of Healing Arts

HAWAII
Aisen Shiatsu School

MARYLAND
Baltimore School of Massage

MASSACHUSETTS
East West Institute of Alternative Medicine

MINNESOTA
The Minnesota Center for Shiatsu Study

NEW JERSEY
Our Lady of Lourdes Institute of Wholistic Studies
School of Asian Healing Arts

PENNSYLVANIA
Career Training Academy
East-West School of Massage Therapy
Meridian Shiatsu Institute

Canada
BRITISH COLUMBIA
Canadian Acupressure Institute

ONTARIO
Centennial College
Shiatsu Academy of Tokyo
Shiatsu School of Canada

SPIRITUALITY, HEALTH, AND MEDICINE

WASHINGTON
Bastyr University

TAI CHI TEACHER TRAINING

FLORIDA
Seminar Network International

TUI NA

(See Acupressure)

VEDIC MEDICINE/VEDIC PSYCHOLOGY

IOWA
Maharishi University of Management

VETERINARY HEALTH CARE

ARIZONA
Southwest Institute of Healing Arts

COLORADO
Boulder College of Massage Therapy

OHIO
Integrated Touch Therapy for Animals

OREGON
Animal Natural Health Center

VIRGINIA
Equissage

Canada

ONTARIO
D'Arcy Lane Institute School of Massage Therapy

Multiple State Locations

International Veterinary Acupuncture Society

YOGA TEACHER TRAINING

ARIZONA
Southwest Institute of Healing Arts

CALIFORNIA
BKS Iyengar Yoga Center of Southern California
The Expanding Light
Iyengar Yoga Institute of San Francisco
Mount Madonna Center
United States Yoga Association
Yoga College of India
Yoga Works

COLORADO
Day-Star Method of Yoga
Rocky Mountain Institute of Yoga and Ayurveda
Shambhava School of Yoga

FLORIDA
Yogi Hari's Ashram

MARYLAND
The Yoga Center

MASSACHUSETTS
Kripalu Center for Yoga and Health

NEW JERSEY
Our Lady of Lourdes Institute of Wholistic Studies
School of Asian Healing Arts
Studio Yoga

NEW YORK
Omega Institute

PENNSYLVANIA
The Himalayan International Institute of Yoga Science and
    Philosophy

VIRGINIA
Aromatherapy Center
Satchidananda Ashram—Yogaville

WASHINGTON
Yoga Centers

Canada

BRITISH COLUMBIA
Yasodhara Ashram

Multiple State Locations

American Viniyoga Institute
American Yoga Association
DoveStar Institute
Integrative Yoga Therapy
International Alliance of Healthcare Educators
International Yoga Studies
Kali Ray TriYoga
Phoenix Rising Yoga Therapy
3HO International Kundalini Yoga Teachers Association
Sivananda Ashram Yoga Camp

Profiles of Schools and Programs

ARIZONA

Arizona School of Integrative Studies

753 North Main Street
Cottonwood, Arizona 86326
PHONE: (520) 639-3455
FAX: (520) 639-3694
E-MAIL: asis@wildapache.net
WEBSITE: www.wildapache.net/asis

The Arizona School of Integrative Studies (ASIS) was founded in January 1996 by Jamie and Joseph Rongo and Nancy Matthews. There are twelve instructors, with a maximum of twenty students per class.

Accreditation and Approvals
ASIS is licensed by the State of Arizona, a member of the AMTA Council of Schools, and approved by the National Certification Board for Therapeutic Massage and Bodywork (NCBTMB) as a continuing education provider. Graduates are qualified to take the National Certification Examination for Therapeutic Massage and Bodywork (NCETMB).

Program Description
The 750-hour Massage and Hydrotherapy Training Program consists of 366 hours of massage modalities, 244 hours of conjunctive course studies, and 140 additional hours. Massage modalities include Swedish Massage, Connective Tissue Massage, Reflexology, Neuromuscular Therapy, Shiatsu, Integration, Polarity Therapy, Sports Massage, Connective Tissue Therapy, Awareness and Integrative Massage, and Review. Conjunctive course studies include Anatomy and Physiology, Kinesiology and Palpation, Hydrotherapy, Nutrition, Herbology, Homeopathy, Communication Skills, Life Skills (CPR, First Aid, and HIV), Business and Arizona Law, and Review. Orientation, massage journals, and community outreach require additional hours. Classes are held five days per week.

Continuing Education
Continuing education workshops for massage and bodywork professionals include Present Centered Awareness Therapy, Connective Tissue Therapy, Aromatic Impressions: The Art and Science of Aromatherapy, Soft Tissue Injuries for Runners, Orthobionomy, Advanced Sports Massage, Process Oriented Polarity Therapy, Structural Integration, Spa Director Certification, and others.

Admission Requirements
Applicants must be at least 18 years of age (this requirement may be waived through a personal interview), have a high school diploma or equivalent, submit a self-recommendation, and have a personal interview.

Tuition and Fees
Application fee, $50; student packet and books, $300; tuition, $5,500; optional massage table, $300 to $600; oils and linens are additional.

Financial Assistance
Payment plans may be arranged.

Desert Institute of the Healing Arts

639 North Sixth Avenue
Tucson, Arizona 85705
PHONE: (520) 882-0899 / (800) 733-8098

FAX: (520) 624-2996
E-MAIL: info@diha.org
website: www.diha.org

The Desert Institute of the Healing Arts was founded in 1982. There are forty instructors, with a maximum of twenty-eight students per class.

Accreditation and Approvals

The Desert Institute's massage and shiatsu programs are both accredited by the Commission on Massage Training Accreditation (COMTA). The school is accredited by the Accrediting Commission of Career Schools and Colleges of Technology (ACCSCT) and a member of the AOBTA Council of Schools and Programs. Graduates are qualified to take the National Certification Examination for Therapeutic Massage and Bodywork (NCETMB).

Program Description

The Desert Institute offers certificate programs in Massage Therapy and Zen Shiatsu.

The 1,000-hour Massage Therapy Certificate Program consists of courses in Massage Theory and Practice (including hydrotherapy), Anatomy and Physiology, Communication Skills, Business and Professionalism, and Benefits of Massage Therapy, plus electives in Massage Practicums (including addictions recovery, massage and HIV/AIDS, physically challenged, prenatal massage, senior massage, and sports massage), Professional Development (including movement integration, stretching and joint mobilization, tai chi chuan, and yoga), Classroom Lab/Clinic (including Anatomiken and palpatory integration), Beginning Shiatsu, On-Site Chair Massage, and others. CPR/First Aid certification is required and must be arranged by the student. Students are expected to receive two professional massages per trimester.

The 650-hour Zen Shiatsu Certificate Program includes Western Anatomy and Physiology, Zen Shiatsu Technique, Qi Dance, Foundations of Eastern Medicine, Communications, Business and Professionalism, Shiatsu Clinic, Practicum, and Survey of Bodywork Modalities. CPR/First Aid certification is required and must be arranged by the student. Students are expected to receive two professional shiatsu treatments per trimester.

Admission Requirements

Applicants must be at least 21 years of age (exceptions will be made with parental consent), have a high school diploma or equivalent, interview with an admissions representative, and agree to adhere to codes of conduct and ethics. Anyone who has been convicted of a felony may not be eligible for city licensing, which is a requirement for the massage therapy practicums (check with the City of Tucson prior to applying).

Tuition and Fees

There is a $25 application fee.

Fees for the Massage Therapy program are as follows: tuition, $9,180; books and supplies, $700; City Student Trainee License fee, $25; massage table (average cost), $600; AMTA student membership (optional), $168; CPR/First Aid, up to $35; and six professional massages (two per trimester), $150 to $250.

Fees for the Zen Shiatsu program are as follows: tuition, $6,030; books and supplies, $400; futon, $50 to $100; AOBTA student membership (optional), $40; and six professional shiatsu treatments, $150 to $250.

Financial Assistance

Federal grants and loans are available.

International Yoga Studies

(See Multiple State Locations, page 399)

Jin Shin Jyutsu®

(See Multiple State Locations, page 400)

Phoenix Institute of Herbal Medicine and Acupuncture

P.O. Box 2659
Scottsdale, Arizona 85252
PHONE: (480) 994-3648
FAX: (602) 439-1511
E-MAIL: contactus@pihma.com
WEBSITE: www.pihma.com

Phoenix Institute of Herbal Medicine and Acupuncture (PIHMA) was founded in 1996 by Catherine Niemiec. There are twenty-four instructors, with an average of fifteen students per class.

Accreditation

PIHMA has conditional degree-granting status from the Arizona State Board for Private Postsecondary Education, and is in the process of applying for accreditation with the Accreditation Commission for Acupuncture and Oriental Medicine (ACAOM). Graduates are qualified to sit for the National Certification Commission for Acupuncture and Oriental Medicine (NC-CAOM) exam.

Program Description

PIHMA offers Master of Sciences degrees and certification in Acupuncture, Chinese Herbology, and Oriental Medicine.

The four-year, 2,835-hour Oriental Medicine Certification Program consists of 162 semester units. Courses include Oriental Medical Theory, Point Energetics, OM Diagnosis and Practicum, Point Location/Surface Anatomy, Acupressure and Meridians, Materials and Methods of Oriental Medicine, Clinic Technique and Observation, Qi Gong/Tai Chi, Acupuncture Practicum, Oriental Medicine, Acu-Microsystems Practicum, Oriental Nutrition, Clinic, Oriental Medical Pathology, Classics Seminar and Thesis, Advanced Clinical Techniques, Ethics, Practice Management, Externship/Internship, and Electives (which may include Five Element Training, Japanese Acupuncture, Touch for Health, Korean Acupuncture, Oriental and Western Herbology, Tibetan Herbology, Ayurvedic Medicine, Introduction to Homeopathy, Chinese Medical and Conversational Language, and others). Courses in the Western Sciences include Anatomy and Physiology, Medical Terminology and History, Biology/Microbiology, Chemistry, CPR/First Aid, Bio-Pharmacology, Psychology, Western Clinical Sciences, Western Nutrition, Western Pathology and Diagnosis, Advanced Western Pathology, Comparative Clinical Sciences, Botany, and Physics.

The 2,280-hour Acupuncture Certification Program consists of 120 semester units from those listed above.

The 1,500-hour Herbology Certification Program consists of 100 semester units, and may be studied separately or as part of the Oriental Medicine program. The program is designed for acupuncturists or other health professionals who would like to have more confidence in using Chinese herbs, or who have not yet studied the Chinese herbal system. Each segment covers a review of syndromes and practical diagnostics related to the herbs and formulas presented; a thorough discussion of individual herbs and formulas; major Chinese patent products and American-made Chinese herbal products; how to modify basic formulas according to differentiation of symptoms and signs; case studies; and home review exercises.

Community and Continuing Education

Courses open to the community include a 100-hour Herbal Primer, 12-hour Basic Oriental Herbology, and Introduction to Oriental Medicine. Mini-classes are also offered in such areas as Oriental Medicine and Chinese Culture, Tai Chi, Qi Gong, Feng Shui, Acupressure, and others.

Continuing education courses for health professionals include a fifty-hour Gatekeeper training, 200-hour Intermediate Practitioner Level, Acupuncture in Dentistry, Emergency Acupuncture, and Pulse Diagnosis.

Admission Requirements

Applicants must have a high school diploma or equivalent, plus two years (sixty semester hours/ninety quarter units) of classes at the baccalaureate level or equivalent from a regionally accredited college or university. Applicants must also submit two letters of reference and a short essay.

Tuition and Fees

Classes are generally offered at $10 per hour (may vary). Estimated tuition for completion of the Oriental Medicine Certification is $28,350; for Acupuncture Certification, $22,800; and for Herbal Certification, $15,000. Tuition is reduced when Western Science prerequisites are waived in.

Financial Assistance

Payment plans and work-study are available.

Phoenix Therapeutic Massage College

609 North Scottsdale Road
Scottsdale, Arizona 85257
PHONE: (602) 945-9461

FAX: (602) 425-8247
E-MAIL: ptmc@impulsedata.com
WEBSITE: ptmcaz.com

Phoenix Therapeutic Massage College (PTMC) was founded in 1981 and purchased by K. C. Miller and Wayne Schmeeckle in 1998. There are twenty-one instructors; classes average fifteen to twenty-four students.

Accreditation and Approvals
PTMC is accredited by the Accrediting Council for Continuing Education and Training (ACCET). Graduates are qualified to take the National Certification Examination for Therapeutic Massage and Bodywork (NCETMB).

Program Description
PTMC offers two science-based massage programs: a 750-hour Therapeutic Massage Program and a 1,125-hour Professional Certification Program for Therapeutic Massage.

The 750-hour Therapeutic Massage Program offers basic education in therapeutic massage. Courses include Anatomy, Physiology, Massage, Health Care, Nutrition, Career Development, and Externship.

The 1,125-hour program consists of the 750-hour Therapeutic Massage Program followed by 375 hours of specialty classes including Advanced Sports, Deep Tissue, Traditional Chinese, Lymphatic, Pregnancy, and Geriatric massage; Kinesiology; Pathology; Hydrotherapy; and Chiropractic Assistant training.

Programs are offered mornings, afternoons evenings and weekends.

Admission Requirements
Applicants must have a high school diploma or equivalent; be physically, mentally, and emotionally capable of performing massage therapy; pass the entrance exam; and interview with an admissions representative.

Tuition and Fees
Total charges are $6,506 for the 750-hour program and $9,316 for the 1,125-hour program; these figures include application fee, tuition, books, supplies, college shirts, and massage table.

Financial Assistance
Federal grants and loans, payment plans, and veterans' benefits are available; PTMC is also approved by Vocational Rehabilitation.

Program in Integrative Medicine

University of Arizona
P.O. Box 245153
Tucson, Arizona 85724-5153
PHONE: (520) 626-7222
FAX: (520) 626-6484
WEBSITE: www.integrativemedicine.arizona.edu

The Program in Integrative Medicine at the University of Arizona College of Medicine was founded by Dr. Andrew Weil, M.D., an internationally recognized expert on holistic medicine. There are fifteen to twenty local instructors and ten to fifteen national contributors. Four fellows are selected each year.

Accreditation and Approvals
The Program in Integrative Medicine is not accredited, as there does not yet exist an accrediting body in Integrative Medicine. The Program is working with other medical schools around the country which are interested in implementing integrative medicine programs, and hopes to create an accrediting body through these associations. The Program in Integrative Medicine is housed within the Department of Medicine at the University of Arizona College of Medicine, which is an accredited program.

Program Description
The Program in Integrative Medicine at the University of Arizona College of Medicine is a new approach to medical education. The program consists of a fellowship, a teaching clinic, a professional development/continuing education program for individuals in practice, and a research program.

The fellowship component is a two-year intensive program for M.D.s and D.O.s who have completed residencies in primary care specialties. As part of the training, an Integrative Medicine Clinic was established where the doctors begin to practice the new approach and learn to develop integrative treatment plans. The fellowship program includes a core curriculum of twelve subject areas, clinical training, and a commitment to self-care, personal awareness, and change. The core curriculum includes Healing-Oriented Medicine, The Philosophy of Science, Research Education, Nutritional Medicine, Botanical Medicine, Mind-Body Medicine, Spirituality and Medicine, Energy Medicine, Complementary and Alternative Medicine, Medicine and Culture, The Art of Medicine, and Leadership, Medicine and Society. In the clinical training, fellows see patients four half-days per week and present new patients in an interdisciplinary patient conference. The conference includes the program director, medical director, and clinicians representing Oriental medicine, homeopathy, mind/body medicine, osteopathy, pharmacy, nutrition and spirituality. A "container for change" is established at the beginning of the fellowship and supported over the two-year course of the fellowship: fellows have no clinical responsibilities during their first two months; attend retreats led by a psychologist and Zen teacher; are taught meditation techniques; receive mutual support through personal reflection in a group; and read, write and discuss poetry.

A 1,000-hour Associate Fellowship in Integrative Medicine is scheduled to begin in fall 2000 and extend over two years. This program will be offered in a predominantly distance learning format via the Internet, with an on-site component that will address those areas not suitable for the distance learning format. The program will address the needs of physicians and nurse practitioners who wish to remain in their practices and learn to incorporate Integrative Medicine.

Admission Requirements

The fellowship is open only to M.D.s and D.O.s who have completed residencies in primary care specialties. The Certificate Program in Integrative Medicine is designed for physicians, clinicians, nurse practitioners, nurses, pharmacists, and other health care providers.

Tuition and Fees

Contact the university for tuition information.

Financial Assistance

Each of the four fellows selected receives a stipend of $35,716 per year.

RainStar College

4110-4130 North Goldwater Boulevard
Scottsdale, Arizona 85251
PHONE: (602) 423-0375 / (888) RAINSTAR
FAX: (602) 945-9824
E-MAIL: info@rainstargroup.com
WEBSITE: www.rainstargroup.com

RainStar College (previously the RainStar School of Therapeutic Massage, the New Life Therapy Center and A Touch of Health) was founded in 1988 by Jody Russell. There are sixty instructors, with ten to twenty-five students per class.

Accreditation and Approvals

RainStar College is accredited by the Integrative Massage and Somatic Therapies Accreditation Council (IMSTAC) and is approved by the National Certification Board for Therapeutic Massage and Bodywork (NCBTMB) as a continuing education provider. Graduates of all but the 200-hour program are qualified to take the National Certification Examination for Therapeutic Massage and Bodywork (NCETMB).

Program Description

RainStar offers several levels of massage therapy training: the Basics Program (200 hours), the Graduate Program (500 hours), the Advanced Graduate Program (750 hours), and the Master's Program (1,000 hours). Each program covers topics in Massage; Anatomy, Physiology and Kinesiology; Health Awareness; and Opportunities in Business.

The Basics Program may be completed in two months full- or part-time. Topics covered include Swedish Therapeutic Massage, Introduction to Craniosacral Therapy, Basic Reflexology, Principles of Advanced Techniques, and Basic Pregnancy Massage.

The Graduate Program may be completed in three months full-time, six months part-time, or two months accelerated. Topics covered Swedish Therapeutic Massage, Advanced Techniques, Lymphatic Drainage, Mineral Body Wrap, Craniosacral Therapy, Pulsing, Shiatsu, Hydrotherapy, Sports Massage, Infant/Child Therapy, Clinical Practicum, and more.

The Advanced Graduate Program offers additional instruction and practice in advanced topics. The program may be completed in five months full-time, ten months part-time, or four months accelerated.

The Master's Graduate Program offers additional instruction and practice in advanced topics. The program may be completed in seven months full-time, fourteen months part-time, or five months accelerated.

Community and Continuing Education

A wide variety of continuing, introductory, and advanced certifications are offered on a regular basis and are open to the public. Topics include Acupressure, Aromatherapy, Ayurveda, Geriatric Massage, Chinese Herbs, Essential Elements of Nutrition, Iridology, Reiki, Sports Massage, and many more.

Admission Requirements

Applicants must be at least 18 years of age; have a high school diploma or equivalent and have a minimum GPA of 2.5; have the physical and emotional ability to perform as a massage therapist; and have a personal interview.

Tuition and Fees

Tuition is as follows: Basics Program, $2,495; Graduate Program, $5,995; Advanced Graduate Program, $7,295; Master's Program, $8,895. Books, manuals, oil, lotion, and linens are additional.

Financial Assistance

A payment plan, loans, partial scholarships, and veterans' benefits are available.

Southwest College of Naturopathic Medicine and Health Sciences

2140 East Broadway
Tempe, Arizona 85282
PHONE: (602) 858-9100
FAX: (602) 858-9116
E-MAIL: admissions@scnm.edu
WEBSITE: www.scnm.edu

Southwest College of Naturopathic Medicine and Health Sciences was founded by Michael Cronin, N.D., and Kyle Cronin,

N.D., in 1993. There are thirty-nine faculty members; class sizes average twenty to thirty in spring, fifty to seventy in fall.

Accreditation and Approvals

Southwest College is accredited by the Council on Naturopathic Medical Education (CNME) and has approval to operate from the State of Arizona Naturopathic Physicians Board of Medical Examiners. Southwest College is licensed by the Arizona State Board of Private Postsecondary Education to offer the Doctor of Naturopathic Medicine degree and was granted a Regular Vocational Program License to offer the Certificate in Acupuncture Program. Graduates of the Professional Master's-Level Program in Acupuncture are eligible to take the National Certification Commission for Acupuncture and Oriental Medicine (NCCAOM) national board exams.

Program Description

The four-year graduate program leading to the Doctor of Naturopathic Medicine degree may be completed in sixteen quarters by a full-time, year-round student. Students are prepared to take the licensing examinations necessary to practice as naturopathic physicians.

Courses offered in the basic sciences include Anatomy with Lab, Biochemistry, Embryology, Histology, Medical Genetics, Medical Microbiology, Physiology, and Pathology. Diagnostic courses include Physical Diagnosis, Clinical Diagnosis, Laboratory Diagnosis, and Diagnostic Imaging. Other related courses include Public Health and Environmental Medicine, Psychology and Counseling, and Research.

Clinical courses include Naturopathic Manipulative Therapies, Hydrotherapy, Orthopedic and Sports Medicine, Acupuncture and Oriental Medicine, Emergency Medicine, Minor Surgery, Pharmacology and Pharmacognosy, Botanical Medicine, Homeopathic Medicine, Nutritional Medicine, History and Philosophy of Naturopathic Medicine, Naturopathic Standards of Care, Medical Ethics, Jurisprudence, Business Practices, and Clinical Practice.

The Clinical Competency Program (clinical training) takes place at the Southwest Naturopathic Medical Center. This program allows students the opportunity to build clinical skills.

The Professional Master's-Level Program in Acupuncture is a three-year, 2,232-hour program designed using national standards. Courses offered include Anatomy and Physiology, Biochemistry, Living Anatomy, Western Psychology, Research Methodologies, Physical Diagnosis, Western Pathology, Fundamentals of Oriental Medicine, Basic Acupuncture Techniques, Western Nutrition, Point Location and Pathology, Traditional Chinese Medicine (TCM) Diagnosis, Ethics/Practice Management, Auricular Acupuncture, Pharmacology, Clinic Observation, TCM Therapeutics, Clinic Internship, Meridian and Points, Chinese Prepared Medicines, Qigong (TCM meditation), Tui Na (TCM massage), TCM Gynecology, and Master's Project.

In their eighth quarter, students enter the Clinic Internship Program at the medical center. Students are required to take the Clean Needle Techniques Course (CNT) of the Council of Colleges of Acupuncture and Oriental Medicine (CCAOM) prior to entering the clinic to ensure their knowledge of clean needle techniques for the safety of the patients. A maximum of eight credits of clinical training may be earned by taking part in an optional externship trip to China.

Admission Requirements

Applicants must submit three letters of recommendation; those with complete files are invited to the campus for a series of interviews. The college follows the rolling admissions model. In addition, each program has specific requirements.

For the N.D. program, applicants are required to have a bachelor's degree with a GPA of 2.5 or greater. Specific course requirements include English (six semester hours, at least three of which must be English composition), psychology (six semester hours), humanities (six semester hours), general chemistry with lab (eight semester hours), organic chemistry with lab (four semester hours), and general biology with lab (twelve semester hours). The student must have a GPA of 3.0 or greater in prerequisite courses.

For the acupuncture program, applicants must have completed sixty semester hours with a GPA of 2.5 or greater. Specific course requirements include English composition (three semester hours), psychology (six semester hours), general biology with lab (eight semester hours), and general chemistry with lab (eight semester hours). The student must have a GPA of 3.0 or greater in prerequisite courses.

Tuition and Fees

Tuition and fees for the N.D. program is $14,500 per year. Tuition and fees for a full-time acupuncture student average $7,700 per year.

Financial Assistance

For the N.D. program, subsidized and unsubsidized Stafford Loans are available, up to a maximum of $18,500 for each three-quarter period. No federal financial aid is available for the acupuncture program at this time.

Southwest Institute of Healing Arts

1402 North Miller Road
Scottsdale, Arizona 85257
PHONE: (602) 994-9244
E-MAIL: doyourdream@swiha.org
WEBSITE: www.swiha.org

Southwest Institute of Healing Arts was founded in 1992 by Brian and K. C. Miller. There are fifteen core instructors with over 100 part-time instructors. Over 300 students have graduated from the massage therapy programs, and over 2,000 students have enrolled in continuing education classes. In addition to the programs described here, the institute offers a 200-hour Massage Technician program.

Accreditation and Approvals

Southwest Institute of Healing Arts is licensed by the Arizona State Board of Private Postsecondary Education. Graduates of massage therapy programs of 500 hours or more are qualified to take the National Certification Examination for Therapeutic Massage and Bodywork (NCETMB). Graduates of the Reflexology Program who complete the required outside documented sessions are eligible to sit for the International Reflexology Therapy Examination Council test. In Arizona, reflexologists are required to be licensed massage therapists; students who complete the 500-hour Reflexology Program are eligible for licensure. A.P.P. and R.P.P. graduates are eligible for certification with the American Polarity Therapy Association (APTA). Graduates of the 500-hour Oriental Studies Program are eligible for national certification with the American Oriental Bodywork Therapy Association (AOBTA). Graduates of the 100-hour Hypnotherapy Program are eligible for registration with the American Board of Hypnotherapy.

Program Description

The 500-hour Therapeutic Massage Program consists of core requirements of Applied Anatomy, Physiology, First Aid and CPR, and Business Practices and Ethics. Beyond this, students may substitute classes for any scheduled classes other than the core requirements. Recommended electives are Applied Myotherapy, Breast Health, Carpal Tunnel/Thoracic Outlet Release, Corporate Chair Intro, Deep Tissue Sculpting, Energetic Acupressure, Fibromyalgia Therapy, Hand and Wrist Repair, Lower Back Pain Release, Lymphatic Massage, Modified Myotherapy, Myotherapy, Neck Release, Reflexology, Rock and Unlock, Sports Massage Intro, Swedish Massage, Therapeutic Touch Intro, TMJ Release, Polarity Cranial Unwinding, and Swedish Esalen.

Specialty Track programs of 500 hours are also offered in Sports Therapy, Energy Work, and Spa Treatments. These programs have the same four core requirements as the Therapeutic Massage Program, with electives chosen in each specialty. Sports Therapy electives include Competitive Edge Nutrition, Exercise Physiology, Endurance Training, Sports Therapy, Fitness Program Design, Intro to Supplements, Sports Injury Management, Sports Nutrition, and others. Energy Work electives include Aromatherapy, Acupressure, Aura, Balancing Male and Female Energy, Hatha Inner Dance, Holographic Repatterning, Magnet Therapy, Polarity, and more. Spa Treatment electives include Spa Therapies Intro, Face-lift Acupressure, Reiki, Aromatherapy Massage, Ayurvedic Bindi Herbal, and others.

Programs of 300 and 500 hours are offered in Reflexology. The 300-hour Reflexology Program consists of required classes in Applied Anatomy, Physiology, First Aid and CPR, Business Practices and Ethics, and four levels of Reflexology. Students choose an additional 100 hours of electives from Auriculotherapy, Auriculotherapy Advanced, Emotional Reflexology, Face-Lift Acupressure, Face Reflexology, Meridian Reflexology, Aromatherapy and Five Element Acupressure, Introduction to Reflexology, Toe Reading, or Face Reading. For the 500-hour Reflexology Program, students choose a total of 300 hours of electives.

Both Associate Polarity Practitioner (A.P.P.) and Registered Polarity Practitioner (R.P.P.) Programs are offered; the A.P.P. Program may be taken for 175 or 500 hours; the R.P.P. Program is 706 hours.

The 175-hour A.P.P. Program consists of Polarity Basic I and II, Polarity Reflexology, Polarity Communication, Anatomy, documented polarity sessions, Clinical Supervision, and five documented R.P.P. sessions.

For the 500-hour A.P.P. Program, students add courses in Applied Anatomy, Physiology, First Aid and CPR, and Business Practices and Ethics.

The 706-hour R.P.P. Program consists of the A.P.P. Program (less Anatomy), plus Spinal Balancing, Polarity Exercise, Six Point Star and Colon, Autonomic Nervous System, Communications, Cleanse Group, Energetic Nutrition, Business Professional Ethics, Advanced Study Group, Five Point Star and Lymphatic, Internship, Advanced Supervision, Cranial Unwinding, Anatomy, seventy documented sessions, and ten one-hour sessions with an R.P.P.

A 500-hour Oriental Studies Program consists of a major in either Tui Na, Zen Shiatsu, Qigong Tui Na, or Jin Shin Jyutsu®, plus courses in Applied Anatomy, Business Practices and Ethics, Dragon and Tiger Qigong or Yoga, CPR/First Aid, Oriental Theory, Oriental Therapy Clinic, and sixty hours of hands-on Oriental electives chosen from Anma, Aromatherapy Five Element Acupressure, Qigong Healing, Internal Organ Massage, Oriental First Aid, Thai Massage, Energetic Acupressure, Yoga, or others.

The 300- and 500-hour Equine Massage Therapy Programs are offered to licensed massage therapists or those pursuing licensure by completing a state recognized human massage therapy program. The 300-hour Equine Massage Therapy Program consists of Basic Equine Anatomy, Physiology, and Pathology; Equine Massage Techniques; Equine Massage Practices and Ethics; Equine Massage Movement and Performance; Equine Massage Therapy Internship; Field Experience; and electives chosen from Equine Lameness, Saddlefitting Techniques, Proper Shoeing Evaluation, Equine Acupressure, Stretching Exercises for the Rider, Equine Stretches, Equine Deep Tissue Sculpting, Introduction to Equine Alternative Therapies, and Equine Sports Massage Techniques. For the 500-hour Equine Massage Therapy program, students add courses in Applied Anatomy, Physiology, First Aid, CPR, Business Practices and Ethics, and additional equine electives. Electives to be offered in the future include Equine Myofascial Release, Equine Kinesiology, Equine Cranial Sacral Techniques, Performance Horse Analysis, Equine Nutrition, and Equine Behavior.

The 500-hour Western Herbalism Program is open to students who have completed Foundations of American Herbal Studies. The one-year hands-on course offers intensive training in herbal studies with a science core requirement. The program consists of four Herbal Modules, three Comprehensive Bio Sciences modules, Botany, Clinical Externship, and electives.

The 200-hour Hatha Yoga Teacher Training consists of courses in Hatha, Pranayama, Strength, All Body, Twelve Systems, Pregnancy, All That Jazz, Inner Dance, CPR, electives, and class prep.

The 100-hour Hypnotherapy Program consists of three levels of Hypnotherapy classes plus eight hours of electives chosen from Love Yourself, Heal Your Life; Boundaries and Ethics; and Alchemical Hypnotherapy.

The 300-hour Holistic Nutrition Specialist Program consists of Foundations of Holistic Nutrition, Stress Management, Support Group Facilitation, Survey of Contemporary Nutrition Therapies, Whole Food Cuisine, Foundations of Holistic Nutrition, Strategies for Weight Disorders, Intro to Supplements, Optimum Health in a Toxic World, Public Speaking and Presentation, Practice Development Portfolio, and Ethics and Boundaries in Nutrition.

Associate of Occupational Science Degree Programs are offered in Holistic Health Care, Clinical Nutrition, Body-Mind Transformational Psychology, Chinese Herbology, and Oriental Bodywork. Each requires a minimum of sixty credit hours.

The Associate of Occupational Studies in Holistic Health Care is open to those holding a certificate in therapeutic massage, nursing, or equivalent therapeutic modality. Required core courses are Applied Psychology, Healing the Healer, Psychology of Health and Healing, Psychoneuroimmunology, Optimum Health in a Toxic World, Exercise Physiology, Breast Health and Counseling Skills, Foundations for Holistic Nutrition, Polarity, Body/Mind Therapy Training, Plant-Based Technologies, Hypnotherapy, Practice Development Portfolio, Public Speaking and Presentation, and Writing for Publication. Students then choose an area of specialty from among Holistic Nutrition, Polarity Certification, Hypnotherapy, Western Herbalism, Aromatherapy, or Oriental Specialty.

The Associate of Occupational Studies in Clinical Nutrition is open to those who have completed the 300-hour Holistic Nutrition Therapist Program (above). Additional courses include Applied Psychology/Body-Mind Class, Comprehensive Biosciences, Fundamentals of Nutritional Assessment, Nutrition for Life's Different Stages, Energetic Nutrition, Therapeutic Diet Planning, Foundations of American Herbalism, and others.

It is highly recommended that students entering the Associate of Occupational Studies in Body-Mind Transformational Psychology Program have a massage therapist license as they will need the licensing to do hands-on work with their clients. Topics covered in this program include Body Centered Modalities (Polarity, Body Centered Psychology, Intuitive Massage, and Oriental Bodywork); Mind Technologies (Hypnotherapy, NLP, Gestalt, and Body Centered Coaching); and Spiritual Exploration (Aikido, Qigong or Yoga, Meditation, and Comparative Spiritual Traditions), plus required courses in such areas as Psychology, Medical Astrology, Intuitive Studies, Hypnotherapy, Polarity, and others.

The Associate of Occupational Studies in Chinese Herbology includes courses in Oriental Nutrition Therapy, Comprehensive Biosciences, Oriental Theory, Intro to Chinese Patent Herbs, Five Element Psychology and Counseling, Chinese Materia Medica, Herbal Formulas, and others.

The Associate of Occupational Studies in Oriental Bodywork includes courses in TCM Nutrition, Intro to Chinese Patent Herbs, Advanced Oriental Theory, Point Location, Spirit of Points, Five Element Personality, and others.

Admission Requirements

Prerequisites, if any, are listed at the beginning of each program description.

Community and Continuing Education

Courses may be taken individually outside of a planned diploma, certificate, or degree program.

Tuition and Fees

Tuition for the 500-hour Therapeutic Massage, Specialty Track, Oriental Studies, or A.P.P. Program is $3,750 or $7.50 per hour; additional hours after 500 are $7.50 per hour.

Tuition for the 300-hour Equine Massage Therapy Program is $2,250; additional hours are $7.50 each.

Tuition for the 500-hour Western Herbalism Program is $4,050 or $7.50 to $8.50 per hour.

Tuition for the 100-hour Hypnotherapy Program is $910, or

$7.50 to $9.50 per hour. Tuition for Associate of Occupational Science Degree programs is as follows: Holistic Health Practitioner, $9,638; Body-Mind Psychology, $8,085; Clinical Nutrition, $6,975; Oriental Bodywork, $10,243; Chinese Herbology, $9,000.

Most individual courses are $7.50 to $9.50 per hour.

Financial Assistance

Payment plans and work-study are available.

Southwest School of Botanical Medicine

P.O. Box 4565
Bisbee, Arizona 85603
PHONE: (520) 432-5855
E-MAIL: hrbmoore@primenet.com
WEBSITE: chili.rt66.com/hrbmoore/HOMEPAGE/

The training program at the Southwest School of Botanical Medicine is now in its nineteenth year. Director Michael Moore has been a practicing herbalist since 1968 and has written several books about the medicinal plants of the southwest. The program is limited to twenty-eight students.

Program Description

An annual 500-hour, twenty-week rigorous training program is offered in Professional Herbology. Classes include Botanical Materia Medica, Physiology for the Herbalist, Herbal Pharmacy, Herbal Therapeutics, Botany for the Herbalist, Constitutional Medicine, Clinical Practicum, Business Practicum, Herbal Formulating, Random Acts (various classes with visiting and local experts), Q&A and Review, and Field Work/Wildcrafting.

Classes are held Monday through Thursday from January to May.

Tuition and Fees

Tuition is $2,500 and includes the primary texts. Additional costs include books, up to $100; supplies, $100 to $300; and field trips, $400 to $800.

Wesland Institute

3367 North Country Club Road
Tucson, Arizona 85716
PHONE/FAX: (520) 881-1530
E-MAIL: ninoc@primenet.com
WEBSITE: www.weslandinstitute.com

The Wesland Institute was established in 1988. There is one instructor, with an average of eight students per class. The Hypnotherapy Certification Program is also available in a home-study format (see page 485).

Accreditation and Approvals

Wesland Institute is licensed by the Arizona State Board for Private Postsecondary Education, and is endorsed by the International Medical and Dental Hypnotherapy Association (IMDHA).

Program Description

The Hypnotherapy Program consists of 100 hours of in-class instruction and 130 hours in an externship program. Topics covered include Introduction, Glossary of Terms, Historical Overview, Overview of Current Psychotherapies, Basic Physiology, Patterns of Programming, Laws of Suggestion, Experiential Suggestibility Tests, Types of Suggestibility, Preinduction Interview, Traditional Inductions, Deepening Techniques, Visualizations, NLP Theories and Techniques, Smoking Cessation, Weight Control, Analytical Hypnotherapy, Age Regression, Past Life Regression, Phobias, Anesthesiology, Ericksonian Hypnosis, Hypnotherapy and Children, Marketing, and Law. The supervised externship allows the student to work with clients in a simulated office or clinical situation.

Classes may be completed in four weeks in the accelerated, Tuesday-through-Friday program, or in twelve weeks of Saturday classes.

Continuing Education

Continuing education classes are held periodically throughout the year.

Admission Requirements

Applicants must be at least 18 years of age and have a high school diploma or equivalent.

Tuition and Fees

Tuition is $1,200, including a $100 preregistration fee.

Financial Assistance

Payment plans are available.

ARKANSAS

White River School of Massage

48 Colt Square, Suite B
Fayetteville, Arkansas 72703
PHONE: (501) 521-2550
FAX: (501) 521-2558
WEBSITE: www.wrsm.com

The White River School of Massage was founded in 1991 by Ellen May and Michael Avenoso. There are thirteen instructors, with an average of twenty-four students per class.

Accreditation and Approvals

White River School of Massage has been approved by the Arkansas State Board of Massage Therapy and is a member of the American Massage Therapy Association (AMTA) Council of Schools. Graduates are qualified to take the National Certification Examination for Therapeutic Massage and Bodywork (NCETMB). White River School of Massage is approved by the National Certification Board for Therapeutic Massage and Bodywork (NCBTMB) as a continuing education provider.

Program Description

The 500-hour Professional Massage Training Program includes Anatomy and Physiology, Swedish Massage, Sports Massage, Myofascial Therapy, Neuromuscular Therapy, Shiatsu, Craniosacral Therapy, Reflexology, Therapeutic Modalities, Spa Services, Hygiene/First Aid/CPR, Business Management and Marketing, Body Mechanics/Self-Care, Clinical Practice, and Assessment Skills. A Special Hospital Internship is available. Optional electives are also offered in such areas as herbology, aromatherapy, yoga, and others at additional cost. Students may take weekday, weekend, or summer intensive courses.

Continuing Education

White River School of Massage sponsors nationally recognized leaders in the field of therapeutic massage and bodywork in special seminars for both students and practicing professionals.

Admission Requirements

Applicants must be at least 18 years of age, have a high school diploma or equivalent, and interview with an admissions representative.

Tuition and Fees

Tuition is $3,500. Additional expenses include a $100 application fee and approximately $80 for books.

Financial Assistance

Several types of financial assistance are offered, including payment plans, a 5 percent prepayment discount, veterans' benefits, and some state assistance.

CALIFORNIA

Academy for Guided Imagery

P.O. Box 2070
Mill Valley, California 94942
PHONE: (415) 389-9324 / (800) 726-2070
FAX: (415) 389-9342
E-MAIL: agi1996@aol.com
WEBSITE: www.interactiveimagery.com

The Academy for Guided Imagery was founded in 1989 by Martin Rossman, M.D., and David E. Bresler, Ph.D. The directors and faculty have taught Interactive Guided Imagery[SM] at hundreds of organizations including Columbia University, Disney, University of Illinois, University of California, the American Holistic Medical Association, and others. There are forty-five instructors, with an average of twenty-five students per class. (See page 472 for the Interactive Guided Imagery self-paced study program.)

Accreditation and Approvals

The academy has been approved for continuing education credits by the American Psychological Association, the California Board of Behavioral Sciences, the California Board of Registered Nursing, and the California Alcoholism and Drug Counselors Education Program.

Program Description

The 150-hour Professional Certification Program offers in-depth training in Interactive Guided Imagery[SM] to professional health care providers over a period of fourteen to twenty-four months. Home study modules are combined with fifty-two hours of small group supervision.

The home study modules consist of Interactive Guided Imagery: Clinical Training for Brief Therapy and Mind/Body Medicine; Advanced Tools for Success I, which includes The Role of the Imagery Guide and Advanced Work with the Inner Advisor; Advanced Tools for Success II, which includes Resistance and Parts Work and Parts, Polarities and Conflict Resolution; Advanced Tools for Success III, which includes Interactive Guided Imagery with Children, and Adult Survivors of Childhood Abuse; Advanced Tools for Success IV, consisting of Physical, Chronic and Life-threatening Illness, and Death, Dying, Loss and Transformation. Candidates also complete thirty-three hours of Independent Study and fifty-two hours of Preceptorship I and II, in which certification candidates gain a working understanding of techniques and principles.

Admission Requirements

The applicant must be a practicing health care professional (usually in a counseling field).

Tuition and Fees

Tuition for the entire program is $2,995.

Financial Assistance

A monthly payment plan is available.

Academy of Chinese Culture and Health Sciences

1601 Clay Street
Oakland, California 94612

PHONE: (510) 763-7787
FAX: (510) 834-8646
E-MAIL: acchs@best.com
WEBSITE: www.acchs.edu

The Academy of Chinese Culture and Health Sciences was founded in 1982 by Dr. Wei Tsuei. There are forty-seven instructors, with an average of twenty-five students per class.

Accreditation and Approvals

The academy's Master of Science in Traditional Chinese Medicine degree program is accredited by the Accreditation Commission for Acupuncture and Oriental Medicine (ACAOM). Graduates are eligible to take the acupuncture licensure examination given by the California State Acupuncture Committee, and are eligible for licensure in other states. The academy is approved by the California Acupuncture Committee as a continuing education provider for licensed acupuncturists, and by the California Board of Registered Nursing as a provider of continuing education for registered nurses.

Program Description

The academy offers a four-year Master of Science in Traditional Chinese Medicine program that may be completed in three calendar years of full-time study (a student may elect part-time study with the approval of the administration). The curriculum is divided into two portions: the preprofessional courses of the first two calendar years and the graduate courses of the final calendar year. The preprofessional courses are considered equivalent to the latter two upper-division years of a baccalaureate program. Comprehensive exams are given at the beginning of the fifth and ninth trimesters to determine a student's eligibility for the next level of study.

The 2,992-hour curriculum includes History of Medicine, Medical Chinese, Foundations of TCM, Taiji Philosophy, Tui Na (Acupressure Technique), Ethics, Acupuncture, Herbology, Western Pathology, TCM Diagnosis, Western Pharmacology, Herbology-Formulas, Western Physical and Lab Diagnosis, Clinic (Observer), Research Methodology, Western Medical Sciences, Combined Western and Chinese Nutrition, TCM External Medicine, TCM Internal Medicine, TCM Pediatrics, Practice Management, Clinic (Internship), TCM Gynecology Plus, TCM Traumatology, Research Seminar, Classics, and Clinical

Applications of TCM. Optional electives that may be taken during the final three trimesters include Advanced Taiji Quan, Comparative Medical Sciences, Drug Detoxification, Tui Na II, Chinese Herbal Dietetics, TCM Geriatrics, Psychology in TCM, Advanced Herb and Formula, Chinese Medicine and AIDS, Medical Sexology, TCM Pharmacology, TCM Treatment of Modern Disease, TCM English Terminology, TCM Otolaryngology, TCM Internal Medicine III, and Selected Classics of Acupuncture.

The academy's curriculum is presented in English, Chinese and Korean language sections. Students attend lectures two days per week for the entire three-year program.

Continuing Education

The academy offers a special graduate-level program for California licensed acupuncturists who wish to earn a master's-level degree. The Special Master of Science in Traditional Chinese Medicine—Degree Program for Licensed Acupuncturists consists of a minimum of sixty graduate trimester units from the graduate curriculum, as well as special electives that vary from term to term, and 210 clinic hours.

Admission Requirements

Applicants must have completed at least sixty semester units of general education at any accredited college or university and attained a GPA of at least 2.3 (C+) in all prerequisite work and a 2.0 (C) in any individual course. Prerequisites include thirty-eight semester units of general education plus twenty-two semester units in Western Medical Terminology, General Psychology, General Biology, General Chemistry, General Physics, Human Anatomy, and Human Physiology. Applicants must also submit an essay and résumé, three personal references, and have a personal interview.

Tuition and Fees

Tuition for the Master of Science in TCM program is $25,936 plus approximately $1,000 in fees; books and supplies additional. Tuition for the Special Degree Program for Licensed Acupuncturists is $7,300 to $8,600 plus approximately $500 in fees; books and supplies additional.

Financial Assistance

Payment plans, loans, and veterans' benefits are available.

Academy of Professional Careers

6784 El Cajon Boulevard C
San Diego, California 92115
PHONE: (619) 461-5100 / (800) 400-1005
FAX: (619) 461-5100

The Academy of Professional Careers was founded in 1995 as an auxiliary of the Academy of Court Reporting (La Mesa). The number of instructors varies; class sizes average forty students.

Accreditation and Approvals

The Academy of Court Reporting d/b/a Academy of Health Professions is accredited by the Accrediting Council for Continuing Education and Training (ACCET). Graduates are qualified to take the National Certification Examination for Therapeutic Massage and Bodywork (NCETMB).

Program Description

The 730-hour Massage Therapy Program includes Essentials of Massage Therapy, Thailand Medical Massage, Physiology, Touch for Health/Applied Kinesiology, Chair Massage, Reflexology, Anatomy, Swedish Massage, Body Mechanics, Kinesiology, Sports Massage, Therapeutic Exercises, Shiatsu, Pathology, Deep Tissue Massage, Injury Care, Passive Joint Movement, Business Management, Jin Shin Acutouch, CranioSacral Therapy, Polarity Therapy, CPR/First Aid, Nutrition, Clinical Practice, and Externship.

The 1,000-hour Holistic Health Practitioner Program includes all of the courses in the 730-hour Massage Therapy program plus Psychic Awareness, Herbology, Pregnancy Massage, Clinical Counseling, Point Location, Tui Na Medical Massage, Advanced Jin Shin Energywork, Structural Alignment, and Ayurveda.

Admission Requirements

Applicants must have a high school diploma or equivalent or demonstrated ability to benefit from training by passing the academy's entrance exam. All applicants must take an entrance exam. Classes are taught in English only.

Tuition and Fees

Tuition for the Massage Therapy Program is $7,138; additional expenses include registration fee, $100; transcript fee, $5;

books, $456; and massage table, $500. Tuition for the Holistic Health Practitioner Program is $9,502. Additional expenses include registration fee, $100; transcript fee, $5; books, $503; and massage table, $500.

Financial Assistance
Federal grants, loans, and veterans' benefits are available.

Acupressure Institute

1533 Shattuck Avenue
Berkeley, California 94709
PHONE: (510) 845-1059 / (800) 442-2232
FAX: (510) 845-1496
E-MAIL: info@acupressure.com
WEBSITE: www.acupressure.com

The Acupressure Institute was founded in 1976. Founder and author Michael Reed Gach, Ph.D., has practiced acupressure for over twenty years. There are thirty instructors, with an average of sixteen (maximum twenty-two) students per class. The institute also has a catalog featuring healing books, charts, cassette tapes, and instructional videos (see pages 464–65).

Accreditation and Approvals
The Acupressure Institute is an approved provider of continuing education credits for registered nurses and physical therapists, and has been granted institutional approval by the Bureau for Private Postsecondary and Vocational Education. Upon completion of the Basic Acupressure and Shiatsu Training Program, students may practice acupressure and massage in California, and may legally charge a fee for sessions.

Program Description
The 150-hour Basic Acupressure and Shiatsu Training Program leads to certification as an acupressure or shiatsu technician. Students study over seventy-five acupressure points and ten styles of acupressure, as well as the twelve organ meridians. Classes include Fundamentals of Acupressure; Basic, Intermediate, and Advanced Acupressure; Anatomy and Physiology; Business Practice and Ethics; Supervised Sessions; Documented Practice; and three electives chosen from Reflexology and Acupressure, Touch for Health, Zen Shiatsu, Barefoot Shi-

atsu, Tui Na: Chinese Massage, Acu-Yoga Self-Help Techniques, and Acupressure Oil Massage. The program may be completed in six months to one year of part-time study, or in one-month intensives. Classes may be taken individually without enrollment in the certificate program.

The 200-hour Advanced Training Acupressure Specialization Programs allow students to further their skills and knowledge of acupressure in such areas as Women's Health, Advanced Shiatsu, Sports Acupressure, Emotional Balancing, Arthritis and Pain Relief, Traditional Oriental Therapy, and Acupressure Stress Management. Programs may be completed in eighteen months to two years of part-time study, or in one-month intensives.

The 850-hour Acupressure Therapy Program is designed for those who wish to practice as professional acupressure therapists, and may fulfill requirements in other states for massage therapy. Students may complete the program within one year of full-time study, or two to four years of part-time study. Course work includes 350 hours of advanced training classes, plus Anatomy and Physiology, Self-Development (including Tai Chi, Qigong, or another internal healing art), Apprenticeship Training Classes, Documented Practice, Advanced Practice, and Teacher Training and/or Project.

Some of the classes offered as part of the Advanced Training and Acupressure Therapy Programs include Acupressure First Aid, On-Site Acupressure, Arthritis Relief: Self-Help, Table Shiatsu, Advanced Five Elements, Intuitive Acupressure and Self-Awareness, Pulse and Tongue Assessment, Traditional Oriental Theory, Sports Applications, Body Psychology, Counseling Skills, the Chakras, Emotional Balancing Using the Meridians, Major Medical Disorders, Western Herbology, Chinese Herbal Patent Remedies, Acu-Yoga Teacher Training, and others. Students in the four-day Acu-Yoga Teacher Training class receive a diploma upon completion.

Admission Requirements
Applicants must be at least 18 years of age and in good health. Acupressure Therapy Program applicants must have taken courses in anatomy/physiology and business practice and ethics.

Tuition and Fees
Tuition for the 150-hour Basic Acupressure and Shiatsu Training Program is $1,175; there is a registration fee of $75. Tuition

for the 200-hour Advanced Training Acupressure Specialization Program is $1,575; there is a registration fee of $75. Tuition for the 850-hour Acupressure Therapy Program is $5,500, plus a $100 registration fee. Books average $75 per program.

Financial Assistance

A payment plan and full payment discount is available. Work-trade is available to a limited number of students; request an application for work-trade. Housing resources are available upon request.

Alchemy Institute of Healing Arts

2310 Warwick Drive
Santa Rosa, California 95405
PHONE: (707) 579-4984 / (800) 950-4984
E-MAIL: quigley@sonic.net

The Alchemy Institute of Healing Arts was founded in 1986 as the Alchemical Hypnotherapy Institute, for the purpose of preparing students to work as hypnotherapists. Alchemical hypnotherapy is a therapeutic process that assists clients in accessing and using their inner guides—autonomous beings that live within the subconscious mind—to change their lives. This type of hypnotherapy includes techniques from many schools of hypnotherapy and psychology, including gestalt, regression therapy, neurolinguistic programming (NLP), and others.

The institute was founded by David Quigley, a state-approved hypnosis trainer since 1983 and a member of the advisory board of the American Council of Hypnotist Examiners (ACHE). There are two instructors, with an average of ten to fifteen (maximum thirty) students per class.

Accreditation and Approvals

All courses offered by the Alchemy Institute of Healing Arts are approved by American Council of Hypnotist Examiners (ACHE). The school is authorized by the California Board of Registered Nursing to provide continuing education credits for nurses, and is approved by the Bureau for Private Postsecondary and Vocational Education.

Program Description

AIHA offers three levels of hypnosis certification, each building on the one before.

The 150-hour Master Hypnotist Training Program qualifies the student for certification as a Master Hypnotist. Students will make contact with their inner child and inner mate, and will learn techniques applied to smoking, weight loss, addictions, and phobias, along with instruction in establishing a professional practice. Completion of certification requires four evaluated alchemical sessions as a client; completion of two professional sessions with an assistant or an alchemical hypnotherapist concurrent with the training program; and two (for resident students) or three (for weekend students) hypnotherapy practice sessions with a fellow student.

The Certified Hypnotherapist Training (200 hours total) builds upon the basic training with an additional 50 hours of study, and leads to certification as a Certified Hypnotherapist.

The Alchemical Hypnotherapist Training (350 hours total) leads to certification as an Alchemical Hypnotherapist. Students must complete the basic training and receive the Alchemical Hypnosis certification; complete one hundred hours of further instruction at any AIHA-approved school (400-level courses); complete 90 hours of assisting at a basic alchemical training; and receive five documented alchemical sessions.

Core courses offered in the three programs include Introduction to Hypnotherapy and Post-Hypnotic Suggestion, Emotional Clearing Work, Past Life Regression and Inner Guides, Conference Room Therapy, Specific Regimens, and Establishing a Professional Practice. Advanced electives include Pain and Disease Control, Advanced Alchemical Techniques, Touch Skills for the Hypnotherapist, NLP for the Alchemist, Ericksonian Hypnosis, Weight Management, Clearing the Trauma of Sexual Abuse, Wilderness Intensive, and others.

Instruction is offered in both residential and weekend formats.

Continuing Education

The 85-hour Alchemical Package for Hypnotherapists is offered to those who have completed at least one hundred hours of hypnosis study.

Admission Requirements

The Master Hypnotist, Certified Hypnotherapist, and Alchemical Hypnotherapist Certification Programs were designed to accommodate the entry-level student. Applicants must complete an application form, be fluent in the English language, pass the Wonderlic Basic Skills test (a standardized test of basic math and verbal skills), and have a personal interview.

Tuition and Fees

Costs for the Master Hypnotist Certification (150 hours) are as follows: registration fee, $75; tuition, $1,980 to $2,640 (depending on payment plan); books, $75; two alchemical sessions, $200; ACHE membership, $125; AIHA membership, $100; and practicums, $15 to $120.

Costs for the Certified Hypnotist Certification (200 hours) are the same as for Master Hypnotist Certification, plus an additional $660 to $720 in electives.

Costs for the Alchemical Hypnotherapist Certification are the same as for Certified Hypnotist Certification, plus an additional $660 to $720 in electives, $75 for an apprenticeship program, and $500 for additional alchemical sessions.

Facility and residence fees for residential intensives vary with the program and type of accommodation, and range from $144 for commuter fee without lunch to $1,585 for private room.

Financial Assistance

A payment plan, scholarships, and loans are available.

Alive and Well! Institute of Conscious BodyWork

100 Shaw Drive
San Anselmo, California 94960
PHONE: (415) 258-0402
FAX: (415) 258-0635
E-MAIL: Alive@alivewell.com
WEBSITE: alivewell.com

Alive and Well! was founded in 1987 by Jocelyn Olivier, whose creation of Conscious BodyWork was influenced by her studies in neuromuscular reeducation, educational and applied kinesiology, American Indian and Hawaiian shamanism, and Tui Na. There are thirty instructors, with a maximum of twenty-two students for hands-on classes.

Accreditation and Approvals

The certification programs at Alive and Well! meet the minimum education requirements for the State of California. Graduates of programs of 500 or more hours are qualified to take the National Certification Examination for Therapeutic Massage and Bodywork (NCETMB).

Continued Education Units (CEUs), including Nursing CEUs for the State of California, are available for most of the courses offered. Alive and Well! is approved by the National Certification Board for Therapeutic Massage and Bodywork (NCBTMB) as a continuing education provider.

Program Description

Alive and Well! offers state-approved certification courses for Certified Massage Technician, Advanced BodyWorker, Conscious BodyWorker, and Master BodyWorker.

The 140-hour Certified Massage Technician (CMT) Program may be completed in as little as four months or as long as one year. The curriculum consists of Anatomy, Conscious BodyWork Level I, a choice of Principles of Polarity or Conscious BodyWork Level II, Massage Ergonomics, Establishing a Business, Kinesiology, Nutritional Physiology, Reflexology, a choice of Counseling for Bodyworkers or Conscious Breathwork, and supervised clinical practice. A summer intensive allows completion of this program in just three weeks.

The 300-hour Advanced Bodyworker (ABW) Program includes the 140-hour CMT program and allows for the development of either a structural or energetic focus, with additional courses in Advanced Palpatory Anatomy, a choice of Conscious BodyWork Level II or Principles of Polarity (whichever has not yet been taken), Deep Tissue, Ethics and Communication, Integrative Lymph-Visceral Massage, Somatic Process and Integration, and supervised clinical practice. For an energetic focus, the Deep Tissue and Integrative Lymph-Visceral Massage classes are replaced with Brain Function Facilitation, Emotional Energetic Tune-Ups, Principles of Polarity II, and Physiology of Stress Management.

The 570-hour Conscious BodyWorker (CBW) Program offers, in addition to the 140-hour CMT training (or equivalent) and the 160-hour ABW training, courses such as Sports Injury and Chronic Pain, Cranio-Sacral Therapy, Acupressure, Trigger Points and Pain Release, Reiki, Qigong, On-Site Massage, and other classes, with a program emphasis in either structural work, energetic work, or integrated work.

The 1,000-hour Master BodyWorker (MBW) Program includes the CMT and ABW structural training plus an additional 700 hours of instruction in such areas as Acupressure, Biomechanics of Ergonomics, Brain Function Facilitation, Building Your Practice, NeuroMuscular Reprogramming, Qigong, Cranio-Sacral Therapy, Touch for Health, On-Site Massage, Sports Injury and Chronic Pain, Personal Nutrition, Trigger Points and Pain Release, and more, including electives and supervised practice.

Community and Continuing Education
Free introductory evenings provide a discussion and demonstration of the programs offered at the school. Other free lectures open to the public focus on a wide variety of bodywork and massage-related topics.

A seventy-two hour professional development course unique to Alive and Well! is offered in Conscious BodyWork NeuroMuscular Reprogramming. In addition, most classes may be taken individually for CEUs.

Admission Requirements
The State of California requires that students enrolling in the 140-hour CMT program take an Ability to Benefit Assessment test (a test of basic math and verbal skills).

Tuition and Fees
Tuition for the CMT program is $1,400; for the ABW program, $3,185; for the CBW program, $6,480; and for the MBW program, $12,155. Tuition for the seventy-two-hour Conscious BodyWork NeuroMuscular Reprogramming program is $1,240. Tuition figures do not include books and supplies.

Financial Assistance
Payment plans, prepayment discounts, work-study, and veterans' benefits are available. One free 140-hour CMT training is offered per year to a person working with populations or groups who cannot afford or do not know the value of massage and bodywork.

American Academy of Medical Acupuncture
(See Multiple State Locations, pages 384–85)

American College of Traditional Chinese Medicine

455 Arkansas Street
San Francisco, California 94107
PHONE: (415) 282-7600
FAX: (415) 282-0856
E-MAIL: lhuang@actcm.org
WEBSITE: www.actcm.org

The American College of Traditional Chinese Medicine was founded in 1980 as a not-for-profit corporation. In 1981, the college opened its Community Clinic, which provides low-cost health care to an average of 800 patients per month. The clinic operates a program for HIV-positive patients funded by the Ryan White Comprehensive AIDS Resources Emergency Act. There are forty-two instructors with an average of fifteen to twenty students per class.

Accreditation and Approvals
The Master of Science degree program in Traditional Chinese Medicine is accredited by the Accreditation Commission for Acupuncture and Oriental Medicine (ACAOM).

Program Description
The four-year Master of Science in Traditional Chinese Medicine Degree Program may be completed in three calendar years.

First-year courses include History of Healing Symposium, Fundamental Theory of TCM, Point Location and Indications, Meridian Structure and Point Systems, Medical Chinese, Tai Chi, Differential Diagnosis, the Pharmacopoeia, Medical Terminology, Qigong, Pathophysiology, Clinical Practicum, Supervised Observation, Clinical Procedures, and others.

Second-year courses include Intermedical Communications, Advanced Diagnosis and Treatment Principles, Meridian Structure and Point Systems, Herbal Prescriptions, Clinic:

Close Supervision, Chinese Physio-massage and Therapy, Advanced Acupuncture, Nutrition and the Treatment of Disease, Pathophysiology: Shang Han Lun, Clinic: Partial Supervision, and others.

Third-year courses include Professional Issues and Bioethics, Survey of Biomedical Pharmacology, Pathophysiology: Wen Bing, Grand Clinical Rounds, Classical Prescriptions, Introduction to Clinical Research Methodology, Proseminars, Internship, and others.

The curriculum requirements of either the eleventh or twelfth quarters may be met through the study abroad program.

Classes are held both days and evenings.

Admission Requirements

Applicants should have a bachelor's degree or equivalent and have completed the preprofessional general education requirements, which consist of specific courses in language communication (thirteen quarter credits), comparative studies (six quarter credits), reasoning (six quarter credits), and general science (twenty-two quarter credits). Students who have deficiencies in these requirements will be considered on an individual basis and may be admitted provisionally. In addition, applicants must submit two letters of recommendation (one from a health care practitioner), a health certificate, and a statement of purpose.

Tuition and Fees

Tuition is $134 per credit. Additional expenses include an application fee of $50 for full-time students and $100 for part-time students; graduation fee, $75; and books and supplies.

Financial Assistance

A payment plan is available.

American Institute of Massage Therapy

2156 Newport Boulevard
Costa Mesa, California 92627-1710
PHONE: (949) 642-0735
FAX: (949) 642-1729
E-MAIL: AIMT1Inc@aol.com
WEBSITE: members.aol.com/AIMT1Inc/index.html

Dr. Myk Hungerford, AIMT's founder, served as the National Director of Education for the American Massage Therapy Association from 1981 to 1984 and began offering instruction in 1983. There are three instructors, with an average of twelve to eighteen students per class.

Accreditation and Approvals

The AIMT program is accredited by the Commission on Massage Training Accreditation (COMTA). Graduates are qualified to take the National Certification Examination for Therapeutic Massage and Bodywork (NCETMB). AIMT is approved and recognized by the International Myomassethics Federation (IMF), the Alberta (Canada) Massage Therapy Association, and the International Sports Massage Federation, and is approved for continuing education by the California Board of Registered Nursing.

Program Description

The forty-eight week, 1,029-hour Scientific Swedish Massage and Sports Massage Program includes 615 classroom hours, nine hours of testing, and 405 hour of clinical internship, plus supervised hours working at sporting events and taking field trips. The program consists of both massage therapy and sports massage components, taught simultaneously. The massage therapy program is based on Swedish massage and includes Anatomy and Physiology, Pathology, Nutrition (including herbology), Hydrotherapy, Specialized Modalities (which may include acupressure, Chinese/Russian techniques, reflexology, remedial exercise, and lymphatic drainage, and are subject to change), Psychology and Philosophy, and Supplementary Basic Courses (including Hygiene, CPR, First Aid, Medical Ethics, Clinical Practice, and Didactic Studies of other manipulative therapies). The sports massage component emphasizes Sports Kinesiology, Functional Muscle Testing, Counterstrain, PNF Stretches, Sports Pathology and Psychology, and Immediate Injury Care. Pre-event massage, post-event massage, training and conditioning, and restoration/rehabilitation are also covered. Graduates receive a certification/diploma as both a massage therapist and sports massage specialist.

Admission Requirements

Applicants must be a high school graduate or equivalent, pass the entrance exam, and submit two letters of recommendation.

Tuition and Fees

Tuition is $7,000. Other fees include application/registration fee, $60; books (approximate), $95; and massage table, $200 to $800.

Financial Assistance

Monthly and trimester payment plans are available.

American University of Complementary Medicine

11543 Olympic Boulevard
Los Angeles, California 90064
PHONE: (310) 914-4116
FAX: (310) 479-3376
E-MAIL: Mail@aucm.org
WEBSITE: www.aucm.org

American University of Complementary Medicine (AUCM) was founded in 1995 as Curentur University by Terry S. Jacobs. There are thirty-one instructors, with ten to thirty students per class.

Accreditation and Approvals

AUCM is a nonprofit university licensed by the State of California as a degree-granting institution.

Program Description

Certification programs are offered in Clinical Homeopathy and in Holistic Health. Master of Arts degree programs are offered in Homeopathy and Holistic Studies. Additional programs are being developed in the fields of Herbology, Mind-Body Medicine, Oriental Bodywork, Tui Na, and Ayurvedic and Botanical Medicine. Contact the university or consult the website for the latest offerings.

The 240-hour Certificate Program in Homeopathy consists of four levels: Principles of Clinical Homeopathy, Homeopathic First Aid in Acute Situations, Homeopathy for Chronic or Long-Term Situations, and Homeopathy for Internal and External Disorders.

The 240-hour Certificate Program in Holistic Health consists of Mind-Body Healing Techniques, Principles of Nutri-

tional Medicine, Introduction to Ayurveda, Principles of Clinical Homeopathy, and Introduction to Oriental Medicine.

The Master of Arts in Homeopathy consists of sixty-one units and includes such courses as Principles of Homeopathy, Homeopathic Case Taking, Homeopathic First Aid and Acute Prescribing, Miasms and Chronic Diseases, Gemmotherapy, Cell Salts, Flower Essences, Homeopathic External/Internal Medicine, Homeopathy Internship/ Externship, Clinical Diagnosis and Laboratory Test Analysis, and others.

The Master of Arts in Holistic Studies consists of forty units of core courses, including Holistic Psychology and Psychopathology, Comparative Nutrition, Pathology and the Nature of Disease, Intro to Psychoneuroimmunology, Epistemology and the Scientific Method, and Master's Thesis in Holistic Studies. In addition, there are ten units of specialty courses required, which may be taken in one of the following areas: Mind-Body Medicine, Nutritional Medicine, Ayurvedic Medicine, Chinese Medicine, or Homeopathy.

Admission Requirements

Certificate program applicants should have a high school diploma or equivalent and a personal interview.

Master of Arts degree program applicants must have a bachelor's, submit two letters of recommendation and an application essay, and have a personal interview.

Tuition and Fees

Tuition for the Certificate programs is $3,540 and includes books and materials. Tuition for the Master of Arts degree in Homeopathy is $15,219; tuition for the Master of Arts degree in Holistic Studies is $9,203.

Additional expenses include application fee, $75; annual library fee, $30; annual student association fee, $24; and petition to graduate fee, $75.

Financial Assistance

Payment for all programs can be made on a per-course basis, through payment plans, financial assistance, or by securing student lending through private institutions.

Aromatherapy Institute and Research

P.O. Box 2354
Fair Oaks, California 95628
PHONE: (916) 965-7546
FAX: (916) 962-3292
E-MAIL: victoria@leydet.com
WEBSITE: leydet.com

Aromatherapy Institute and Research was founded in 1990 by Victoria Edwards, who has been offering classes since 1977 and currently serves as advisor to NAHA educational committees. There are three instructors, with an average of twelve to twenty students per class.

Program Description
The 120-hour Aromatherapy Training Course Level I consists of eighty classroom hours and forty hours of independent home study; classes meet for five three-day weekends. Topics covered include Phytotherapy, Herbs and Plant Identification, Distillation and Extraction Methods, Caring and Storing of Essential Oils, Historical Data, Functional Groups and Families, Therapeutic Properties, Adulteration, Chemistry, Carrier Oils and Hydrosols, Anatomy and Physiology, Applications and Treatments, Safety and Toxicity Data, Olfactory System, Emotional and Psychological Studies, Client Consultation, Designing a Program, Ethics, Case Histories, Business Practices and Legalities, Setting Up a Practice, and more.

Community and Continuing Education
In 1997 Victoria Edwards began Aroma Camp, an annual Joint Studying Project with people in southern France and from England, Germany, the United States, and Japan. The 1999 seminar was a ten-day travel study tour of France covering French Medical Aromatherapy, identification of wild aromatics, lectures, and more. A video is available for interested students.

Advanced courses are offered in such areas as subtle energy work, anointing and aroma points, color and aromas, chakra balancing, or in other areas of interest to the student; courses may be offered as weekend seminars or as independent study. Contact the institute for details.

Tuition and Fees
Tuition is $1,995; books and some materials are additional. Tuition for Aroma Camp is approximately $2,500 (airfare not included). Tuition for advanced courses may range from $300 to $1,000, depending on length.

Financial Assistance
A payment plan and prepayment discount are available.

Biofeedback Institute of Los Angeles

3710 South Robertson Boulevard, Suite 216
Culver City, California 90232-2351
PHONE: (310) 841-4970 / (800) 246-3526
FAX: (310) 841-0923

Biofeedback Institute of Los Angeles, a nonprofit organization, was founded in 1970 as a stress-management center. The institute has conducted professional biofeedback training programs under the direction of Marjorie K. Toomim, Ph.D., since 1973. There are five instructors; class sizes vary from one or two to ten or more. In addition to the program described here, the institute offers shorter training programs and a home study course (see page 471).

Accreditation and Approvals
The twenty-one-week program at Biofeedback Institute of Los Angeles prepares students for the Biofeedback Certification Institute of America (BCIA) examination and for Certification in Neurofeedback. The institute is approved for continuing education credit by the Biofeedback Certification Institute of America, the Biofeedback Society of California, the Board of Professional Nursing, the American Dental Association, and the California Post Secondary Educational Institute.

Program Description
The twenty-one-week Comprehensive Biofeedback Training Course consists of five three-day seminars and a sixteen-week practicum. The seminars are Introduction to Clinical Biofeedback and Relaxation Training, Stress Management and Advanced Treatment Procedures, Conditions Commonly Referred for Clinical Biofeedback, BCIA Examination Review: Instrumentation and Electronics, and BCIA Examination Review:

Clinical Biofeedback. The sixteen-week practicum consists of sixteen evening classes covering Advanced Clinical Biofeedback Training, Advanced Instrumentation Training, sixteen hours of Case Conference, ninety hours of work with Clinic Patients, fifteen hours of Supervision, and ten hours of Personal Biofeedback Training. Comprehensive Course participants may repeat all classes except the Personal Biofeedback Training as often as desired until they pass the BCIA exam.

Admission Requirements
Enrollment is open to psychologists, physicians, nurses, chiropractors, medical assistants, teachers, and others who have a professional background that involves interpersonal communication and a helping role. Applicants without a bachelor's degree in a health care–related field need special permission to enroll.

Tuition and Fees
Tuition is $2,450 for the entire twenty-one-week training.

Financial Assistance
Payment plans and discounts are available.

B.K.S. Iyengar Yoga Association of Southern California

8119 La Mesa Boulevard
La Mesa, California 91941
PHONE: (619) 469-9642
E-MAIL: yogagold@aol.com

The B.K.S. Iyengar Yoga Training Program was founded in 1992 with direct input from B.K.S. Iyengar. Gloria Goldberg is the training coordinator. The institute has programs in both Los Angeles and San Diego. There are five instructors; class sizes vary from two to thirty or more.

Program Description
A three-year comprehensive Iyengar Yoga Training Program is offered for teachers and serious students and includes over 500 hours of training. The program is created with direct and continuous input from B.K.S. Iyengar. The curriculum covers Fundamental Asanas and Pranayama, Yoga Philosophy, Anatomy and Physiology of Yoga Poses, Teaching Asanas and Pranayama, Basic Adjustments, Therapeutics (Special Issues), and Ayurveda and Yoga. The program includes weekly classes, weekend workshops, a three-day residential intensive, practice and teaching principles, and more.

Admission Requirements
Applicants should have practiced Iyengar yoga for at least two years with a certified Iyengar yoga teacher. Students with less than two years' experience who feel ready for this program should contact the program coordinator.

Tuition and Fees
Tuition for entire three-year program is $6,000; there is a $25 application fee, and books are approximately $150.

Financial Assistance
Payment plans and some scholarships are available

Body Therapy Center

368 California Avenue
Palo Alto, California 94306
PHONE: (650) 328-9400
FAX: (650) 328-9478
E-MAIL: btcbdywrk1@aol.com
WEBSITE: www.bodymindspirit.net

Body Therapy Center was founded in 1981. Lucia Miracchi, co-founder, has been involved in the healing arts for over thirty years. There are thirty instructors, with an average of twenty-two students per class.

Accreditation and Approvals
Body Therapy Center is approved by the State of California, and approved as a continuing education provider by the National Certification Board for Therapeutic Massage and Bodywork (NCBTMB) and the Board of Registered Nurses. Graduates of massage therapy programs of 500 or more hours are qualified to take the National Certification Examination for Therapeutic Massage and Bodywork (NCETMB).

Program Description

The center offers 1,000 hours of professional certification courses comprised of eight classes of 125 hours each. These courses may be taken individually as desired or combined for a 500-hour certificate.

The 125-hour Fundamentals of Massage Course includes Anatomy and Physiology; Ethics; History, Business Issues & When to Refer; Movement Awareness; and Demonstration and Practice. In addition to classroom instruction, students are required to complete and document sixteen body massages outside of class, receive one outside professional massage, and complete reading and exam requirements.

The 125-hour Fundamentals of Shiatsu Course includes Demonstration and Practice, Anatomy and Physiology, Ethics, and Theory. In addition to classroom instruction, students are required to complete and document sixteen body massages outside of class, receive two outside Shiatsu massages, and complete reading and exam requirements.

The 125-hour Advanced Shiatsu Course includes Demonstration and Practice, Anatomy and Physiology, Clinical Application of Theory/Meridians, and Ethics. Students are also required to complete twenty practice massages and receive one Shiatsu session from a list of approved practitioners.

The 125-hour Jin Shin Do Acupressure Course consists of three sections. Basic JSD includes thirty main JSD points and a color-coded release method; the segmental release method; body-focusing techniques; the eight Strange Flows; and a total of fifty-five acu-points. Intermediate JSD includes bodymind function of the twelve organ meridians, assessment skills, breathing techniques, and an additional fifty-five acu-points. Advanced JSD covers Five Elements, relationships between meridians, tonification and sedation points and techniques, pulse reading, and specific acu-point combinations. Students must also receive two JSD sessions from a registered JSD practitioner or authorized JSD teacher.

The 125-hour Advanced Bodywork Symposium includes seminars in Alchemy of Anatomy and Movement, Movement and Manipulation, Muscle Meridian Massage, Body of Emotion: Explorations in Rosen Method, and the Hakomi Approach.

The 125-hour Advanced Massage and Bodywork Training Course includes Anatomy and Physiology, Demonstration and Practice, Movement Awareness, and Communication Skills and Ethics. Training covers deep tissue techniques in conjunction with anatomy, gentle joint manipulation and mobilization, energy work, and pressure points. Students are also required to complete and document twenty-four bodywork sessions, attend a 1.5-hour tutorial with an instructor and classmate, receive two bodywork sessions, and complete reading and exam requirements.

The 125-hour Sports Massage Course includes Stretching, Event Sports Massage, Preventive Sports Massage, and Sports Massage Following Injuries. Students are also required to complete and document ten one-hour, full-body massages, complete twelve hours of supervised event massage, and complete a research paper, reading, and exam requirements.

The 125-hour Clinical Deep Tissue Massage Course covers such topics as anatomy, physiology, and kinesiology; different theories and techniques; body mechanics and self-care; looking and thinking strategically; soft-tissue injuries; contraindications; bodywork philosophy; and myomassethics. Students must also complete twenty-four practice massages.

Community and Continuing Education

Community workshops are open to the public; no prior experience is required. Topics include Basic Shiatsu, Beginning Massage, Body Balancing, Couples Massage, Introduction to Massage, Reflexology, and others.

Continuing education courses are offered to professional bodyworkers and include such topics as Advanced Jin Shin Do; Ethics for Bodyworkers; Introduction to Trager®; Onsite Seated Massage; Dynamics of Working with Abuse Survivors; Massaging the Sick, Injured, and Dying; Reiki; Taxes for Bodyworkers; and others.

Admission Requirements

Applicants must be at least 18 years of age and interview with the school administrator.

Tuition and Fees

Tuition for Fundamentals courses is $1,050 per course; tuition for Advanced courses is $1,275 per course. Books and supplies are additional.

Tuition for community workshops ranges from $60 to $220; continuing education courses range from $35 to $385.

Financial Assistance
Payment plans are available.

The Breema Center

6076 Claremont Avenue
Oakland, California 94618
PHONE: (510) 428-0937
WEBSITE: www.breema.com

The Breema Center (formerly the Institute for Health Improvement) was founded in 1980 to introduce Breema bodywork to the West. Breema is an ancient bodywork system that emphasizes nonjudgmental treatment and practitioner's comfort; treatments, performed comfortably clothed on a padded floor, release tension and create vibrant health, mental clarity, and emotional balance for both practitioner and recipient. Director Jon Schreiber, D.C., has been practicing and teaching Breema bodywork for over twenty years and directs the Breema Health and Wellness Center, where Breema bodywork is the primary healing modality.

Accreditation and Approvals
The Breema Center is a vocational school licensed by the Bureau for Private Postsecondary and Vocational Education, and is approved by the National Certification Board for Therapeutic Massage and Bodywork (NCBTMB) as a continuing education provider.

Program Description
The center offers a 165-hour Practitioner Certificate in Breema bodywork. The requirements for certification include Breema bodywork classes and workshops, supervised practicum sessions, Practitioner Colloquium, Anatomy and Physiology, Nutrition and Cleansing Workshop, Self-Breema classes, and fifteen hours of electives. Students may choose from weekly classes, weekend workshops, and longer intensive programs in order to accrue the required number of Breema bodywork hours. The program requires at least six months to complete. Graduates are prepared to establish a private Breema bodywork practice.

Admission Requirements
Students applying for the Certificate Program must have a sincere interest in Breema and the ability to do basic sequences comfortably.

Tuition and Fees
Total tuition varies with the courses chosen. Five-week modules cost $140 for one module, $230 for two modules, and $315 for three modules. A ten-day Breema Intensive is offered for $550. Weekend workshop packages are offered for $250.

Financial Assistance
Early registration and multiple class discounts, and some work exchange positions are available.

California College of Ayurveda

1117A East Main Street
Grass Valley, California 95945
PHONE: (530) 274-9100
FAX: (530) 274-7350
E-MAIL: info@ayurvedacollege.com
WEBSITE: www.ayurvedacollege.com

The California College of Ayurveda (CCA) was founded in 1995 by Dr. Marc Halpern. There are four instructors, with a maximum of forty students per class. Classes are held at the main campus in Grass Valley as well as at satellite locations in southern California and the Bay Area.

Accreditation and Approvals
CCA is a California State–approved college for the study of Ayurvedic medicine. Certification as a Clinical Ayurvedic Specialist is recognized in the State of California.

Program Description
The Clinical Ayurvedic Specialist Program consists of 500 hours of classroom education and supervised clinical internship and an additional 250 hours of independent study. The certification program consists of sixteen three-day weekend classes held once per month along with a six-month clinical internship. The curriculum covers Principles of Ayurveda; Ayurveda and the Emotions; Spirit, Herbs, and Pancha Karma;

Clinical Management of Disease; Ayurvedic Psychology; and Pulse Diagnoses, Aromatherapy, Color Therapy, and Mantra Therapy.

Admission Requirements

Applicants must have a high school diploma or equivalent and submit a short essay. Students who are not already licensed health care professionals will be required to take Anatomy, Physiology, and Medical Terminology, and General Western Diagnostics and Medical Communication (offered at the college in a one-weekend format); students who have taken college-level Anatomy and Physiology may waive this requirement.

Tuition and Fees

Tuition for the two-year program is $6,250 paid prior to the start of class. Additional expenses include application fee, $55; registration fee, $45; books, $440; and equipment, $70.

Financial Assistance

Payment plans and limited work-study positions are available.

California College of Physical Arts

Huntington Beach Campus
18582 Beach Boulevard, Suite 14
Huntington Beach, California 92648
PHONE: (714) 964-7744 / (800) 884-7744
FAX: (714) 962-3934
E-MAIL: calcopa@gte.net

California College of Physical Arts (CAL COPA) was founded in 1980. There are seven instructors, with a maximum class size of twelve students. In addition to the programs described here, CAL COPA also offers massage programs of shorter duration.

Accreditation and Approvals

CAL COPA is approved by the Bureau for Private Postsecondary and Vocational Education. Graduates of massage therapy programs of 500 or more hours are eligible to take the National Certification Examination for Therapeutic Massage and Bodywork (NCETMB).

Program Description

CAL COPA offers three programs of 500 or more hours: Massage Practitioner, Myotherapist, and Holistic Health Practitioner.

The 500-hour Massage Practitioner program consists of a 300-hour program covering Swedish Massage, Theory, Anatomy, Physiology, Ethics, Professionalism, Nutrition, Trigger Points, Joint Movement, PNF Stretching, Formula Massage, Injury Care, Internship/Externship, and more, plus 100 hours of Sports/Medical Massage, and an additional 100 hours that includes fifty hours of Acupuressure or Shiatsu plus an additional fifty hours in electives chosen from Reflexology, Advance Sports, Bowen Technique, Geriatric Massage, Aromatherapy, Spa Services, and Business and Billing for the Massage Therapist. Attendance of an outside documented and supervised community service event is required.

The 600-hour Myotherapist program consists of the 500-hour Massage Practitioner program above, plus an additional fifty hours of Acupressure or Shiatsu (whichever was not taken previously) and fifty hours of electives chosen from the options above which were not taken previously.

The 1,000-hour Holistic Health Practitioner program consists of the 600-hour Myotherapist program described above with an additional 400 hours of electives chosen from Acupressure, Aromatherapy, Bowen Technique, Chair Massage, Geriatric Massage, Hawaiian Lomi Lomi, Herbal, Nutrition, Pregnancy and Infant, Oriental Health Systems, Canine and Feline Massage, Equestrian Massage and Treatment, Reflexology, Shiatsu, Reconstructive Massage Therapy, Advance Sports Massage, Spa Services, Business and Billing for the Massage Therapist, Reiki, Iridology, and Magnetic Therapy.

Classes are offered mornings and evenings.

Admission Requirements

Applicants may be required to complete an entrance exam; a high school diploma or equivalent is desirable but not required. Applicants must demonstrate proficiency in English and submit four names as personal references.

Tuition and Fees

Tuition for the 500-hour Massage Practitioner program is $4,125; for the 600-hour Myotherapist program, $4,950; and for the 1,000-hour Holistic Health Practitioner program, $8,250.

Additional expenses include registration fee, $75; materials fee, $25; books and supplies are additional.

California Institute of Integral Studies

1453 Mission Street
San Francisco, California 94103
PHONE: (415) 575-6150
FAX: (415) 575-1264
E-MAIL: info@ciis.edu
WEBSITE: www.ciis.edu

The California Institute of Integral Studies (formerly the California Institute of Asian Studies) was founded in 1968 by Haridas Chaudhuri. In addition to the programs described here, the institute offers many academic programs, most of which are postgraduate master's degree– or Ph.D.-level programs dealing with various aspects of psychology, philosophy, religion, and/or business; these are described in detail on their website. There are eighty-three instructors, with an average of fifteen to twenty students per class.

Accreditation and Approvals
The institute is accredited by the Western Association of Schools and Colleges.

Program Description
A ninety-unit master's degree in Counseling Psychology with Emphasis in Integral Health program prepares graduates to pass the national certifying examination for health educators and includes coursework in health education, core integral health studies, health education practicum (fieldwork), electives, and thesis preparation and writing. The curriculum includes Body/Mind Practices in Various Cultures; Anatomy, Experience, and Healing Practices; Body Movement; Multicultural Approaches to Health, Sexuality, and Body Movement; and more.

A Bachelor of Arts Completion Program consists of twelve months (four quarters) of weekend seminars covering such areas as Ecology and the Environment, Social Change, and Integral Learning.

Community and Continuing Education
Public lectures and continuing education workshops are offered in a variety of topics, including Shamanic Extraction Healing Training, Korean Shamanic Transformation, and Kirtan: The Art of Devotional Yoga.

Admission Requirements
The master's degree in Counseling Psychology with Emphasis in Integral Health program requires a bachelor's degree (preferably in the health sciences), two letters of recommendation, and a writing sample.

Bachelor of Arts Completion Program applicants must have earned 75 to 120 quarter units of transferable credit, submit a personal statement, and participate in a full-day workshop, An Introduction to Integral Learning.

Tuition and Fees
Tuition is $9,650 per year for full-time study or $567 per unit for part-time study for the master's degree program; $13,740 or $370 per unit for the Bachelor of Arts Completion Program. Additional expenses for all programs include a $135 per-semester registration fee.

Financial Assistance
Payment plans and federal loans are available to eligible students.

California Institute of Massage and Spa Services

730 Broadway
P.O. Box 673
Sonoma, California 95476
PHONE: (707) 939-9431

The California Institute of Massage and Spa Services (CIMSS) was founded in 1992 by director Kate Alves. There are four core faculty members with numerous guest instructors; the maximum class size is twelve students.

Accreditation
CIMSS is licensed by the Bureau for Private Postsecondary and Vocational Education. Graduates of programs of 500 or more

hours are qualified to take the National Certification Examination for Therapeutic Massage and Bodywork (NCETMB). CIMSS is approved by the California Board of Registered Nursing for continuing education credits.

Program Description

The five programs described here total over 600 hours of Massage Therapy instruction. The Massage Technician Program must be taken first; additional programs may be taken in any sequence.

The 165-hour Massage Technician Program includes Swedish Massage, Anatomy and Physiology, Reflexology, Body Mechanics, Breath Work, Aromatherapy, Joint Mobilization, Business Skills, Ethics, and Communication.

The 100-hour Advanced Massage I Program covers Trigger Point Therapy, Energy Balancing, Pre-Natal and Side-Lying Massage, Seated Massage, Facial Massage, and Advanced Anatomy.

In the Advanced Massage II Program, students choose 135 hours from such electives as Shiatsu, Spa Massage, Geriatric Massage, Therapeutic Touch, Lymphatic Massage, Sports Massage, Practice-Building Skills, and Deep Tissue Massage.

The 100-hour Spa Services Program covers Hydrotherapy, Aromatherapy, Mud Wraps, Dry Seaweed Wraps, Indian Herbal Treatment, Body Scrubs, Seaweed Wraps, Paraffin Baths, Lymphatic Dry Brushing, and Setting Up the Spa Environment.

The 100-hour Shiatsu Program covers both table and floor treatments in traditional Shiatsu/Acupressure.

Admission Requirements

Applicants must be at least 18 years of age (those younger than 18 may be accepted with permission of a parent or guardian).

Tuition and Fees

Tuition for the Massage Technician Program is $1,150. Tuition for Advanced Massage I is $895. Tuition for Advanced Massage II depends on courses selected. Tuition for the Spa Services Certification is $950. Tuition for the Shiatsu program is $895. Registration, books, and materials are included in tuition figures; required student liability insurance is an additional $39.

Financial Assistance

A payment plan is available.

California School of Herbal Studies

P.O. Box 39
Forestville, California 95436
PHONE: (707) 887-7457
FAX: (707) 887-1654
E-MAIL: cshs@sirius.com
WEBSITE: www.cshs.com

Founded in 1978 by Rosemary Gladstar, California School of Herbal Studies (CSHS) is America's oldest school for herbalists. The school is located on eighty acres in Sonoma County and includes a working garden of medicinal and native plants. There are twelve instructors, with an average of thirty students.

Program Description

The eight-month, 480-hour Foundations and Therapeutic Herbalism Program includes two separate, semester-long programs: Foundations of Herbalism (240 hours) and Therapeutic Herbalism (240 hours). The two semesters may be taken separately, although the Therapeutic Herbalism Program requires previous herbal or therapeutic experience.

The 240-hour Foundations of Herbalism curriculum includes Materia Medica: Anatomy, Physiology, and Body Systems; Introduction to Herbal Actions; Medicine Making and Lab; Botany and Field Identification; Introduction to Global Healing Traditions; Aromatherapy; Herb Cultivation; Harvesting Techniques; Principles of Ethical Wildcrafting; Basics of Therapeutics; Principles of Bioregionalism; Nutrition and Healing Foods; Herbal Information Gathering; Herbal First Aid; Natural Cosmetics and Crafts; Green Politics; Bach Flower Essences; History and Mythology; the Business of Herbalism; Student Projects; and Medicine Show.

The 240-hour Therapeutic Herbalism curriculum includes System and Actions Model of Western Herbalism; Western Constitutional Herbalism; Materia Medica; Herbal Dispensatory; Phytochemistry; Phytopharmacology; Case Studies; Therapeutic Aromatherapy; Botany and Field Identification; Herb Cultivation; Informed Consent Issues; Interview Techniques; Student Projects; and Student Case Studies.

Classes meet Tuesday through Thursday in the daytime; students spend additional time outside class in medicine making, special projects, and overnight identification and wildcrafting trips.

A six-month, sixty-hour weekend course, Body Systems and Herbal Wellness, meets one weekend per month and explores physiology, materia medica, and therapeutics.

Another six-month, sixty-hour weekend course, The Technology of Independence, bases its curriculum on plants within a half-day's drive of San Francisco. The curriculum includes Plant Identification, Field Trips, Medicine Making, and Materia Medica.

One-day workshops are held spring through fall in Herbal Medicine Making, Therapeutic Applications of Essential Oils, Food as Medicine, Herbal Ways for Women, Plant Energetics, and Herbs for Winter Health. Spring and summer herb walks include Plants of Pomo Canyon, Berkeley Botanical Gardens, Springtime in Emerald Valley, and Summer at Shell Beach.

Admission Requirements

Students must complete an application questionnaire.

Tuition and Fees

There is a $15 application fee. Tuition for the Foundation and Therapeutic Herbalism Program is $2,600 per semester or $4,995 for the entire program, plus $300 to $500 for books and materials. Tuition for Body Systems and Herbal Wellness, Therapeutic Intensive, and Technology of Independence is $475; register with a friend for $425 each. The one-day workshops are $40. Herb Walks are $20.

California School of Traditional Hispanic Herbalism

Charles Garcia
2810 Lincoln Avenue
Richmond, California 94804
PHONE: (510) 233-5837
E-MAIL: cgarcia@dnai.com
      clh_2554@hotmail.com

California School of Traditional Hispanic Herbalism was founded in 1998 by Charles Garcia to preserve the healing traditions of the Hispanic curanderos and curanderas (folk healers) of California. Garcia is a third-generation curandero who has lectured at universities and health care consortiums, and teaches a section for the Red Cross Wilderness First Aid

Course. Classes are usually taught by two instructors and one aide; class sizes range from seven to twelve students. For online classes, see pages 473-74.

Program Description

Introduction to Hispanic Herbalism is a four-week course in beginning herbalism that includes a history of California Hispanic herbalism, herbal remedies for everyday ailments, easy preparations, folklore, and foods.

Traditional Hispanic Herbalism and Magic is a seven-week course covering medicinal and magic herbs, infusions, decoctions, poultices, wines, vinegars, concepts of illness, the use of poisons in healing, the hierarchy of Hispanic lay healers, cross-cultural healing influences, and more.

The Hispanic Materia Medica meets two evenings per week for one month. The course covers native, European, and some Asian plants as used by folk healers in treating specific ailments, health maintenance, and spiritual healing.

Community and Continuing Education

One-day intensives are offered on such topics as Hispanic Mysticism, Magic, and Ritual; Survival Herbs; Intuitive Diagnosis; and Herbal Dyes and Dying Techniques.

Admission Requirements

Applicants must be at least 18 years of age (under 18 with parental permission). Students must spend some time outdoors for successful completion of these courses; individuals with mobility problems can discuss options with the instructor.

Tuition and Fees

Introduction to Hispanic Herbalism is $85. Traditional Hispanic Herbalism and Magic is $150. Hispanic Materia Medica is $170. One-day intensives are $35 to $65.

Financial Assistance

Payment plans may be created for students in need; in extreme cases, payment may be waived completely.

Center for Hypnotherapy Certification

OFFICE:
455 Newton Avenue #1
Oakland, California 94606
PHONE: (510) 839-4800 / (800) 398-0034
FAX: (510) 836-0477
E-MAIL: mgordon@hypnotherapycenter.com
WEBSITE: www.hypnotherapycenter.com

CENTER:
401 Grand Avenue, #210
Oakland, California 94610

The Center for Hypnotherapy Certification was founded in 1995 by Marilyn Gordon. There are four to six instructors; class sizes range from ten to thirty-nine students.

Accreditation and Approvals
The training is approved by the Bureau for Private Postsecondary and Vocational Education, and approved for continuing education credit for nurses and by the National Guild of Hypnotists.

Program Description
The 100-hour, twelve-day Core Training Certification Program covers Terminology, Rapport, Habit Control, Making Hypnosis Tapes, Pre-Hypnosis Techniques, Levels of Hypnosis Depth Testing, Self-Hypnosis, Regression Therapy, Inner Guidance Techniques, Transformational Healing, Hypnoanesthesia, How to Give Workshops and Hypnosis Demonstrations, How to Teach Self-Hypnosis, Ethics, Marketing and Business, Intuition Training, Emotional Clearing, Trauma Release, Past-Life Regression, Phobias, Neurolinguistic Programming, Ericksonian Hypnotherapy, Chakras, Mind-Body Healing, and more.

The Advanced Certified Hypnotherapist program consists of an additional fifty hours of training taken over six classes. Classes may be chosen from EFT, The Emotional Freedom Technique; Medical Hypnotherapy; The Spirit of Shamanism; Hypnotherapeutic Dreamwork; Breakthroughs in the Energy Therapies; Death and Healing: Looking at the Other Side of Life; Chakras and Healing; and others.

Students may acquire another fifty hours of training through participation in the Center's low-fee clinic.

Admission Requirements
Admission is open to everyone upon approval.

Tuition and Fees
Tuition for the Core Training is $1,600. Individual advanced classes are $70 each.

Financial Assistance
Interest-free payment plans are available.

Central California School of Body Therapy

Administration:
1330 Southwood # 7
San Luis Obispo, California 93401
PHONE/FAX: (805) 783-2200
E-MAIL: siouxsun1@aol.com

CLASSROOM FACILITY:
265 Prado Road, Suite 4
San Luis Obispo, California 93401

The Central California School of Body Therapy was established in 1991 by Susan E. Stocks and Dr. Marie Moore. There are nine instructors, with an average of twenty students per class.

Accreditation and Approvals
The 550-hour Massage Therapist Program is accredited by the Commission on Massage Training Accreditation (COMTA); graduates of this program are qualified to take the National Certification Examination for Therapeutic Massage and Bodywork (NCETMB).

Program Description
The curriculum for the 550-hour Massage Therapist Program consists of Circulatory Massage, Lymphatic Massage, Deep Tissue Therapies, Anatomy/Physiology for Massage Professionals, Natural Therapeutics, Kinesiology, Acupressure/Shiatsu, Jin Shin Jyutsu, Therapeutic Massage, Reflexology, Sports Massage, Health in the 90s, Business Management, and supervised practice.

The 200-hour Massage Practitioner Course concentrates on contemporary and sports massage, and is transferable into the Massage Therapist Program.

Continuing Education

Continuing education is offered in structural integration, sports massage, cranial sacral, and other topics.

Admission Requirements

Prospective students must submit an application, scores from a standardized test of basic manual and verbal skills, and a personal interview. Reading and writing at the eleventh-grade level is required.

Tuition and Fees

There is a $75 registration fee for both courses

Tuition for the Massage Therapist Program is $4,500. Additional expenses include a massage table, $200 to $660, and books, $500.

Tuition for the Massage Practitioner Course is $725. Additional expenses include a massage table, $200 to $660, and books, $65.

Cleveland Chiropractic College of Los Angeles

590 North Vermont Avenue
Los Angeles, California 90004-2196
PHONE: (323) 660-6166 / (800) 466-CCLA
FAX: (323) 660-4195
E-MAIL: cclaadm@aol.com
WEBSITE: www.clevelandchiropractic.edu

Dr. C. S. Cleveland Sr., Dr. Ruth R. Cleveland, and Dr. Perl B. Griffin founded Cleveland Chiropractic College of Kansas City in 1922. In the 1940s, the Board of Trustees acquired Ratledge Chiropractic College in Southern California. Ratledge was rechartered as Cleveland Chiropractic College of Los Angeles in 1950, and in 1992, the college joined with its sister school, Cleveland Chiropractic College of Kansas City, to form a multicampus system. There are twenty-eight full-time and forty-three part-time instructors, with an average of sixty students per class.

Accreditation and Approvals

Cleveland Chiropractic College of Los Angeles is accredited by the North Central Association of Colleges and Schools and by the Council on Chiropractic Education (CCE).

Program Description

The 4,410-hour Doctor of Chiropractic degree program may be completed in three or four years. The program consists of courses taken from each of several departments: the Department of Human Life and Sciences (Anatomy, Physiology, Pathology, Microbiology, Chemistry, and Public Health courses); the Department of Diagnostic Sciences (including Diagnosis, X-Ray Interpretation, X-Ray Procedure, and Public Health); the Department of Chiropractic Sciences (Chiropractic Orientation, Philosophy, Technique, Physiotherapy, Clinic Management, and Practice Management courses); Research; and Clinical Internship.

CCC-LA also offers a B.S. in Human Biology degree, as well as all eight preprofessional health sciences courses in Chemistry, Physics, Biology, and Anatomy/Physiology.

Continuing Education

The Office of Continuing Education presents relicensing seminars in various subject areas that have included clinical nutrition, sports injury technique, X-ray, neurology, workers' compensation, infectious diseases including AIDS, and others.

Admission Requirements

Applicants must have completed at least sixty semester units of prechiropractic courses at a regionally accredited college with a cumulative GPA of 2.5 or higher. Candidates having a bachelor's degree are preferred. Specific numbers of prerequisite semester units are required in biological science, general chemistry, organic chemistry, general physics, general psychology, social sciences/humanities, and English/communications. Applicants must also submit and essay and two letters of recommendation; ideally, one should be from a chiropractor or other health care professional.

Tuition and Fees

Tuition is $185 per contact hour. Additional expenses include application fee, $50; malpractice insurance, $20 per trimester; and books and supplies, approximately $300 per trimester.

Financial Assistance

Payment plans, federal and nonfederal scholarships, grants, loans, and work-study programs are available.

College of the Botanical Healing Arts

1821 17th Avenue
Santa Cruz, California 95062
PHONE: (831) 462-1807
FAX: (831) 425-8258
E-MAIL: cobha@cruzio.com
WEBSITE: www.cobha.com

The College of Botanical Healing Arts (COBHA) was founded in 1997 by Elizabeth Jones and is a nonprofit institution. There are five instructors; class sizes average twelve to fifteen students for classes, twelve to twenty-five for workshops and guest lectures.

Accreditation and Approvals

COBHA is in the process of applying for California State certification through the Bureau for Private Postsecondary and Vocational Education.

Program Description

The 300-hour Aromatherapy Practitioner Certification Program consists of Level One: Foundation Course, ten Level Two classes, and four elective classes and/or workshops.

Level One: Foundation Course is an introduction to aroma science and aroma intuition. Level Two courses include The History of Medicine, Aroma Botany, Physiology Part One and Two, Essential Oil Chemistry, Mind & Body, Clinical Science, Energetic Healing, Communication and Business Skills, Clinical Practice Theory, and Clinical Internship.

Admission Requirements

Applicants must be at least 18 years of age, have a high school diploma or equivalent, and have a personal or telephone interview with a school administrator.

Community and Continuing Education

Workshops and guest lecture series are open to the public and include such topics as Introduction to Chinese Tonic Herbs, Advanced Aromatherapy Science, and Aromatherapy and Herbs.

Tuition and Fees

Tuition for Level One is $384 and includes textbook. The total cost for all ten classes of Level Two, excluding electives, is $3,096 (tuition based on $12 per hour); Level Two textbooks are additional and in some classes optional.

Financial Assistance

Payment plans and prepayment discounts are available.

Creativity Learning Institute

(See Multiple State Locations, page 390)

Curentur University

(See American University of Complementary Medicine, page 67)

Dandelion Herbal Center

4803 Greenwood Heights Drive
Kneeland, California 95549
PHONE: (707) 442-8157
FAX: (707) 442-8157
E-MAIL: discover@northcoast.com

The Dandelion Herbal Center was founded in 1988 by Jane Bothwell. There are twelve instructors, with an average of twenty-five students per class.

Program Description

Beginning with Herbs is a prerequisite course for the Ten-Month Apprenticeship Program (below). The class meets one evening per week for two months and covers herbal first aid, preparation and use of herbs, wild plant identification, herbal remedies for common imbalances, herbal formulation, and wild foods.

The Ten-Month Herbal Apprenticeship Program is offered each year from February to November and meets one weekend per month. Topics covered include History of Herbal Medicine, Traditions of Healing, Herbs for the Nervous System, Percolation Method of Tincturing, Herb Gardening, Dandelion Harvest, Herbs for the Liver and Digestive Herbs, Using Herbs with

Children, Basics of Botany, Herbs for the Urinary System, Herbs for the Skin, Muscles and Bones, Exploring the Flower Essence System of Healing, Herb Harvesting and Medicine Making, Herbs for the Reproductive System, Herbs for the Respiratory System, Natural Immunity, Herbs for the Endocrine and Lymphatic Systems, plus field trips.

Community and Continuing Education
Herb Walks are offered throughout the year and focus on edible, medicinal, and traditional uses of plants.

Festival of Herbs meets one weekend per month from August to April and offers an opportunity to study with renowned herbal teachers such as Michael Moore, Rosemary Gladstar, and others. Each month will feature a different teacher, and all classes include Herb Walks.

The Herbal Clinic class meets twice per month for six months. This is an advanced class for herbalists to practice and refine their counseling skills. Students evaluate case studies, practice with actual clients, and discuss current herbal news and research.

Admission Requirements
Applicants must complete an application form.

Tuition and Fees
Tuition for Beginning with Herbs is $225. Tuition for the Ten-Month Apprenticeship is $1,200 plus $25 materials fee.

Herb Walks are $15. Tuition for Festival of Herbs is $1,200. Tuition for the Herbal Clinic class is $300.

Financial Assistance
Limited work-trade is available.

The Day-Break Geriatric Massage Project

(See Multiple State Locations, pages 390–91)

Desert Resorts School of Somatherapy

13090 Palm Drive
Desert Hot Springs, California 92240
PHONE: (760) 329-1175 / (800) 270-1175
FAX: (760) 329-5925

E-MAIL: ramonam@somatherapy.com
WEBSITE: www.somatherapy.com

The Desert Resorts School of Somatherapy was founded in 1991 by Ramona Moody French, who was an instructor at Mueller College in San Diego for eight years. There are eight instructors, with an average of ten to twenty-four students per class.

Accreditation and Approvals
Desert Resorts School of Somatherapy is approved by the Bureau for Private Postsecondary and Vocational Education, and is approved as a continuing education provider by the National Certification Board for Therapeutic Massage and Bodywork (NCBTMB) and by the California Bureau of Registered Nurses. Graduates of the 600- and 1,000-hour programs are eligible to take the National Certification Examination for Therapeutic Massage and Bodywork (NCETMB).

Program Description
The 300-hour Massage Technician Program consists of classes in Swedish Massage, Acupressure, Anatomy, Business and Ethics, Aromatherapy, and Spa Services.

The 600-hour Massage Therapist Program consists of the 300-hour Massage Technician Program followed by an additional 300 hours in Acupressure II, Sports Massage, Deep Tissue Massage, Polarity, Advanced Anatomy, and Nutrition.

The 1,000-hour Holistic Health Practitioner Program consists of the 600-hour Massage Therapist Program followed by an additional 400 hours in Acupressure III, Sports Massage II, Deep Tissue II, Holistic Theory, Pathology, and Physiology.

The 160-hour Comprehensive Decongestive Therapy Course provides instruction in performing manual lymph drainage. The curriculum includes Anatomy and Physiology, Pathology, Indications and Contraindications, Additional Techniques, Bandaging/Exercises, Practice, review, and testing.

Admission Requirements
Applicants must be at least 18 years of age; in good health with no communicable disease; be U.S. residents; and have a personal interview.

Tuition and Fees
Tuition and fees are as follows: Massage Technician, $1,815;

Massage Therapist, $3,885; Holistic Health Practitioner, $5,790; Comprehensive Decongestive Therapy, $1,995. Books and supplies are additional.

Financial Assistance
Payment plans, veterans' benefits, and vocational rehabilitation assistance are available.

Diamond Light School of Massage and Healing Arts

45 San Clemente Drive
Corte Madera, California 94925
PHONE: (415) 454-6651
FAX: (415) 459-2804
E-MAIL: diamondlight@earthlink.net
WEBSITE: www.diamondlight.com

MAILING ADDRESS:
P.O. Box 5443
Mill Valley, CA 94942

Diamond Light School of Massage and Healing Arts was founded in 1987 by Vajra Matusow, who has been practicing and teaching bodywork and healing for over twenty-six years. There are six instructors; class sizes average twelve to twenty students. Classes are held in Corte Madera and in San Anselmo.

Accreditation and Approvals
Diamond Light is accredited by the California State Bureau of Private Postsecondary and Vocational Education. Graduates of the 500-hour Advanced Bodywork Practitioner Course are qualified to take the National Certification Examination for Therapeutic Massage and Bodywork (NCETMB).

Program Description
The 150-hour Massage Certification Course consists of 100 hours of training and fifty hours of practice. Courses include Swedish/Esalen Massage; Foot Reflexology; Business, Hygiene, and Ethics; Massage Theory and History; Lymphatic Massage; Anatomy and Physiology; Survey of Massage Technique; and Supervised Practicum.

The fifty-six-hour Deep Bodywork Certification Program offers instruction in techniques developed to address core patterns underlying chronic, functional, and structural problems of the musculoskeletal system. Courses include Theory of Deep Bodywork, Demonstration and Practice of Deep Bodywork Technique, and Anatomy.

A 100-hour Hypnotherapy Course offers instruction in Advanced Hypnotic Induction Methods, Advanced Verbal Skills Development, Intuitive Abilities Development, Advanced Past Life Regression Therapies, Dealing with Bizarre Hypnotic Phenomena, Treatment Strategies for Complex Cases, and Business and Ethical Issues.

A 100-hour Energetic Healing Course focuses on such topics as Energy and Chakra Work, Laying On of Hands, Working with the Elements, Meditation and Healing Practices from Various Traditions, Sound Healing, Reiki Certification, and Subtle Sense Perception.

A 500-hour Advanced Bodywork Practitioner Course offers instruction in Anatomy, Deep Tissue Massage, Meditation, Advanced Healing Techniques, and Supervised Practicum.

Other programs include Reiki Levels I and II certification, offered over a two-day weekend, and a one-day seminar in Hypnotherapy for Bodyworkers.

Classes are offered evenings and weekends.

Admission Requirements
Applicants must be at least 16 years of age or have parental permission.

Tuition and Fees
Tuition is as follows: Massage Certification, $1,295; Deep Bodywork, $625; Advanced Bodywork, $4,500; Hypnotherapy, $1,450; Energetic Healing, approximately $1,200 (depending on courses chosen); Reiki Levels I and II, $225; and Hypnotherapy for Bodyworkers, $85.

Financial Assistance
A discount is given for early payment; payment plans and work-study are available.

Dongguk Royal University

School of Oriental Medicine and Acupuncture
440 Shatto Place
Los Angeles, California 90020
PHONE: (213) 487-0110 / (800) 303-1800
FAX: (213) 487-0527
E-MAIL: dru@pdc.net
WEBSITE: www.dru.edu

In 1997, Royal University of America (founded in 1979) merged with Dongguk University, one of the top ten colleges and universities in South Korea. Collectively, the two institutions have been educating students for more than 110 years. There are fifty-one instructors and an average of fifteen to twenty students per class.

Accreditation and Approvals

The Master of Science in Oriental Medicine degree program is accredited by the Accreditation Commission for Acupuncture and Oriental Medicine (ACAOM) and approved by the Medical Board of California Acupuncture Board.

Program Description

The four-year, 2,700-hour Master of Science in Oriental Medicine Program may be completed in thirty-six months in an accelerated program. Courses are conducted in English, Korean, and Chinese. The program consists of 400 hours of Basic and Applied Science (including Anatomy and Physiology, Equipment and Safety Code Review, and Pathophysiology); 710 hours of Oriental Medicine Theory, Acupuncture, and Tui Na Therapy (including History of Eastern/Western Medicine, Introduction to Oriental Medicine, General Pathology, Basic Diagnosis, Zangfu Diagnosis, Internal Medicine, Gynecology, Pediatrics, Acupuncture Anatomy, Meridian Theory, Acupuncture Physiology, Acupuncture Therapeutics, Tai Chi Chuan, Qi Gong, Tui Na, and others); 450 hours of Herbology (Botany, Nutrition, Herbs, Applied Herbology, Advanced Formula, and others); 180 hours of Western Medicine (Western Medical Terminology, Survey of Clinical Medicine, Western Medical Tests and Labs, Internal Medicine, and First Aid/ CPR); thirty hours of Terminology and History of Medicine; thirty hours of Management and Ethics; ninety hours of Electives (a minimum of three chosen from Chinese Medical Language, English Medical Language, Tui Na, Auricular and Electro Acupuncture, Sa-sang Constitutional Medicine, and Medical Billing); and 810 hours of Clinical Training (Practice Observation, Case Seminar, Diagnosis and Evaluation, and Supervised Practice).

Admission Requirements

Applicants must have completed a minimum of two academic years (sixty semester units or ninety quarter units) of education at the baccalaureate level with a minimum GPA of 2.0, and must demonstrate English-language competency. Applicants must also submit two letters of recommendation and a personal essay.

Tuition and Fees

Tuition is $100 per didactic unit and $70 per clinical unit; total tuition for the program is approximately $25,000. Additional expenses include a $100 application fee; graduation evaluation fee, $200; comprehensive graduation exam fee, $100; malpractice insurance, $30 per quarter; CPR, $30; First Aid, $30; books are additional.

Financial Assistance

Federal grants, loans, work-study, scholarships, and veterans' benefits are available.

Dry Creek Herb Farm and Learning Center

13935 Dry Creek Road
Auburn, California 95602
PHONE: (530) 878-2441
FAX: (530) 878-6772

Dry Creek Herb Farm and Learning Center was founded in 1988 by Shatoiya de la Tour. In addition to apprenticeships and classes, the center offers garden tours and sells organically grown herbs and herb products, books, and skin-care products in their gift shop and by mail order. There are eighteen instructors, with an average of eighteen students per class.

Accreditation and Approvals

Nursing CEUs are available for some classes.

Program Description

The nine-month Earth-Centered Apprenticeship Program meets one weekend per month or one Thursday per week. The course combines Rosemary Gladstar's correspondence course, The Science and Art of Herbology, with extensive hands-on herbal instruction, usage, and much more. Topics covered include Herbal Philosophies; Herb Walks and Plant Identification; Harvesting Roots; Healing Through the Seasons; Spiritual Attunement with the Plants; Tea and Tincture Formulation; Herb Actions and Body Systems; Making Tinctures, Liniments, Salves, Poultices, Compresses, and Capsules; Herbal First Aid; Essential Oils, Infused Oils, and Aromatherapy; Herb Gardening; Wildcrafting; Herb Crafts and Cosmetics; Trends in Herbalism, Legal Herbalism, and Herbal Careers; and much more.

Community and Continuing Education

Individual classes and workshops are held evenings and weekends throughout the year on a wide variety of topics that have included Herb Gardening, Herbal Brewing, Aromatherapy, Aura Soma, Herbal First Aid, Soapmaking, Basic Herb Usage, Medicinal Herb Garden Tour, Feng Shui, and more.

A Labor Day Intensive offers instruction in the tradition of herbs through lectures and hands-on participation.

Advanced and progressive study programs are offered annually. Each provides an opportunity to study with a variety of teachers from around the country.

Tuition and Fees

Tuition for the Earth-Centered Apprenticeship Program is $1,495; students should budget an additional $300 for books and materials. Classes and workshops are $15 to $75. The Labor Day Intensive is $175. Advanced programs are $600 to $1,150.

Financial Assistance

Work-study is available for the Apprenticeship Program.

East West Academy of Healing Arts/Qigong Institute

(See Multiple State Locations, page 393)

East West School of Herbology

Box 275
Ben Lomond, California 95005
PHONE: (800) 717-5010
FAX: (831) 336-4548
E-MAIL: herbcourse@planetherbs.com
WEBSITE: www.planetherbs.com

The East West School of Herbology was founded by Michael Tierra, L.Ac., O.M.D., who maintains an herb and acupuncture clinic in Santa Cruz, teaches, writes, and creates a line of herbal products. The East West School's primary method of instruction is through three correspondence courses in herbalism (see page 475), plus the seminar described here. There are over 3,000 students worldwide. (The Tierras also teach a five-day seminar each fall at the Omega Institute in New York; see pages 266–67.)

Accreditation and Approvals

The East West School of Herbology is approved by the California Board of Registered Nursing to provide continuing education credits for 400 contact hours.

Program Description

A week-long seminar is offered each year in the mountains outside Santa Cruz. Topics covered in the past include the Five Stagnations: The Mother of All Diseases; Treating Skin Diseases with Herbs; Biomagnet Healing; Treatment of Stress, Anxiety, and Insomnia with Herbs; Herb Walks; Preparations; Pulse and Tongue Diagnosis; and Planetary Formulas. Mornings begin with Pranayama, yoga, qigong, tai chi, or meditation.

Admission Requirements

There are no minimum age or educational requirements.

Tuition and Fees

Tuition is $575, plus room and board fees of $360.

Financial Assistance

There are a limited number of partial scholarships.

Emperor's College of Traditional Oriental Medicine

1807-B Wilshire Boulevard
Santa Monica, California 90403
PHONE: (310) 453-8300
FAX: (310) 829-3838
E-MAIL: outreach@emperors.edu
WEBSITE: www.emperors.edu

The Emperor's College of Traditional Oriental Medicine was founded in 1983. There are forty-five instructors; the average class size is twenty students.

Accreditation and Approvals

The Master of Traditional Oriental Medicine Program (MTOM) is accredited by the Accreditation Commission for Acupuncture and Oriental Medicine (ACAOM) and approved by the California State Department of Education. Graduates are qualified to take the California Acupuncture Licensing Examination, as well as the national certification examinations in Acupuncture and Chinese Herbology administered by the National Certification Commission for Acupuncture and Oriental Medicine (NCCAOM).

Program Description

The 2,955-hour Master of Traditional Oriental Medicine Program consists of 2,005 academic hours and 950 clinical hours and may be completed in four years. The program is composed of an intensive study of Traditional Oriental Medicine that includes didactic and clinical training in Acupuncture and Herbology, as well as Tai Chi and Qi Gong, Acupressure, and Western Medical Sciences. A partnership with Daniel Freeman Marina Hospital allows interns to treat an acute-care in-patient population at a major Western hospital and interact with Western medical health care professionals, providing greater integration with modern Western health care.

The master's program consists of 685 hours of Western Sciences (including Chemistry, Anatomy/Physiology, Biochemistry, Physics for Acupuncturists, Pathology, General Psychology, Basic Nutrition, East/West Medical History, Western Physical Assessment, Western Medical Terminology, Clinical Nutrition, Western Pharmacology, Clinical Diagnosis by Lab Data, Introduction to Medical Imaging Procedures, and others); 410 hours of Acupuncture (including Introduction to Meridians, Acupuncture Energetics, Acupuncture Anatomy, Acupuncture Therapeutics, Tui Na, Acupressure, Acupuncture Technique, Microsystems, Secondary Vessels, and others); 460 hours of Oriental Medicine (including Philosophy, Chinese Medical Language, Zang-Fu Syndromes, Oriental Diagnosis, Five Elements, Tai Chi, Medical Qi Gong, Chinese Internal Medicine, Principles of Treatment, and Composite Diagnosis); 410 hours of Herbology (including Introduction to Herbology, Herb Pharmacopoeia, Herb Formulae, Advanced Formulas, Formulae Writing, Herb Pharmacy, Patent Medicines, Chinese Nutrition, and Shang Han/Wen Bing); 950 hours of Clinical Training (including Clinical Observation, Pre-Clinical Course, Internship, and Case Review/Presentation); and forty hours of electives chosen from Introduction to Ayurvedic Medicine, Shiatsu, Reflexology, Kinesiology, Feng Shui, Korean Hand Acupuncture, Pediatrics, Drug Detoxification, and others. Extracurricular course offerings include Mediation, Yoga, Martial Arts, and San Do.

Admission Requirements

Applicants for admission to the MTOM degree program must have completed sixty semester units of undergraduate course work from an accredited college, submit two letters of recommendation and a personal essay, and have a personal interview.

Tuition and Fees

Tuition is $108 per unit; clinical courses are $9 per hour. The approximate total cost for the master's program is $33,000, plus an additional $1,200 for books, herb samples, and supplies. The application fee is $50.

Financial Assistance

Federal student aid and direct loans are available.

Esalen Institute

Highway 1
Big Sur, California 93920-9616
PHONE: (831) 644-8476 / (831) 667-3000

FAX: (831) 667-2724
E-MAIL: group2000@esalen.org
WEBSITE: www.esalen.org

The Esalen Institute was founded in 1962 as an educational center devoted to exploring unrealized human capacities through East/West philosophies and didactic/experiential workshops. There are about 500 instructors, with eight to forty students per class.

Accreditation and Approvals
A number of workshops may be taken for continuing education credit by nurses and psychologists, and are approved by the California Board of Registered Nursing and the California Psychological Association. Two-day workshops offer ten hours of CEU credit; five-day workshops offer thirty hours of CEU credit for nurses, and twenty-six hours for psychologists.

Program Description
The twenty-eight-day Massage Practitioner Certification Program is a professional training program that, coupled with thirty documented massage sessions, leads to a California State–approved Certificate of Completion. The training includes Anatomy, Movement, Meditation, Gestalt Awareness, Ethics and Business Practices, and Self-Care. Training is held in month-long workshops or in three- and twelve-day workshops over the course of three to six months.

Continuing Education
Workshops that provide continuing education credit for nurses are offered throughout the year. Some topics include Adventures in Bodywork, the Subtle Art of Meditation, Psychoneuroimmunology and Its Implications, Weekend Massage Intensive, Sports Massage: Keeping the Player Playing, Hanna Somatics: Mastery of Muscles and Emotions, Religious and Spiritual Problems: A Paradigm Shift in Mental Health, Gestalt Practice, Polarity Massage Intensive, Zero Balancing® Open Forum, Five-Day Massage Intensive, Birth Experience: A Pathway to Life, the Heart of the Shaman, Caring for the Dying: What Really Works?, Practical Herbology: An Esalen Garden Workshop, and many others.

Workshops that offer continuing education credit for psychologists have not been outlined at this writing.

Tuition and Fees
Tuition for the Massage Practitioner Certification Program is $3,325 with standard accommodations, or $2,350 with bunk bed room, if available. Tuition for continuing education programs is $1,110 for seven days, $740 for five days, and $380 per weekend with standard accommodations; tuition with bunk bed room, if available, is $845, $550, and $300, respectively. Lower rates are available for sleeping bag space and those with their own accommodations. All rates include meals.

Financial Assistance
Work-study is available, and a discount is offered for senior citizens.

EverGreen Herb Garden and School of Integrative Herbology

P.O. Box 1445
Placerville, California 95667
PHONE/FAX: (530) 626-9288
E-MAIL: evrgreen@innercite.com

Founded in 1984 by Candis Cantin Packard and Lonnie Packard, the EverGreen Herb Garden and School of Integrative Herbology is an auxiliary of EverGreen Wholistic Ministry, a nonprofit ministry dedicated to gentle healing of body, mind, and spirit. There are four instructors, with twenty to twenty-five students per class.

Program Description
The forty-five-hour, three-month Beginning Integrative Herbology Study Program (Part 1) covers such topics as determining the Ayurvedic constitutional types, lifestyle considerations, harmonizing diet and lifestyle with the seasons, identification and use of local and traditional Western herbs, introduction to Chinese and Ayurvedic herbs, and making herbal preparations.

The forty-five-hour, three-month Intermediate Integrative Herbology Study Program (Part 2) includes such topics as the Ayurvedic view of the six stages of disease manifestation, Ayurvedic anatomy, deeper understanding of the constitutional types, continuing herb identification and applications, advanced herbal formulations for acute and chronic conditions, Chinese tongue diagnosis, and the use of Chinese tonic herbs.

The 120-hour, nine-month Integrative Herbology—Advanced Wholistic Lifestyle Counseling Program (Part 3) covers the Chinese system of diagnosis, aromatherapy, advanced tongue and pulse diagnosis, communications training, comparative religion and mythology, and advanced herbology (including herb gardening, wildcrafting, flower essence, and herbal formulations), plus personal studies, ten client case studies, and required reading.

Admission Requirements

There are no admission requirements for Part 1 or 2. Part 3 requires the successful completion of Part 1 and 2 plus completion of an application form to determine eligibility.

Tuition and Fees

The suggested donation for Part 1 is $450; for Part 2, $450; and for Part 3, $1,600.

Financial Assistance

Exceptions to the standard terms and payment plans can be considered.

The Expanding Light

Ananda's Retreat Center
Ananda Church of Self-Realization
14618 Tyler Foote Road
Nevada City, California 95959
PHONE: (530) 478-7518 / (800) 346-5350
FAX: (530) 478-7519
E-MAIL: info@expandinglight.org
WEBSITE: www.expandinglight.org

Founded in 1968, The Expanding Light offers a variety of retreats and programs based on the teachings of Paramhansa Yogananda, author of *Autobiography of a Yogi*. Programs are offered in yoga, meditation, self-discovery, and healthy living. There are about ten instructors, with an average of twenty students per class.

Program Description

The twenty-six-day Ananda Yoga Teacher Training Program is a total immersion program with a full schedule. The program covers a wide range of asanas, getting beyond the body mechanics into a deeper transformational experience, anatomy and physiology for yoga teachers, pranayama techniques, designing routines and teaching asanas, teaching yoga to seniors and pregnant women, and organizing and marketing classes effectively.

Admission Requirements

Applicants should have a regular hatha yoga practice.

Tuition and Fees

Tuition varies with type of accommodation from $1,770 (your own tent or RV) to $3,804 (private deluxe room). Costs include meals and all program activities.

Financial Assistance

A limited number of partial scholarships are available for low-income individuals. Discounts are available for seniors and groups.

Feldenkrais® Resources

(See Multiple State Locations, pages 393-94)

Five Branches Institute

200 Seventh Avenue
Santa Cruz, California 95062
PHONE: (831) 476-9424
FAX: (831) 476-8928
E-MAIL: tcm@fivebranches.edu
WEBSITE: www.fivebranches.edu

Five Branches Institute was founded in 1984 and is a nonprofit corporation. The institute is named for the five branches of traditional Chinese medicine: energetics, dietary medicine, acupuncture, herbology, and bone medicine. There are twenty-five instructors; entry-level core classes average twenty-five students, lab sections no more than fifteen.

Accreditation and Approvals

The master's degree program offered at Five Branches Institute is accredited by the Accreditation Commission for Acupuncture and Oriental Medicine (ACAOM), and fulfills the requirements for students wishing to take the California State Licensing Exam and the National Certification Commission for Acupuncture and Oriental Medicine (NCCAOM) Exam.

ACAOM is developing standards and criteria for the final approval of the doctorate degree from the U.S. Department of Education, which is expected in 1999.

Program Description

The 2,800-hour, three-and-a-half year Master's Degree in Traditional Chinese Medicine (MTCM) includes courses from six departments: Traditional Chinese Medical Theory, Acupuncture, Chinese Herbology, Auxiliary Studies, Modern Sciences, and Clinical Training.

First-year courses include Theory, Acupuncture, Philosophy/History, Qigong, Medical Terminology, Herbology, and Clinical Theater.

Second-year courses include continuing studies in Theory, Acupuncture, Herbology, Pathophysiology, and Clinical Theater, as well as Bodywork, Dietetics, Clinical Sciences, and Clinical Rounds.

Third-year courses continue to build on Theory, Acupuncture, Herbology, and Bodywork, and also include Ethics/Business Management, Pharmacology, electives, Clinical Rounds, and Supervised Practice.

In the fourth year, students take TCM seminars, electives, Medical Research, Psychology, Clinical Rounds, and Supervised Practice.

Electives include classes in such specialties as Ob/Gyn, Pediatrics, Internal Medicine, and Neurology, among others.

Continuing Education

While continuing to offer a postgraduate study program in China and postgraduate elective courses in TCM specializations in Santa Cruz, the Institute will be integrating these courses into a formal doctorate program being developed for the profession. The doctorate degree will have a clinical emphasis and will include advanced courses in both TCM classics and in TCM specializations such as gynecology, pediatrics, oncology, neurology, and internal medicine. The doctorate will add 1,200 to 1,500 hours to the MTCM program and students will be able to take the doctorate either as a continuation of their master's degree or as returning professionals. It is expected that doctorate-level students will be able to take part of their doctoral requirements in China.

Admission Requirements

Applicants must have completed at least sixty semester units of general education from a nationally accredited college, including college-level courses in human anatomy and physiology, physics, chemistry, and biology. In addition, applicants must submit a statement of purpose and three letters of personal reference, and have a personal interview.

Tuition and Fees

Tuition for academic units is $175 per semester unit; for clinical units, $350 per semester unit. The estimated total for the program, including tuition, fees, and books, is $28,000.

Financial Assistance

Federally funded financial aid (Stafford loans), payment plans and a Founder's Scholarship are available.

Five Element Training Program

8950 Villa La Jolla Drive, Suite 2162
La Jolla, California 92037
PHONE: (858) 457-1314
FAX: (858) 457-3615
The Five Element Training Program has been offered since 1987. There are two instructors; class size is limited to forty. The 1999 program was held in San Diego.

Accreditation

The program is accredited by the American Academy of Medical Acupuncture for fifty hours of continuing education.

Program Description

The Five Element Acupuncture for Physicians Training Program is presented over ten days. The program includes three days (twenty hours) of videotaped instruction followed by seven days of direct formal instruction. Topics covered include Identifying Causative Factors, Levels of Illness (including spirit level), Five Element Laws, Diagnostic Skills (including pulse diagnosis and emotion testing), Function and Spirit of the Acupuncture Points, Five Element Treatment Organization, and Patient Self-Care.

Admission Requirements

The program is designed to provide further training for physician graduates of the UCLA acupuncture training program as well as other physicians with previous acupuncture training.

Tuition and Fees

Tuition is $2,100, which includes videotapes, syllabus, continental breakfast daily, and lunch on the first day.

Flower Essence Society

P.O. Box 459
Nevada City, California 95959
PHONE: (530) 265-9163 / (800) 736-9222
FAX: (530) 265-0584
E-MAIL: fes@floweressence.com / info@flowersociety.org
WEBSITE: www.floweressence.com / www.flowersociety.org

The Flower Essence Society is a division of Earth-Spirit, a non-profit educational and research organization dedicated to the development of flower essence therapy (see page 448 for membership and page 466 for catalog information). The society has been offering its Practitioner Intensive for over fourteen years.

Program Description

Introductory weekends offer a comprehensive overview of flower essence theory and practice, including flower essence selection techniques and the study of live plant specimens.

The Practitioner Intensive is a week-long program open to those who have completed the weekend program or its equivalent. The program presents extensive profiles of major flower remedies, including typical combinations, case studies, and remedies for special populations; counseling; selection techniques; key "meta-levels" of in-depth flower essence therapy; essence combining; and distinctions between flower essences

and other remedies such as homeopathic or psychiatric drugs. Features include plant observation, artistic sessions, and a field trip with optional overnight camping to the Sierra Nevada mountains to prepare a flower essence. Practitioner certification is available to those who complete all the assignments and submit three in-depth case studies and a related paper within seven months after the program.

Tuition and Fees

Tuition varies depending on program and location. In 1999, the cost for an introductory weekend was $250; the Practitioner Intensive was $1,658 (double occupancy) to $2,053 (single occupancy) and included tuition, meals, lodging, and fees.

Hahnemann College of Homeopathy

80 Nicholl Avenue
Pt. Richmond, California 94801
PHONE: (510) 232-2079
FAX: (510) 412-9044
E-MAIL: hahnemann@igc.apc.org
WEBSITE: www.hahnemanncollege.com

The Hahnemann College of Homeopathy began its educational program in 1986. The college is located in a modern medical facility, along with the Hahnemann Medical Clinic and Hahnemann Pharmacy. There are six instructors, with an average of thirty-five students per class. A home study program will be added in summer 2000; see website for details.

Accreditation and Approvals

The Hahnemann College of Homeopathy has been accredited by the Bureau for Private Postsecondary and Vocational Education, and by the Council on Homeopathic Education (CHE) as an advanced-level postgraduate course.

Program Description

The 864-hour Comprehensive Professional Course in Classical Homeopathy is open to all licensed health care practitioners. The course meets in four-day sessions nine times per year for four years. A new course begins every two years, usually in January. The curriculum includes History, Philosophy, and Theory; Materia Medica: Comparative Materia Medica; Case Analysis; Case Taking and Management; and additional topics. In addition to classes, students are responsible for ten to twenty hours per week of home study, and are required to analyze and treat twenty-four chronic cases. Each student is assigned to a preceptor in the community who assists with case analysis.

Admission Requirements

Admission is open to licensed health care professionals—M.D., D.O., D.C., N.D., D.D.S., P.A., N.P., L.Ac., D.P.M., or D.V.M.—from accredited, residential schools. Applicants must submit a copy of their medical license. Prior background in homeopathy is not required.

Tuition and Fees

Tuition is $16,000. Additional expenses include an application fee, $50, and books, approximately $500. Students must also have a video camera for making videotapes for review and critique.

Healing Hands School of Holistic Health

11064 Pala Loma Drive
Valley Center, California
PHONE: (760) 746-9364 / (800) 355-6463

Healing Hands School of Holistic Health was founded by Paula and Neha Curtiss. There are nineteen instructors. Classes are offered in Escondido and Laguna Hills. In addition to the programs described here, Healing Hands offers a 100-hour Massage Technician Training Program.

Accreditation and Approvals

Healing Hands School of Holistic Health is certified by the Bureau of Private and Post-Secondary Education. Graduates of massage therapy programs of 500 or more hours are qualified to take the National Certification Examination for Therapeutic Massage and Bodywork (NCETMB). Healing Hands is approved by the California Board of Registered Nursing to offer continuing education credits to health care professionals.

Program Description

The 500-hour Massage Therapist Program consists of their 100-hour Massage Technician Training Program (focusing on anatomy, massage strokes, and body mechanics), 100 hours of Human Anatomy for Bodyworkers, and 300 hours chosen from Advanced Circulatory and Sports Massage, Shiatsu and Oriental Healing Techniques, Tui Na, Deep Tissue/Introduction to Structural Integration, Structural Organization, Geriatric Massage, and Recovery Practical.

The 1,000-hour Holistic Health Practitioner Program builds upon the 500-hour Massage Therapist Program with an additional 500 hours of electives chosen from Aromatherapy, Breath Therapy, Chair Massage, Cranio-Sacral Therapy, Exploring Meditation, Healing from Within, Herbology, Homeopathy, Hydrotherapy, Jin Shin, Myofascial Release, Neuromuscular Therapy, Nutrition, Passive Joint Movement, Reflexology, Repetitive Posture Stress Patterns, Seichim/Reiki, Sports Injuries, Structural Analysis, Subtle Touch, Tai Chi Chuan, Thai Massage, Touch for Health, and Yoga.

Admission Requirements

Applicants must complete a registration form.

Tuition and Fees

Tuition for the 500-hour Massage Therapist Program is $2,750. Tuition for the 1,000-hour Holistic Health Practitioner Program is $5,500. Books, linens, and massage table are additional.

Financial Assistance

Payment plans are available.

Heartwood Institute

220 Harmony Lane
Garberville, California 95542
PHONE: (707) 923-5002 / (707) 923-5000
FAX: (707) 923-5010
E-MAIL: admission@heartwoodinstitute.com
WEBSITE: www.heartwoodinstitute.com

Heartwood Institute, founded in 1978, is located on 240 remote acres in the mountains of California's North Coast. Students live on campus in simple rooms and enjoy organic and largely vegetarian meals in a log lodge surrounded by forests and meadows. There are ten instructors, with an average of sixteen to twenty students per class. In addition to the programs described here, Heartwood also offers a 100-hour Heartwood Massage Certification program.

Accreditation and Approvals

Heartwood is licensed to operate by the Bureau for Private Postsecondary and Vocational Education. All programs are accredited by the Accrediting Council for Continuing Education and Training (ACCET). The Polarity Therapy program is approved by the American Polarity Therapy Association (APTA). Heartwood is member of the AMTA Council of Schools. The Oriental Healing Arts and Whole Foods Nutrition program is approved by the American Oriental Bodywork Therapy Association (AOBTA). Graduates of massage therapy programs of 500 or more hours are qualified to take the National Certification Examination for Therapeutic Massage and Bodywork (NCETMB). Heartwood is approved as an NCBTMB continuing education provider.

Program Description

Heartwood offers three massage therapy programs: a 575-hour Massage Therapist Program, a 750-hour Advanced Massage Therapist Program, and a 1,000-hour Holistic Health Practitioner program.

The curriculum for the 575-hour Massage Therapist Program includes Massage Theory and Technique, Deep Tissue Massage, Musculoskeletal Anatomy, Introduction to Body Systems, Body Systems 2, Kinesiology, Pathology, Successful Business Practices, Therapeutic and Professional Skills, Clinical Practicum in Massage Therapy, Tai Chi or Yoga, Exercise Therapy, Hydrotherapy, Standard First Aid, CPR, and Communicable Disease Guidelines for Bodyworkers.

The 750-hour Advanced Massage Therapist Program includes all classes taught in the 575-hour program plus electives chosen from Polarity Therapy, NMT, Myofascial and Craniosacral Techniques, Seated Massage, Fragile Care Massage, Foot Reflexology, and more.

The twelve-month, 1,000-hour Holistic Health Practitioner Program includes all classes taught in the 750-hour Advanced Massage Therapist Program plus 250 additional hours in courses such as Integrating Hypnotherapy with Bodywork, Communication Skills, Spa Services, Breath and Transformation, or a combination of intensives that include Energy Work, Oriental Techniques, Neuromuscular Therapy, Sports Massage, Structural Bodywork, and others.

Students who complete the 240-hour Polarity Therapy Massage Practitioner Training and receive five professional sessions may join APTA as an Associate Polarity Practitioner; they may then become Registered Polarity Practitioners by completing the Polarity Internship, Polarity Diet, Craniosacral Therapy, and Somatic Emotional Clearing intensives, and receiving five professional sessions.

The two-quarter, 620-hour Oriental Healing Arts and Whole Foods Nutrition Program offers a comprehensive approach to the healing arts, integrating whole-foods nutrition, herbology, Zen Shiatsu acupressure, Traditional Chinese Medicine assessment and treatment tools, and awareness and movement practices.

Continuing Education

Heartwood Institute offers intensive trainings throughout the year that may be taken as continuing and advanced education by massage practitioners and other professionals, as entry-level trainings, or for personal growth and spiritual development. Such intensives include Neuromuscular Therapy, Craniosacral Therapy, Zen Shiatsu Acupressure, Orthopedic Massage, Sports Massage, TMJ Dysfunction, and more.

Admission Requirements

Applicants must have a high school diploma or equivalent, be committed to completing their training and seeking employment after graduation, supply two personal references, and be interviewed by admissions personnel.

Tuition and Fees

Tuition for the 575-hour Massage Therapist Program is $5,570; for the 750-hour Advanced Massage Therapist Program, $7,375; and for the 1,000-hour Holistic Health Practitioner Program, $9,825. Tuition for the Oriental Healing Arts and Whole Foods Nutrition program is $6,200.

Room and board is $2,260 per quarter double occupancy, $3,500 per quarter single occupancy, $2,020 per quarter camping space (available summer and fall quarters).

Hellerwork International

(See Multiple State Locations, page 395)

Hypnosis Motivation Institute

18607 Ventura Boulevard, Suite 310
Tarzana, California 91356
PHONE: (818) 758-2747 / (818) 344-4464, ext. 747
WEBSITE: www.hypnosismotivation.com

The Hypnosis Motivation Institute, founded in 1967 by Dr. John G. Kappas, has over fifty therapists on its staff and serves several hundred clients per week. In addition to its resident program, HMI Extension School offers a Foundations in Hypnotherapy course on video (see pages 484–85).

Accreditation and Approvals

HMI is nationally accredited by the Accrediting Council for Continuing Education and Training (ACCET). HMI is approved by the California Board of Registered Nursing as a provider of continuing education units, and by the Board of Behavioral Science Examiners for the hypnosis training of licensed marriage and family therapists.

Program Description

The 720-hour Hypnotherapy Program consists of Hypnosis 101 (which covers such topics as History of Hypnosis, Theory of Mind, Environmental Hypnosis and Hypersuggestibility, Various Hypnotic Inductions, Deepening Techniques, Postsuggestion to Re-Hypnosis, Three Stages of Somnambulism, Self-Hypnosis, Group Hypnosis, and more); Clinical Hypnosis 201 (which covers Hypnotic Modalities, Neurolinguistic Programming, Ericksonian Hypnosis, Hypnotic Regressions, Dream Therapy, Hypnotic Extinction of Fears and Phobias, Kappasinian Hypnosis, Medical Model of Hypnosis, Child Hypnosis, Hypnodiagnostic Tools, Hypnodrama, and Practice Law and Ethics); Hypnotherapy 301 (covering Physical and Emotional Sexuality, Systems Approach, Clinical Case Presentation, Low Blood Sugar Symptoms, Eating Disorders, Substance Abuse, Residency Orientation, Advertising and Promotion, First Consultation, Advanced Child Hypnosis, Adult Children of Dysfunctional Families, Crisis Intervention, Defense Mechanisms, Mental Bank, Sexual Dysfunction, General Self-Improvement, Habit Control, and Counseling and Interviewing); Handwriting Analysis; Clinical Applications 401; and Clinical Internship 501.

Admission Requirements

Applicants must be at least 18 years of age; have a high school diploma or equivalent or pass the Wonderlic Basic Skills test (a standardized test of basic math and verbal skills); and have a personal interview. The Taylor-Johnson Temperament Analysis Profile will also be administered to every applicant, and results must fall within a range deemed acceptable by HMI.

Tuition and Fees

Tuition for the entire program is $9,360.

Financial Assistance

Payment plans and federal financial aid are available. Clinical Internship 501 students may earn money working in the clinic.

Hypnotherapy Training Institute

4730 Alta Vista Avenue
Santa Rosa, California 95404
PHONE: (707) 579-9023
FAX: (707) 578-1033
E-MAIL: hypno@sonic.net
WEBSITE: www.sonic.net/hypno

Hypnotherapy Training Institute (HTI) was founded in 1978 by Randal Churchill; Marleen Mulder is the current director. The institute is one of the original four licensed hypnotherapy schools in the world. Churchill and Mulder are the primary instructors and teach 80 percent of the program, assisted by occasional guest instructors; the average class size is thirty students.

Accreditation and Approvals

Hypnotherapy Training Institute is licensed and diplomas authorized by the Bureau for Private Postsecondary and Vocational Education. Graduates are eligible for American Council of Hypnotist Examiners (ACHE) certification upon completion of Level Four.

Program Description

The Hypnotherapy Training program consists of five fifty-hour levels.

Level One covers Historical Overview of Hypnosis, Pre-Induction Interview, Establishing Realistic Goals, Induction and Deepening Techniques, Developing Hypnotic Rapport, Suggestibility Testing, Awakening Techniques, Post-Hypnotic Reinduction, Semantics of Hypnosis, Stress Reduction Strategies, Addiction and Habit Control, How to Teach Self-Hypnosis, Hypnotizing Children, Indirect Suggestion, Ericksonian Techniques, Shamanism (including Huna), Grounding and Centering Methods, and more.

Level Two covers Quantum Cellular Hypnotherapy, Discovering Underlying Issues, NLP Overview, Pacing and Leading, Producing Analgesia/Anesthesia, Emergency Uses of Hypnosis, Post-Hypnotic Amnesia, Intuitive Hypnotherapy, Overcoming Fears and Phobias, Hypnosis in Childbirth, Systematic Desensitization, Hypnosis and Dentistry, Spiritual Hypnosis, Transpersonal Hypnosis, Ethics, Semantics and the Law, and more.

Level Three is an advanced course emphasizing live demonstrations. Topics covered include Regression Strategies, Integrating Modalities, Gestalt, Transactional Analysis, Inner Child Work, Hypnoanalysis, Hypnotic Dreamwork™, and Business and Marketing Strategies.

Level Four continues to develop major themes from Level Three. Topics covered include Advanced Ideomotor Techniques including the Churchill Imprint Method, Comprehensive Regression Strategies, Advanced Hypno-Healing Methods, Bioenergetics, Experiential Holotropic Breathing Sessions, Creative Business and Marketing Strategies, and more.

A Level Five class is offered to HTI graduates; contact the institute for details.

Admission Requirements

Applicants must have a high school diploma or equivalent and have a personal interview.

Tuition and Fees

Tuition for each level is $695; books for each level average $35.

Financial Assistance

The institute is approved by Vocational Rehabilitation; private sources of assistance may be available.

Hypnotism Training Institute of Los Angeles

700 South Central Avenue
Glendale, California 91204
PHONE: (818) 242-1159
FAX: (818) 247-9379
WEBSITE: www.GilBoyne.com

Hypnotism Training Institute of Los Angeles (HTI) was founded in 1956. All classes are taught by Gil Boyne; class sizes average ten to twelve students. Home study courses and training videos are available; see pages 484 and 485.

Accreditation and Approvals

HTI is licensed by the California Board of Education as a vocational/professional school and approved for continuing education credits by the California Board of Registered Nursing.

Program Description

Course 101: Professional Hypnotism Training Course is a fifty-hour learn-by-doing program that includes History of Hypnosis, Nature of Hypnosis, Suggestibility Training, Induction Techniques, Programming the Subconscious, Hypnotic Age Regression, Post-Hypnotic Suggestions, Group Hypnosis, Instantaneous Hypnosis, Developing a Successful Practice, and much more. Students will be hypnotized to deep trance level and will hypnotize other class members. Classes meet on three consecutive weekends or for five consecutive days.

In the fifty-hour Course 201: Hypnotherapy: Principle and Practice, students view videotapes of therapies conducted by Gil Boyne using unique therapy techniques.

Course 301: Advanced Clinical Hypnotherapy is a fifty-hour continuation and expansion of Course 201. Case histories are more complex, and explanation of concepts and therapeutic choices is given after each therapy session. Courses 201 and 301 both teach uncovering techniques such as age regression, emotional ventilation, subconscious reeducation, and the reprogramming of fixed ideas from childhood.

Course 401: Hypnotherapy in Healing and Pain Control is a fifty-hour program that focuses on all aspects of healing and controlling and eliminating pain. Video case histories are shown and include techniques for First Emergency Responders and utilization of pain control by nurses, extraordinary treatment by hypnosis of burns and other major injuries, and more.

A four-month Clinical Hypnotherapy Residency is offered to those who have completed the above 200 hours of hypnotherapy training. Students gain clinical experience in a supervised setting at the HTI clinic.

Tuition and Fees
Tuition for each course is $750.

Institute of Classical Homoeopathy

1336-D Oak Avenue
St. Helena, California 94574
PHONE: (707) 963-7796
FAX: (707) 963-6131
VOICE MAIL: (415) 248-1632
E-MAIL: ICHinfo@classicalhomoeopathy.org
WEBSITE: www.classicalhomoeopathy.org

The Institute of Classical Homoeopathy (ICH) is a nonprofit educational institution founded in 1992. Classes are held at Fort Mason Center in San Francisco. The average class size is fifteen; there are four faculty members.

Accreditation and Approvals
ICH is approved by the Bureau for Private Postsecondary and Vocational Education. Continuing education credits are available for Registered Nurses.

Program Description
The four-year Classical Homeopathy curriculum consists of Philosophy and Principles of Classical Homeopathy, Materia Medica, Medical Sciences and Case Analysis (which includes classes in Anatomy and Physiology, Pathology, Clinical Science and Medical Terminology, and Psychology), Clinical Practice and Case Analysis, and Practice Management and Ethics. Home study is an important aspect of the training program; regular reading and writing assignments include a major written as-

signment every four weeks. Classes meet thirteen weekends per year. Red Cross First Aid and CPR are required for graduation.

Admission Requirements
Applicants must have a high school diploma or equivalent (two years of college is preferable), submit a written application and personal interview, and demonstrate emotional maturity.

Tuition and Fees
Tuition ranges from $3,600 to $4,200, depending on the payment plan selected and whether science classes are needed; tuition may be increased, if necessary, for subsequent years. There is a $50 registration fee.

Financial Assistance
Payment plans are available.

Institute of Integrative Aromatherapy

(See Multiple State Locations, pages 395–96)

Institute of Psycho-Structural Balancing

3767 Overland Avenue, Suite 105
Los Angeles, California 90034
PHONE: (310) 815-3675
FAX: (310) 815-3670
E-MAIL: ipsb@concentric.net
WEBSITE: www.ipsb.com

The Institute of Psycho-Structural Balancing (IPSB) was founded in 1978. There are twenty-eight instructors; enrollment is limited to twenty-four students per class.

Accreditation and Approvals
IPSB has been granted institutional approval by the Bureau of Postsecondary and Vocational Education. Graduates of massage therapy programs of 500 or more hours are qualified to take the National Certification Examination for Therapeutic Massage and Bodywork (NCETMB). IPSB is approved by the California Board of Registered Nursing as a continuing education provider.

Program Description

The 150-hour Massage Technician Program is a prerequisite for the 539-hour Massage Therapist Program; it may also be taken independently. The program consists of Tai Chi Chuan, Swedish/Esalen Massage Techniques, Body Psychology, Self-Massage, Anatomy, Joint Mobilizations, Energy Balancing, Introduction to Deep Tissue, Chiropractic Massage, Spa Massage, Seated Massage, Business Practices, and Philosophy of a Holistic Practitioner.

For the 539-hour Massage Therapist Program, students are required to complete the Massage Technician Program plus 389 hours of additional studies. Courses include Acupressure Theory, Basic Acupressure for Bodyworkers, Advanced Circulatory Massage, Anatomy/Physiology, Business for Bodyworkers, CPR/First Aid, Deep Tissue, Healthy Boundaries for Bodywork, Human Energy Systems, Hydrotherapy, Hygiene, Pathology, and fourteen hours of electives chosen from such courses as Cranial, Lymphatic Clearing, Polarity, Pregnancy Massage, Reflexology, Aromatherapy, Sports Massage, Psychology of Muscles, and others.

Classes are held days, evenings, and weekends.

Continuing Education

All classes may be taken individually provided any prerequisites are met; some classes require Massage Technician training or Massage Technician training and some advanced classes.

Admission Requirements

Applicants must be at least 18 years of age and successfully complete the IPSB application and interview process.

Tuition and Fees

Tuition for the Massage Technician program is $1,275. Tuition for the Massage Therapist program is $5,068. There is a $75 registration fee.

Financial Assistance

Installment arrangements and tuition financing are available. There is a 5 percent discount for payment in full at time of contract.

Integrative Yoga Therapy

(See Multiple State Locations, page 396)

International Professional School of Bodywork

1366 Hornblend Street
San Diego, California 92109
PHONE: (858) 272-4142 / (800) 748-6497
FAX: (858) 272-4772
E-MAIL: beingipsb@aol.com
WEBSITE: www.ipsb.edu

The International Professional School of Bodywork (IPSB) was founded in 1977. Dr. Edward W. Maupin, president of IPSB and licensed clinical psychologist, has practiced the Rolf method of structural integration since 1968. There are thirty instructors, with a maximum of twenty-six students per class.

Accreditation and Approvals

IPSB is approved by the Bureau for Private Postsecondary and Vocational Education as a degree-granting school. In addition, the school is accredited by the Commission on Massage Training Accreditation (COMTA), is a member of the AOBTA Council of Schools and Programs, and is approved by the California Board of Registered Nursing for continuing education credits. Graduates of massage therapy programs of 500 or more hours are qualified to take the National Certification Examination for Therapeutic Massage and Bodywork (NCETMB).

Program Description

The 120-hour (twelve-credit-unit) Essentials of Massage and Bodywork certificate program covers theory and practice of circulatory massage (including Swedish and Esalen massage), deep tissue work, passive joint movement, and muscle sculpting, along with tai chi and the IPSB movement form. Classes include Anatomy, Physiology, and Hygiene; Massage Techniques; Somatic Psychology; Support and Maintenance Systems; Ethics, Business, and Legal Issues; Practice Session; and a Portfolio.

The 150-hour (fifteen-credit-unit) Contemporary Methods of Massage and Bodywork Certificate Program offers instruction in six specialized areas of advanced bodywork to those who have completed the Essentials. Courses include Circulatory Massage Applications, Deep Tissue Sculpting, Oriental Theories and Healing Massage, Somatic Assimilation, Somatic Psychology, and Passive Joint Movement.

Additional certificate programs are offered in specialized internships that range from ninety to 250 hours (nine to twenty-five credit units). These include Relational Somatics, Sensory Repatterning, Somato-Emotional Integration, Structural Integration, Sports Massage, Neuromuscular Therapy, Circulatory Massage Therapeutics, Tui Na Massage, Jin Shin Acutouch, Thailand Medical Massage, Seitai Shiatsu, and Teacher Training.

The Associate of Science degree is a diploma program of 104 credit units (approximately 1,200 hours), with a major course of study in massage and bodywork. It includes the Essentials and Contemporary Methods of Massage and Bodywork Programs above, along with studies in anatomy, physiology, massage electives (which may include Alexander Technique, Feldenkrais Awareness Through Movement®, Sports Massage, Foot Reflexology, Tui Na Massage, Lymphatic Massage, Jin Shin Acutouch, Thailand Massage, and others), electives in kinesiology, creating a professional practice, neuromuscular therapy, principles of structural integration (Rolfing), clinical applications, supervised practice, and other courses, plus one internship in a specialized form of advanced techniques of massage and bodywork.

The Associate of Arts degree is a diploma program of 132½ credit units (approximately 1,470 hours), with a major course of study in massage and bodywork that may be taken in Clinical Methods, Integrative Somatic Methods, Oriental Methods, or Individualized Methods. All of the courses listed in the Associate of Occupational Studies Program above are included in this program, plus four internships in a specialized form of advanced techniques of massage and bodywork.

The Bachelor of Arts degree in humanities is a diploma program of 224 credit units (approximately 2,400 hours), with its major course of study in massage and bodywork. It includes one of the four Associate of Arts degrees or their equivalents, plus additional classes in humanities. Courses include Learning Seminars, Language and Communication, Biology, Nutrition, History, Mathematics and Numbers, Music Appreciation, Physics, Psychology, Great Books, Anthropology/Sociology, Self-Directed Learning, Other Humanities, and a Portfolio of Learning.

The Master of Arts degree in somatics is a diploma program of fifty credit units (approximately 650 hours) that has a prerequisite of the IPSB bachelor's degree or its equivalent. The major course of study is in massage and bodywork. The master's degree includes Learning Seminars, Advanced Specializations, Self-Directed Specialization, Self-Directed Comprehensive Studies, Self-Directed Studies, Seminars in Advanced Specializations, Portfolio of Logs and Learning, and a thesis, project, or dissertation.

Classes are held both days and evenings. Full-time, all-day intensive programs are available to those who wish to minimize the time required for training. All students are required to complete First Aid/CPR training.

Admission Requirements

Applicants must be at least 18 years of age, have a high school diploma or equivalent, be free of any diseases or disabilities that would limit physical exertion, have the ability to apply techniques or breathing, and show no evidence of mental instability. Applicants who do not have a high school diploma or equivalent may enroll in certificate programs or individual classes, and may be eligible to continue after taking an approved test to demonstrate their ability to benefit from the program.

Tuition and Fees

Tuition costs are as follows: for the Essentials of Massage and Bodywork Program, $900; for the Contemporary Methods of Massage and Bodywork Program, $1,125; for the Associate of Science Program, $8,860; for the Associate of Arts in Clinical Methods, Integrative Somatic Methods, Oriental Methods, or Individualized Methods Programs, $11,305 to $11,475; for the Bachelor of Arts degree, $22,105; and for the Master of Arts degree, $10,450. Other fees include an application fee of $100 and a supply fee of $50 per quarter; books are additional.

Financial Assistance

Payment plans, limited work-study, veterans' benefits, and Vocational Rehabilitation are available. Residents of some Canadian provinces may finance their training through Canadian Government Student Loans.

Iyengar Yoga Institute of San Francisco

2404 27th Avenue
San Francisco, California 94116
PHONE: (415) 753-0909
FAX: (415) 753-0913
E-MAIL: iyisf@sirius.com
WEBSITE: www.iyisf.org

Founded in 1974, the Iyengar Yoga Institute of San Francisco (IYISF) has the oldest Iyengar teaching program in the United States. IYISF is owned and operated by the B.K.S. Iyengar Yoga Association of Northern California, a nonprofit membership organization. There are eleven faculty members.

Accreditation and Approvals

The program is approved by the California Bureau for Private Postsecondary and Vocational Education and prepares students to take the Iyengar Yoga National Association of U.S. Introductory Certificate Assessment.

Program Description

The Advanced Studies Teacher Training Program may be completed in two years. The Year One curriculum includes Asana I through III, Anatomy I and II, The Sutras, Intro to Pranayama, Physiology, Bhagavad Gita, and electives. Year Two includes Teaching Asana I through III, Pranayama I and II, Asana IV, Apprenticeship, and Student Teaching.

The program may be taken for credit toward a Yoga Instructor Certificate of Completion or on a noncredit basis. Students who intend to receive a Yoga Instructor Certificate of Completion must enroll in classes for credit and take classes sequentially. To receive credit, a student must attend a minimum of 80 percent of class hours; papers and/or final exams will be required.

Community and Continuing Education

The institute offers a full range of educational programs on yoga with the study of Western sciences, including introductory classes, workshops, intensives, and retreats.

Admission Requirements

Teacher Training applicants should have practiced Iyengar Yoga with a certified Iyengar yoga teacher for a minimum of two years on a consistent basis before starting Asana I. In cases where there are no certified Iyengar yoga teachers, an in-person assessment is necessary. There are no prerequisites for entering Anatomy I, Physiology, or Philosophy classes.

Tuition and Fees

Tuition is $90 per unit for the forty-eight-unit program. Additional expenses include the application fee, $20; association membership, $45 per year; required texts, $220; recommended reading, $60; props, $150; and graduation fee, $25. Total cost for the program is approximately $4,885.

Financial Assistance

Two scholarships are awarded annually.

Jin Shin Do Foundation for Bodymind Acupressure

FACILITY AND MAILING ADDRESS:
1084G San Miguel Canyon Road
Watsonville, California 95076
PHONE: (831) 763-7702
FAX: (831) 763-1551
E-MAIL: Iona@JinShinDo.org
WEBSITE: www.JinShinDo.org

ALTERNATE MAILING ADDRESS:
P.O. Box 1097
Felton, California 95018

Jin Shin Do Foundation for Bodymind Acupressure was founded in 1982 by Marsaa Teeguarden, the current director. Jin Shin Do acupressure combines deep finger pressure on acupoints with simple body-focusing techniques to release physical and emotional tension and produce a pleasurable trance state. A typical session lasts one to one and a half hours and may be effective in relieving headaches, back and shoulder pain, sinus pain, allergies, and other conditions.

Accreditation and Approvals

The Jin Shin Do Foundation is a member of the American Oriental Bodywork Therapy Association (AOBTA) Council of

Schools and Programs and is approved by the National Certification Board for Therapeutic Massage and Bodywork (NCBTMB) as a continuing education provider.

Registered JSD practitioners with a 500-hour transcript can meet education eligibility requirements for taking the national Oriental Bodywork Therapy exam given by the National Commission for the Certification of Acupuncture and Oriental Medicine (NCCAOM).

Program Description

Jin Shin Do Introductory, Module I, and Module II classes are taught by authorized JSD teachers located throughout the country and around the world. Students may contact the foundation for a directory of authorized JSD teachers and registered JSD acupressurists.

Classes offered by registered JSD acupressurists and authorized JSD teachers include short introductory classes such as Five-Step JSD Neck-Shoulder Release (three hours), Fundamentals of Self-Acupressure (twelve to sixteen hours), and JSD Acupressure Facial (six hours).

Module I consists of 150 hours of theory and technique necessary for effective practice of Jin Shin Do, including locating over 200 acupoints, identifying the eight strange flows or extraordinary meridians, the twelve organ meridians, pressure technique, Five Phases theory, and more. Module I is divided into Basic, Intermediate, and Advanced JSD, and Bodymind Processing Skills.

Module II consists of 100 hours of modality technique and practice, including an in-depth study of strange flows, organ meridians, zang-fu, causes of imbalance, precise point location and angle of pressure, point combining, and more.

Module III consists of seventy hours of clinical experience, either as an internship at a bodywork school or as an externship with supervision from an authorized JSD teacher, acupuncturist, or other health professional.

An Intensive Teacher Training Program with Iona Marsaa Teeguarden is offered periodically, and includes in-depth training and practice teaching.

Requirements for registered Jin Shin Do acupressurists include Modules I and II, plus Module III or 125 logged experience hours, along with ten private sessions, practical examination, and compliance with local licensing requirements, if any. To become a certified practitioner with AOBTA requires completion of Module III plus an additional seventy hours of study (of JSD or any recognized Oriental modality), 100 hours of anatomy and physiology, and an eight-hour CPR class.

To become authorized to teach the Jin Shin Do basic class, practitioners must have taken Module I and Module II, be a registered JSD acupressurist, take the Intensive Teacher Training Program, log a total of 300 experience hours, take a practical exam, and assist two classes; to teach the intermediate class, practitioners must have a total of 600 experience hours, have taught three Basic JSD classes, assist with two intermediate classes, and take a practical exam; to teach the advanced class requires a special project and practical exam with Iona.

When authorized JSD teachers have been actively practicing for five years and teaching for two, they may be accepted as candidates for AOBTA certified instructor in the style of Jin Shin Do. The certifying process includes an interview with three certified instructors.

Admission Requirements

Classes are open to anyone who has met the prerequisites (i.e., has taken the preceding classes with an authorized JSD teacher).

Tuition and Fees

Fees for classes vary according to the area and class setting. Fees for Modules I and II generally range from $10 to $15 per class hour.

Financial Assistance

Payment plans and work-study may be available from individual instructors.

John F. Kennedy University

Graduate School for Holistic Studies
12 Altarinda Road
Orinda, California 94563
PHONE: (925) 254-0105
FAX: (925) 254-3322
WEBSITE: www.jfku.edu

John F. Kennedy University was founded in 1964 as one of the first universities in the United States dedicated solely to adult education, and has since expanded to meet the full range of student needs. Today, undergraduate and graduate programs in liberal arts, management, psychology, holistic studies, and law enroll approximately 2,000 students, 80 percent of whom are in the graduate program.

Accreditation and Approvals
John F. Kennedy University is accredited by the Western Association of Schools and Colleges.

Program Description
The Graduate School for Holistic Studies offers Master of Arts (M.A.) and Master of Fine Arts (M.F.A.) degrees in arts and consciousness, with specializations in Transformative Arts and Studio Arts; Counseling Psychology, with specializations in Transpersonal and Somatic Psychology; Holistic Health Education; Interdisciplinary Consciousness Studies; and Transpersonal Psychology.

The M.A. in Counseling Psychology with Holistic Studies specialization meets the educational requirements for California Marriage and Family Therapist (M.F.T.) licensure. Courses offered in Holistic Studies include Principles of Holistic Health, Psychology of Nutrition and Eating Disorders, Diet in Health and Disease, Physiology and Psychology of Stress, and Mind/Body Approach to Self-Care.

Admission Requirements
Students entering the Master of Arts in Holistic Health Education program are required to fulfill a writing competency requirement. All students in the Holistic Health specialization are required to complete at least twelve months or forty-eight hours of individual psychotherapy with a licensed counselor.

Graduate applicants who have not completed their Bachelor of Arts degree may enroll in the school's articulated studies option, which allows up to eighteen to twenty-four graduate-level units to apply to both a B.A. and M.A. degree concurrently.

Tuition and Fees
Graduate tuition is $287 per unit; books are additional. There is a $50 application fee.

Financial Assistance
Federal grants and loans, California State Graduate Fellowships and California grants, university scholarships, and payment plans are available.

Kali Ray TriYoga®

(See Multiple State Locations, pages 400–401)

Kyung San University

8322 Garden Grove Boulevard
Garden Grove, California 92644
PHONE: (714) 636-0337
FAX: (714) 636-8459
E-MAIL: admin@kyungsan.edu
WEBSITE: www.cerfnet.com/kyungsan/

Kyung San University (KSU) was founded in 1994 by Kwee Ja Ohm, Ilan Kwang Ohm, and others. There are approximately twenty instructors, with an average of ten students per class. KSU has not yet had a graduating class.

Accreditation and Approvals
KSU is a candidate for accreditation with the Accreditation Commission for Acupuncture and Oriental Medicine (ACAOM) and approved by the California Acupuncture Committee. The university is recognized by the Bureau for Private Postsecondary and Vocational Education.

Program Description
The four-year Master of Science in Oriental Medicine Degree Program includes courses in the areas of Basic Studies and General Science (including Human Biology, Topographic Anatomy, Basic Physics, Basic Chemistry, Organic and Biochemistry, Principles of Nutrition, Anatomy and Physiology, Chinese Nutrition, General Psychology, Western Pathology, History of Medicine and Acupuncture, and Western Medical Terminology); Exercise and Massage (including Chinese Philosophy (Qi Gong), Tai Chi, and Acupressure); Herbology (including Botany and Introduction to Herbology, Oriental Medicine: Herbology, Herbal Prescriptions, and Herbal Pharmacy); Acupuncture and Acupuncture Techniques (including Introduction to Acupuncture, Points Location and Theory, Acupuncture Techniques, and Auricular/Scalp Acupuncture); Theory Dan Practice of

Oriental Medicine (Oriental Medicine Terminology, Fundamental Theories of Oriental Medicine, Diagnostic Methods of Oriental Medicine, Essentials of Oriental Medicine, Internal Medicine, and Oriental Doctor's Treasured Reference); Western Clinical Science (including Pharmacology, CPR, Survey of Health Care Systems, and Clinical Aspects of Western Medicine); Clinical Training (including Observation and Internship); Practice Management (including Ethics and Professional Issues, and Clinic Management); Graduation Assessment Test (GAT); and Thesis. Electives are offered when there is sufficient interest in a given topic; courses may include Conversational Chinese, Conversational Korean, Psychology of Patient Care, Tui Na, Principles of Homeopathy, and others. Students are required to complete a minimum of 800 hours in clinical internship, 75 percent of that total at KSU. Courses are taught in Korean and English.

Admission Requirements

Applicants must be at least 18 years of age and in good health, with the mental capacity and emotional stability necessary to succeed; have completed at least two academic years (sixty semester units or ninety quarter units) at an accredited school or college of general education courses and technical courses related to the health sciences and Oriental medicine, and have a cumulative GPA of 2.0 or better; and demonstrate their ability to read and write English or Korean at the college-entrance level.

Tuition and Fees

Tuition for the four-year program is $21,070. There is a $100 application fee.

Life Chiropractic College West

25001 Industrial Boulevard
Hayward, California 94545
PHONE: (510) 276-9013 / (800) 788-4476
FAX: (510) 276-4893
E-MAIL: admissions@lifewest.edu
WEBSITE: www.lifewest.edu

Life West was originally incorporated as Pacific States Chiropractic College in 1976, and reorganized as Life Chiropractic College West in 1981. There are nearly 800 students, with ninety-four instructors and an average class size of thirty-five students.

Accreditation and Approvals

Life Chiropractic College West is accredited by the Council on Chiropractic Education (CCE).

Program Description

The 4,862-hour Doctor of Chiropractic (D.C.) degree program features an integrated emphasis on chiropractic philosophy and technique. The program may be completed in as few as thirteen quarters. Classroom and clinic experience provides students with a strong background in the sciences, a deep understanding of chiropractic philosophy, and training in twelve leading techniques, including Diversified Gonstead, Toggle, Drop-Table, NUCCA, Extremity, SOT, Biophysics, Activator, Motion Palpation, BEST, and Logan.

Admission Requirements

Applications for admission are accepted up to two years prior to a student's intended term of entry. Applicants must have completed, or be working toward, a total of at least sixty semester units of college-level work (ninety semester units as of fall 2001) divided among the basic sciences (biology, general chemistry, organic chemistry, and physics), social sciences/humanities, English/communication skills, and psychology. There is also a minimum GPA requirement as well as a number of required documents; contact the admissions office for detailed information on prerequisites and needed application materials.

Tuition and Fees

Tuition is $4,250 per quarter; for students who choose an extended schedule, there are reduced tuition rates for the extra quarters of study. Total tuition for the thirteen-quarter program is $55,250, plus an estimated $750 for books and supplies per academic year.

Financial Assistance

Forms of financial assistance include federal grants and loans; state grants; Bureau of Indian Affairs grants; scholarships; ChiroLoan and other loan programs; federal and institutional work-study; and veterans' benefits. International students are eligible for a 25 percent tuition discount.

Los Angeles College of Chiropractic

16200 East Amber Valley Drive
Whittier, California 90609-1166
PHONE: (562) 947-8755 / (800) 221-5222
E-MAIL: lacc@deltanet.com
WEBSITE: www.deltanet.com/lacc

The Los Angeles College of Chiropractic was founded by Dr. Charles Cale and his wife Linnie in 1911; the first classes of their nine-month program were held in their home. The college moved several times before arriving at its present site in 1981. The ADVANTAGE program was added to the curriculum in 1990. There are seventy-three faculty of the college and eighty-nine faculty of the Division of Postgraduate Education; class sizes vary.

Accreditation and Approvals
The Doctor of Chiropractic degree program at the Los Angeles College of Chiropractic is accredited by the Council on Chiropractic Education (CCE) and the Accrediting Commission for Senior Colleges and Universities of the Western Association of Schools and Colleges.

Program Description
The 4,860-hour Doctor of Chiropractic degree program is based on the ADVANTAGE program of chiropractic education. This program is an innovative approach that aims at acquiring competencies, rather than learning subjects, and begins skill development on day one. The program integrates patient care with the basic sciences, and increases lab and hands-on experiences. The twenty chiropractic competencies that drive the ADVANTAGE program are History Taking, Physical Examination, Neuromusculoskeletal Exam, Radiological Exam, Clinical Lab Exam, Special Studies, Diagnosis and Clinical Impression, Referral/Collaborative Care, Treatment Plan, Spinal Adjusting, Extra Spinal Adjusting, Non-Adjustive Physical Procedures, Psychosocial Exam, Emergency Care, Case Follow-Up and Review, Record Keeping, Nutritional Consulting, Practice Management, Research, and Professional Responsibilities.

As students progress through the ADVANTAGE curriculum, they will be involved with four divisions: Basic Sciences (including the departments of Anatomy, Physiology, Biochemistry and Nutrition, and Pathology/Microbiology); Clinical Sciences (including the departments of Principles and Practice, Chiropractic Procedures, Diagnosis, and Radiology); Clinical Internship; and Research.

Continuing Education
The college offers postgraduate educational programs leading to professional certification and/or eligibility to take a board examination in a specialty area, as well as continuing education programs for paraprofessionals. Postgraduate courses include Chiropractic Neurology, Chiropractic Orthopedics, Chiropractic Rehabilitation, and Sports and Recreational Injuries: Prevention, Evaluation, and Treatment. Residency programs are offered in clinical sciences and radiology. A series of postgraduate seminars for license-renewal credit is offered throughout the state.

Admission Requirements
Applicants must have completed at least eighty-five semester units leading to a baccalaureate degree; prechiropractic credits must have been earned at an accredited institution. No fewer than six semester units each must have been taken in Biological Sciences, General Chemistry, Organic Chemistry, and General Physics; other prerequisites include six semester units of English and/or Communications, three semester units of Psychology, and fifteen semester units in Social Sciences or Humanities with a minimum grade of C in each. Applicants should have attained a cumulative GPA of 2.5 or better; graduates with a minimum cumulative GPA of 2.75 will be given preferential consideration for admissions. Additionally, applicants must submit three letters of recommendation (at least one should be from a Doctor of Chiropractic or other health care professional) and have a personal interview.

Tuition and Fees
Tuition for the Doctor of Chiropractic degree program is $5,523 per trimester. Additional expenses include an application fee of $50; an associated student body fee of $30 per trimester; books (approximate), $600 per trimester; and equipment (approximate), $1,200.

Financial Assistance

Payment plans, federal and private scholarships, grants, loans, and work-study are available.

Los Angeles East West Center Institute for Macrobiotic Studies

11215 Hannum Avenue
Culver City, California 90230
PHONE/FAX: (310) 398-2228

The Los Angeles East West Center Institute for Macrobiotic Studies was founded in 1973 by Cecile Tovah Levin, an internationally known and MEA accredited Senior Teacher and Senior Counselor, author, and speaker who has been a student and teacher of the macrobiotic way of life since 1960. Levin is the only instructor; the average class size is six students.

Program Description

A series of courses is offered that provides an in-depth study of macrobiotics for both beginning and advanced students, and for those who simply want to improve their own health and that of their families. Certificates will be given to students who complete all the courses.

Fundamentals of Macrobiotic Cooking is a one-year series of seasonal cooking courses designed to guide beginners making the transition to macrobiotic cooking. Topics covered include Fundamentals of Nutrition, Cutting and Cooking Techniques, Cooking with the Seasons, Cooking for Regeneration, Cooking for One, and Family Cooking. Students must complete at least one course in this series as a prerequisite for the Macrobiotic Life seminars.

The Macrobiotic Life seminars are a one-year series of seasonal courses consisting of day-long participatory seminars. They include Advanced Macrobiotic Cooking Classes, Luncheon, Special Foods Processing Workshops, Home Remedies and Healing Workshops, and Way of Life Studies.

The Macrobiotic Study Intensive is an advanced course following the Macrobiotic Life Seminars. The intensive offers a one-year, in-depth exploration of life, healing, and personal development according to macrobiotic principles. Topics covered in fireside lectures include the nature of disease and health, the mechanism and function of universal order, how to improve mental clarity, developing judgment and consciousness, and applying the laws of nature to everyday life.

The Classic Macrobiotic Cuisine Gourmet Cooking Courses and Gourmet Dinners help students to elevate their macrobiotic cooking repertoire to a level of elegance and sophistication. The course is an extension of the Macrobiotic Life seminars.

Tuition and Fees

Prepaid tuition for the Fundamentals of Macrobiotic Cooking course is $495 per ten-week course or $50 per individual class. Prepaid tuition for the Macrobiotic Life seminars is $650 per nine-week course or $75 per seminar. Prepaid tuition for the Macrobiotic Study Intensive is $285 per twelve-week course or $25 per individual class. The cost of the Classic Macrobiotic Cuisine Gourmet Cooking Course/Fundraising Dinners is $75 for the workshop and dinners, or $50 for the Dinners only.

Financial Assistance

Course payment may be made in two installments.

McKinnon Institute

2940 Webster Street
Oakland, California 94609-3407
PHONE: (510) 465-3488
E-MAIL: mckinnon@aol.com

The McKinnon Institute was founded in 1973 by Judith McKinnon. There are twenty-nine instructors; massage classes average ten students, anatomy and business classes average twenty-two. See page 487 for video information.

Accreditation and Approvals

McKinnon Institute is approved by the Bureau of Private Postsecondary and Vocational Education, and by the California Board of Registered Nurses and Respiratory Care Practitioners as a continuing education provider. Those wishing to take the National Certification Examination for Therapeutic Massage and Bodywork (NCETMB) must have 100 hours of Anatomy and Physiology and 400 hours of massage; courses and certificate programs at McKinnon may be combined to meet or exceed these requirements.

Program Description

McKinnon's seven certificate programs may be combined in an individually designed program in order to meet the National Certification Exam requirements (see above).

The 100-hour Swedish/Esalen Certificate consists of Swedish/Esalen Massage, Anatomy and Physiology, and Business, Ethics, and Hygiene.

The 142-hour Asian Systems Level I Certificate includes Shiatsu I, Acupressure I, and Anatomy and Physiology.

The 132-hour Asian Systems Level II Certificate includes Shiatsu II, Acupressure II, Anatomy and Physiology, and Business, Ethics, and Hygiene.

The 142-hour Sports/Deep Tissue Level I Certificate includes Sports Massage I, Deep Tissue, I, Reflexology I, and Anatomy and Physiology.

The 142-hour Sports/Deep Tissue Level II Certificate includes Sports Massage II, Deep Tissue II, Trigger Point, Exercise Physiology, and Anatomy and Physiology.

The 136-hour Subtle Systems Certificate consists of Craniosacral Therapy, Subtle Touch, Specialized Settings, and Anatomy and Physiology.

The 126-hour Advanced Modalities Certificate consists of Advanced Business, On-Site Massage, Somatics, Reflexology II, Pregnant Woman/Infant Massage, and Anatomy and Physiology.

Admission Requirements

Applicants must have a high school diploma or equivalent and understand the English language.

Tuition and Fees

Tuition for each certificate program is as follows: Swedish/Esalen, $999; Asian Systems Level I, $1,350; Asian Systems Level II, $1,254; Sports/Deep Tissue Level I, $1,254; Sports/Deep Tissue Level II, $1,350; Subtle Systems, $1,400; and Advanced Modalities, $1,197.

Financial Assistance

Veterans' benefits are available.

Meiji College of Oriental Medicine

2550 Shattuck Avenue
Berkeley, California 94704

PHONE: (510) 666-8248
FAX: (510) 666-0111
E-MAIL: meiji@pacbell.net
WEBSITE: www.meijicollege.org

Meiji College of Oriental Medicine (MCOM) was founded in 1990 by alumni of Japan's Meiji Institute of Oriental Medicine and moved to their current address in December 1998. MCOM integrates Western clinical sciences with acupuncture and herbology, and emphasizes the contributions of the Japanese tradition to Oriental medicine. There are five full-time and twenty part-time instructors; class sizes average twenty students (maximum thirty).

Accreditation and Approvals

The program at MCOM is accredited by the Accreditation Commission for Acupuncture and Oriental Medicine (ACAOM). The curriculum meets both the didactic and clinical requirements of the California Acupuncture Committee. Graduates are qualified to take the California State Licensing Exam and the National Certification Commission for Acupuncture and Oriental Medicine (NCCAOM) exam. MCOM has also been granted institutional approval from the Bureau for Private Postsecondary and Vocational Education.

Program Description

MCOM offers a full-time, 2,520-hour program leading to the Master of Science degree in Oriental medicine. The curriculum consists of 1,410 lecture hours and 1,110 clinical practice hours. The three-year course of study is equivalent to four academic years. Students who wish to attend part-time are asked to submit a plan demonstrating how they will complete the program in six years (90 percent of students are full-time).

Year One courses include History of Healing, Western Medical Terminology, Anatomy, Moxibustion and Cupping, Traditional Chinese Medicine Theory, Fundamentals of Acupuncture Technique, Oriental Herbology, Meridian Points, Observation, Physiology, Acupuncture Hygiene, Acupuncture Technique, Auricular and Scalp Acupuncture, Pathology, Theory of Meridians, Nutrition and Vitamins, Pulse Examination and Palpation Technique, Oriental Herbology and Dispensary, and Herb Identification.

Year Two courses include Herbal Prescription, Western

Clinical Science, Pharmacology, Electrical Acupuncture, TCM Diagnosis, Acupuncture Treatment Points, Pathways and Crossing Points, Observation, Meridian Point Anatomy, Research Methodology, Extraordinary Meridians and Points, Extra Points and Hand and Foot Acupuncture, Tongue Diagnosis, Western Physical Examination, Guided Practice, Practice Management and Ethics, Classic Texts, CPR and First Aid, and Oriental Medical Review.

Year Three courses include Oriental Clinical Medicine, Partial Supervision, Proximal Supervision, Research, and Oriental Medical Review.

Admission Requirements

Applicants must hold a bachelor's degree from an accredited postsecondary institution with a cumulative GPA of 2.5 or higher, and must have completed undergraduate courses in biology, chemistry, physics, and psychology; submit two letters of recommendation, an essay, a résumé, and a health certificate; and have a personal interview.

Tuition and Fees

Tuition is $8,200 per year ($24,600 total). There is an application fee of $50 and a graduation fee of $50; books, supplies, and other fees are additional.

Financial Assistance

Federal financial aid is available in the form of Stafford Loans.

Mendocino School of Holistic Massage and Advanced Healing Arts

2680 Road B
Redwood Valley, California 95470
PHONE: (707) 485-8197
FAX: (707) 462-0879
E-MAIL: rammpack@pacific.net
WEBSITE: www.pacific.net/~rammpack

The Mendocino School of Holistic Massage and Advanced Healing Arts was founded in 1993 by Theresa and Clark Ramm. There is one instructor; classes are limited to ten students.

Accreditation and Approvals

Mendocino School of Holistic Massage and Advanced Healing Arts is licensed and regulated by the Bureau for Private Postsecondary and Vocational Education. The Certified Holistic Massage Therapist, Certified Rebirther, and Holistic Health Practitioner programs are approved for continuing education units by the California Board of Registered Nurses. Graduates of the 500-hour program are qualified to take the National Certification Examination for Therapeutic Massage and Bodywork (NCETMB).

Program Description

The 500-hour Holistic Health Practitioner Certification Program requires completion of three programs: the 220-hour Advanced Holistic Massage Therapist (AHMT) Program, the 180-hour Certified Master Rebirther (CMR) Program, and the 100-hour Holistic Health Practitioner (HHP) Program.

The 220-hour AHMT Program covers such topics as Polarity Energy Balancing Massage; Energy Field Anatomy, Theory and Practice; Relaxation and Balancing Techniques; Organ Revitalization; Conscious Breathwork; Intuitive Development for Bodyworkers; Emotional Point Release; Core Foot Reflexology; Polarity Yoga; Lymphatic Drainage Massage; Swedish/Esalen Relaxation Techniques; Pressure Point Techniques; Body Mapping; Polarity Spine Balancing Massage; Counseling for Holistic Bodyworkers; Yoga and Stretching; Pathology; Mind-Body Hypnosis/ Gestalt; Practicum; and more.

The 180-hour CMR Program includes Overview of Pre- and Perinatal Trauma; Imprinting and Core Assumptions; Prenate and Neonate Capabilities; Codependency and the Need for Love and Touch; Cellular Memory and Early Imprinting; Primal Health; Conception and Before; Practicum; and more.

The 100-hour HHP Program includes Self-Awareness and Change: Principles and Practices; Holistic Health: Principles and Practices; Stress Prevention/Management; Building Self-Esteem; Inner Dialogue and Self-Care; Holistic Nutrition and Fitness; Goals and Milestones; Lifestyle Balancing; Forgiveness and Healthy Boundary Systems; Aromatherapy; Somatic Psychology; Transforming the Emotional Body; Herbalism; Applied Kinesiology; Anger Release Work; Introduction to Homeopathy; Creative Counseling Skills; and more.

The AHMT and CMR Programs may also be taken alone, as may their 100-hour Certified Trained Rebirther, 120-hour Certified Holistic Massage Therapist, and forty-hour Energy Medicine Training programs (not described here).

Other programs offered include a 100-hour Holistic Hypnosis Certification program, with lectures, demonstrations, and supervised practice in therapeutic hypnosis.

Admission Requirements
Applicants must be at least 16 years of age. Everyone is invited (subject to student interview and permission of the instructor) to participate in classes.

Tuition and Fees
Total tuition for the HHP Program is $5,250, broken down as follows: 220-hour AHMT Program, $2,500; 180-hour CMR Program, $1,550; 100-hour HHP Program, $1,200. Books are additional.

Tuition for the 100-hour Holistic Hypnosis Program is $895.

Financial Assistance
Discounts and installment plans are available.

The Michael Scholes School for Aromatic Studies

(See Multiple State Locations, pages 401–2)

Midwifery Institute of California

Administrative Office:
P.O. Box 128
Bristol, Vermont 05443
PHONE: (802) 453-3332
California Address:
P.O. Box 1558
Sebastopol, California 95473-1558
E-MAIL: edavis@birth-sex.com
WEBSITE: www.birth-sex.com

Midwifery Institute of California (MIC) was founded by Elizabeth Davis and Shannon Anton. The Heart and Hands Midwifery Intensives began in 1982, and the Study Group started in 1994. There are twenty-five instructors, with a maximum of sixteen students per class.

Accreditation and Approvals
MIC is in the pre-accreditation period with the Midwifery Education Accreditation Council (MEAC). The curriculum prepares students to meet MANA Core Competencies and meets the requirements of California law. Pending approval by the Medical Board of California, MIC graduates will be qualified to take the California licensing exam.

Program Description
The eighty-four-semester-unit Midwifery Program is divided into three academic years and may be taken on-site or through distance learning. The program incorporates antepartum, intrapartum, postpartum, newborn, and well-woman care, plus beginning, intermediate, and advanced practica. Unit credit is granted as follows: eighteen units of Heart and Hands course work (beginning and advanced); twenty-four units of Study Group course work; two units of approved elective course work and credit for life experience; and forty units of supervised apprenticeship providing instruction and requisite clinical experiences. Students may complete the course work at their own pace.

Heart and Hands Midwifery Intensives are offered on-site or at a distance. The course work includes History and Politics of Midwifery, Prenatal Care and Complications, Counseling and Communication Skills, Sexuality in the Childbearing Cycle, Facilitating Labor and Assisting Delivery, Labor/Delivery Complications and Transport, Perineal Assessment and Repair, Newborn Complications and Neonatal Testing, Postpartum Care, Breastfeeding and Maternal Adjustment, and Homeopathy and Herbs in Pregnancy and Birth.

Study Group is composed of fifty-three modules, each of which takes an average of six hours to complete. Sample module topics include Breastfeeding, Breech Presentation, Brow and Face Presentations, Charting, Digestion, Female Sexuality, Fertility and Conception, Fetal Heart Rate Patterns, Hemorrhage, Miscarriage and Stillbirth, Nutrition, Pre-eclampsia, Prenatal Genetic Screening, Suturing, Well Woman Care, and others.

Admission Requirements
Applicants must have a high school diploma or equivalent.

Tuition and Fees

The Heart and Hands and Study Group course work fees, application and administrative fees, and preceptor fees total $7,100 on-site or $7,320 at a distance. Electives are chosen from outside the program for additional fees.

Financial Assistance

Payment plans are available.

Monterey Institute of Touch

27820 Dorris Drive
Carmel, California 93923
PHONE: (831) 624-1006
FAX: (831) 626-6916
E-MAIL: mit@redshift.com

The Monterey Institute of Touch (MIT) was founded in 1983; since 1985, the institute has been headed by Birgit Ball Eisner and her daughter, Barbara Ball, both certified Rolfers. There are approximately twenty instructors, with an average of twenty students per class (minimum eight, maximum twenty-two).

Accreditation and Approvals

Courses at MIT are approved for continuing education units (CEUs) by the National Certification Board for Therapeutic Massage and Bodywork (NCBTMB) and by the California Board of Registered Nursing. Course approval is granted by the Bureau for Private Postsecondary and Vocational Education. Graduates of programs of 500 or more hours are qualified to take the National Certification Examination for Therapeutic Massage and Bodywork (NCETMB).

Program Description

The 200-hour Massage Practitioner Program includes courses in Therapeutic Massage Techniques, Anatomy, Physiology, Polarity, Shiatsu, Self-Care and Movement Awareness, Reflexology, Sports Massage, Intuitive Massage, Business Practice and Ethics, and Supervised Internship Sessions. Students are required to have completed MIT's fourteen-hour Introduction to Massage class prior to enrollment. This program is offered as a fourteen-week day class, a twenty-week evening class, a twenty-week weekend class, and a five-week intensive.

The 500-hour Massage Therapist Program is open to students who have completed the 200-hour Massage Practitioner Program and may be completed in a minimum of twelve months. The program follows AMTA guidelines and includes 100 hours of Intermediate Massage (Anatomy, Massage, Clinical Massage, and Movement), 100 hours of Advanced Massage (Anatomy, Body Handling, Massage, Hand/Wrist and Forearm Care, and CPR/Emergency Medical Practice), and 100 hours of specialization in areas such as sports massage, craniosacral therapy, prenatal massage, and Swedish massage.

Continuing Education

A variety of courses are offered, to both professional massage practitioners and the general public. Offerings typically include Chair Massage, Prenatal Massage, Soft Tissue Release, Aromatherapy, Lymphatic and Visceral Massage, Range of Motion/Body Handling, Movement Awareness, Trigger Point, and others.

Admission Requirements

Applicants must be at least 18 years of age; have a high school diploma or equivalent; be physically capable of performing and receiving massage; have a personal interview; complete MIT's Introduction to Massage class; and submit a short autobiography and two letters of recommendation.

Tuition and Fees

There is an application/registration fee of $75. The Introduction to Massage course costs $85. Tuition for the 200-hour program is $975, plus a final fee of $45; books are approximately $55. Tuition for the 500-hour program is approximately $3,000 to $5,000, depending on the electives chosen.

Financial Assistance

Payment plans are available.

Mount Madonna Center

445 Summit Road
Watsonville, California 95076
PHONE: (408) 847-0406
FAX: (408) 847-2683

E-MAIL: programs@mountmadonna.org
WEBSITE: www.mountmadonna.org

The Mount Madonna Center, founded in 1978, is a community dedicated to the daily living of spiritual ideals through the practice of yoga. The mountaintop facility is surrounded by redwood groves and serves vegetarian meals.

Accreditation and Approvals
Many workshops offered at the center may be taken by nurses, LMFCCs, and LCSWs for continuing education credit.

Program Description
The Mount Madonna Center offers a variety of workshops, many focusing on yoga, but also including psychology, personal growth, spiritual pathways, and related topics. Many offer a blend of the ancient wisdom of yoga with contemporary approaches to body/mind therapy.

The Ashtanga Yoga Teacher Training Intensive runs twenty to twenty-five days (those without experience in Ashtanga, or eight-limbed, yoga are required to attend the entire twenty-five days). Training focuses on methods of body/mind purification, asana, pranayama, mudra (energy-raising techniques), and meditation, and provides opportunities for student teaching.

A three-week class is offered in Ayurveda, Ancient Health Science of India. The course focuses on Functional Assessment of Doshic Subtypes; Clinical Evaluation of Thirteen Main Srotamsi (body energy channels); the Ancient Art of Balancing Your Agni (metabolic fire); First Aid Management of Common Elements According to Ayurveda; and Etiology, Symptomatology, and Management of Psychological Disorders, as well as Ayurveda in daily life, diet and sex in relation to constitution, and more.

Tuition and Fees
Tuition for a typical weekend program is $150 plus meals and lodging.

The Ashtanga Yoga Teacher Training Intensive costs $645, plus a meals/lodging fee of $19 (commuting) to $78 (single room) per day.

Tuition for the Ayurveda, Ancient Health Science of India program is $1,325 for the full program, $475 for a week, or $150 for a weekend, plus a meals/lodging fee of $19 (commuting) to $78 (single room) per day.

Financial Assistance
Work-study is available. Discounts are offered for stays of a week or longer.

Mueller College of Holistic Studies

4607 Park Boulevard
San Diego, California 92116-1243
PHONE: (619) 291-9811 / (800) 245-1976
FAX: (619) 543-1113
E-MAIL: info@muellercollege.com
WEBSITE: www.muellercollege.com

Mueller College was founded in 1976 by E. W. "Bill" Mueller. There are twenty instructors, with an average of sixteen to twenty-four students per class; the teacher: student ratio is 1:6 when performing bodywork.

Accreditation and Approvals
The 512-hour Massage Therapist Course is accredited by the Commission on Massage Training Accreditation (COMTA); graduates are qualified to take the National Certification Examination for Therapeutic Massage and Bodywork (NCETMB). The Acupressurist Course is approved by the American Oriental Bodywork Therapy Association (AOBTA). The school is approved by the California Board of Registered Nursing and by the National Certification Board for Therapeutic Massage and Bodywork (NCBTMB) as a continuing education provider.

Program Description
In the "Mueller Method" 100-hour Massage Technician Certificate Program, students are taught circulatory massage techniques and practice assessment, centering, breathing, and body mechanics. Courses include Introduction to the Body Systems, History and Theory, Business and Ethics, and Demonstration and Practice. This course is a prerequisite for all of the other programs.

The 620-hour Massage Therapist Certificate Program includes Anatomy and Physiology, Business and Ethics, Cellular Biology (Nutrition), Kinesiology, CPR, Professional Bodywork, Teaching Assistant, Pathology, Acupressure I and II, Advanced Techniques: Active (Sports), Advanced Techniques: Passive, and Massage Technician Lab.

The 734-hour Acupressurist Certificate includes Anatomy and Physiology, Business and Ethics, Kinesiology, Acupressure I and II, Acupressure III: Types of Qi, Acupressure IV: Point Selection Concepts, Acupressure V: Chi Nei Tsang and Micro-Circuits, Acupressure VI: Syndromes and Traditional Functions, Clinical Applications (Lab Internship), and Acupressure VII: Comparison of Oriental and Western Techniques.

The 1,000-hour Holistic Health Practitioner Certificate may be taken in either a Massage Therapist (Western Studies) or Acupressurist (Oriental Studies) format. The Western Studies program consists of the 620-hour Massage Therapist Certification followed by Advanced Applications I and II, Community Event, eighty hours of electives, Peer Review, Professional Bodywork, Social Psychology, Teaching Assistant, and Workshops. The Oriental Studies program consists of the 734-hour Acupressurist Certification followed by Advanced Applications I or II, Community Event, sixty-four hours of electives, Peer Review, Professional Bodywork, Teaching Assistant, and Workshops.

Each program may be taken in an accelerated format.

Admission Requirements

Applicants must be at least 18 years of age and in good health. A qualifying process is required for each course of study and must be completed at the school.

Tuition and Fees

Tuition and fees for the Massage Technician Course are $695 (ongoing) or $750 (accelerated), plus $95 for books and supplies. Tuition and fees for the Massage Therapist Course are $4,410 (ongoing) or $4,640 (accelerated), plus approximately $357 for books and supplies. Tuition and fees for the Acupressurist Course are $5,435 (ongoing) or $5,715 (accelerated), plus approximately $347 for books and supplies. Tuition and fees for the Holistic Health Practitioner Course/Western Studies are $5,770 (ongoing) or $6,050 (accelerated), plus approximately $380 for books and supplies. Tuition and fees for the Holistic Health Practitioner Course/Oriental Studies are $6,065 (ongoing) or $6,370 (accelerated), plus approximately $370 for books and supplies.

Financial Assistance

Payment plans, veterans' benefits, and California Vocational Rehabilitation are available.

National Holistic Institute

5900 Hollis Street, Suite J
Emeryville, California 94608-2008
PHONE: (510) 547-6442 / (800) 315-3552
FAX: (510) 547-6621
E-MAIL: nhi@nhimassage.com
WEBSITE: www.nhimassage.com

The National Holistic Institute was founded in 1979 by Carol Carpenter. Since its founding, NHI has graduated over 4,500 students. There are thirty instructors, with an average of twenty-five students per class.

Accreditation and Approvals

NHI is accredited by the Accrediting Council for Continuing Education and Training (ACCET). Graduates are qualified to take the National Certification Examination for Therapeutic Massage and Bodywork (NCETMB).

Program Description

The Massage Therapist and Health Educator Program consists of thirty-six quarter-credit hours. The curriculum consists of Massage Theory and Practice (including Swedish massage, acupressure/shiatsu, seated massage, foot reflexology, deep tissue massage, hydrotherapy, stress management, and more), Anatomy, Physiology, Kinesiology and Pathology, Practice Management, Student Clinic, and Externship/Community Service. The full-time day program takes approximately ten months to complete; the evening/weekend program, one year; and the weekend class, seventeen months.

Admission Requirements

Prospective students must have a high school diploma or equivalent or successfully complete an entrance exam, and be interviewed on campus or by phone.

Tuition and Fees

Tuition is $9,260. Additional expenses include books and supplies, $294; massage table, face rest, and case, $550; and registration fee, $75.

Financial Assistance
Federal grants, loans, and work-study are available.

Natural Healing Institute of Naturopathy

MAILING ADDRESS:
P.O. Box 230294
Encinitas, California 92023-0294
PHONE: (760) 943-8485 / (800) 559-4325
FAX: (760) 943-9477
E-MAIL: NHI@inetworld.net

CLASSROOM LOCATION:
2146 Encinitas Boulevard, Suite 105
Encinitas, California

The Natural Healing Institute (NHI) was founded in 1997. Director Steve Schechter, N.D., H.H.P., has founded and directed three schools of natural healing. The faculty consists of thirty-two full- and part-time members. Class size is limited to sixteen students for massage and twenty students for all other classes. (Distance learning programs are also offered; see page 463.)

Accreditation and Approvals
The Natural Healing Institute is licensed and certified to operate by the Bureau for Private Postsecondary and Vocational Education and the Department of Consumer Affairs. Graduates of programs of 500 or more hours are qualified to take the National Certification Examination for Therapeutic Massage and Bodywork (NCETMB). NHI is approved by the California Board of Registered Nurses for continuing education credits.

Program Description
Programs are offered in Clinical Herbology, Clinical Nutrition, Professional Hypnotherapy, Massage Therapies, Holistic Health Practitioner (HHP), and Body-Mind Integrative Therapies.

The Certified Clinical Herbalist Program consists of 150 hours. Classes include Introductory Herbology I and II, Preparing Herbal Remedies, Eastern and Western Herbs Intermediate

I through IV, and Herb Identification Classes. A Certified Master Clinical Herbalist program requires an additional 150 hours for a total of 300 hours; these additional hours are taken in Herb Identification Classes, Creating an Herb Garden, Advanced Herbology, and Supervised Practicum.

The 200-hour Certified Clinical Nutritionist Program consists of Introduction to Nutrition, Major Dietary Systems, Vitamins and Minerals, Nutrient-Dense Superfoods, Antioxidants, Specialty Programs, Environmental Nutrition and Detoxification, Fasting, Sports Nutrition Programs, Maternal Child Nutrition, Health and Dental Connection, and Individualized Programs and Supervised Clinic.

The 200-hour Certified Professional Hypnotherapy Program consists of Introduction to Hypnosis I and II, Principles and Practices of Hypnotherapy I and II, and Hypnosis for Change I and II.

The 500-hour Massage Therapist Program is designed to meet the training requirements of locales and states having 500-hour standards. The program consists of a 100-hour Massage Technician Program plus an additional 400 hours in electives. NHI offers 766 hours of Massage Therapy training, from which students can choose a minimum of 500 hours. Required Massage Therapist Program classes (370 hours) include the 100-hour Massage Technician Program plus courses in Traditional Oriental Medicine, the 12 Organ Meridians, Basics of Acupoint Location, Tui Na I, Shiatsu/Acupressure I, Sports/Athletic Massage, Freeing Touch/Active and Passive Joint Rotation, Business Practices, Supervised Massage Practicum and Student Clinic, Introduction to Hypnosis I, Introduction to Herbology I, Introduction to Nutrition I, and Anatomy, Physiology, Kinesiology and Pathology I. Electives include Introduction to Herbology II, Introduction to Nutrition II, Introduction to Hypnotherapy II, Tui Na II, Shiatsu/Acupressure II, Chair Massage, Hawaiian Healing Arts/Lomi Lomi, Chinese Cranial Sacral Balancing, Visceral Release Massage, Reichean Deep Tissue and Myofascial Massage, Immune Boosting Lymph Massage, Traditional Thai Medical Massage I and II, Reflexology and Applied Kinesiology, Pregnant, Post-Partum and Infant Massage, Advanced Massage Techniques, Energetic Healing/Energy Massage Therapy I, II, and III, and Body Reading, Assessment, and Analysis.

The 1,000-hour Holistic Health Practitioner (HHP) Program consists of 192 required hours in Introduction to Herbology I and II, Introduction to Nutrition I and II, Introduction to Professional Hypnotherapy I and II, Anatomy, Physiology, Kinesiology and Pathology I and II, Business Practices, Communication Skills I, and Advanced Supervised Practicum. An additional 808 hours of electives may be chosen from any other classes in the Massage Technician, Massage Therapy, Nutrition, Herbology, Hypnotherapy, and Body-Mind Integrative Therapies programs.

In the 250-hour Body-Mind Integrative Therapies (Spiritual Counseling) Program, students choose from courses in Hydrotherapy, Aromatherapy, Boundary Issues, Paradigms of Healing, Opening the Heart, Communication Skills, Let the Body Lead, The Healing Relationship, Enneagram, Health Analysis, Iridology, Rayid Iris Analysis, Bach Flower Remedies, Sound and Music in Healing, Introduction to the Inca Medicine Wheel, Lifestyle Integrative Therapies, Intimacy and the Body-Mind Connection, Shamanic Healer, Compassionate Communication, Sacred Healing Space, Natural Healing Seminar, and Advanced Supervised Practicum.

Community and Continuing Education
Courses listed above may be taken individually for personal growth without enrollment in a certificate program.

Admission Requirements
Applicants must be at least 18 years of age, have a high school diploma or equivalent, be in good health, and complete a short written assignment. Applicants enrolling in one or more full programs to receive a diploma, certificate, and license must be a U.S. citizen or have a valid student visa or green card.

Tuition and Fees
Tuition for the Certified Clinical Herbalist Program is $1,425; the Certified Master Clinical Herbalist Program is an additional $1,240.

Tuition for the Clinical Nutritionist Program is $1,792.

Tuition for the Certified Professional Hypnotherapy Program is $1,495.

Tuition for the 370 required Massage Therapist hours is $2,268; additional courses range from $90 to $215 each.

Tuition for the 192 required Holistic Health Practitioner hours is $1,318; additional courses range from $5 to $10 per class hour. Cost of the total HHP Program is approximately $7,500 to $8,500, depending on electives.

Tuition for the Body-Mind Integrative Therapies Program varies with courses chosen; courses range from eight to fifty-two hours and cost from $72 to $468 each.

Financial Assistance
Payment plans and "Earn As You Learn" programs (in which students are credited $10 per practicum hour) are available.

Ohlone Center for Herbal Studies

924 San Miguel Road
Concord, California 94518
PHONE: (925) 691-4756
E-MAIL: pamela@dnai.com

Ohlone Center for Herbal Studies was founded in 1993 by Pam Fischer. There are ten instructors, with an average of ten to fifteen students per class.

Program Description
The Ten-Month Apprenticeship Program is designed for advanced beginner to intermediate-level students, and combines Pam Fischer's clinical work with Rosemary Gladstar's The Science and Art of Herbology for a comprehensive foundation. Classes meet one evening per week and one Sunday per month from September to June. The program covers medicinal herbology, advanced herbal preparation and formulation, materia medica and herbal research, herbal first aid and home health care, natural cosmetic and skin care, constitutional therapy, wildcrafting, Earth awareness and plant identification, organ systems and physiology, and clinical case studies.

Upon completion of the Apprenticeship Program (or instructor's consent), students may enroll in Herbal Therapeutics, which meets one evening per week and one Sunday per month from September to June. This program covers alternative diagnostic techniques, nutrition, counseling skills, clinical record keeping, advanced herbal formulation, case review, and more. Many guest herbalists will lecture about their cases. Two extended weekend classes are included in the course, one in the foothills and one in the high Sierras.

Upon completion of both the Apprenticeship and Therapeutic Programs (or instructor's consent), students may enroll in the Clinical Internship. Students will see clients, make herbal assessments, prepare and formulate herbal products, and evaluate client progress. Also included are basic record keeping, business accounting, budgeting, and advertising. The class will begin to write and publish their work in the Ohlone Center Wellness Letter and develop personal wildcrafting grounds.

Community and Continuing Education
Short courses are offered in a variety of topics, including Introduction to Herbalism, Herbs for Women, Herbs for Children, Herbs for Animals, Spring and Fall Tonics, Health and Abundance: A Wellness Class for Large Women, Wild About Mushrooms, Herbs for Seniors, Herbal Holidays, Asthma Workshop, Herbs for Bodyworkers, and others.

Tuition and Fees
Tuition for the Ten-Month Apprenticeship is $1,500; for Herbal Therapeutics, $1,500; and for Clinical Internship, $1,500.

Pacific Academy of Homeopathy

1199 Sanchez Street
San Francisco, California 94114
PHONE: (415) 458-8238
FAX: (415) 695-8220
E-MAIL: health@homeopathy-academy.org
WEBSITE: www.homeopathy-academy.org

The Pacific Academy of Homeopathy was founded in 1985 as a nonprofit educational organization. The academy supports a low-cost student clinic in Marin County, San Francisco, and Berkeley. There are eight instructors; classes average fifteen to thirty students.

Accreditation and Approvals
The academy has been certified by the Bureau for Private Postsecondary and Vocational Education. The academy is applying for accreditation by the Council on Homeopathic Education (CHE). CEUs are available for nurses and other licensed health practitioners.

Program Description
The 660-hour, three-year Professional Training Program gives students a thorough understanding of homeopathic principles and practice through an experiential curriculum. In addition to classroom hours, the student is required to do substantial home study. The program consists of ten weekends per year and a five-day intensive each summer. Over 300 hours of extra clinical supervision is offered over the three years. This is designed to integrate and assess the student's knowledge in a clinical setting.

Anatomy and Pathology courses are offered for those without medical training.

Community and Continuing Education
Ongoing seminars are offered to those interested in learning the basic principles of homeopathy and how to use homeopathy in acute conditions.

Admission Requirements
Admission is open to both medically licensed and nonmedically licensed students. Questions regarding academic qualifications should be directed to the admissions committee.

Tuition and Fees
Tuition is $3,900 per year. Other costs include an application fee of $25; Anatomy and Physiology, $275; Pathology for Alternative Practitioners, $375; and books, approximately $300 per year for two years.

Financial Assistance
Payment plans are available.

Pacific College of Oriental Medicine

(See Multiple State Locations, pages 405–6)

Pacific Institute of Aromatherapy

(See Multiple State Locations, page 407)

Palmer College of Chiropractic West

90 East Tasman Drive
San Jose, California 95134
PHONE: (408) 944-6024 / (800) 442-4476
FAX: (408) 944-6032
E-MAIL: pccw-admiss@palmer.edu
WEBSITE: www.palmer.edu

The Palmer Chiropractic University System includes both Palmer College of Chiropractic West and Palmer College of Chiropractic (Davenport, Iowa). Palmer College of Chiropractic West (PCCW) was established in 1980. There are thirty-nine full-time and thirty-four part-time instructors; classes have a teacher: student ratio of 1:10.

Accreditation and Approvals

PCCW is accredited by the Council on Chiropractic Education (CCE).

Program Description

The Doctor of Chiropractic (DC) four-year degree program consists of thirteen quarters. The Clinical Practice Curriculum, introduced in 1995, standardizes the students' first ten quarters to an average of six or seven classes (approximately 32.5 hours). Tracks of courses emphasize specific areas of instruction and are linked by common subject matter over several successive quarters: Chiropractic Clinical Evaluation, Chiropractic Technique and Management, Foundations of Chiropractic Practice, Problem Solving in Differential Diagnosis, Radiographic Interpretation, and a series of courses that emphasize the development of primary care skills.

Emphasis is placed on the basic sciences in the first half of the program, followed by a corresponding focus on the clinical sciences in the last half. Study of chiropractic principles and procedures is followed throughout the curriculum. Students spend their ninth through twelfth quarters of study treating patients at the Palmer West Community Clinics in San Jose and Santa Clara.

Continuing Education

Palmer West offers seminars, symposia, and conferences for Doctors of Chiropractic seeking additional education to meet relicensure requirements.

Admission Requirements

Applicants must have completed at least sixty semester units of college or university credit leading to an associate's or bachelor's degree, including a minimum of six semester units of biology, general chemistry, organic chemistry, physics, and English or communications, three semester units of psychology, and fifteen semester units of humanities or social sciences. Beginning fall 1999, applicants must have earned a minimum GPA of 2.5. Additionally, applicants must submit two letters of recommendation and an essay, and have a personal interview.

Tuition and Fees

Tuition is $13,095 per year. Additional expenses include a $50 application fee and approximately $1,439 per year for books.

Financial Assistance

Federal and private grants, loans, scholarships, and work-study are available.

Phillips School of Massage

101 Broad Street
P.O. Box 1999
Nevada City, California 95959
PHONE: (530) 265-4645
FAX: (530) 265-9485
E-MAIL: psm@jps.net
WEBSITE: www.jps.net/psm/

Judy Phillips founded the Phillips School of Massage in 1983. The school takes a holistic view of treatment, with emphasis on balancing the body structure and energy flow of both therapist and client. There are eight instructors, with one instructor or assistant to every two to eight students. In addition to the program described here, massage programs of shorter duration are also offered.

Accreditation and Approvals

Phillips School of Massage has been licensed by the California State Board of Education since 1983, and is also approved by the California Board of Registered Nursing for continuing education. Graduates are qualified to take the National Certification Examination for Therapeutic Massage and Bodywork (NCETMB).

Program Description

The 600-hour Massage Therapy Certificate Program consists of Level I: Basic, Level II: Advanced, and Continuing Education workshops. The 230-hour Level I Program covers Anatomy and Physiology, Bodywork Techniques (including Swedish, Circulatory, Lymphatic, Sports, Deep Tissue, Ortho-Bionomy, Reflexology, Shiatsu, and Acupressure), Sensory Awareness, Practical Application (including Community Outreach), and Self Care and Development. The 230-hour Level II program covers Assisting, Assistant Training and Review, Clinic Experience, Injury Prevention, Deep Tissue Bodywork, Acupressure, Structural Assessment, and Community Outreach. Required Continuing Education workshops include Anatomy Intensive and Chakras, Body Memory, and Massage. Students also choose seventy additional hours of electives from those described under Continuing Education (below).

Continuing Education

Continuing education workshops are offered on a regular basis and have included Acupressure, Anatomy, Aromatherapy, Body Reading, Chakra Exploration and Massage, Compassionate Touch, Cranial-Sacral Introduction, Deep Tissue Bodywork, Injury and Trauma Resolution, Muscle Neurology, Ortho-Bionomy, Reflexology, and Sports Massage.

Admission Requirements

Applicants must be in good health.

Tuition and Fees

Tuition for Level I is $1,600; tuition for Level II is $3,700 to $4,200; tuition for Continuing Education workshops ranges from $100 to $550. Books and supplies are additional.

Financial Assistance

Payment plans, prepayment discounts, and limited work scholarships are available.

Polarity Healing Arts

19600 Cave Way
Topanga, California 90290
Phone (310) 455-7873 / (877) 455-7873
FAX: (310) 455-9832
E-MAIL: Phasm3@aol.com
WEBSITE: www.polarityhealingarts.com

Polarity Healing Arts was founded in 1986 by Gary B. Strauss, R.P.P. and past board member of the American Polarity Therapy Association. There are ten instructors, with an average of six to twenty students per class. Retreat-style trainings are also offered in Hawaii, Switzerland, and Ireland.

Accreditation and Approvals

The A.P.P. (Associate Polarity Practitioner) and R.P.P. (Registered Polarity Practitioner) training programs are approved by the American Polarity Therapy Association (APTA).

Program Description

The 179-hour A.P.P. Certification Course consists of five courses, each seventeen to forty-two hours in length: Polarity I and II (which cover basic principles of energy flow, the polarity general session, an exploration of polarity energetics and the expression of life energy through the Five Elements, bodywork sessions for balancing each element, and polarity exercises), Communication, Evaluation, and Study Group (which constitutes professional clinical development in the polarity healing arts). Students must also receive five and give thirty sessions. Courses may also be taken individually.

The seventy-two-hour Craniosacral Unwinding Program offers specialty training for bodyworkers and other health care professionals in using palpation skills to get into harmony, resonance, and rapport with the fluid nature of the body. Three courses (Cranial I through III) cover an introduction to the craniosacral rhythm, concepts, and motion; developing palpation skills; and physical and energetic techniques for working with the connective tissue system of the body, focusing extensively on the cranium. Courses may be taken individually.

The R.P.P. Program adds approximately 500 to 550 hours to the A.P.P. training above and takes twelve to eighteen months to complete. Classes will include Cranial I through III, Intermediate IA, IB, and II (covering the autonomic nervous system, organ systems, and integration), Spinal/Structural Balancing, Advanced Communication, Nutrition, Business and Professional Ethics, Cleanse Group, Fire Into Water, Advanced Supervision, Polarity Exercise, Advanced Study Group, Internship, and elective classes taught by visiting instructors. Classes may also be taken individually.

Admission Requirements

There are no specific admission requirements for the A.P.P. Program. R.P.P. applicants must have completed an A.P.P. Program.

Tuition and Fees

Tuition for the entire A.P.P. Course is $1,988; individual courses range from $294 to $588. Tuition for the entire Craniosacral Unwinding Program is $1,088; individual courses are $336. Tuition for the R.P.P. Course is $3,794.

Financial Assistance

Payment plans and combination discounts are available.

Polarity Therapy Center of Marin

P.O. Box 23
Tomales, California 94971
PHONE: (707) 878-2278

The Polarity Therapy Center of Marin was founded in 1991 by Hanna Hammerli, a Registered Polarity Practitioner (R.P.P.) and certified polarity instructor with over twenty years of experience as a bodyworker. Trainings are held in a rural, scenic area on a small organic farm. There are two instructors, with an average of three to four students per class.

Accreditation and Approvals

Trainings are approved by the American Polarity Therapy Association (APTA).

Program Description

The 155-hour A.P.P. Training consists of five three-day intensives that offer instruction in methods of physical, mental, and spiritual healing through Polarity Therapy, Polarity Yoga, Polarity Reflexology, the Five-Pointed Star, Structural Balance, Client Communication, Nutritional Counseling, and Business Management. A.P.P. Training is also available as private instruction. Intensives may also be taken separately.

The 615-hour R.P.P. Training, which consists of the A.P.P.

Training above and an additional 460-hour segment, is taught over a two-year period. Segments are devoted to Ether, Air, Fire, Water, and Earth, as well as orthodox Anatomy and Physiology. The R.P.P. Training is available as private instruction, or as an intensive if four or more students participate in the program.

Community and Continuing Education

The center offers events such as Polarity Process days, Inner Bonding workshops, and Silent Meditation. Free half-hour interviews with Hanna are available upon request.

Admission Requirements

The A.P.P. Training is open to everyone. The R.P.P. Training is open to those who have completed a 155-hour A.P.P. course and are certified through APTA as an A.P.P.

Tuition and Fees

The A.P.P. Training costs $1,650 total for five intensives. These intensives are $325 to $350 each if taken separately. Private instruction is $90 per two-hour class (minimum forty classes for entire program).

The R.P.P. Training costs $4,800 as an intensive, somewhat more for private instruction; please call for details.

Financial Assistance

Limited work-study is available.

Quantum-Veritas International University Systems

International College of Homeopathy
Veritas Institute of Homeopathy
8306 Wilshire Boulevard, # 728
Beverly Hills, California 90211
PHONE: (310) 645-0443
FAX: (310) 645-1814
E-MAIL: registrar@qvius.edu
WEBSITE: www.qvius.edu

The International College of Homeopathy is a ten-year-old school that offers postgraduate instruction to health care professionals within the Quantum-Veritas International University Systems (QVIUS) organization; there are six instructors. The Veritas Institute of Homeopathy offers training in homeopathy to nonmedical students; classes will be offered in Los Angeles and Orlando, Florida, in January 2000. Founded in 1998 by Dr. Edwin C. Floyd, QVIUS is a nonprofit institution with a focus on teaching from a vitalistic perspective. Many courses are still in the development stage.

Accreditation and Approvals
The International College of Homeopathy is applying for accreditation with the Council on Homeopathic Education (CHE). Graduates are eligible to sit for the Certification Examination with the National Board of Homeopathic Examiners.

Program Description
The International School of Homeopathy offers 600 postgraduate training hours in Classic Homeopathy. The 300-hour Level I program consists of six modules: Classical Homeopathy; Introduction to Miasms and Homeopathic Materia Medica; Introduction to Case Taking, Case Analysis, and Case Management; Case Taking, Case Analysis, Case Management, and Smaller Remedies; and Comprehensive Review of Vitalistic Healing and Review and Preparation for National Board Examination. Classes are held one weekend per month over two years. The 300-hour Level II program covers the Fundamental Principles of Homeopathy, Materia Medica and Families of Remedies, Repertory Exercises, Case Analysis, Case Taking Technique, and Case Analysis.

The Veritas Institute of Homeopathy offers a 600-hour training in Classical Homeopathy to nonmedical students. Classes meet one weekend per month.

Programs are under development in the departments of Ayurveda, Ethnic and Energy Healing, Astrocybernetic Institute (studying the effects of Astrology, Meditation, and Biofeedback), the School of Bio-Functional Medicine, Botanical Medicine, Dietary Therapeutics, Homeotherapeutics, Meridian Therapy, and Somiatry Institute.

Admission Requirements
The International School of Homeopathy Program is open to health care professionals. The Veritas Institute of Homeopathy Program requires applicants to have completed two years of specific college courses, including Biology, Chemistry, Physics, and others; contact the school for details.

Tuition and Fees
Tuition for the International School of Homeopathy program is $325 per weekend or $1,170 per four-month quarter. Tuition for the Veritas Institute of Homeopathy program is $275 per weekend.

Financial Assistance
Payment plans are available.

Reese Movement Institute, Inc.

Feldenkrais Southern California
2187 Newcastle Avenue, Suite 102
Cardiff-by-the-Sea, California 92007
PHONE: (619) 436-9087 / (800) 500-9087
FAX: (619) 436-9141
E-MAIL: RMIMoves@aol.com

The Reese Movement Institute will begin a new Feldenkrais Professional Training Program® in San Diego Beginning in February 2001. Previous trainings have been held in Los Angeles, West Virginia, Italy, and Germany. The institute's directors are Mark Reese, Ph.D., and Donna Ray-Reese. Mark Reese is one of the world's foremost authorities on the Feldenkrais method and graduated from the first United States Feldenkrais training program in 1977. There are two to four instructors, with an average of thirty students per class.

Accreditation and Approvals
Reese Movement Institute San Diego Feldenkrais Professional Training Program is fully accredited by the Feldenkrais Guild and is recognized as a private postsecondary educational institution by the state of California.

Program Description
The four-year Feldenkrais Professional Training Program spans 160 teaching days. After satisfactory learning of Awareness Through Movement®, Functional Integration, and Feldenkrais Theory, graduates are awarded certificates as Guild Certified

Feldenkrais Practitioners® or Guild Certified Feldenkrais Teachers®. Those who do not wish to become certified practitioners but wish to study for their own personal growth may also participate; in this case it is not necessary to satisfy the same graduation requirements.

Admission Requirements
There are no specific educational prerequisites. Applicants must submit three letters of recommendation.

Tuition and Fees
There is a $50 application fee. Tuition is $3,600 per year.

Financial Assistance
Payment plans are available.

reSource

Box 5398
Berkeley, California 94705
PHONE: (510) 433-7917
FAX: (510) 841-3258
WEBSITE: www.re-source.to

reSource was founded in 1982 by Gail Stewart, the current director. There are five instructors, with an average of twelve students per class.

Accreditation and Approvals
reSource is approved by the Bureau for Private Postsecondary and Vocational Education. Graduates of programs of 500 or more hours are qualified to take the National Certification Examination for Therapeutic Massage and Bodywork (NCETMB).

Program Description
The 200-hour Massage Practitioner Program covers the fundamentals of massage and bodywork, anatomy, physiology, and professional development in core classes; electives include Massage Review, Body Reading, and Bodymind Survey.

The 500-hour Bodywork Practitioner Program offers continuing education for massage and bodywork practitioners interested in upgrading their certification to 500 hours. The core professional support and practice group is open to massage and bodywork practitioners in their first two years of professional practice. Credit toward certification may be earned by taking electives at reSource or other state-approved schools.

The 1,000-hour Advanced Bodywork Practitioner Program is a program of continuing support, supervision, and practice for massage and bodywork practitioners with at least two years of professional experience. Classes are selected from a list of required and elective subjects that include the Trager® approach, Rosen method, deep tissue, bodyreading, and others.

Admission Requirements
Those applying to the Massage Practitioner Program must be at least 18 years of age and be able to read, write, and speak English. All applicants must have a personal interview.

Tuition and Fees
Tuition for core classes in the Massage Practitioner Course is $1,072; recommended electives are $400. Tuition for other programs varies with the courses selected.

Samra University of Oriental Medicine

3000 South Robertson Boulevard, 4th Floor
Los Angeles, California 90034
PHONE: (310) 202-6444
FAX: (310) 202-6007
E-MAIL: admissions@samra.edu
WEBSITE: www.samra.edu

Samra University derives its name from the acronym of its parent, the Sino-American Medical Rehabilitation Association, chartered in 1969. There are approximately sixty-five instructors, with an average of fifteen to twenty students per class.

Accreditation and Approvals
The Master of Science in Oriental Medicine degree program is accredited by the Accreditation Commission for Acupuncture and Oriental Medicine (ACAOM). Graduates are qualified to take the California State Acupuncture Licensing Examinations as well as the acupuncture and Chinese herbology exams given by the National Certification Commission for Acupuncture and Oriental Medicine (NCCAOM).

Program Description

The entire academic program of Samra University is given, in separate classes, in English, Korean, and Mandarin Chinese.

The Master of Science in Oriental Medicine Degree Program is a four-academic-year course of study that may be completed in thirty-six months of full-time study. The program includes 800 hours of clinical training as well as 1,700 hours of didactic courses from the departments of Oriental Medical Theory, Acupuncture, Chinese Herbology, and Western Clinical Sciences. Students may elect to complete part of their pre-master's internship and/or postgraduate studies at Beijing University of Chinese Medicine in China.

Samra University is currently developing an advanced program of study leading to the Doctor of Oriental Medicine degree.

Continuing Education

Samra University offers a three-month advanced internship in cooperation with the Zhejiang College of Traditional Chinese Medicine in Hangzhou, China. This program is designed to meet the needs of American students who have completed their formal training.

Admission Requirements

Applicants must have earned grades of C or better in at least sixty semester units in general education and/or technical courses from an accredited college or university, and must demonstrate an ability to read and write English, Mandarin Chinese, or Korean at the college-entrance level. In addition, applicants may be required to submit letters of recommendation, a short essay, or other materials as requested by the admissions office.

Tuition and Fees

The application fee is $75. Total tuition for the Master of Science degree is $25,520 ($105 per quarter unit); books and medical supplies are approximately $2,100 for the program.

Financial Assistance

Payment plans and federal grants and loans are available.

Santa Barbara College of Oriental Medicine

1919 State Street, Suite 207
Santa Barbara, California 93101
PHONE: (805) 898-1180 / (800) 549-6299
FAX: (805) 682-1864
E-MAIL: admissions@sbcom.edu
WEBSITE: www.sbcom.edu

The Santa Barbara College of Oriental Medicine (SBCOM), founded in 1986, grew out of the Santa Barbara branch of the California Acupuncture College, which was established in 1981. There are nineteen instructors, plus guest lecturers; class sizes average twenty students.

Accreditation and Approvals

The Master of Acupuncture and Oriental Medicine degree program is accredited by the Accreditation Commission for Acupuncture and Oriental Medicine (ACAOM); graduates are eligible to take the California Acupuncture Licensing Exam as well as the National Acupuncture and Herbology exams. SBCOM is approved by the State of California Acupuncture Board as a continuing education provider.

Program Description

The 2,680-hour, four-academic-year Master of Acupuncture and Oriental Medicine degree program may be completed in as little as three calendar years. Courses are offered in the areas of Acupuncture Science: Theories, Acupuncture Science: Techniques, Western Medical Science, Eastern Medical Heritage, Herbology: Chinese Herbal Medicine, Practice Management, Clinical Practice, and Master's Degree Project. Classes are held day and evening.

SBCOM is in the process of initiating pilot programs for teacher and student exchange with Osaka College of Acupuncture and Moxabustion.

Admission Requirements

Applicants must have completed at least sixty semester units of postsecondary education (including human anatomy with lab and physiology), with a minimum cumulative GPA of 2.0. In addition, applicants must submit two letters of recommendation and have a personal interview.

Tuition and Fees

Tuition for the Master of Acupuncture and Oriental Medicine Program is $150 per trimester unit. Additional expenses include application fee, $75; registration, $25; intern malpractice insurance, approximately $140 per trimester; and books, supplies, and lab fees, approximately $500 per year. Total estimated expense for the three-year program is $27,700.

Financial Assistance

Federal grants and loans are available.

School for Self-Healing

(See Multiple State Locations, pages 411–12)

School of Healing Arts

1001 Garnet Avenue #200
San Diego, California 92109
PHONE: (619) 581-9429
FAX: (619) 490-2555
E-MAIL: sha@adnc.com
WEBSITE: www.schoolhealingarts.com

The School of Healing Arts was founded in 1984 as the Institute of Health Sciences. In 1990, Seymour Koblin took over the school and turned it into a nonprofit organization. There are thirty instructors, with an average of fifteen students per class.

Accreditation and Approvals

The School of Healing Arts offers state-certified vocational training. The school is approved as a continuing education provider by the National Certification Board for Therapeutic Massage and Bodywork (NCBTMB), by the California Board of Registered Nursing, by the American Board of Hypnotherapy, and by Associated Bodywork Massage Professionals (ABMP). The Massage Technician, Zen-Touch™ Technician, Clinical Massage Therapist, and Holistic Health Practitioner programs meet or exceed San Diego licensing requirements; graduates of programs of 500 or more hours are qualified to take the National Certification Examination for Therapeutic Massage and Bodywork (NCETMB).

Program Description

The 110-hour Massage Technician Course may be taken over fourteen days or eight to eleven weeks. The curriculum includes Anatomy and Physiology, Massage Techniques: Parasympathetic, Massage Techniques: Zen-Touch, Introduction to Advanced Techniques, and Ethics and Licensing. This program is also offered in a Spanish-speaking section.

The 130-hour Zen-Touch Technician Program may be completed in three to four months. It includes instruction in Zen-Touch, Traditional Home Remedies, Oriental Health Assessment, and Destiny Studies.

A 300-hour Whole Foods Nutritional Consultant Program may be completed in six to nine months. Courses include Basic Nutrition, Comparative Nutrition, Herbology, Oriental Health Assessment, Food Preparation, Communication for Counselors, Anatomy and Physiology, Nutritional Studies, Traditional Home Remedies, Electives, Business Practices, First Aid and CPR, and Nutritional Counselor Internship.

Hypnosis and Mind-Body Therapy is a 200-hour program that may be completed in six to nine months. Courses include Introduction to Mind/Body Healing, Hypnosis Strategies and Structures, Working with Clients and Hypnosis Techniques, and Hypnosis Internship.

The 500-hour Clinical Massage Therapist Program takes six to twelve months to complete. Course work begins with the 110-hour Massage Technician Program, then adds additional classes in Anatomy and Physiology, Hydrotherapy, Basic or Comparative Nutrition, Movement Therapy, Oriental Health Assessment, Counseling, First Aid and CPR, Business Practices, and Massage Methods and Body Therapy electives. The Zen-Touch Practitioner/Instructor Certification may be included in this program for an additional $500 and with approval of Seymour Koblin.

The 1,000-hour Holistic Health Practitioner Program takes one to two years to complete. This is the most versatile program, as it may include any of the modalities and/or certifications offered at the school. A typical program includes courses in Anatomy and Physiology, Massage Technician, Hydrotherapy, Basic or Comparative Nutrition, Herbology Introduction, Movement Therapy, Oriental Health Assessment, Counseling, First Aid and CPR, Business Practices, and Massage Methods and Body Therapy electives. Hypnotherapy certification may be included in the program for an additional $200.

Community and Continuing Education
One-day and longer individual courses are offered throughout the year in many areas of holistic health. Subjects include Destiny and Intuition Studies, Holistic Care for Pets, Shamanic Counseling, Soul Retrieval Workshop, Watsu®, Yoga, Herbology, Tui Na Massage, Ayurveda: Introduction to Principles, Meditation, Biodynamic Gardening, Whole Foods Cooking, Macrobiotics, Herbology, Feng Shui, Tai Chi, and many others.

Tuition and Fees
Tuition for each program is as follows: Massage Technician, $750; Zen-Touch Technician, $795; Nutritional Counselor, $2,250; Hypnosis and Mind/Body Therapy, $1,700; Clinical Massage Therapist, $3,750; and Holistic Health Practitioner, $7,500. Any course may be taken on an individual basis at the rate of $9 per hour.

Financial Assistance
Payment plans are available. CMT and HHP students may work in the student clinic after 110 hours of massage technician training; a San Diego work permit is required.

School of Shiatsu and Massage at Harbin Hot Springs

P.O. Box 889
Middletown, California 95461
PHONE: (707) 987-3801
FAX: (707) 987-9638
E-MAIL: info@waba.edu
WEBSITE: www.waba.edu

The School of Shiatsu and Massage at Harbin Hot Springs is owned by the Worldwide Aquatic Bodywork Association. Watsu®, or water shiatsu, was developed here by the school's director, Harold Dull, and has been used as a tool for rehabilitation by the physical therapy community. There are twenty instructors, with an average of sixteen to twenty-four students per class.

Accreditation and Approvals
The School of Shiatsu and Massage is a nonprofit institution and was granted approval from the Bureau for Private Postsecondary and Vocational Education. It is also approved by the California Board of Registered Nursing as a continuing education provider. Graduates of programs of 500 or more hours are qualified to take the National Certification Examination for Therapeutic Massage and Bodywork (NCETMB).

Program Description
The School of Shiatsu and Massage offers a 100-hour Practitioner Certificate Course that provides a foundation for additional independent fifty- and 100-hour modules. After completing 300 hours, students receive an Advanced Bodywork Practitioner certificate; after 500 hours, a Therapist certificate; and after 1,000 hours, an Advanced Body Therapist certificate.

Massage 100, an eleven-day, 100-hour intensive, provides training in a comprehensive massage that includes Swedish, Deep Tissue, Shiatsu, Rebalancing, and Esalen techniques, along with an introduction to Watsu.

Other entry-level bodywork intensives open to beginners include Watsu, Introduction to Massage, Shiatsu, Tantsu, Rebalancing, Acupressure, and CranioSacral.

Intensives that require previous bodywork intensives or experience include Therapeutic Massage, Lymphatic Massage, Deep Tissue, Pain Relief, Living Anatomy, Watsu Body Wave, Waterdance, Sports Massage, Diving into the Self, and others.

Admission Requirements
Applicants should be at least 18 years of age, have a high school diploma or equivalent, and have the physical ability and emotional maturity to perform bodywork.

Tuition and Fees
Students pay for each class as they take it. Total tuition and fees for programs are as follows: Week-long fifty-hour intensive, $600; Practitioner, $1,200; Advanced Bodywork Practitioner, $3,600; Therapist, $6,000; and Advanced Body Therapy, $12,000. Prices include lodging in the form of indoor or outdoor camping.

Shiatsu Massage School of California

2309 Main Street
Santa Monica, California 90405
PHONE: (310) 396-4877 / (310) 396-2130

FAX: (310) 396-4502
E-MAIL: shiatsanma@aol.com
WEBSITE: home.earthlink.net/~shiatsuanma

In 1976, Dr. DoAnn T. Kaneko, a licensed acupuncturist and Doctor of Oriental Medicine, established shiatsu-anma workshops for foreigners in Tokyo; later, Dr. Kaneko developed the Shiatsu Massage School of California (SMSC), which began offering its 500-hour curriculum in 1986. There are eleven instructors, with an average of twelve (maximum twenty-four) students per class.

Accreditation and Approvals
SMSC is approved by the Bureau for Private Postsecondary and Vocational Education. Its programs are approved by the California Board of Nursing for continuing education units.

Program Description
SMSC offers a certification course and three diploma courses in Shiatsu-Anma that may be taken successively for a total of 500 hours. Classes are offered days, nights, and weekends.

The 104-hour Shiatsu-Anma Technician Course covers Shiatsu-Anma Theory and Practice, Traditional Chinese Medicine, Anatomy and Physiology, CPR/First Aid, Ethics: Legal and Business, and Do-In.

The Program A Diploma Course is a 150-hour, six-month Shiatsu-Anma Practitioner program covering the same curriculum as the Certification course with the addition of Pain and Orthopedic Evaluation, and Intern Clinical Study.

The Program B Diploma Course is a 150-hour, six-month Shiatsu-Anma Therapist course that may be taken concurrently with or after the completion of Program A. Program B includes Shiatsu-Anma Theory and Practice, Traditional Chinese Medicine, Anatomy and Physiology, and Clinical Study.

The Program C Diploma Course is a 200-hour, seven-month Shiatsu-Anma Specialist course that may be taken after the completion of Programs A and B. Program C includes Shiatsu-Anma Theory and Practice, Traditional Chinese Medicine, Anatomy and Physiology, Clinical Study, and twenty-four additional hours in electives.

Community and Continuing Education
Shiatsu-Anma weekend workshops and a Summer Shiatsu Short Course are open to high school graduates. Healing Arts weekend workshops may also be taken by nurses for continuing education credit and include such topics as Tui Na Chinese Massage, Postural Integration, Reflexology, Thai Massage, Chair Massage, Emotional Anatomy, and others.

Admission Requirements
Certificate Course or Program A Diploma Course applicants must have a high school diploma (Program B and C prerequisites are listed above). All new students should attend an orientation program or make special arrangements to meet with the director.

Tuition and Fees
Paid-in-full tuition for the Certification Course is $830; for the Program A Diploma Course, $1,150 for the Program B Diploma Course, $1,150; and for the Program C Diploma Course, $1,525. Additional expenses include a $75 registration fee; books for Diploma A are $46.

Financial Assistance
Payment plans are available.

Sierra Institute of Herbal Studies

P.O. Box 426
Big Oak Flat, California 95305
PHONE: (209) 962-7425
E-MAIL: sierrain@lodelink.com
WEBSITE: www.lodelink.com/sierrain

Sierra Institute of Herbal Studies was founded in 1996 by Dodie Heiny, who cofounded Havasu Hills Herb Farm and teaches herb classes at Merced College and Modesto Junior College. Dodie is the primary instructor, with occasional guest instructors; class sizes average twenty students.

Accreditation and Approvals
Sierra Institute is applying for certification to offer some of its classes for CEUs; contact the Institute for further information.

Program Description
In the Herbal Intensive Program, classes meet one weekend per

month for eight months. Students are immersed in hands-on herbal medicine-making, herb walks, wildcrafting excursions, planting and propagating herbs, discussions about starting an herb business, wild food preparation, and plant identification. The Intensive also includes Rosemary Gladstar's correspondence course, The Science and Art of Herbalism.

Community and Continuing Education

One-day courses are offered in a variety of herb-related subjects. Courses previously offered include Herbal Medicine Chest, Herbs for Women's Health, Herbs for Summertime Health, Herbal Resources for the Health Care Provider, Wreath Making with Fresh Herbs, herb walks, and others.

Tuition and Fees

Tuition for the 2000 Herbal Intensive was $795; prices may vary. Tuition for short courses ranges from $20 to $45.

Sivananda Ashram Yoga Camp

(See Multiple State Locations, pages 423–24)

South Baylo University

MAIN CAMPUS:
1126 North Brookhurst Street
Anaheim, California 92801-1701
PHONE: (714) 533-1495
FAX: (714) 533-6040

LOS ANGELES CAMPUS:
2727 West 6th Street
Los Angeles, California 90057-3139
PHONE: (213) 738-0712
FAX: (213) 480-1332
E-MAIL: song@southbaylo.edu
WEBSITE: www.southbaylo.edu

South Baylo University was founded in 1977 as the Academy of Political Economy and Management for the purpose of redirecting the deterioration of the values of modern society. The academy was authorized to grant academic degrees in 1978, and moved to Anaheim in 1994. There are seventy-eight faculty members; the average class size is ten to fifteen students.

Accreditation and Approvals

The master's degree program in Acupuncture and Oriental Medicine is accredited by the Accreditation Commission for Acupuncture and Oriental Medicine (ACAOM).

Program Description

The master's degree program in Acupuncture and Oriental Medicine consists of 194 units in didactic courses and 840 hours of internship. Required courses include Biology, General Chemistry, Physics, Psychology, Medical Terminology, Anatomy/Physiology, History of Medicine, Oriental Medicine Principles, Herbal Principles, Herbology, Acupuncture, Oriental Medicine Diagnosis, Pharmacology, Pathology, Nutrition and Therapeutic Diet, Herbal Prescription, Acupressure/Breath Exercise, Herbal Practice, Oriental Medicine Internal Medicine, Western Diagnosis, Practice Management, Clinical Medicine, Clinical Sciences, Clinical Training, Acupuncture Theory/Therapy, Oriental Medicine Infectious Diseases, Oriental Medicine Gynecology, Research Methodology, Direct Management, and more. Classes are conducted in English, Chinese, and Korean.

Admission Requirements

Applicants must have completed at least sixty semester units at an accredited institution and be proficient in the English language (students wishing to take instruction in Chinese or Korean will not need to show English proficiency). An oral or written examination may be given to applicants whose qualifications are questionable.

Tuition and Fees

Tuition is $100 per unit. Other fees include: application fee, $100; internship fee, $7 per hour; malpractice insurance for intern, $50 per quarter; and evaluation for graduation, $180.

Financial Assistance

Federal grants, loans, work-study, and state grants are available.

Stens Corporation

(See Multiple State Locations, pages 414–15)

Taoist Sanctuary of San Diego

4229 Park Boulevard
San Diego, California 92103
PHONE: (619) 692-1155
FAX: (619) 692-0428
E-MAIL: taosanct@cts.com
WEBSITE: taoistsanctuary.org

The Taoist Sanctuary of San Diego was founded in 1975. Tui Na is an ancient Chinese system of healing bodywork that uses soft-tissue manipulation, structural alignment, and traditional Chinese medical theory. Director Bill Helm has taught Tui Na since 1978 and is also Dean of Allied Arts at Pacific College of Oriental Medicine. There is one instructor, with two or three assistants per class; classes average fifteen students.

Accreditation and Approvals

The Taoist Sanctuary is approved by the California Acupuncture Committee for its Tui Na courses.

Program Description

The fifty-hour Structural Disorders Tui Na Intensive certificate program includes Oscillating Hand Techniques, Pressure Hand Techniques, Passive Joint Movement, and Traditional Chinese Medical Theory, which includes Eight Principles of Differentiation, Theory of Trauma/Blood Stasis-Qi Stagnation, Painful Obstruction Syndrome, Theory and Uses of Herbal Preparations, Major Acupoints, Channel Palpation, Qigong, and more.

The forty-hour Qi Gong Therapeutics Intensive certificate program includes exercises for balancing and strengthening the practitioner's own body and energy system, exercises and self-massage prescribed for patients for specific signs and symptoms, and the use of the practitioner's own energy projected into the patient for healing (Nei Gong Gee Liao).

One-day workshops are offered throughout the year in Upper Extremity, Lower Extremity, Tonification Dispersion Treatments, and Spine Treatments.

Admission Requirements

The workshops and certificate programs are designed for acupuncturists, massage therapists, and other health professionals.

Tuition and Fees

Tuition for the Structural Disorders Tui Na Intensive is $600 each. Tuition for Qi Gong Therapeutics is $500. Books, linens, and optional massage table are additional. Tuition for the one-day workshops is $110 in advance or $125 at the door.

Touch for Health Kinesiology Association

(See Multiple State Locations, pages 415-16)

The Touch Therapy Institute®

15720 Ventura Boulevard, Suite 101
Encino, California 91436
PHONE: (818) 788-0824
FAX: (818) 788-0875
E-MAIL: touch@touchtherapyinstitute.com
WEBSITE: www.touchtherapyinstitute.com

The Touch Therapy Institute® was founded in 1989. There are twenty instructors for the 500- and 1,000-hour programs. Class sizes are limited to thirty-four students in practice sessions and sixty students in lecture; for hands-on classes, the teacher: student ratio is 1:6. In addition to the programs described here, the institute offers a 200-hour Massage Technician course and a 100-hour supplemental course.

Accreditation

The Touch Therapy Institute has been granted course approval by the Bureau for Private Postsecondary and Vocational Education. Graduates of the 500- and 1,000-hours programs are qualified to take the National Certification Examination for Therapeutic Massage and Bodywork (NCETMB). CEUs are available for nurses.

Program Description

The 500-hour Massage Therapist Program consists of the 200-hour Massage Technician Course (which includes Anatomy, Physiology and Kinesiology; Basic Swedish Massage, Deep Tissue, Massage for Young Children, and 30-Minute Full Body Massage; Body Mechanics; CPR and First Aid; Energy and Color Therapy; Ethics; How To Start Your Own Massage Business; Nutrition; and Massage Practicum), plus an additional

300 hours of courses that include Advanced Anatomy, Physiology and Kinesiology; Advanced Swedish Strokes; Aromatherapy; Body Awareness and Seeing; Chair Massage; Myofascial Trigger Points; Palpation Series; Rotator Cuff Solutions; Pregnancy and Doula Massage; Therapeutic Stretching; and 138 hours of electives.

The 1,000-hour Advanced Massage Therapist Program consists of the 500-hour program described above plus an additional 500 hours of electives.

Elective courses include Acupressure, Alexander Technique, Aromatherapy, Ascending and Transcending the Chakras, Basic Reflexology, Cranial-Sacral Basics, Deep Tissue Integration, Doula Training, Elements of Psycho-Physical Integration, Emotions for Muscles, Fibromyalgia and Muscle Pain, Field Work, Geriatric Massage, Hand Reflexology, Lomi Lomi, Lymphatics for Immune Response, Massage for Parents, Naturopathic Approaches to Common Ailments, Personal Training Course, Polarity Therapy, Qi Gong, Reflexology, Relieving TMJ Pain, Sports Massage, Therapeutic Stretching, Therapeutic Touch, Volunteer Work, Yoga for the Eyes, and others.

Classes are offered days, evenings, and weekends.

Admission Requirements

Applicants must be at least 18 years of age and be evaluated favorably at an interview or an Open House to determine their likely success as a massage professional (Open Houses are held twice each month). Applicants must be emotionally stable and physically capable of performing massage.

Tuition and Fees

Tuition for the 500-hour Massage Therapist Program is $2,400 to $4,225, depending on electives chosen. Tuition for the 1,000-hour Advanced Massage Therapist program is $2,940 to $6,418 depending on electives chosen. Additional expenses for either program include an $80 registration fee, books, and class handouts.

Financial Assistance

Students may pay by the class. Veterans' benefits and early payment discounts are available. The institute is in the process of obtaining federal funding.

Touching for Health Center

School of Professional Bodywork
628 Lincoln Center
Stockton, California 95207
PHONE: (209) 474-9559 / (800) 474-9559
FAX: (209) 474-9559
E-MAIL: tfhc@inreach.com

Touching for Health Center (TFHC) was founded in 1990. There are eight instructors, with an average of ten to twelve students per class. In addition to the program described here, the center offers certificate programs in Massage Technician (105 hours), Home Health Aide (forty hours), and Holistic Health Massage Practitioner (225 hours).

Accreditation and Approvals

TFHC is approved to operate by the Bureau of Private Postsecondary Vocational Education. Graduates of the 500-hour program are qualified to take the National Certification Examination for Therapeutic Massage and Bodywork (NCETMB).

Program Description

The 500-hour Therapeutic Massage Practitioner Program consists of 105 hours of core subjects plus 395 hours additional required hours. Core subjects include Anatomy, Physiology, Business Ethics and Documentation, History and Psychology of Massage, Massage Theory and Hygiene, and Massage Demonstration and Practice. The additional 395 hours includes courses in Acupressure, Advanced Anatomy and Physiology, Assessment and Treatment Planning, Business Practice, Clinical Treatments, CPR, Deep Tissue, Human Behavior, Hydrotherapy, Indications/Contraindications, Introduction to Other Modalities, Kinesiology, Lymph Drainage, Massage Theory Practice, Medical Terminology, Polarity, Reflexology, and Sports Massage.

Admission Requirements

Applicants must be at least eighteen years of age and in good health.

Tuition and Fees

Tuition, books, and fees for the 105 core hours totals $900; tuition, books, and fees for the additional 395 hours totals $3,982.

Financial Assistance

Payment plans are available.

The Trager® Institute

(See Multiple State Locations, pages 416–17)

Trinity College

SAN FRANCISCO LOCATION
939 Market Street, 2nd Floor
San Francisco, California 94103
PHONE/FAX: (415) 541-7777

SAN JOSE LOCATION
1150 North First Street
San Jose, California 95112
PHONE: (408) 287-5100

Trinity College was founded in 1988 by GSBC Inc. The Massage Therapy program was first offered in 1997. The number of instructors varies; classes average forty students.

Accreditation and Approvals

Trinity College is accredited by the Accrediting Council for Continuing Education and Training (ACCET). Graduates are qualified to take the National Certification Examination for Therapeutic Massage and Bodywork (NCETMB).

Program Description

The 730-hour Massage Therapy program includes Essentials of Massage Therapy, Anatomy, Swedish Massage/Aromatherapy, Functional Anatomy, Body Mechanics/Therapeutic Exercises, Kinesiology, Sports Massage/Basic Injury Care, Dynamic Practicum, Shiatsu, Practical Physiology, Deep Tissue Massage, Passive Joint Movement, Business Management, Jin Shin, Energetic Techniques (Reiki), Professional Development, CPR/First Aid, Nutrition, Chair Massage, Strategic Swedish Massage,

Physiology, Massage Practicum, Hydrotherapy, Reflexology, Clinical Practice: Internship, and Clinical Practice: Externship.

Admission Requirements

Applicants must have a high school diploma or equivalent or demonstrated ability to benefit from training by passing Trinity's entrance exam. All applicants must take an entrance exam.

Tuition and Fees

Tuition is $7,053. Additional expenses include registration fee, $100; transcript fee, $5; books, $443; and massage table, $525.

Financial Assistance

Federal grants, loans, work-study, and veterans' benefits are available.

Twin Lakes College of the Healing Arts

1210 Brommer Street
Santa Cruz, California 95062
PHONE: (831) 476-2152
FAX: (831) 476-6048

Twin Lakes College of the Healing Arts was founded in 1982. The current director, Becky Williams, has been teaching in the health field since 1977. There are thirty to thirty-five instructors, with an average of eight to fourteen (maximum sixteen) students per class.

Accreditation and Approvals

Graduates of massage therapist programs of 500 or more hours are qualified to take the National Certification Examination for Therapeutic Massage and Bodywork (NCETMB). All courses at Twin Lakes College are approved for continuing education units for nurses.

Program Description

The 200-hour Level I Massage Practitioner Certificate program exceeds the minimum requirements for practicing in California and serves as the basis for the longer massage programs. The 200-hour program includes 100 hours of massage classes (chosen from Integrative Swedish Massage, Polarity Therapy

Energy Balancing, Acupressure or Shiatsu), plus Anatomy I and Physiology for Bodyworkers, Professional Studies I (which includes Communication and Counseling Skills, Business Practices, and Ethics), Internship/Practice Sessions, and completion of the Massage-A-Thon event. Courses are offered day and evening.

A 200-hour Women's Massage Practitioner Certificate Program is offered once each year to women only. The curriculum includes Swedish Massage along with the other Level I Massage requirements of Anatomy I, Professional Studies, and a Massage-A-Thon event.

The 300-hour Level II Intermediate Massage Practitioner Program consists of the 200-hour Level I program plus Anatomy II, Biomechanics, and sixty hours of Bodywork electives.

The 500-hour Level III Professional Massage Therapist Program consists of the 300-hour Level II program plus Professional Studies II, Anatomy III, CPR, at least thirty-four hours of Bodywork choices, and 100 hours of electives (which may include Additional Bodywork, Hypnotherapy, Essential Oils, Dream Studies and other classes offered).

The 750-hour Level IV Professional Massage Therapist and Natural Health Counselor consists of the 500-hour Level III program plus Advanced Professional Studies III, 120 hours of Bodywork choices and 100 hours of electives (which may include Additional Bodywork, Hypnotherapy, Essential Oils, Dream Studies, and other classes offered).

Courses offered as bodywork choices or electives include Jin Shin Jyutsu, Reiki, Clinical Applications, Acupressure, Foot Focus Workshop, Breema, Sports Massage, Structural Balance, Ayurvedic Theory and Principles, Ayurvedic Full Body Oil Massage, Pre- and Post-Natal, Infant Massage, and others.

Two certificates are offered in Hypnotherapy:

The 100-hour Level I Hypnosis Practitioner Certificate Program includes Self Hypnosis, Direct and Indirect Suggestion, and Client Management Skills.

The 200-hour Professional Hypnotherapist Program consists of Level I (above), followed by Level II: Transpersonal and Spiritual Perspectives of Hypnosis (seventy hours), which draws upon Eastern, Western and Shamanic traditions, and Level III: Advanced Professional Studies (thirty hours), which focuses on the process of becoming a professional hypnotherapist.

A thirty-hour Essential Oils Therapy Program teaches students to work with essential oils either in an aromatherapy practice or in combination with other healing modalities. This class is a prerequisite for Essential Oils Massage.

A 150-hour Essential Oils and Aromatherapy Program consists of the thirty-hour Essential Oils Therapy I followed by the 120-hour Essential Oils Therapy II: Applications for the Health Professional. Topics covered include blending, theory and history, and both classical and contemporary approaches.

Continuing Education
Open to Certified Massage Practitioners, a twenty-five-hour, five-day Subtle Body EnergyWork intensive combines Hypnosis, Touch, and Aromatherapy.

A twenty-five-hour Touch Pro® Chair Massage Technique and Business Skills Workshop is open to Certified Massage Practitioners or students currently enrolled in a licensed massage school.

Additional continuing education courses are offered to the public and to massage professionals.

Admission Requirements
Applicants must have a high school diploma or the equivalent and have a personal interview.

Tuition and Fees
Depending on courses chosen, tuition for the 200-hour Massage Program is $1,300 to $1,600; for the Intermediate and Advanced Massage Programs, $4,500 to $5,500; books and supplies are additional.

Tuition for the 100-hour Hypnotherapy Program is $2,600 for the complete three-level program.

Tuition for Essential Oils Therapy I is $300; for Essential Oils Therapy II, $875.

Financial Assistance
Payment plans, early-bird discounts, and student referral incentives are available.

United States Yoga Association

2159 Filbert Street
San Francisco, California 94123
PHONE: (415) 931-YOGA
FAX: (415) 921-6676
E-MAIL: tony@usyoga.org
WEBSITE: www.usyoga.org

The United States Yoga Association was founded in 1984. Instructors at the United States Yoga Association come from a lineage of yogis in India who are not vegetarian and do not advocate particular spiritual beliefs; one's lifestyle and spiritual evolution are considered personal choices. There is one instructor; classes average ten to fifteen students.

Accreditation and Approvals
The Yoga Challenge® * I Instructor Training Program is endorsed by the Yoga Alliance.

Program Description
The three-month Yoga Challenge I Instructor Training Program is geared for those who want to enhance a career in physical fitness, health, or alternative medicine. The program includes ten two-hour lecture/workshops covering hatha yoga philosophy and history and the benefits and principles of the Yoga Challenge I system; thirty classes/hours of practice; and a thirty-class internship teaching at a school or community center. Independent study requirements include a reading list, completion of an accredited, college-level anatomy course, and twenty hours of yoga philosophy classes and CPR.

Admission Requirements
Anyone who is willing to learn and practice yoga regularly, has the gift to teach, and enjoys seeing people benefit from it is encouraged to become an instructor. Students should have a basic knowledge about yoga and physical health; vegetarianism is not required.

Tuition and Fees
Tuition is $2,000; independent study expenses are additional.

Financial Assistance
A payment plan is available.

Valley Hypnosis Center

3705 Sunnyside Drive
Riverside, California 92506
PHONE: (909) 781-0282
E-MAIL: cernie@pe.net
WEBSITE: www.wordpr.com/cernie/

The Valley Hypnosis Center, founded in 1982 by Sally Cernie, Ph.D., has a spiritual focus that allows hypnotherapists to reach clients beyond the physical realm. In 1998, the center added classes in homeopathy taught by Dr. M. Iqbal. There are two instructors and two aides; classes average six students (maximum twelve).

Accreditation and Approvals
The Valley Hypnosis Center is approved by the Bureau for Private Postsecondary and Vocational Education, and by the California Board of Registered Nursing and the Academy of General Dentistry as a provider of continuing education units.

Program Description
Principles of Hypnosis 100 is designed for students with no prior hypnosis experience. Topics covered include Preinduction Techniques, Reflexive Exercises for Suggestibility, Awakening Procedures, Post-Hypnotic Suggestion, Automatic Writing, Pain Alleviation, Memory and Concentration, Self-Confidence Building, Obesity and Weight Control, and Age Regression. The course is given in two formats: three hours per week for sixteen weeks, or one three-day weekend intensive.

Principles of Hypnosis 100A is a fast-paced, intensive training in the art and science of hypnotism, from history to modern uses. Students will learn how to hypnotize themselves and others.

Hypnotherapy 101 is an accelerated course in psychology and advanced hypnotic techniques for those who have completed Principles of Hypnosis 100 or 100A. Subjects include Psychosexual Development, Defense Mechanisms, Psychopathology, Insight vs. Supportive Treatment, Transference and Counter

Transference, Behavior Modification Techniques, Biofeedback and Autogenic Training, and Interviewing and Communication Skills. The course consists of seventy-two hours of training: twelve weeks of classroom work for three hours per week, and thirty-six hours of clinical work under the supervision of a trained health care professional.

Clinical Applications of Alchemical Hypnotherapy 201 is an advanced form of hypnotherapy connecting us with our spiritual roots. The fifty-four-hour course is divided into three sixteen-hour weekend intensives: Emotional Clearing and Inner Child Work, Inner Guides and Past Life Regression, and Conference Room Therapy.

The Homeopathic Program is designed for students with no prior training or exposure to homeopathy and is divided into three six-week sessions. Session One consists of basic principles and theories of homeopathy; Session Two covers common uses of various remedies; and Session Three covers the therapeutic uses of remedies for specific problems.

Other programs offered include a two-day course in Iridology, and two three-hour Reiki trainings.

Tuition and Fees

Tuition for the Hypnosis courses is as follows: for Principles of Hypnosis 100, $750; for Principles of Hypnosis 100A, $495; for Hypnotherapy 101, $750; and for Clinical Applications of Hypnotherapy 201, $750.

Tuition for the Homeopathic Program is $300 per session.

Tuition for Iridology is $295. Tuition for Reiki I is $100; for Reiki II, $150.

Financial Assistance

Weekly payments may be arranged per agreement between the student and the director.

Vega Institute

1511 Robinson Street
Oroville, California 95965
PHONE: (530) 533-4777
FAX: (530) 533-4999

The Vega Institute, founded in 1974 by Herman and Cornellia Aihara, is the world's oldest macrobiotic residential school, teaching concepts in macrobiotic nutrition, healing, cooking, and outlook that are unavailable elsewhere.

Program Description

The three-week Cooking Teachers' Training Foundations Program prepares students to teach macrobiotic cooking classes. Topics covered include Developing the Spirit of a Macrobiotic Cooking Teacher, Macrobiotic Nutrition and Food Products, Macrobiotic Cooking Techniques, Design Macrobiotic Cooking Courses, Balance Between Service and Business, and Student-Teacher Practice Demonstration.

The four-week Counselor Training Foundations I Program prepares students to become macrobiotic counselors. Topics covered include Personal Development, How to Begin Macrobiotic Counseling, Food Selection and Preparation Theory, Herman Aihara's Acid/Alkaline Theory, Macrobiotic Recommendations, Yin/Yang Principle in Diet and Healing, Natural Healing From Head to Toe, How to Read the Body, Practice Sessions and Constructive Critique, and final exam.

Macrobiotic Counselor Training II offers continued development of macrobiotic counseling skills. The four-week program consists of one week discussing the macrobiotic needs of individuals with major health concerns; two weeks attending the Cancer and Healing Program, during which students assist with private and group consultation sessions; a fourth week of exploration into the counseling process; and completion of projects and special assignments.

Macrobiotic Counselor Training III is a three-month apprenticeship. Students assist the experienced counselors, do their own practice sessions and projects, and help in the day-to-day operations of the Vega Study Center.

Reading the Body: A Holistic Diagnosis Intensive is a one-week course in macrobiotic visual diagnosis techniques. This course is part of the four-week Counselor Training Foundations program, but may also be taken separately. Topics include determining strengths and weaknesses of a person's constitution, seeing how the external reflects the internal, the relationship between facial features and specific internal organs, and more.

In the six-month Kitchen Apprentice Program, students work forty hours per week in the Vega Study Center's kitchen and learn macrobiotic kitchen organization and maintenance skills, Vega-style macrobiotic cooking skills, traditional pickle making, macrobiotic foods processing, quantity cooking and menu mastery, and more; students also learn independently through projects, written assignments, and lectures.

Students may also earn study credits worth two weeks of free courses at Vega through the six-month residency Front Office Personnel Program. In exchange for forty hours per week of front office responsibilities that include light secretarial work, mail-order sales, and assigning guest rooms, students receive room and board, macrobiotic meals and community support, staff outings, and guided independent study through written assignments.

Community Education

A wide variety of additional courses and programs are offered to the public, including two-week Cancer and Healing, Macrobiotic Lifestyle Essential, and Arthritis: Living Without It Programs; a one-week Natural Healing From Head to Toe intensive; and programs in cooking, internal cleansing, diabetes and hypoglycemia, qigong healing, meditation, and more.

Admission Requirements

Counselor Training Foundations I or its equivalent is a prerequisite for the Macrobiotic Counselor Training II, and Macrobiotic Counselor Training II is a prerequisite for Macrobiotic Counselor Training III.

Tuition and Fees

Tuition is as follows: for Cooking Teachers' Training, $1,980; for Counselor Training, $2,100; for Macrobiotic Counselor II, $2,100; for Macrobiotic Counselor III, $500; and for Reading the Body, $645. Tuition includes meals and all class fees. Accommodations are additional and range from $95 to $425 per week, depending on the type of housing and number of occupants.

Tuition for the six-month Kitchen Apprentice program is $1,500 and includes accommodations. Tuition for the six-month Front Office Personnel Program is $1,200 and includes accommodations.

Financial Assistance

Discounts are available for couples or for early registration.

Western Institute of Neuromuscular Therapy

22981 Mill Creek Drive, Suite A
Laguna Hills, California 92653
PHONE: (949) 830-6151
FAX: (949) 830-1729
E-MAIL: director@wintherapy.com
WEBSITE: www.wintherapy.com

Western Institute of Neuromuscular Therapy (WIN) was founded in 1994 by Cynthia Ribeiro and Maryalice Bourdelais. There are seven instructors, with an average of twenty students per class.

Accreditation and Approvals

WIN has been granted approval to operate by the Bureau for Private Postsecondary and Vocational Education. WIN is a member of the AMTA Council of Schools; graduates are qualified to take the National Certification Examination for Therapeutic Massage and Bodywork (NCETMB). WIN is approved by the NCBTMB as a continuing education provider.

Program Description

WIN is currently undergoing curriculum revision. While the core of the program will remain in place, classroom instruction will be offered in a wider range of massage and bodywork theory and technique. Contact the institute for additional information.

The 500-hour Professional Massage Therapist Course is offered in three fifteen-week terms. Classes include Anatomy and Physiology, Kinesiology and Pathology; Introduction to Massage; Professional Development; Therapy Techniques; Event Participation; and Clinical/Practicum. Techniques introduced in the program include Swedish Massage, Pre- and Post-Event Sports Massage, Deep Transverse Friction, Myofascial Release, Trigger Point Therapy, Proprioceptive Neuromuscular Facilitation, and Strain/Counterstrain.

The 1,000-hour Professional Therapeutic and Sports Massage Therapist Course is offered in four fifteen-week terms. After completing the three terms described above, students explore anatomy, physiology, kinesiology and pathology for specific sports injuries; injury evaluation; therapeutic stretching techniques; and continue participation on the sports massage team of athletic events and their involvement in the Supervised Clinical Program.

Continuing Education

A variety of workshops are offered to students, graduates, and other massage professionals in addition to the core program.

Admission Requirements

Applicants must be at least 18 years of age; have a high school diploma or equivalent (those without a high school diploma will be considered on an individual basis); be in sound mental and physical health; and be physically able to perform massage; submit three letters of reference and a health examination form; and have a personal interview. Applicants must be of good character and free from drug and chemical dependency, and must have had at least one professional massage prior to admission.

Tuition and Fees

Tuition for the 500-hour program is $5,000, plus $465 for books and supplies. Tuition for the 1,000-hour program is $8,000, plus $601 for books and supplies. Additional expenses for either program include a massage table, $300 to $700, and liability insurance, approximately $35 per year.

Financial Assistance

Payment plans are available.

Wyrick Institute for European Manual Lymph Drainage

(See Multiple State Locations, page 420)

Yo San University

1314 Second Street
Santa Monica, California 90401-1103
PHONE: (310) 917-2202
FAX: (310) 917-2203
E-MAIL: info@yosan.edu
WEBSITE: www.yosan.edu

Founded by Taoist Master Hua-Ching Ni in 1989, Yo San University is a Taoist school dedicated to the principles of harmony and balance. There are thirty-five instructors, with an average of twenty-five students per class.

Accreditation and Approvals

YSU's Master of Acupuncture and Traditional Chinese Medicine Program is accredited by the Accreditation Commission for Acupuncture and Oriental Medicine (ACAOM). YSU graduates are eligible to take the California State Licensing Examination and the National Certification Commission for Acupuncture and Oriental Medicine (NCCAOM) exam. YSU is approved by the California State Acupuncture Committee as a provider of continuing education certification for licensure renewal for licensed acupuncturists.

Program Description

The four-year Master of Acupuncture and Traditional Chinese Medicine Program enables full-time students to graduate in four years, spending the last year as a practice intern in the teaching clinic, a full-service, low-cost facility open to the public, which includes a complete herbal pharmacy. The program may also be taken on a part-time basis.

Courses in the first year typically include General Biology, Western Medical Terminology, Fundamentals of Taoism, Principles and Theories of TCM, Herbal Pharmacopoeia, Qigong/Eight Treasures, Introduction to Chinese Herbology, Fundamentals of Natural Healing, Human Anatomy and Physiology, General Chemistry, Fundamentals of the Health Practitioner, Biochemistry, and others.

Topics covered in the second year include Acupuncture Anatomy and Therapeutics, Herbal Prescriptions, TCM Diagnosis, Western Nutrition, Pathophysiology, Chinese Nutrition, Chinese Medical Terminology, Introduction to Botany, Practice Management, Psychology and Counseling, and a continuation of topics begun the first year.

Courses introduced in the third year include TCM Internal Medicine, Western Clinical Medicine, Acupuncture Techniques, General Physics, Tui Na/Acupressure, Tai Chi Chuan, Western Pharmacology, TCM Gynecology and Pediatrics, Biomedical Understanding of Acupuncture, Shang han/Wen bing, Auricular/Scalp Acupuncture, Survey of Health Professions, Laws and Ethics, Introduction to TCM and Acupuncture Classics, Medical History, and Observation Internship, followed by a preclinical examination.

The fourth year consists of Practice Internship and Tai Chi Chuan, followed by the graduation examination.

Community and Continuing Education

Laypersons, professionals, and students at other schools may enroll as special students and take some courses for enrichment without enrolling in the master's degree program. Introductory courses are offered to the public in such topics as Introduction to TCM, Introduction to Herbology, and Qigong. In addition, public workshops and seminars are scheduled on a periodic basis.

Advanced seminars and workshops are offered for the refinement of skills of the licensed acupuncturist.

Admission Requirements

Applicants must have completed at least two years (sixty semester units or ninety quarter units) at an accredited undergraduate institution. Applicants must submit two letters of recommendation, interview with an admissions representative, and submit a personal essay. The essay and academic training must demonstrate the applicant's desire to become a healer and the ability to successfully complete the medical curriculum.

Tuition and Fees

Tuition for the Master's Program is $160 per unit; tuition for the Qi Development Program is $80 per unit. Additional expenses include: application fee, $50; new student registration, $100; continuing student registration, $25; student association fee, $10 per trimester; clinic hours, $6 per hour; herb pharmacy lab fee, $25 per 14 hours; clinic malpractice insurance, $60 per trimester enrolled; and graduation fee, $100. The total estimated tuition is $29,485 ($2,450 per trimester); books and clinic supplies are approximately $1,000 per year.

Financial Assistance

Partial scholarships, federal loans, and work-study are available.

Yoga College of India

8800 Wilshire Boulevard, 2nd Floor
Beverly Hills, California 90211
PHONE: (310) 854-5800
FAX: (310) 854-6200
E-MAIL: Bikramc@aol.com
WEBSITE: www.bikramyoga.com

The Yoga College of India was founded over twenty years ago by Bikram Choudhury; its Teacher Training Program began in 1994.

Program Description

The intensive two-month Accelerated Yoga Teacher Training Program requires over 500 hours of study. The course includes Yoga Philosophy, Theory and Practice of Bikram's Hatha Yoga System (eighty-four poses), Allopathic Physical Systems (taught by guest doctors), Yogic Physical Systems (energy fields, energy flow, and energy regeneration), Integration of Medical and Yogic Systems, Yoga Therapy (the application of asanas to diseases and disorders), and Marketing (promotion, setting up a yoga studio, and administration). Classes are held all day Monday through Friday, and Saturday morning, with an optional Sunday morning class.

Tuition and Fees

Tuition is $4,000; room and board are available for not more than $1,250.

Yoga Works

1426 Montana Avenue, 2nd Floor
Santa Monica, California 90403
PHONE: (310) 393-5150
FAX: (310) 656-5892
Additional location:
2215 Main Street
Santa Monica, California 90405

Yoga Works was founded in 1987. The Teacher Training Program runs twice a year and accepts thirty-six people per session. Maty Ezraty and Lisa Walford are the primary instructors.

Program Description

The six-week Yoga Works Teacher Training and In-Depth Study Course is designed to train students in the fundamentals of teaching yoga. The course offers detailed instruction in the theory and practice of yoga asanas, breath, the art of teaching, and a basic overview of yoga philosophy.

Additional requirements for Teacher Training Certification include six months of Teacher Assistance; observing one weekend Intro course; assisting in two weekend intro courses; eighty hours of workshop attendance (including at least one Iyengar Teacher's Intensive and one workshop on either Meditation, Pranayama or Philosophy); attendance at two Easy Does It classes, five Level One classes, five Prenatal classes, one Menstrual Cycle class, and one Restorative class; thirty hours of Philosophy course work; and twenty hours of Anatomy course work. Yoga Works is in the process of implementing these new courses.

Admission Requirements

In addition to completing an application form, applicants must take at least one class with either Lisa or Maty.

Tuition and Fees

Tuition for the six-week Teacher Training program is $1,195 ($995 when paid in advance).

COLORADO

Academy of Natural Therapy

P.O. Box 237
123 Elm Avenue
Eaton, Colorado 80615
PHONE: (970) 454-2224
FAX: (303) 454-3147
E-MAIL: naturaltherapy@juno.com
WEBSITE: www.naturaltherapy.com

The Academy of Natural Therapy was founded in 1989 by Dorothy Mongan. There are seven instructors; classes are limited to ten students, with two to four classes per year.

Accreditation and Approvals

The Academy of Natural Therapy is approved and regulated by the Division of Private Occupational Schools, State of Colorado Department of Higher Education. Graduates are qualified to take the National Certification Examination for Therapeutic Massage and Bodywork (NCETMB).

Program Description

The 1,100-hour, twelve-month Massage Therapy Program includes classes in History of Massage, Interpersonal Communication, Pathology for Massage Practitioners, Reflexology, Anatomy and Physiology, Swedish Massage, Counseling Techniques, Infant Massage, CPR, Kinesiology, Neuromuscular Reeducation, Shiatsu, Clinical Practice, Career Development and Professional Ethics, Field Experience, Nutrition, Hydrotherapy, Sports Massage, Yoga, and Tai Chi. The program may also be taken on a part-time basis.

Admission Requirements

Applicants must be at least 18 years of age, have a high school diploma or equivalent, be physically able to perform massage, have a physical exam and submit a medical history, and provide three letters of reference. A college background in the sciences is encouraged but not required.

Tuition and Fees

Tuition is $5,000, and includes books, supplies, and liability insurance.

Financial Assistance

Payment plans and scholarships are available.

Artemis Institute of Natural Therapies

P.O. Box 1824
Boulder, Colorado 80306
PHONE: (303) 443-9289
FAX: (303) 443-6361

The Artemis Institute of Natural Therapies was founded in 1990 by Peter Holmes, a medical herbalist and licensed acupuncturist. The institute is named for the Greek goddess Artemis, Lady of the Wild Things and protector of plant life.

Program Description

The institute offers an annual five-day Herbal Medicine Intensive, two-day seminars in clinical aromatherapy, and part-time professional programs in clinical aromatherapy and herbal medicine.

The five-day, thirty-five-hour Herbal Medicine Intensive includes classroom training in the holistic and energetic principles of herbal medicine; constitutional typing according to the four elements; herbal formulas for common ailments; herb and weed walks in and around Boulder; hands-on experience preparing herbal extracts; and slide shows and videos covering various aspects of herbal medicine.

A two-day seminar in clinical aromatherapy is offered to both students and health professionals, and covers clinical aromatherapy for health care, massage, emotional balancing, and first aid. Topics include the hands-on formulation of essential oils, concepts of quality, scent psychology, types of applications, and much more.

The 150-hour Professional Certification Program in Clinical Aromatherapy includes the basics of self-help and symptom relief, in-depth clinical and health evaluation skills, theory, and hands-on direction. The program is suitable for both the beginner and the health professional wishing to add aromatherapy to his or her practice.

A 400-hour Professional Certification Program in Herbal Medicine meets three days per month for sixteen months. This program is designed for the serious student of botanical medicine and covers natural medicine, herbology, pathology, diagnostics, and therapeutics in a holistic integration of traditional herbal energetics and science. Students learn skills in health maintenance and disease prevention, plant identification and collection, herb extract making and formulating, treatment of simple and complex conditions, and how to conduct a health evaluation.

Admission Requirements

Applicants must have a personal interview.

Tuition and Fees

Tuition for the Herbal Medicine Intensive is $375; an optional certification test costs $20. Tuition for the Clinical Aromatherapy Seminar is $185; for the Professional Certification Program

in Clinical Aromatherapy, $1,200; and for the Professional Program in Herbal Medicine, $2,500.

Financial Assistance

Payment plans are available by special arrangement.

BioSomatics

(See Multiple State Locations, pages 387–88)

Boulder College of Massage Therapy

6255 Longbow Drive
Boulder, Colorado 80301
PHONE: (303) 530-2100 / (800) 442-5131
FAX: (303) 530-2204
E-MAIL: cstanke@bcmt.org
        gknippa@bcmt.org
WEBSITE: www.bcmt.org

Boulder College of Massage Therapy (BCMT), a not-for-profit institution, enrolled its first class in 1976; over 2,500 students have since graduated from its 1,000-hour program. The Student Clinic provides over 6,000 massages per year to the greater Boulder community. There are thirty-four instructors. The maximum teacher: student ratio is 1:20 for hands-on courses, 1:54 for lecture courses.

Accreditation and Approvals

BCMT is accredited by the Accrediting Commission of Career Schools and Colleges of Technology (ACCSCT). Graduates are qualified to take the National Certification Examination for Therapeutic Massage and Bodywork (NCETMB). BCMT is approved as a continuing education provider by the National Certification Board for Therapeutic Massage and Bodywork (NCBTMB).

Program Description

The 1,000-hour Diploma Program in Massage Therapy consists of 850 classroom hours, seventy-five hours in Clinic Practicum, forty-five hours in electives, and thirty hours of Internship activities. Classes include four hands-on massage therapy techniques: Zen Shiatsu, Swedish Therapeutic Massage, Normalization of Soft Tissue, and Integrative Therapeutic Massage. Other classes include Anatomy and Physiology, Kinesthetic Anatomy in Clay: Zoologik System, Client Communication Skills, Movement, Structural Kinesiology, Professional Ethics, Pathophysiology, Career Development, Professional Development, Clinical Kinesiology, and Hydrotherapy. Electives include Sports Massage, Orthopedic Massage, Reflexology, Prenatal Massage, Labor and Postpartum Massage, Infant Massage, Table Shiatsu, Advanced Anatomiken, Chair Massage, Energy Medicine, and Herbology.

Classes are offered on both a day and evening schedule. Full-time students attend classes five days per week and complete the program in one year; part-time students attend classes four evenings per week and occasional Saturdays, and complete the program in two years.

Continuing Education

Advanced Bodywork Studies (ABS) courses are offered throughout the year to professional massage therapists. Programs offered include a 200-hour Orthopedic and Sports Massage Certification Program and a 200-hour Equine Massage Certification Program.

Admission Requirements

Diploma Program applicants must be at least 21 years of age (exceptions may be made on an individual basis); have a high school diploma or equivalent; submit two letters of recommendation, three essay questions, a health history form, a financial plan, and documentation of a negative TB test taken within one year; have received at least two professional massages; and interview with a faculty member. Long-distance applicants may interview by telephone.

Tuition and Fees

Tuition for the Diploma Program is $8,800. Additional expenses include a $75 application fee; lab fees, $540; books and supplies, approximately $950; massage table, approximately $700; required professional massages, approximately $350; and graduation fee, $35.

Advanced Bodywork Studies courses vary in price; please call for current catalog.

Financial Assistance

Federal grants and loans, veterans' benefits, and state loans and grants are available to those who qualify.

Colorado Institute for Classical Homeopathy

MAILING ADDRESS:
2299 Pearl Street, #400
Boulder, Colorado 80302
PHONE: (303) 440-3717
FAX: (303) 440-6526
E-MAIL: bseideneck@aol.com
WEBSITE: www.coloradohomeopathy.org

CLASSROOM:
3107 28th Street
Boulder, Colorado 80302

The Colorado Institute for Classical Homeopathy was founded in 1991 by Barbara Seideneck Chom, C.C.H., and Mark Manton, N.D., Lic.Ac. It is a nonprofit organization, approved and regulated by the State of Colorado. There are six instructors and a maximum class size of twenty-six.

Accreditation and Approvals

The institute is approved and regulated by the Division of Private Occupational Schools, State of Colorado Department of Higher Education.

Program Description

The institute offers a two-year, 450-hour program in Classical Homeopathy; classes are held one weekend a month. The second year of study prepares students to take the examination for national certification in classical homeopathy given by the Council for Homeopathic Certification.

The curriculum includes History and Philosophy, Study of the Repertories, Materia Medica, Principles of Homeopathic Practice, Case Taking, Case Analysis, Supervision of Study, Clinical Training, and Practice Management. Classes are held on weekends.

Admission Requirements

Applicants should be over 21 years of age, have taken (or be taking concurrently) college-level anatomy and physiology, and have an entrance interview.

Tuition and Fees

Tuition is $3,500 per year. Other expenses include a $25 registration fee and approximately $250 per year for books.

Financial Assistance

A payment plan is available.

Colorado Institute of Massage Therapy

2601 East St. Vrain
Colorado Springs, Colorado 80909
PHONE: (719) 634-7347 / (888) 634-7347
FAX: (719) 447-9198
E-MAIL: info@coimt.com
WEBSITE: coimt.com

Colorado Institute of Massage Therapy (CIMT) was founded in 1985 by Mrs. Togi Kinnaman, a nationally recognized workshop leader in trigger point release therapy. CIMT is currently affiliated with the Penrose–St. Francis Health Care System and is working to develop one of the first hospital-based massage therapy certification programs in the United States. There are seventeen instructors, with an average of thirty-two students per class.

Accreditation and Approvals

CIMT is a member of the American Massage Therapy Association (AMTA) Council of Schools and is approved by the Colorado Department of Private Occupational Schools. Graduates are qualified to take the National Certification Examination for Therapeutic Massage and Bodywork (NCETMB).

Program Description

The 1,150-hour Massage Therapy Program prepares students for careers as licensed massage therapists specializing in neuromuscular therapy (CIMT method). Courses include Massage Ethics, History, Equipment, Hygiene, Business Practices, Wholistic Health and Bodywork Concepts, Theories and Methods of Healing, Muscle Tension Release, Massage Theory and Movements in Swedish Massage, Deep Tissue Massage, Foot Reflexology, Anatomy and Physiology, Structural Kinesiology, Pathology, Applied Massage: Athletic and Sports Massage, Elderly, Arthritic, Bedridden, Intuitive Massage, Applied Massage for Common Physical Complaints, Psychological Aspects of Massage and Support Group Discussion, Related Therapies: Hydrotherapy, Exercise/Stretching, Muscle Testing, Nutrition, Motion Pressure Point Therapy, Foot Reflexology, Definitions and Discussion of Various Bodywork Disciplines in the Health Care Field Today, Self-Care Practices, and Clinical Practice of Swedish and Neuromuscular Therapy, Deep Tissue Massage (CIMT System), and Foot Reflexology.

Students prepare for private practice by performing one hundred full-body massages, forty-eight massage appointments in the student clinic, thirty chair massages, ten foot reflexology charted sessions, thirteen trigger point therapy charted sessions, six preceptor evaluation massages (outside class), three instructor evaluation massages, and record keeping on each massage, as well as receiving twenty massages. In addition, twelve hours each are spent outside the classroom in marketing, sports massage, and research.

Community and Continuing Education

Introduction to Massage Therapy workshops are offered monthly for prospective students at no charge.

A series of courses in neuromuscular therapy (NMT) are offered through the International Academy of NMT of St. Petersburg, Florida. Independent workshops are offered in Spinal Muscles, Upper Extremity, Lower Extremity, and Cranium/Core Muscles. Classes may be taken in any order.

Admission Requirements

Applicants must be at least 21 years old (but may be younger with permission of the admissions committee) and have a high school diploma or equivalent.

Tuition and Fees

The program cost, including application, registration, tuition, clinic, and other expenses is $7,700. Other costs include: massage table, $60 to $500; oils, $25 to $50; linens, $30 to $50; student clinic uniform, $50 to $100; and graduation dinner, $15 to

$25. NMT workshops cost $275 per weekend (review $215), plus an extra $25 if registered less than three weeks prior to the event.

Financial Assistance

Payment plans and veterans' benefits are available.

Colorado School of Healing Arts

7655 West Mississippi, Suite 100
Lakewood, Colorado 80226
PHONE: (303) 986-2320 / (800) 233-7114
FAX: (303) 980-6594

The Colorado School of Healing Arts has been owned and operated by Health Care Associates, Inc., since 1986.

Accreditation and Approvals

CSHA is accredited by the Accrediting Commission of Career Schools and Colleges of Technology (ACCSCT). CSHA is approved by the Integrative Massage and Somatic Therapies Accreditation Council (IMSTAC); by the State of Washington Department of Health; and by the Colorado Department of Higher Education, Division of Private Occupational Schools. Graduates are qualified to take the National Certification Examination for Therapeutic Massage and Bodywork (NCETMB). CSHA is approved by the National Certification Board for Therapeutic Massage and Bodywork (NCBTMB) as a continuing education provider.

Program Description

The 670-hour Certified Massage Therapist Program may be completed in as little as twelve months; fifteen- and eighteen-month programs are also available. Courses include Massage Levels I, II, and III; Anatomy; Physiology; Body-Centered Therapy; Integrative Massage Lab; Applied Kinesiology; Diet and Nutrition; Business; Sports Massage I; and Clinical Massage. A current CPR card is required upon graduation.

A CMT Program for nurses is designed to train R.N.s and L.P.N.s as massage therapists. Students must transfer in 330 hours of previous educational and occupational experience and complete the 670-hour Certified Massage Therapist Program to receive 1,000-hour certification.

The 1,000-hour CMT program offers an additional 330 hours of advanced instruction beyond the 670-hour program. Students may select 330 hours from advanced training programs and electives such as Table Shiatsu, Cranial Sacral Therapy, Neuromuscular Therapy, Trauma Touch Therapy, Sports Massage, Reflexology, Teaching Assistant, Internship, Palpation of Anatomy, Natural Alternatives to Chronic Disease, Herbology, Prenatal Massage, Aromatherapy, Seated Massage, Introduction to Polarity, Neuroanatomy, and others.

Community and Continuing Education

Introduction to Massage Therapy is an optional introductory survey class for those considering a career in massage therapy. The $50 fee may be applied toward the full program tuition upon enrollment.

Advanced training certificate programs in Cranial-Sacral Therapy, Neuromuscular Therapy, Reflexology, Sports Massage, Table Shiatsu, and Trauma Touch Therapy may also be taken independently of the 1,000-hour program.

The 530-hour Cranial-Sacral Therapy Program consists of 160 hours of anatomy, physiology and neuroanatomy, plus 240 hours of practical training.

The 300-hour Neuromuscular Massage Therapy Program consists of Advanced Neuromuscular Techniques, Comprehensive Review/Assessment Practicum, Massage Level III, Neuroanatomy, and Palpation of Anatomy.

The 230-hour Reflexology Certificate curriculum includes Reflexology I and II, Anatomy, Physiology, and Business; thirty hours of documented sessions with clients are also required.

The 100-hour Sports Massage Certificate Program consists of three levels of sports massage course work. Students are also required to provide sports massage at several outside events.

The 500-hour Table Shiatsu Program consists of Table Shiatsu I and II, Qigong, and Oriental Medical Theory.

The 100-hour Trauma Touch Therapy Certificate Program consists of two fifty-hour courses. These programs are designed for health care professionals who are incorporating consciously applied touch into their work with individuals who have experienced trauma or abuse.

Courses are also offered in such areas as CPR/First Aid for Bodyworkers, Infant Massage, Insurance Billing, and many others.

Admission Requirements

Applicants must be at least 18 years of age; have a high school diploma or equivalent; be emotionally stable and physically able to perform and receive massage; have a personal interview; and submit three personal references.

Tuition and Fees

There is a $50 application fee for all courses.

Tuition for the 670-hour Certified Massage Therapist Program is $4,850. Additional expenses include books, $350; two professional massages, $100; uniform, $25; and massage table, approximately $475.

Tuition for the 1,000-hour CMT Program varies with courses selected.

Tuition for the Introduction to Massage Therapy Class is $50.

Tuition for the Cranial-Sacral Therapy Program is $4,090; additional expenses include books, $200, materials fee, $50, and two professional massages, $100.

Tuition for the Neuromuscular Massage Therapy Program is $2,235; additional expenses include books, $200, and materials fee, $45.

Tuition for the Reflexology Certificate Program is $1,715; additional expenses include books, $160, materials fee, $10, and one professional treatment, $50.

Tuition for the Sports Massage Certificate Program is $770 plus $10 for books.

Tuition for the Table Shiatsu Program is $3,695 plus $200 for books.

Tuition for the Trauma Touch Therapy I Program is $495, plus $45 for books; tuition for the Trauma Touch Therapy II Program is $295, plus $15 for books.

Financial Assistance

Payment plans are available.

Colorado School of Traditional Chinese Medicine

1441 York Street, Suite 202
Denver, Colorado 80206-2127
PHONE: (303) 329-6355
FAX: (303) 388-8165

The Colorado School of Traditional Chinese Medicine (CSTCM) was founded in 1984 by Dr. George Kitchie, Dr. Mark Manton, and Dr. Cheng Shi. The school offers a faculty of both Chinese and Western instructors, providing a well-rounded experience representing several modalities of diagnosis and treatment.

Accreditation and Approvals

CSTCM is approved and regulated by the Department of Higher Education, Division of Private Occupational Schools, for the State of Colorado. In Spring/ Summer 1999, CSTCM will begin the Eligibility Process, with the objective of candidacy for accreditation and eventually accreditation with the Accreditation Commission for Acupuncture and Oriental Medicine (ACAOM). CSTCM is applying to the Colorado Department of Education for degree-granting privileges in fall 1999. After this approval, CSTCM will then offer a Master of Science in Traditional Chinese Medicine.

The curriculum at CSTCM has been designed to prepare students for the National Certification Commission for Acupuncture and Oriental Medicine (NCCAOM) exam and follows the guidelines set by NCCA and the Council of Colleges of Acupuncture and Oriental Medicine (CCAOM).

Program Description

CSTCM currently offers a three and one-half year, 2,475-hour program in Traditional Chinese Medicine. Students may enroll on a full- or part-time basis.

Year One includes Basic Theory of TCM, Acupuncture Meridian and Point Theory and Practicum, Chinese Herbal Medicine, Acumoxa Technique, TCM Diagnosis, TCM Differentiation, Clinical Diagnosis, Clinical Observation, and Western Medical Subjects.

In Year Two, the curriculum covers such topics as Acupuncture Treatment of Disease, Chinese Herbal Medicine Prescriptionology, Clinical Diagnosis Forum, Clinical Acupuncture Internship, Chinese Herbal Patent Medicine, Advanced Acupuncture Techniques, Allopathic Pathology and Physical Diagnosis, Professional Ethics and Human Services, Clinical Observation, and Student Acupuncture Clinic.

Year Three covers Advanced Student Acupuncture Clinic, Chinese Herbal Medicine Clinical Internship, TCM Internal

Medicine, Clinical Diagnosis Forum, and Business Management.

Specialty electives include Aesthetic Acupuncture, Basic Chinese Language, Feng Shui, Integrating Oriental and Western Medicine, Qigong, Tai Chi Chuan, TCM and Dermatology, TCM and Nutrition, TCM and Tui Na, Tibetan Medicine, Wen Bing Lun/Shang Han Lun, and others.

Students must also complete training in First Aid/CPR prior to graduation.

Admission Requirements

Applicants must be at least 21 years of age and have completed a minimum of sixty credit hours at an accredited college or university. All applicants must sit for a formal interview and must have completed the application process outlined in the school catalog.

Tuition and Fees

Tuition is $6,700 per academic year. Additional expenses are outlined in the school catalog.

Financial Assistance

Monthly payment plans and interest-free loans are available.

Cottonwood School of Massage Therapy

11100 East Mississippi Avenue, #B-100
Aurora, Colorado 80012
PHONE: (303) 745-7725
FAX: (303) 751-1861

The Cottonwood School of Massage Therapy was founded in 1993 by Jackie Odey. There are six instructors, with an average of fifteen students per class. In addition to the programs described below, Cottonwood also offers an Associate Polarity Practitioner (A.P.P.) Training, taught by Gary Peterson.

Accreditation and Approvals

The Cottonwood School of Massage Therapy is approved and regulated by the Division of Private Occupational Schools, Department of Higher Education, and is a member of the American Massage Therapy Association (AMTA) Council of Schools.

Graduates are qualified to take the National Certification Examination for Therapeutic Massage and Bodywork (NCETMB).

Program Description

Cottonwood offers three massage therapy programs:

The 500-hour, twelve-month Basic Massage Therapist Program consists of three fifteen-week trimesters. Classes include Musculoskeletal Anatomy and Myology; Massage Theory and Practice (Swedish); Myology, Systemic Anatomy/Physiology; Deep Tissue Massage; and Neuromuscular Therapy and Muscle Energy Procedures/Clinical Massage Practicum.

The 750-hour Intermediate Massage Therapist Program is typically completed within eighteen months. Classes include Business 101 for Massage Therapists; Ethics; NCBTMB Review and Prep; Shiatsu; Musculoskeletal Anatomy and Myology; Massage Theory and Practice; Myology, Systemic Anatomy/Physiology; Deep Tissue Massage; Therapeutic Massage; Clinical Massage Practicum; Positional Release Techniques; plus 104 hours of the student's choosing from Specialty Focus classes. Completion of the program is at the student's own pace.

The 1,000-hour Advanced Massage Therapist Program is typically completed within twenty-four months. Classes include Musculoskeletal Anatomy and Myology; Massage Theory and Practice; Myology, Systemic Anatomy/Physiology; Deep Tissue Massage; Therapeutic Massage; Clinical Massage Practicum; Business 101; NCBTMB Review; Ethics; Shiatsu; Positional Release; Advanced Neuromuscular Therapy; Advanced Pathology; Sports Massage; Classical Massage; plus 202 hours of the student's choosing from Specialty Focus classes. Completion of the program is at the student's own pace.

Specialty Focus classes that may be chosen as part of the 750-hour and 1,000-hour programs include Advanced Neuromuscular Therapy, Advanced Pathology, Aromatherapy, Classical Massage Techniques, Contemplative Massage, Cranial Sacral Therapy, Day Spa Procedures, Facilitating Inner Peace, Geriatric Massage, Herbology, Integrated Approach to Holistic Wellness Care, Intuitive Communications, Korean Reflexology, Massage Therapy for Pregnancy, Massage Therapy for Labor and Delivery, Massage Therapy for Postpartum, Movement in Massage, Reflexology, Reiki, Save Your Thumbs, Seated Massage, Sports Massage, and Tui Na.

Admission Requirements

Applicants must be at least 18 years of age, have a high school diploma or equivalent, be physically able and emotionally stable, and have an admissions interview.

Tuition and Fees

Tuition for the 500-hour program is $4,000; for the 750-hour program, $5,625; and for the 1,000-hour program, $7,250. Additional expenses include application fee, $40; *Graf's Anatomy*, $100 per year; clinic clothing, $20 per year; student liability insurance, $35 per year; sheets and oil, $10 per month; required massages by teachers (two per trimester), $70 per trimester; CPR class, $25 per year; and massage table, $500 and up.

Financial Assistance

Bank financing, veterans' benefits, and other forms of financing are available.

Crestone Healing Arts Center

P.O. Box 156
Crestone, Colorado 81131
PHONE: (719) 256-4036
FAX: (719) 256-4036
E-MAIL: retuta@crestonehac.com

At Crestone Healing Arts Center, founded in 1994 by Dan Retuta, massage is seen as a spiritual as well as a technical discipline. The school is an experiment in community, as students live, study, and train together in a retreat-style environment. There is one instructor, with an average of seven students per class.

Accreditation and Approvals

Graduates are qualified to take the National Certification Examination for Therapeutic Massage and Bodywork (NCETMB).

Program Description

A twelve-week, 520-hour in-residence Massage Therapy Certification Program divides instruction into Massage and Support courses. Massage courses comprise 279 hours and include Acupressure, Reflexology, Shiatsu, Swedish Massage, Integrated Massage, Prenatal Massage, Emotional Balancing Techniques, and On-Site Stress Relief. Support courses take up the remaining 241 hours and include Group Dynamics and Open Forum, Movement and Qi Development, Herbology for Massage Therapists, Business Practice, Basic Oriental Healing Philosophy, CPR/First Aid, Community Massage Practicum, and Anatomy and Physiology.

Admission Requirements

Applicants must be at least 18 years of age, have a high school diploma or equivalent, have received at least one professional massage, and have an interview. Students must also be ready to engage in all aspects of CHAC programs.

Tuition and Fees

Tuition is $3,950. Additional expenses include a $40 application fee; in-residence housing, $850; books, $375; CPR training, text, and certification, $45; herbology training, $180; supplies and materials, $75 to $150; and student liability insurance, $45.

Financial Assistance

Payment plans are available.

Day-Star Method of Yoga

2565 South Meade Street
Denver, Colorado 80219
PHONE: (303) 934-6309
FAX: (303) 975-9381
E-MAIL: solsiren@aol.com

Susan Flanders, director and instructor of Day-Star Yoga, has been teaching yoga for twenty-six years and training classical yoga teachers for over fifteen years. There are two instructors, with an average of six to ten students per class.

Program Description

The 100-hour Hatha Yoga Teacher's Course is a purely classical system. The thirteen-class program meets one Sunday per month and includes Yogic Thought, Basic Principles of Classic Hatha Yoga, Asana, Breath, Teaching Techniques, Body-Mind, Five Ways of Bending, Working with the Body, Body Work, Student Teaching, Lesson Plans, Stress, Relaxation, Meditation,

Special Populations, Business, Advertising, and more. Students are required to read and report on six books, take seven quizzes, teach eight student teaching sessions, submit a final exam, attend a full semester of standard yoga classes (as a student teacher), teach a mini-class to a group of friends, and make a relaxation tape.

Admission Requirements

Applicants should have the desire to teach; it is recommended, but not required, that students have two years of yoga practice.

Tuition and Fees

Tuition is $1,000; books are additional.

Financial Assistance

A payment plan is available.

Institute of Integrative Aromatherapy

(See Multiple State Locations, pages 395-96)

International Veterinary Acupuncture Society

(See Multiple State Locations, pages 398-99)

Massage Therapy Institute of Colorado

1441 York Street, Suite 301
Denver, Colorado 80206-2127
PHONE: (303) 329-6345

The Massage Therapy Institute of Colorado (MTIC) was founded in 1986 by Mark H. Manton. MTIC has developed a unique style of clinically effective massage techniques that integrate information from several massage and healing disciplines. MTIC shares space with the Colorado School of Traditional Chinese Medicine.

Accreditation and Approvals

MTIC is approved and regulated by the Division of Private Occupational Schools, State of Colorado Department of Higher Education. Graduates are qualified to take the National Certification Examination for Therapeutic Massage and Bodywork (NCETMB).

Program Description

A 1,060-hour program is offered in Western clinical massage that emphasizes the use of Swedish massage, deep tissue massage, neuromuscular therapy, reflexology, and allied massage methods such as myofascial techniques and abdominal organ manipulation. Courses include General Anatomy and Pathology, Anatomy Project Lab, Kinesiology I and II, General Pathology, Allied Modalities—Hydro- and Heliotherapy, Business Management, Basic Student Massage Clinic, Advanced Student Massage Clinic, Swedish Massage, Deep Tissue, Neuromuscular Therapy, Reflexology, Myofascial Therapy, and 100 hours of required modules that include Asian I and II, Myofascial, Posture Lab, Sports Massage, Psychology Bodywork, Ethics, Self-Care for Massage Therapists, and Insurance Billing. In addition, in Practicum I—Giving, students perform 350 program hours of massage; in Practicum II—Receiving, students receive 100 hours of massage; in Practicum III—Private Evaluations, which is scheduled quarterly, students' progress in hand skills and massage techniques is assessed. Students must also complete a CPR certification course in order to be certified as massage therapists. Day and evening programs are available.

Continuing Education

Second-year advanced training is offered in myofascial therapy and remedial massotherapy.

Admission Requirements

Applicants must be at least 21 years of age and preferably have completed an A.A., B.S., or B.A. degree. Age and degree requirements may be waived providing the applicant has equivalent life experiences and demonstrates a desire and aptitude for massage therapy training.

Tuition and Fees

Tuition is $5900. Other costs include: application fee, $25; books, $300 prepared literature, $35; student liability insurance, $95 per year; table and accessories, $450 to $750; four to six optional massages, $140 to $200; Banya session (hydrotherapy session at Izba Spa), $70; clinic polo shirt, $20; and documentation notebook, $15.

Financial Assistance
A payment plan is available.

MountainHeart School of Bodywork and Transformational Therapy

P.O. Box 575
Crested Butte, Colorado 81224
PHONE: (970) 349-0473 / (800) 673-0539
FAX: (970) 349-0473
E-MAIL: cragmc@crestedbutte.net
WEBSITE: user.gunnison.com/~cragmc/MtnHrtSchlHm.html

MountainHeart was founded in 1997 by Christine and Craig McLaughlin. There are four instructors, with an average of ten students per class.

Accreditation and Approvals
MountainHeart is approved and regulated by the Colorado Division of Private Occupational Schools. Graduates of massage therapy programs of 500 hours or more are qualified to take the National Certification Examination for Therapeutic Massage and Bodywork (NCETMB).

Program Description
Courses in the 850-hour Certified Massage Therapist (CMT) Program include Aligning with Purpose, Learning Strategies, Awareness and Transformation, Business and Marketing, Therapeutic Massage, Experiential Anatomy and Physiology, Therapeutic Relationships, Therapy Integration, Assessment Skills, The Body Metaphoric, Transformational Neuromuscular Therapy, Assisted Stretching, Internal Organ Massage and Balancing, The Language of Dreams, Transforming Trauma, and BodyGuide Energy Work. Classes are held days, evenings, and/or weekends.

The 1,000-hour Massage Therapy Program consists of the 850-hour CMT program along with an additional 150 hours of course work selected from their other programs or continuing education courses (see below). This may be completed while in the CMT program or after graduation.

The 218-hour Reflexology Program includes courses in Business and Marketing, Experiential Anatomy and Physiology, Introduction to Reflexology, and Basic, Intermediate and Advanced Reflexology. There are no prerequisites.

The forty-two-hour Spa Therapy Program is open to CMT students or graduates, or with permission. Courses include Spa Therapies 1 and 2, and Hydrotherapy; topics include essential oils, dry brushing, scalp massage, exfoliation and mud treatments.

The eighty-hour Sports Massage Program is open to CMT students or graduates, or with permission. Courses include Therapeutic Massage 3, Sports Massage: Injury Free Training and Competition, and Sports Rehabilitation Massage.

A ninety-six-hour Instructors Program is open to CMT graduates, licensed professionals or with permission. Courses include Learning Strategies, Learning Strategies for Instructors, and Classroom Facilitation.

Continuing Education
Many of the courses for all of MountainHeart's programs are also available as CEUs or electives. Other continuing education courses that may be offered include Aromatherapy, Allergy Re-Scripting, Beliefs and Health, Cranium Reflex Therapy, Developing Your Intuitive Abilities, Holistic Healing Through Herbs and Nutrition, Massage for the Elderly, Infant and Toddler Massage, Meditation, On-Site Massage, Shiatsu, Tai Chi, Therapeutic Yoga, and others.

Admission Requirements
Applicants must be at least 18 years of age, mentally and emotionally healthy, and physically able to perform and receive massage, and must interview with an admissions representative.

Tuition and Fees
Tuition is as follows: 850-hour CMT Program, $6,163; Reflexology, $1,799; Spa Therapy, $347; Sports Massage, $660; Instructors, $888. Tuition for the 1,000-hour Massage Therapy Program depends on electives chosen. Fees for continuing education/elective courses range from $132 to $330, depending on hours.

Approximate additional expenses include a $50 application fee; books, $250; supplies, $100; professional massages, $45; massage table, $400; student liability insurance, $39.

Financial Assistance
Private student loans are available

Polarity Center of Colorado

1721 Redwood Avenue
Boulder, Colorado 80304
PHONE: (303) 443-9847
FAX: (303) 415-1839
E-MAIL: chittyj@aol.com
WEBSITE: www.polaritycolorado.com

The Polarity Center of Colorado (PCC) was founded in 1991. PCC emphasizes the importance of craniosacral therapy and its integration within polarity, and includes craniosacral training in both its A.P.P. and R.P.P. programs. There are three instructors plus teaching assistants; classes range from six to twenty-six students.

Accreditation and Approvals

PCC is approved and regulated by the Division of Private Educational Schools, Department of Higher Education, State of Colorado. The A.P.P. and R.P.P. programs are approved by the American Polarity Therapy Association (APTA) and by the Craniosacral Therapy Association of North America (CSTA/NA).

Program Description

PCC offers Polarity Level I and Level II training, based on APTA's educational requirements for Associate Polarity Practitioner (A.P.P.) and Registered Polarity Practitioner (R.P.P.), respectively.

The 120-hour Level I Associate Polarity Practitioner training includes such topics as Cranial I and II, Polarity Theory and Practice, Verbal and Theory (practitioner skills to verbally guide and support the client), Nervous Systems, Five Elements, Bodyreading, and Integration. The program may be taken one weekend per month over six months, or in a "Fast Track" format four days per week for four weeks. For APTA certification, students must also give thirty one-hour polarity sessions, receive five sessions from R.P.P.s, and complete ten additional hours of anatomy and physiology.

The 340-hour Level II Registered Polarity Practitioner training deepens the concepts introduced in Level I, refines and develops practitioner skills, and introduces additional advanced approaches. Topics include Craniosacral Therapy, trauma resolution, communication skills, advanced study of energy patterns, and structural and connective tissue applications. The program may be taken one weekend per month for sixteen months, or in a Fast Track format four days per week for twelve consecutive weeks.

The 350-hour modular Craniosacral Training is designed to meet RCST certification requirements of the Craniosacral Association of North America. Topics include accessing the Breath of Life via felt-sense and palpation, gaining in-depth knowledge of the craniosacral system, identifying and resolving tissue shapes and patterns, fluid-based approaches to specific body areas, trauma resolution, and working with specific pathologies and symptoms. The fifty-day program may be taken as five-day "long weekends" every three months for a total of ten modules.

Admission Requirements

Applicants must be at least 18 years of age unless accompanied by a parent and with special permission. A high school diploma or equivalent is required. Advanced trainings require satisfactory completion of entry-level programs.

Tuition and Fees

Tuition for the Level I training is $1,775 in the weekend format or $1,595 in the Fast Track format. Tuition for the Level II training is $4,395 in the weekend format or $4,495 in the Fast Track format. Craniosacral training is $5,450.

Financial Assistance

Prepayment discounts are available.

Rocky Mountain Center for Botanical Studies

P.O. Box 19254
Boulder, Colorado 80308-2254
PHONE: (303) 442-6861
FAX: (303) 442-6294
E-MAIL: sharih@indra.com
WEBSITE: www.herbschool.com

The Rocky Mountain Center for Botanical Studies (RMCBS) was founded in 1992 by herbalist Feather Jones. There are twenty-five instructors plus guest instructors, with an average of thirty-five students per class.

Accreditation and Approvals

RMCBS is approved and regulated by the Colorado Department of Higher Education, Division of Private Occupational Schools. RMCBS meets approval of the Rocky Mountain Herbalists Coalition.

Program Description

The 707-hour Professional Training for Year One, Western Herbalism Program meets three days per week for four ten-week quarters. Courses include Introduction to Herbalism, Herbal Pharmacy, Earth-Centered Herbalism: The Talking Leaves, Materia Medica: Organ Systems and Herbal Therapeutics, Nutrition, Aromatherapy, Anatomy and Physiology, Basic Principles of Botany, Herb Walks and Ethical Wild Harvesting Techniques, Organic Gardening, Field Trips, Ethnobotany, Pharmacognosy, Wild Foods: Gathering and Preparation, Pathology, Physical Assessment, Case Studies Review, Standard Practice Medicine, Herbal Business Management and Tours, Business Ethics and Practice Issues, Communication Skills: Conflict Resolution and Problem Solving, and Project Review and Presentation.

The 422-hour Advanced Herbal Studies Program: Western Herbalism II is a second-year day program open to first-year RMCBS graduates as well as students from other schools with at least 600 hours of herbal education and knowledge of the local materia medica. Courses include Pathophysiology, Aromatherapy, Flower Essences, Earth Centered Herbalism, Clinical Nutrition, Herbal Therapeutics, Pharmacognosy, Clinical Case Studies, Field Trip, Internship/Practicum, Introduction to Clinical Herbalism, Organ Systems Review, Pharmacology, Introduction to Diagnostics, Interview Skills, Clinical Procedures, Referral Skills, Herbal Pharmacy: Formulations and Dosages, Case Analysis, Toxicology, Side-Effects and Drug Interactions, and Practice Development.

A 252-hour Clinical Herbalism Internship is offered to RM-CBS graduates as well as practitioners or advanced students from other schools with at least 800 hours of herbal education or relevant experience. The program consists of a nine-month internship in the student-run Consultation Center. Students perform intakes and follow-up evaluations, then present each case to fellow students and professional herbalists at weekly round table sessions. Each round table is preceded by a short class on advanced herbal topics.

The 600-hour Essence of Herbalism Evening Certificate Program meets two evenings per week and ten Saturdays per year for two years. Courses include Introduction to Herbalism, Materia Medica: Organ Systems and Herbal Therapeutics, Basic Principles of Botany, Anatomy and Physiology, Nutrition, Herb Walks and Ethical Wild Harvesting Techniques, Herbal Pharmacy, Earth Centered Herbalism, Pathology, Case Studies Review, Physical Assessment, Pharmacognosy, Standard Practice Medicine, Ethnobotany, Business Ethics and Practice Issues, Organic Gardening, Field Trips (a four-day trip to Northern New Mexico and a four-day trip to Arizona), Wild Foods Gathering and Preparation, and Communication Skills: Conflict Resolution and Problem Solving.

Community and Continuing Education

RMCBS offers noncertificate programs covering a variety of topics throughout the year. These programs are open to the public as well as RMCBS students and graduates. Topics have included the Herbal Supplements Retail Training Program, Herbal Adventure in the Rockies: An Introductory Hands-On Intensive, Shamanic Herbalism: Ancient Roots of Healing, Clinical Case Studies Conference, and workshops featuring expert herbalists such as Rosemary Gladstar, Michael Moore, and David Winston.

Admission Requirements

Applicants will be accepted with different educational backgrounds. A high school diploma or equivalent is recommended; an interview and two letters of recommendation are required.

Tuition and Fees

The application fee for all programs is $25.

Tuition for the Year One, Western Herbalism Program is $6,900. Additional expenses include books, $250; field trips, $350; and tools and supplies, $175.

Tuition for Western Herbalism II is $4,400. Additional expenses include books, $250; field trips, $350; and tools and supplies, $175.

Tuition for the Clinical Herbalism Internship is $2,600.

Tuition for the Essence of Herbalism Evening Program is $3,050. Additional expenses include books, $250; field trips, $200; and tools and supplies, $175.

Financial Assistance

Payment plans are available.

Rocky Mountain Institute of Yoga and Ayurveda

P.O. Box 1091
Boulder, Colorado 80306-1091
PHONE: (303) 443-6923
FAX: (303) 443-7956

The Rocky Mountain Institute of Yoga and Ayurveda (RMIYA) was founded in 1990 by five instructors; by 1996, the faculty had expanded to a core of seven, with nine guest faculty members. Because each teacher arranges his or her own class space, classes are offered in Allenspark, Boulder, Denver, and Longmont.

Program Description

The Certification Program in Yoga Therapy and Ayurveda requires forty credits, plus 150 prior or concurrently accumulated asana class hours; it is recommended that students take or have taken at least one course in biochemistry, anatomy, or physiology. Courses include Pranayama and Meditation Levels I and II, Ayurvedic Medicine I, Intermediate Ayurveda: Assessment and Treatment, Medicine for Holistic Health Practitioners, Women's Health Care Through Ayurveda, Asana as Therapy, Asana and Anatomy, Principles of Alignment in Yoga Asana Practice, Asana and Ayurveda, Seminars in Ayurveda, Ayurvedic Massage, Ayurvedic Diet/Ayurvedic Cooking, Karma Yoga: The Yoga of Action and Service, Yoga Psychology and Ayurvedic Psychiatry, Diagnostic Skills in Ayurveda, Pancha Karma: The Cleansing Practices of Yoga and Ayurveda, Ayurveda/Yoga Therapy Internship, and others.

The Practice and Teaching of Yoga Certification Program requires thirty-five credits. Courses include Yoga Philosophy and the Yoga Sutras; Pranayama and Meditation Levels I through III; Mantra, Ritual, and the Devotional Practices of Yoga; Asana and Ayurveda; Classical Yoga Asanas; Principles of Alignment in Yoga Asana Practice; Advanced Asana Practice in the Classical Tradition; Shat Karma and Pancha Karma; Asana as Therapy; Karma Yoga and the Bhagavad Gita; Yoga Psychology; Internship/Student Teaching; Asana for Teachers; and others. In addition, a total of ninety to 150 hours of asana practice time must be accumulated, distributed in the three asana lineages of Classical, Structural/Iyengar, and Ashtanga Vinyasa. Previous asana training may be credited toward this requirement. Students with extensive asana background may complete the program in three semesters.

Admission Requirements

It is preferred that applicants have a bachelor's degree.

Tuition and Fees

Tuition is charged on a per-class basis, ranging from $50 to $350 per class; average early registration tuition is approximately $10 per hour.

Financial Assistance

A discount is given for early registration; work exchanges are available.

Rolf Institute of Structural Integration

205 Canyon Boulevard
Boulder, Colorado 80302
PHONE: (303) 449-5903 / (800) 530-8875
FAX: (303) 449-5978
E-MAIL: RolfInst@aol.com
WEBSITE: www.rolf.org

The Rolf Institute was founded in 1972 by Ida P. Rolf, Ph.D., who examined many systems, including osteopathy, yoga, and chiropractic, in her search for an understanding of structural order. She developed a sequence of work called structural integration that releases the body from lifelong patterns of tension and balances the body, leading to improved appearance and relief from neck, back, and other mobility problems. There are thirty instructors; maximum class sizes are twenty-two students in Unit I, sixteen in Units II and III. Rolfing training is also available in Brazil, Europe, and Australia.

Accreditation and Approvals

The Rolf Institute is the sole certifying body for Rolfers. Graduates of the training programs may refer to themselves as Certified Rolfers and Rolf Movement Practitioners, and may offer this work to the public.

Program Description

In order to become Certified Rolfers, students must complete a series of steps:

1. Experience a ten-session Rolfing series and eight Rolfing Movement Integration sessions (a list of area practitioners may be obtained from the institute).

2. Unit One: Foundations of Bodywork (FOB). This six-week course explores skillful touch, therapeutic relationship, anatomy, kinesiology, and physiology as they relate to Rolfing. Those with training in massage or bodywork may skip this step.

3. Complete the admissions packet and take the entrance exam.

4. Principles of Rolfing Through Movement. This five-day course presents the principles of Rolfing and Rolfing Movement Integration.

5. Unit Two: Embodiment of Rolfing and Rolfing Movement. This seven-week course includes the study of fascial anatomy, recognizing simple structural patterns, integrating functional and structural approaches to Rolfing, and gaining a working knowledge of Rolfing principles. Students give and receive a series of ten Rolfing sessions and three Rolfing Movement sessions.

6. Interim Period. Students are assigned a written paper.

7. Unit Three: Clinical Application of Rolfing Theory. In this eight-week course, students take three clients through the ten series of Rolfing and study fascial anatomy, efficient body use, and business skills and ethics. At this point, the student becomes a Certified Rolfer.

8. Rolfing Movement Certification. This optional four-week course permits students to deepen their understanding of Rolfing Movement. At this point, the student is a Certified Rolf Movement Practitioner.

Community and Continuing Education

Once graduates are certified as Rolfers, they must attend a minimum of eighteen days of approved continuing education over a period of three to seven years in preparation for Advanced Rolfing Training. Such continuing education workshops include instruction in specific manipulative techniques, craniosacral therapy, visceral manipulation, and other subjects.

After a minimum of three years in Rolfing practice and eighteen approved continuing education credits, practitioners must complete a 180-hour, six-week Advanced Rolfing Certification course. This course must be completed within seven years of Rolfing Certification in order to maintain membership in the Institute.

Admission Requirements

Applicants must have experienced the benefits of Rolfing; demonstrate an understanding of anatomy, kinesiology, and physiology; have experience with touch in hands-on application; have experience with the therapeutic relationship; and be of sound moral character. Before beginning Unit Two, applicants must have received ten sessions of Rolfing from a Certified Rolfer; have received eight Rolfing Movement Integration sessions from a Rolf Movement Practitioner; submit letters of recommendation from a Rolfer and Rolfing Movement Teacher; have a B.A. or B.S. degree or comparable life experience; successfully complete the Rolf Institute equivalency exam; have documented experience of training and practice of touch; have fieldwork experience evaluated by a Rolfer; complete the application packet; and successfully complete Principles of Rolfing.

Tuition and Fees

There is a $75 application fee. The equivalency exam for those not taking FOB is $225; books are $250 to $500. Tuition for Unit One is $2,500; for Principles of Rolfing and Unit Two, $5,400; for Unit Three, $5,500, and for Rolfing Movement Certification, $2,900.

Shambhava School of Yoga

2875 County Road #67
Boulder, Colorado 80303
PHONE: (303) 494-3051

FAX: (303) 642-0116
E-MAIL: Kailasa@shoshoni.org
WEBSITE: www.shoshoni.org

The Shambhava School of Yoga was founded in 1976; Shoshoni was founded in 1988 as a yoga and health retreat center. There are six instructors, with an average of fifteen students per class.

Program Description

The six-month Hatha Yoga Teacher Training Program is designed to bring a meditative focus to the practice of yoga, transforming the student into the teacher. Classes meet Sundays, Wednesdays, and one additional day per week. Session One emphasizes classical yoga postures and using the elements of yoga to release our inner energy and open within. Principles of anatomy are also taught, and a meditative practice will be established. Session Two develops an understanding of the principles of vinyasa, counterpose, and modification, emphasizing the development of the student as teacher. Students are exposed to various styles and levels of teaching, including, for those interested, advanced teachings of Kundalini yoga. Students also continue meditation classes. Requirements for the certificate include instructor evaluation, completion of a six- to eight-week yoga course outline, participation in a minimum of 180 course hours, and two weekend yoga retreats at Shoshoni Retreat.

A 160-hour, month-long residential Hatha Yoga Teacher's Training is offered at Shoshoni Yoga Retreat. Instructor Sita Davies emphasizes form (asana), breath (pranayama), and focus (dharana) for a union of body, breath, mind and spirit. Students participate in the yogic lifestyle as residents of the ashram community, filling their days with yoga classes and practice, pranayama, meditation, chanting, and seva (selfless service).

Four-week residential Hatha Yoga Teacher Training Programs are available at Shoshoni Yoga Retreat, P.O. Box 410, Rollinsville, Colorado 80474, (303) 642-0116.

Tuition and Fees

Tuition for the six-month program is $1,790. Tuition includes all classes and two weekend retreats with dorm accommodations at Shoshoni Retreat; books and materials are additional.

Tuition for the month-long residential program is $1,950 including accommodations.

Financial Assistance

Payment plans are available.

South West School of Massage

1309 East 3rd Avenue
P.O. Box 4111
Durango, Colorado 81302
PHONE/FAX: (970) 259-6965
E-MAIL: swsm@frontier.net
WEBSITE: www.swsm.com

The South West School of Massage (SWSM) was founded in 1997 by Jill Clark. There are ten instructors, with ten to twenty students per class.

Accreditation and Approvals

The program at SWSM is approved and regulated by the Division of Private Occupational Schools, Department of Higher Education. Graduates are qualified to take the National Certification Examination for Therapeutic Massage and Bodywork (NCETMB).

Program Description

The 850-hour Massage Therapy Program may be completed in seven months of full-time study or thirteen months of part-time study. Courses include Swedish Massage, Movement, Sports Massage, Neuromuscular Therapy, Connective Tissue Therapy, Deep Tissue Massage, Polarity, Reflexology, Anatomy and Physiology, Kinesiology and Pathology, Oriental Theory, Hygiene and Hydrotherapy, Modality Integration, Massage Practicum: Clinic Internship, and sixty-three hours of Additional/Supplemental Courses in such areas as Chair Massage, Communication Skills, Infant and Pregnancy Massage, Law, Business Development and Ethics.

Admission Requirements

Applicants must be at least 18 years of age, have a high school diploma or equivalent, have a personal interview, have the physical ability to perform massage, submit two letters of recommendation and essays, and have received at least two professional massage treatments. SWSM does not discriminate against those with HIV or Hepatitis C, but must be made aware of these situations in advance in order to make proper arrangements.

Tuition and Fees

Tuition is $6,100 and includes books, CPR and First Aid training, and certificate. Additional expenses include a $50 application fee; supplies, approximately $100; and three professional massages received by a therapist of the student's choice. The purchase of a massage table is highly recommended and SWSM offers student discounts.

Southwest Acupuncture College

(See Multiple State Locations, pages 413–14)

Wellness Institute

(See Multiple State Locations, pages 418–19)

CONNECTICUT

Connecticut Center for Massage Therapy

Main School Address:
75 Kitts Lane
Newington, Connecticut 06111-3954
PHONE: (860) 667-1886
FAX: (860) 667-2175

BRANCH ADDRESS:
25 Sylvan Road South
Westport, Connecticut 06880
PHONE: (203) 221-7325
FAX: (203) 221-0144
E-MAIL: info@ccmt.com
WEBSITE: www.ccmt.com

The Connecticut Center for Massage Therapy, Inc. (CCMT), began with small workshop trainings given by cofounder and current owner Steve Kitts and others in the Hartford area in 1978; in 1992, CCMT opened its Westport branch. There are fifty-five instructors, with an average of twenty students per class.

Accreditation and Approvals

CCMT is accredited by the Accrediting Commission of Career Schools and Colleges of Technology (ACCSCT) and by the Commission on Massage Training Accreditation (COMTA). Graduates are qualified to take the National Certification Examination for Therapeutic Massage and Bodywork (NCETMB).

Program Description

The 638-hour, forty-four-credit Massage Therapist Program includes Acupressure, Anatomy and Physiology, Business Practices, Clinic/Internship, Energetic Foundations, Kinesiology, Massage Therapy, Palpation Lab, Pathology, Professional Foundations, and Standard First Aid/CPR.

An 1,100-hour, seventy-five-credit Clinical Massage Therapist Program is currently in development and will be offered in Westport in May 1999 subject to final approval. The program is intended to meet New York State's increased licensing requirements of 1,000 hours.

Classes are held mornings, afternoons, and evenings. A weekend section is started once each year.

Community and Continuing Education

A two-day "Discovery" workshop is offered throughout the year as an introduction to the school and to massage techniques. An open house is offered at each campus once each month.

The Advanced Studies program provides continuing education to practicing massage therapists, bodyworkers, and other health care practitioners. Offerings include one-day and weekend workshops and certification programs in specific techniques.

Admission Requirements

Applicants must be 18 years of age or older, have a high school diploma or equivalent, be proficient in the English language, be physically capable of performing massage techniques, and interview with the admissions director. Prospective students must also show evidence of receiving at least one professional massage within one year prior to application.

Tuition and Fees

There is a $25 application fee and a $150 registration fee. Tuition for the Massage Therapist Program is $9,750; books are $400 to

$700; and an optional massage table costs $400 to $700 and up. The "Discovery" workshop costs $75 per person.

Financial Assistance
Federal grants and loans and payment plans are available for qualified applicants.

Connecticut Institute for Herbal Studies

87 Market Square
Newington, Connecticut 06111
PHONE: (860) 666-5064

The Connecticut Institute for Herbal Studies (CIHS) was founded in 1992 by director Laura Mignosa, a certified Chinese herbologist, vice president of the Connecticut Herbal Association, national lecturer, and columnist on Chinese herbs.

Accreditation and Approvals
Most courses are eligible for continuing educational units granted by the National Certification Commission for Acupuncture and Oriental Medicine (NCCAOM) and the Massachusetts Committee on Acupuncture.

Program Description
A five-month course in traditional Chinese herbology meets one weekend per month and offers instruction in individual herbs, guiding formulas, and diagnostic paradigms used in Chinese medicine. Topics covered include herbs and formulas used for specific organs, shang han lun, wen bing theory, and yin and yang tonics.

A five-month course in Western herbology is also offered. Classes meet one weekend per month and include all organ systems, herb identification, weed walks, and safety of herbs and contraindications, with special attention to formulas for children, women, and the elderly. Students will create their own herbal medicine cabinets.

A five-month Chinese Herbology and Theory Program meets one weekend per month and is accepted by the NCCAOM for credits toward national certification. Students must have completed a course in Oriental medical theory prior to enrollment. The program teaches the fundamentals of Chinese med-icine and the therapeutic use of over one hundred herbs, and includes herb identification, tastes, formulas, usages, contraindications, preparations, and how and where to purchase herbs.

An Accelerated TCM Theory Course may be taken as a prerequisite for Chinese Herbology and Theory (above). This six-week course meets one evening per week and covers such topics as yin/yang, eight principal and five element theories, physiology, pathology, boundaries and ethics, and more.

A two-weekend Aromatherapy Certificate Program teaches laypersons and practitioners the history, uses, and benefits of aromatherapy, and includes hands-on training.

Community and Continuing Education
Evening and weekend community and continuing education courses are offered in a wide variety of topics, including Vegetarian Cooking, Feng Shui, Chinese Herbs and Common Ailments, Jin Shin Do, Qigong, Pulse Diagnosis, Backyard Herbs, and Evening Weed Walks.

Admission Requirements
Applicants must be at least 18 years of age, have a high school diploma or equivalent, and interview with an admissions representative.

Tuition and Fees
Tuition for the Traditional Chinese Herbology course is $1,250. Tuition for the Western Herbology course is $595. Tuition for the community and continuing education courses varies with the length of the course, from $19 for some evening seminars to $189 for weekend seminars. Tuition for the Chinese Herbology and Theory Course is $875; for the Accelerated TCM Theory Course, $259; and for the Aromatherapy Certificate Program, $159.

Financial Assistance
Payment plans may be arranged on an individual basis.

The Connecticut School for Hypnosis and NLP

28 Gravel Street
Meriden, Connecticut 06450
PHONE: (203) 238-3152 / (203) 237-9779
FAX: (203) 639-1231
E-MAIL: donnassen@home.com
WEBSITE: NLPnow

The Connecticut School for Hypnosis and NLP was founded in 1999 by Don Nassen, an NLP Master Practitioner who is the primary instructor.

Accreditation and Approvals
The Connecticut School for Hypnosis and NLP is approved by the International Medical and Dental Hypnotherapy Association (IMDHA) and is in the process of applying for state accreditation.

Program Description
The first class to be offered is a Practitioner Hypnosis Class that meets for two weekends. This is a 40-hour course leading toward a 120-hour certification by the IMDHA. Topics covered include History of Hypnosis, Taking a Personal History, Pretalk, Calibration and Rapport, Suggestibility Tests, Inductions, Deepening Techniques, Scripts, Business, Jurisprudence, Sources of Information, and more.

Additional classes are planned; contact the school for information.

Admission Requirements
Applicants must be at least 18 years of age with a high school diploma or equivalent.

Tuition and Fees
Tuition for the Practitioner Hypnosis Class is $595.

Northwestern Connecticut Community-Technical College

Continuing Education
Park Place East
Winsted, Connecticut 06098-1798
PHONE: (860) 738-6444 / (860) 738-6446
FAX: (860) 738-6439
E-MAIL: nw_conted@commnet.edu
WEBSITE: www.nwctc.commnet.edu

Northwestern Connecticut Community-Technical College (NCCC) was founded in 1965 and offers degree, transfer, certificate, and continuing education programs in a variety of fields, including the Foundations in Herbal Medicine Certificate Program. Class sizes average ten students.

Accreditation and Approvals
NCCC is accredited by the New England Association of Schools and Colleges. The Foundations in Herbal Medicine Certificate Program may be taken for CEUs.

Program Description
The Foundations in Herbal Medicine Certificate Program is an intensive, in-depth study of herbal medicine consisting of an introductory class, required core courses, and electives supplemented with twelve modules of video learning and corresponding text, and facilitated by medical and naturopathic practitioners.

Admission Requirements
Applicants must be at least 18 years of age and have a high school diploma or equivalent.

Tuition and Fees
Tuition for the Introduction to the Foundations in Herbal Medicine program is $10. Each of the 12 modules in the Foundations in Herbal Medicine Certificate Program is $125.

University of Bridgeport

College of Chiropractic
Bridgeport, Connecticut 06601
PHONE: (203) 576-4279 / (888) 822-4476 (admissions)
FAX: (203) 576-4351 / (203) 576-4342 (admissions)
E-MAIL: l.hildreth@snet.net
WEBSITE: www.bridgeport.edu/chiro

Founded in 1990, the University of Bridgeport's College of Chiropractic is the only chiropractic college in New England and the first university-based chiropractic college in North America. The University of Bridgeport was founded in 1927, and its urban campus comprises ninety-one buildings. There are twenty full-time and thirty part-time instructors, with an average of thirty-two students per class.

Accreditation and Approvals

The University of Bridgeport College of Chiropractic is accredited by the Commission on Accreditation of the Council on Chiropractic Education (CCE) to award the Doctor of Chiropractic (D.C.) degree.

Program Description

The 5,118-hour Doctor of Chiropractic Degree Program is a four-year course of study that includes a clinical internship. The program is divided into the following: Basic Sciences (1,422 hours) including Anatomy, Physiology, Biochemistry, Neuroscience, Pathology, and Microbiology and Public Health; Clinical Sciences (2,550 hours), including Chiropractic History and Philosophy, Principles and Practice, Radiology, Research, Physiologic Therapeutics, Differential Diagnosis, Chiropractic Skills and Technique, Diagnosis, Nutrition, Emergency Procedures, and Business Procedures; and Clinical Services (1,140 hours of supervised patient care).

The College of Chiropractic and the Nutrition Institute offer a joint program for those who wish to pursue a Master of Science degree in human nutrition while working toward the D.C. degree. Chiropractic students will enter the master's program at an advanced level, completing seventeen semester hours of required nutrition courses (including Vitamin and Mineral Metabolism, Nutritional Therapeutics, Developmental Nutrition, Research in Nutrition, and Biostatistics) and three semester hours from an elective.

The University of Bridgeport also offers three prechiropractic programs: bachelor's degree programs consisting of a four-year bachelor's degree prior to entering Chiropractic College, or three years of prechiropractic study with credit earned in Chiropractic College for a bachelor's degree in biology or elective studies with a specialization in prechiropractic; the Basic Program (ninety credits), in which students can meet all require-

ments for Chiropractic College in three years of prechiropractic study; and the Accelerated Science Program, designed for students who already have a bachelor's degree, in which students complete all science prerequisites in two semesters.

Admission Requirements

Applicants for the doctoral program must have completed at least three years (ninety semester hours) of study toward a baccalaureate degree from an accredited, degree-granting institution, and must have achieved a cumulative GPA of 2.50 or greater; a baccalaureate degree is recommended. Specific courses in communication/language skills, psychology, humanities, general chemistry, organic chemistry, general physics, and general biology, zoology, or anatomy and physiology are required. Applicants must also submit three letters of recommendation and an essay.

Tuition and Fees

Tuition is $6,200 per semester; books and supplies are additional. Other fees include: application fee, $75; registration fee, $25 per semester; general university fee, $180 per semester; campus ID and security fee, $80 per semester; health insurance, $386 per year; and accident insurance, $54 per year. Chiropractic students may reside in on-campus residence halls for an additional $1,740 to $2,625 per semester.

Financial Assistance

Scholarships, grants, loans and work-study programs are available.

University of Bridgeport

College of Naturopathic Medicine
60 Lafayette Street
Bridgeport, Connecticut 06601
PHONE: (203) 576-4109 / (800) EXCEL-UB
FAX: (203) 576-4107
E-MAIL: natmed@bridgeport.edu
WEBSITE: www.bridgeport.edu

The College of Naturopathic Medicine was first licensed in December 1996. The University of Bridgeport was founded in 1927, and its urban campus comprises ninety-one buildings.

There are twenty-nine instructors, with an average of twenty students per class.

Accreditation and Approvals

The Doctor of Naturopathic Medicine degree program is licensed by the State of Connecticut Department of Higher Education. The program will hold itself to the professional educational standards required by the Council on Naturopathic Medical Education (CNME).

Program Description

The 4,752-contact-hour Doctor of Naturopathic Medicine Degree Program consists of four academic years plus a required summer recess clinical program. The program is offered on a full-time basis with no students admitted to a part-time course of study; there are no correspondence nor distance-learning courses offered.

The program consists of Basic Sciences (738 hours), which includes Anatomy, Histology, Embryology, Biochemistry, Physiology and Microbiology; Botanical Medicine (108 hours); Clinical Nutrition (144 hours); Clinical Sciences (945 hours), which includes Pathology, Clinical/Physical Diagnosis, Laboratory Diagnosis, Public Health/Epidemiology, Clinical Forum, Diagnostic Imaging, Immunology, Emergency Procedure, Medical Genetics, Pharmacology, and Environmental Medicine; Homeopathic Medicine (144 hours); Naturopathic Obstetrics (36 hours); Naturopathic Practice/Organ Systems (378 hours), which includes Gynecology, Pediatrics, Cardiology, Gastroenterology, Minor Surgery, Eye, Ear, Nose and Throat, Endocrinology, Neurology, Geriatrics, Urology/Proctology, Oncology, and Dermatology; Naturopathic Principles and Practice (162 hours), which includes Naturopathic History and Philosophy, Naturopathic Philosophy and Therapeutics, Practice Management, and Medical Jurisprudence and Ethics; Oriental Medicine (72 hours); Physical Medicine (495 hours), which include Living Anatomy, Hydrotherapy, Physiological Therapeutics, Naturopathic Manipulative Therapeutics, Preventive/Therapeutic Exercise, and Orthopedics/ Sports Medicine; Psychology (162 hours), which includes Physician Heal Thyself, Communication Skills, Counseling Skills and Technique, The Doctor/Patient Relationship, Psychological Assessment, and Addictions and Disorders; Research (72 hours), which includes Research Methodology/Statistics and Thesis; and Clinical Education (1,296 hours).

Much of the first two years is devoted to the basic sciences and an introduction to the philosophy, history and principles of naturopathic medicine. The second two years consist largely of the clinical sciences, including instruction in the various modalities of naturopathic medicine, their application to bodily systems, and practical hands-on integration of didactic learning with patient treatment.

Admission Requirements

Applicants must have a baccalaureate degree from an accredited, degree-granting institution and must have completed preprofessional education with a minimum Quality Point Ratio of 2.50 on a 4.00 scale. The following specific courses must have been completed: Communication/Language Skills, six semester hours; Psychology, three semester hours; Social Science, three semester hours; Humanities, three semester hours; Electives (Social Sciences/Humanities), nine semester hours; General Biology/Zoology/Anatomy and Physiology (with Lab), six semester hours; General Chemistry (with lab), six semester hours; Organic Chemistry (with lab), six semester hours; General Physics (with lab), six semester hours. All biology/zoology/anatomy and physiology, chemistry, and physics courses must have been passed with a grade of C or better and with a cumulative science GPA of 2.5 or better, and must have been taken within the last seven years. Applicants must also submit three letters of recommendation.

Tuition and Fees

Tuition is $6,600 per semester; books and supplies are additional. Other fees include: application fee, $75; registration, campus ID and security, and general university fee, $395 per semester; health and accident insurance, $403 per year. Naturopathic students may reside in on-campus residence halls for an additional $2,015 to $2,845 per semester.

Financial Assistance

Scholarships, grants, loans, and work-study programs are available.

DISTRICT OF COLUMBIA
Institute for Integrated Therapies

3000 Connecticut Avenue NW, Suite 104
Washington, DC 20008
PHONE: (202) 387-0469
FAX: (703) 931-8567

The Institute for Integrated Therapies was founded in 1985 by current director Dr. Margaret L. D'Urso. There are two to eight, instructors, with a minimum of twelve and maximum of twenty-four students per class.

Accreditation and Approvals
The Institute is approved by the National Certification Board for Therapeutic Massage and Bodywork (NCBTMB) as a continuing education provider. Licensure and accreditation are pending.

Program Description
The 130-hour Basic Reflexology Certification Program consists of Beginning Reflexology (history, principles, reflexes, mapping, and techniques), Intermediate Reflexology (anatomy and physiology, client-therapist interaction, sensory skills, reflexes and techniques, and reflexology goals, benefits, and contraindications), Advanced Reflexology (advanced application with additional techniques, reflexes and meridian points, business procedures, supplies and equipment, and more), Practicum, Tutorials and Workbook, supervised sessions, and Certification Class, offering student testing and additional study on ethics, business practices, and more.

Two 200-hour Reflexology Advanced Trainings (Levels II and III) are offered to those who have completed the Basic program. The training consists of Reflex Anatomy; Physiology and Therapy; Energy Healing and Attunement; Vibrational Reflexology; Working the Leg in Reflexology; Myotherapy for the Foot and Lower Leg; Fertility, Pregnancy and Childbirth; Total Foot Care; Advanced Reflexology Application, and Externship, Comprehensive, and Certification.

A 400-hour Reflexology Internship Program is offered to those who have completed any total of 200 hours of reflexology training and consists of Introduction to Internship Training, Internship Seminars and Training, and Externship, Outreach, Project Thesis, Presentation, Evaluation, and Testing.

Continuing Education
The institute offers two 200-hour levels of Alternative and Complementary Naturopathic Medicine courses leading to certification, as well as a 300-hour TransFiber Therapy Training program which offers training in total-body deep muscle massage. These courses emphasize an integrated approach to health care as students participate as both patient and therapist.

Admission Requirements
Aside from the prerequisites noted above, there are no admission requirements.

Tuition and Fees
Tuition for the 130-hour Basic Reflexology is $800. Tuition for the Advanced Series in Reflexology and Naturopathic programs is $950 per 100-hour program. Tuition for the 400-hour Reflexology Internship program is $2,000.

Tuition for the 300-hour TransFiber Therapy program is $1,800.

Financial Assistance
Financial assistance or work-study may be available after completion of the Basic program.

Potomac Massage Training Institute

4000 Albemarle Street NW, 5th Floor
Washington, DC 20016
PHONE: (202) 686-7046
FAX: (202) 966-4579

The Potomac Massage Training Institute was founded in 1976. There are forty-five instructors. There is a maximum of forty-four students per lecture and twenty-two per practical class; the teacher:student ratio is 1:8 in practical classes, 1:14 in lectures.

Accreditation and Approvals
The Professional Training Program is accredited by the Commission on Massage Training Accreditation (COMTA), and

graduates are qualified to take the National Certification Examination for Therapeutic Massage and Bodywork (NCETMB). PMTI is approved by the National Certification Board for Therapeutic Massage and Bodywork (NCMTMB) as a continuing education provider.

Program Description

The 500-hour Professional Training Program consists of three levels. In Level One, students learn to give full-body Swedish massage and provide massage and touch therapy at PMTI-scheduled nursing home projects. Level Two students focus on the musculoskeletal system and kinesiology with specialization in deep tissue work, plus field work and the Student Massage Clinic. In Level Three, students focus on integrating their deep tissue and Swedish techniques while incorporating trigger point therapy and a client-centered approach into their work; additional classes include business, communication, and professional skills. Additional program requirements include electives, classes which introduce Eastern- and energy-based bodywork, CPR and First Aid training, professional massage sessions outside of the program, at least two practice massage sessions outside of class per week, and an independent field work project. The part-time program meets two evenings per week over eighteen months; the intensive program meets four mornings per week over eleven months.

Continuing Education

Continuing education programs offered to massage, bodywork, and other health professionals include Sports Massage, Neuromuscular Training, Connective Tissue Massage, Craniosacral Therapy, Massage as a Medical Intervention, Infant Massage Instructor Certification, Bodywork for the Childbearing Years, and Alexander Technique.

Admission Requirements

Applicants must be at least 18 years of age; have a high school diploma, GED, or college transcript; demonstrate literacy in English; and submit a written statement, two personal references, and a medical/health history form. Applicants must have received a professional massage and should be able to articulate their understanding of massage and its meaning to them. Applicants must have a flexible schedule that allows some weekend, daytime, and evening commitments; be able to devote forty hours per week to classes and study time for the intensive program and twenty hours per week for the part-time program; and have the necessary financial resources.

Tuition and Fees

Tuition is $5,520, including registration fee and deposit. Additional expenses include books, approximately $250; clinic shirt, approximately $25; CPR and First Aid classes, $15 to $50; TB test, between $15 and $40 per year; eight outside professional sessions, $40 to $65 each; optional massage table, $500 to $700; and sheets and oil, approximately $100.

Financial Assistance

Payment plans are available. Outside sources of support have included state agencies and personnel departments for continuing education.

FLORIDA

Academy for Five Element Acupuncture

1170-A East Hallandale Beach Boulevard
Hallandale, Florida 33009
PHONE: (954) 456-6336
FAX: (954) 456-3944
E-MAIL: afea@compuserve.com
WEBSITE: www.acupuncturist.com

Academy for Five Element Acupuncture was established in 1988. There are thirty-four faculty members, with fifteen to twenty-five students per class.

Accreditation and Approvals

The Academy for Five Element Acupuncture is accredited by Accreditation Commission for Acupuncture and Oriental Medicine (ACAOM). Graduates are eligible to sit for the National Certification Examinations in Acupuncture and Chinese Herbology administered by the National Certification Commission for Acupuncture and Oriental Medicine (NCCAOM). Graduates who pass the National Certification Exam in Acupuncture are eligible for licensure in Florida.

Program Description

The structure of the three-year, 2,600-hour Licentiate in Acupuncture Program is unique: the first two years of study are two- or three-week intensive sessions in Florida with home study in between. The third year is clinical training in Florida.

The program consists of 725 hours of Acupuncture Studies, 700 hours of Acupuncture Clinic Internship, 300 hours of Chinese Herbal Studies, 200 hours of Herbal Clinic Internship, 435 hours of Western Science, and 240 hours of Adjunctive courses. Pre- and co-requisite courses include sixty hours of Basic Science, 120 hours of Anatomy and Physiology, and thirty hours of Western Medical Terminology. First Year courses include Introduction to Basic Acupuncture Theory, Introduction to Point Location, Introduction to Point Concepts and Functions, Introduction to Pulse Taking, Introduction to Diagnosis and the Concept of Causative Factor, Introduction to Treatment Techniques and Protocols, Point Location Practicum, Qi Gong/Tai Chi, Nutrition, and Surface Anatomy. Second Year courses include Intermediate Point Location, Treatment Planning and Protocols, The Traditional Diagnosis, Foundations of Chinese Herbal Medicine, Chinese Materia Medica, Chinese Herbal Formulas, Chinese Herbal Differential Diagnosis, Acupressure, Zero Balancing®, Survey Class of American Medicine, Infectious Disease, Pathology, and Clinical Observation. Third Year courses include Advanced Point Location, Advanced Treatment Planning, Advanced Pulse Taking, Acupuncture Case Studies, Human Service Skills: Ethics and Patient Management, Professional Practice, Western Clinical Science and Medical Referral, Pharmacology, Chinese Herbal Therapy, Acupuncture Clinic Internship, Chinese Herbal Clinic Internship, Acupuncture Detox, and Final Project.

Admission Requirements

Applicants must have completed two years (sixty semester credits) of general education at the baccalaureate level, have a personal interview, and submit two letters of reference. English-language proficiency is required of all students.

Tuition and Fees

Tuition for the three-year program is $23,500; materials, including books, equipment, and lab coat, are approximately $800. There is a $150 application fee.

Financial Assistance

Flexible tuition payment plans and private student loans are available.

Academy of Chinese Healing Arts

505 South Orange Avenue
Sarasota, Florida 34236
PHONE: (941) 955-4456
FAX: (941) 330-1951
E-MAIL: acha@gte.net
WEBSITE: www.acha.net

The Academy of Chinese Healing Arts was founded in 1994 by Harrey Kaltsas, A.P., and Cynthia O'Donnell, A.P. There are twenty-four instructors with an average class size of eleven students (maximum twenty-five).

Accreditation and Approvals

The professional master's-level diploma program in Oriental Medicine of the Academy of Chinese Healing Arts is a candidate for accreditation with the Accreditation Commission for Acupuncture and Oriental Medicine (ACAOM) and is in the process of seeking accreditation. The curriculum meets the educational requirements of the Florida Board of Acupuncture Licensing Exam.

Program Description

The 2,700-hour, four-academic-year Oriental Medicine Program may be completed in nine terms and consists of 1,125 hours of Acupuncture Theories, Principles and Techniques; 405 hours of Biomedical Sciences; 450 hours of Chinese Herbology; and 720 hours of Clinical Studies.

Courses in Basic Studies include Historical Overview of TCM, Basic TCM Philosophy, Basic TCM Physiology, TCM Etiology and Mechanisms of Disease, Clinical Safety and Clean Needle Technique, Acupuncture Anatomy and Channel Theory, Evaluation and Diagnostic Methods, Human Service Skills, Tui Na, Tai Chi Chuan and Qigong Exercise Therapy, and Clinical Observation and Practice.

Differentiation of Syndromes (DOS) courses include DOS According to Eight Principles, DOS According to Qi-Blood-Body Fluids, DOS According to the Internal Organs, DOS According to Pathogenic Factors, and DOS According to Six Stages, Four Levels, and Three Burners.

Intermediate Studies courses include General Principles of Acupuncture Treatment and Therapy, Principles of Combinations of Points: The Five Command, The Extraordinary Vessel Points and Japanese Acupuncture, Ear, Hand and Scalp Acupuncture, Instruments and Techniques, Ethics and Practice Management, Introduction to Addictionology, and Clinical Practice.

Courses in the Western Sciences include Western Anatomy and Physiology, Western Pathology, Western Biomedical Terminology, Basic Western Diagnostics Skills and Terminology, Introduction to Psychological Terminology, Introduction to Physics Concepts and Terminology, Introduction to Biochemistry and Terminology, Introduction to Orthopedic Evaluation and Terminology, Introduction to Radiology and Terminology, Clinical Nutrition, and Emergency First Aid, CPR and Terminology.

Herbology courses include Herbal Theory, Herbal Diagnostic Theory, Individual Herbs, Herbal Formulas, Herbal Applications, Food Therapy/Nutrition, Herbal Clinic/Dispensary, Practice Management and Ethics Using Herbs, and Western Pharmacology.

Courses in Advanced Studies include Acupuncture Case Studies and Therapy, Internal Medicine, TCM Pediatrics, TCM Gynecology, External Medicine, Sensory Organ Disorders, Florida State/NCCAOM Exam Review, Homeopathy, Clinical Practice, and Clinical Japanese Acupuncture.

Continuing Education
The academy offers continuing education courses available through correspondence at any time. Weekend and evening workshops which grant CEUs are also offered intermittently.

Admission Requirements
Applicants must be at least 18 years of age, have a high school diploma, and have completed two years of postsecondary education from an accredited institution with a GPA of no less than 2.0. Applicants must also have two personal or phone interviews.

Tuition and Fees
Tuition is $22,000. Additional expenses include application fee,

$75; malpractice insurance, $1,000; and books, approximately $1,000.

Financial Assistance
An in-house interest-free payment plan is available.

Academy of Healing Arts

3141 South Military Trail
Lake Worth, Florida 33463
PHONE: (561) 965-5550
FAX: (561) 641-2603
E-MAIL: aharts@bellsouth.net
WEBSITE: www.ahamassage.org

The Academy of Healing Arts was founded in 1979. There are twelve instructors; massage classes average twenty-five students. In addition to the programs described here, the academy offers programs of study in Facial Skin Care and in Beauty Therapy, which combines the massage and facial programs.

Accreditation and Approvals
The Academy of Healing Arts is accredited by the Accrediting Commission of Career Schools and Colleges of Technology (ACCSCT). The Academy is approved by the Florida Board of Massage as a continuing education provider. Graduates of the Massage Therapy programs are eligible to take the Florida State licensing exam and/or the National Certification Examination for Therapeutic Massage and Bodywork (NCETMB).

Program Description
The 500-hour, five-month Massage Therapy Program consists of 275 lecture hours and 225 clinical hours. Courses include Human Anatomy, Human Physiology, Human Immunodeficiency Virus and AIDS, Massage Therapy (Phases 1 through 3), Hydrotherapy, Statutes/Rules/History, and Introduction to Other Modalities (which may include Acupressure, Nutrition, Soma Therapy, Lymphatic Drainage, Sports Massage, Touch for Health, and others).

The 624-hour, six-month Massage Therapy Program consists 375 lecture hours and 225 clinical hours. Courses include all of those listed in the 500-hour program plus Nature of Disease (Pathology), Good Business Practice, Aromatherapy, and Nutritional Health Management.

CPR Certification and Tai Chi may be included in the Massage Therapy course of study.

Continuing Education

Continuing Education courses are presented throughout the year for students, aestheticians, massage therapists, and health care practitioners. Such courses have included Reflexology, Lymphatic Drainage Methods, Arthritis Self-Help, Reiki, Shiatsu, Aromatherapy, Touch for Health, Embodiment Workshop, Facial Massage Techniques, Insurance Billing, European Body Wraps, and others.

Certain continuing education courses are available for rent on video for $65 each. The Board of Massage has set a limit of three hours credit per subject matter on video.

Admission Requirements

Massage applicants must be at least 18 years of age, have a high school diploma or equivalent, be in good health and free of communicable disease, and have a personal or telephone interview.

Tuition and Fees

Tuition for the 500-hour Massage Therapy program is $3,200. Tuition for the 624-hour Massage Therapy program is $4,750. Each program will require an additional $300 to $350 for books and supplies.

Financial Assistance

Federal grants and loans are available for the 600-hour program. Payment plans and veterans' benefits are available for both massage programs.

Acupressure-Acupuncture Institute

10506 North Kendall Drive
Miami, Florida 33176
PHONE: (305) 595-9500
FAX: (305) 595-2622
E-MAIL: aai@acupuncture.pair.com
WEBSITE: www.acupuncture.pair.com

The Acupressure-Acupuncture Institute (AAI) was founded in 1983 and is the oldest acupuncture school in Florida. The Massage Therapy program was established in 1987. There are seventeen instructors, with an average of fifteen to twenty students per class.

Accreditation and Approvals

The professional master's-level diploma program in Oriental medicine is a candidate for accreditation with the Accreditation Commission for Acupuncture and Oriental Medicine (ACAOM) and is in the process of seeking accreditation. AAI graduates are eligible for licensure in Florida and can sit for the NCCAOM National Diplomate exam. The program also qualifies graduates to apply for a Diplomat in Homeopathy from the National Board of Homeopathic Examiners (NBHE). Massage Therapy graduates are eligible for Florida licensure and are qualified to take the National Certification Examination for Therapeutic Massage and Bodywork (NCETMB).

Program Description

The 2,595-hour Oriental Medicine Program may be completed on either a thirty-six-month or forty-eight-month schedule. First Year courses include Essentials of Chinese Medicine, Introduction to Channels, Biochemistry, Musculoskeletal Anatomy, Oriental Bodywork and Qi Kung, TCM Diagnostic Methods, Point Location, Anatomy and Physiology, Medical Terminology, Oriental Bodywork, TCM Diagnostic Systems, Point Indication, Introduction to Needling, HIV/AIDS Education, Microbiology, Pathology, and Supervised Clinic Observation. Second Year courses include Advanced Acupuncture, Physical Examination, Food Therapy and Nutrition, Chinese Herbal Medicine, Orthopedic Assessment, Pharmacology, Chinese Herbal Medicine, Point Review, and Supervised Clinic Practice. Third Year courses include Internal Medicine, Board Review, Homeopathy, Survey of Medicine, Pharmacognosy, Medial Referral, Behavioral Medicine, Practice Management, and Clinical Practice and Herbal Preparation.

The 500-hour, six-month Massage Therapy Program consists of courses in Anatomy and Physiology, Musculoskeletal Anatomy, Basic Massage Therapy and Clinical Practicum, Theory and Practice of Hydrotherapy, State Rules and History of Massage, Oriental Bodywork, and HIV/AIDS Education.

Continuing Education

A postgraduate 685-hour Chinese Herbology and Homeopathy for Licensed Practitioners certificate program is offered to Florida licensed Acupuncture Physicians who have completed sixty semester credits at the baccalaureate level from an accredited institution. The program includes courses in Chinese Herbal Medicine, Internal Medicine, Food Therapy and Nutrition, Homeopathy, Pharmacognosy, and Clinical Herbal Pharmacy.

A postgraduate 100-hour Acupressure and Shiatsu certificate program is offered to Florida licensed health professionals. The program includes courses in Oriental Bodywork and Supervised Clinic.

Admission Requirements

Oriental Medicine applicants must have completed sixty semester credits at the baccalaureate level from an accredited institution. All students must have completed a twelve-hour CPR class by the end of the first semester.

Massage Therapy applicants must be at least 18 years of age and must have a high school diploma or equivalent.

All applicants must submit an essay and two letters of recommendation.

Tuition and Fees

General fees for all programs include application fee, $50; registration fee, $125; and library fee, $25.

Tuition for the Oriental Medicine Program is $18,125 for full-time students, $150 per semester credit for part-time students. Additional expenses include books and supplies, approximately $1,400; clinic fee, $100 per year; and student malpractice insurance, approximately $200 for each year of Internship.

Tuition for the Massage Therapy Program is $3,500 for full-time students, $9 per classroom hour for part-time students. Additional expenses include books and supplies, approximately $750 (including massage table).

Tuition for the postgraduate Chinese Herbology and Homeopathy for Licensed Practitioners certificate program is $5,500; books and supplies are approximately $450.

Tuition for the postgraduate Acupressure and Shiatsu certificate program is $1,200; books are an additional $100.

Financial Assistance

Payment plans and veterans' benefits are available; INS approved.

American Yoga Association

(See Multiple State Locations, pages 385–86)

Atlantic Institute of Aromatherapy

16018 Saddlestring Drive
Tampa, Florida 33618
PHONE/FAX: (813) 265-2222
E-MAIL: Sylla@AtlanticInstitute.com
WEBSITE: AtlanticInstitute.com

The Atlantic Institute of Aromatherapy was founded in 1989 by Sylla Sheppard-Hanger, a licensed massage therapist, cosmetologist, and esthetician who twice served on the Board of Directors for the American Aromatherapy Association. The teacher:student ratio averages 1:5; maximum class size is ten students. Correspondence courses are also offered; see pages 466–67.

Accreditation and Approvals

Some classes and correspondence courses provide state-certified continuing education units (CEUs) for licensed massage therapists.

Program Description

The two-day Basic Aromatherapy class is an introduction to essential oils and their properties. Topics covered include history of aromatherapy, identifying qualities of essences, basic essential oils, chemistry and constituent properties, production processes, a review of twenty-five basic oils, blending and applications, physiological effects, psychotherapeutic effects, toxicity, dosages, and holistic healing.

The two-day Advanced Aromatherapy class is open to those who have taken the Basic Aromatherapy class. Topics covered include study of essence in the natural environment, botanical families, introduction to aromatic chemistry, study of chemical families, Hippocratic approach, Ayurvedic approach, and perfumery introduction.

The Chemistry of Essential Oils is a two-day class taught by Dr. Robert Pappas, Chemist/Perfumer. Topics covered include chemistry, alkanes, alcohols and ethers, functional groups, alkenes and alkynes, physical properties, phenols, esters, diversity of nature, synthetic vs. natural, myths about essential oil chemistry, distillation, tips on detecting adulteration, and more.

The two-day Principles of Natural Perfumery class covers origins of perfumery, the fragrant art, the perfume types, fragrance user groups, fragrance families, personal fragrances using essential oils, essential oils and carrier oils, odor properties of essential oils, quality control of essential oils, chromatograms of essential oils, isolated and synthetic fragrance materials, and custom blending.

Phytotherapy: Natural Beauty Treatments for Face and Body is a three-day class that presents the therapeutic value of plants for beauty care. Topics covered include adverse reactions, plants, essential oils, other ingredients, problems, botanical baths, face, body treatments, hands, and nails.

Tuition and Fees
Tuition for each class is $275 two weeks in advance, $295 at the door.

Atlantic Institute of Oriental Medicine

1057 SE 17th Street
Fort Lauderdale, Florida 33316-2116
PHONE: (954) 463-3888 / (954) 522-6405
FAX: (954) 463-3878
E-MAIL: atom3@ix.netcom.com
WEBSITE: www.atom.edu

The Atlantic Institute of Oriental Medicine (ATOM), a not-for-profit school, was founded in 1994 by Johanna Chu Yen, M.D., C.A., Michael C.J. Carey, M.A., M.P.H., and Betty Z. Shannon, B.A.. The school has clinical training centers at other locations in Fort Lauderdale and Lauderdale Lakes.

The faculty consists of thirteen members, with an average class size of twenty students.

Accreditation and Approvals
ATOM's professional diploma program in traditional Chinese medicine is accredited by the Accreditation Commission for Acupuncture and Oriental Medicine (ACAOM). Graduates are eligible to sit for the Florida Board of Acupuncture state licensure exam and for the National Commission for Certification of Acupuncture and Oriental Medicine (NCCAOM) acupuncture and herbal certification exams.

Program Description
The 2,718-hour Traditional Chinese Medicine Program corresponds to four academic years and may be completed in a minimum of thirty-six months.

Year One classes include Basic Theory of TCM; Basic Concepts of Meridians and Collateral; Basic Concepts of 12 Divergent Meridians and 15 Collaterals; Meridians, Collaterals and Points: Tiayin and Yangming; Meridians, Collaterals and Points: Shaoyin and Taiyang; Meridians, Collaterals and Points: Shaoyang and Jueyin; Diagnosis Methods of TCM; Differentiation of Syndromes; Etiology and Pathogenesis of TCM; Acupuncture and Moxibustion Techniques; Chinese Language; Western Anatomy and Physiology; Universal Precautions and Clean Needle Technique; CPR and Patient Emergency Care; and Western Pathology.

Year Two classes include Meridians, Collaterals and Points: Extra Channels and Points; Meridians, Collaterals and Points: Ear and Scalp; History of Eastern Medicine; Internal Diseases of TCM; External Diseases of TCM; Ear, Nose and Throat of TCM; Gynecology of TCM; Pediatrics of TCM; Practice of Chinese Medicine; Chinese Language; Western Medical Terminology; Introduction to Herbology; Individual Herbs; and Basic Herbal Formulas.

Year Three classes include Dermatology of TCM; State Acupuncture Laws, Rules and Ethics; Tui Na, Tai Chi and Qi Gong; Introduction to Adjunctive Therapy; Special Topics: Detoxification and Stop Smoking Programs; Special Topics: Facials and Weight Loss; Advanced TCM Study: Nei Jing and Shang Han Lun; Physical Examination and Western Diagnosis; Office Management and Insurance Billing; Equipment and Safety; Introduction to Homeopathy; Basic Herbal Formulas; Clinical Herbal Formulas; and Food Therapy.

Clinical training takes the form of Observation (first 240 hours), Practice Under Supervision (next 270 hours), and Acupuncture and Herb Preparation (final 300 hours).

Admission Requirements

Applicants must be at least 18 years of age; be competent in speaking, reading, and writing English and in understanding spoken English; have completed at least two years' accredited baccalaureate education (sixty or more semester credits); and visit the institute and interview with the director of education. Applicants must also submit a physician's statement of health, one to three letters of recommendation, and an essay.

Tuition and Fees

Tuition is $21,000 for the entire three-year program. Additional expenses include a $20 application fee; registration fee, $120; books, approximately $900 per year, and uniforms and supplies, approximately $125 per year.

Financial Assistance

Payment plans are available.

Boca Raton Institute

5499 North Federal Highway
Boca Raton, Florida 33487
PHONE: (561) 241-8105 / (800) 275-6764
FAX: (561) 241-9789
E-MAIL: info@bocaschools.com
WEBSITE: www.bocaschools.com

Boca Raton Institute was founded in 1983 by Executive Director Constance Gregg. There are eleven instructors, with an average of less than twenty students per class. In addition to the program described here, the institute offers programs in Facial Specialist, Make-Up Artistry, Nail Technology, Cosmetology, Salon Management, and Instructor Training.

Accreditation and Approvals

Boca Raton Institute is accredited by the National Accrediting Commission of Cosmetology Arts and Sciences (NACCAS). Graduates are qualified to take the National Certification Examination for Therapeutic Massage and Bodywork (NCETMB). The Institute is approved by the Florida State Board of Massage as a provider of continuing education units.

Program Description

The 605-hour Massage Therapy Program includes courses in Anatomy and Physiology, Practical and Theory of Massage, Required Clinics, Modalities (which introduces Shiatsu, Reflexology, Sports Massage, Kinesiology, Deep Relaxation Techniques, Neuromuscular Therapy, Trager, Rolfing, Exercise Physiology, CPR Certification Training, Stress Management, Infant Massage, Craniosacral Technique, and Aromatherapy), HIV/AIDS Education, Hydrotherapy, and Business Principles and Florida Law.

Admission Requirements

Massage Therapy applicants must be at least 18 years of age, have a high school diploma or equivalent, and provide a health statement.

Tuition and Fees

The total cost of the 605-hour Massage Therapy Program, including tuition, books, uniform, and registration fee, is $5,240.

Financial Assistance

Federal grants and loans are available.

CORE Institute

223 West Carolina Street
Tallahassee, Florida 32301
PHONE: (850) 222-8673
FAX: (850) 561-6160
E-MAIL: admin@coreinstitute.com
WEBSITE: www.coreinstitute.com

The CORE Institute was founded in 1990 by George and Patricia Kousaleos and is owned by GEO Touch. There are thirteen instructors, with an average of twenty students per class.

Accreditation and Approvals

The CORE Institute's Professional Massage Therapy training program is accredited by the Commission on Massage Training Accreditation (COMTA). The institute is approved by the Florida Board of Massage Therapy and is a member of the AMTA Council of Schools. Graduates are qualified to take the National Certification Examination for Therapeutic Massage and Bodywork (NCETMB) and qualify for Florida State licensing.

Program Description

The 650-hour Professional Massage Therapy Training Program consists of Massage Therapy History and Theory (which includes Fundamentals of Swedish Massage, Basic Massage and Muscle Specific Massage Formats, Fundamentals of Neuromuscular Therapy, Deep Tissue Techniques, CORE Myofascial Therapy, and Massage Practical Clinic); Human Anatomy and Physiology; Musculo-Skeletal Anatomy and Kinesiology; The Therapist/Client Relationship; Human Pathology; Hydrotherapy; Business Practices Survey; Florida Massage Therapy Law and Professional Ethics; Oriental Therapies (which include Five Element Theory, Meridian Line Identification, and Shiatsu); AIDS/HIV Education; and Allied Modalities (including Wellness, Sports Massage, Seated Massage, Polarity, Trager® Approach, Pregnancy Massage Techniques, Massage Therapy for Infants and Children, and Community Outreach). Classes are offered as an eight-month Day Intensive Program or a twelve-month evening Extended Program.

Continuing Education

CORE Institute offers advanced certification training in CORE Somatic Therapy, Sportsmassage, Neuromuscular Therapy, TMJ Therapy, and Seated Massage. Continuing education courses are also offered in such areas as Infant Massage, Deep Tissue Massage, Structural Bodywork, PNF Stretching, Beginning and Advanced Reflexology, and others.

Admission Requirements

Applicants must be at least twenty years of age; have at least two years of college or equivalent work/life experience; have completed an Adult CPR and Basic First Aid course; have a high school diploma or equivalent; submit two letters of reference, essays, and a physician's report; and have had at least one full-body massage from a licensed massage therapist.

Tuition and Fees

Tuition is $5,200, plus a $75 registration fee. Additional expenses include books, supplies, student liability insurance, and CPR/First Aid certification.

Financial Assistance

Payment plans, work-study grants, private student loans, and veterans' benefits are available.

Educating Hands School of Massage

120 Southwest 8th Street
Miami, Florida 33130
PHONE: (305) 285-6991 / (800) 999-6991
FAX: (305) 857-0298
E-MAIL: eduhands@aol.com
WEBSITE: www.educatinghands.com

The Educating Hands School of Massage was founded in 1981 by Iris Burman. There are thirteen instructors, with 120 graduates yearly.

Accreditation and Approvals

Educating Hands is accredited by the Commission on Massage Training Accreditation (COMTA) and licensed by the Florida State Board of Non-Public Career Education. Graduates are qualified to take the National Certification Examination for Therapeutic Massage and Bodywork (NCETMB). Educating Hands is approved by the National Certification Board for Therapeutic Massage and Bodywork (NCBTMB) and by the Florida State Board of Massage as a continuing education provider.

Program Description

The 624-hour Therapeutic Massage Training Program includes courses in Human Anatomy and Physiology, Kinesiology and Palpation, TouchAbilities (Therapeutic Massage), Student Clinic, Hydrotherapy, Introduction to Allied Modalities, Pathology, Florida State Law, Business Principles and Development, and HIV/AIDS.

Community and Continuing Education

For those who are seeking an introductory course in massage therapy, Educating Hands offers Massage For Fun, a workshop in full-body massage for nonprofessionals.

Continuing education seminars are offered throughout the year for licensed massage professionals. Topics include Shiatsu,

Reflexology, NMT, Deep Connective Tissue Massage, Infant Massage, Ethics, Sports Massage, and others.

Admission Requirements

Applicants must be at least 18 years of age, have a high school diploma or equivalent, pass an English Comprehension test, and interview with the director of admissions or an associate.

Tuition and Fees

Tuition for the Therapeutic Massage Training Program is $4,900. Additional expenses include registration fee, $150; books, approximately $320; and student supplies, $125.

Financial Assistance

Payment plans and veterans' benefits are available; an extended finance plan is offered through an independent company. If payment is made in full, student supplies will be provided at no charge.

Florida Academy of Massage

8695 College Parkway, Suite 110
Fort Myers, Florida 33919
PHONE: (941) 489-2282 / (800) 324-9543
FAX: (941) 489-4065
WEBSITE: www.floridaacademymassage.com

The Florida Academy of Massage was founded in 1992 and is headed by Ronald D. Gray. There are six primary instructors plus guest instructors, with an average of eighteen students per class.

Accreditation and Approvals

The Florida Academy of Massage is licensed by the State of Florida, Florida Department of Education, State Board of Nonpublic Career Education, and the curriculum is approved by the Florida Department of Health, Board of Massage Therapy. Graduates are eligible to take the Florida State Board Examination and, upon passing, receive both a Florida State Massage Therapist License and certification from the National Certification Board for Therapeutic Massage and Bodywork (NCBTMB).

Program Description

The 540-hour Massage Therapy Program consists of Massage Therapy (including Swedish Massage), Student Clinic Practicum, Anatomy and Physiology (including Pathology), Allied Modalities (including Muscle Kinesiology, CPR, Counseling Techniques and Sexual Ethics, Oriental Studies, Reiki, Shiatsu, Neuromuscular Therapy, Body Mechanics, Sports Massage, Chiropractic Massage, and Reflexology), Hydrotherapy, Florida Massage Law, and AIDS/HIV Education. Programs are offered day or evening.

Continuing Education

Continuing education workshops are offered throughout the year in such areas as Advanced Bodywork Techniques, Touch for Health, AIDS and Ethics, Foot Reflexology, Craniosacral, Neuromuscular Therapy, Psychoneuroimmunology, On-Site Chair Massage, Somatic Therapy, and Insurance Billing and Reimbursement.

Admission Requirements

Applicants must be at least 18 years of age or have a high school diploma or equivalent; be in good health, free of communicable disease, and be able to give and receive massage; and interview with an admissions advisor.

Tuition and Fees

Tuition is $3,100; registration is $150 and books and supplies are $265. Tuition for continuing education workshops ranges from $60 to $495.

Financial Assistance

Payment plans, Division of Blind Services benefits, Division of Vocational Rehabilitation benefits, and Workforce Council of Southwest Florida training are available. Two scholarships per year are provided through the Florida Association of Postsecondary Schools and Colleges.

Florida College of Natural Health

E-MAIL: fcnh@icanet.net
WEBSITE: www.fcnh.com

FORT LAUDERDALE CAMPUS (MAIN CAMPUS):
2001 West Sample Road, Suite 100

Pompano Beach, Florida 33064-1342

PHONE: (954) 975-6400 / (800) 541-9299

FAX: (954) 975-9633

ORLANDO CAMPUS:

887 East Altamonte Drive

Altamonte Springs, Florida 32701-5001

PHONE: (407) 261-0319 / (800) 393-7337

FAX: (407) 261-0342

MIAMI CAMPUS:

7925 NW 12th Street, Suite 201

Miami, Florida 33126-1821

PHONE: (305) 597-9599 / (800) 599-9599

FAX: (305) 597-9110

SARASOTA CAMPUS:

1751 Mound Street

Sarasota, Florida 34236

PHONE: (941) 954-8999 / (800) 966-7117

FAX: (941) 954-8991

Florida College of Natural Health (FCNH) was founded in Fort Lauderdale in 1986 as Florida Institute. There are forty-seven instructors, with an average of thirty to thirty-five students per class. In addition to the programs described here, FCNH offers an Associate of Science Degree in Natural Health with concentrations in Therapeutic Massage and Skin Care, Paramedical Skin Care, and Advanced Therapeutic Massage; a Skin Care Training Program; and a three-year Master's Degree in Acupuncture program (not ACAOM accredited or candidate).

Accreditation and Approvals

FCNH is nationally accredited by the Accrediting Commission of Career Schools and Colleges of Technology (ACCSCT). The Therapeutic Massage Training Program is accredited by the Commission on Massage Training Accreditation (COMTA), and graduates are qualified to take the National Certification Examination for Therapeutic Massage and Bodywork (NCETMB). The College is approved as a provider of continuing education units by the Florida State Board of Massage Therapy and by the National Certification Board for Therapeutic Massage and Bodywork (NCBTMB).

Program Description

The 624-hour Therapeutic Massage Training Program may be completed in five months of day or six months of evening study. Courses include Human Anatomy and Physiology, Therapeutic Massage, Swedish Massage, Introduction to Allied Modalities (covering Shiatsu, Kinesiology, Trager®, Exercise Physiology, Spa Therapy, Reflexology, Deep Relaxation Techniques, Stretching and Flexibility, First Aid and CPR, Craniosacral Technique, Chinese Medicine, Sports Massage, Neuromuscular Therapy, Polarity, Stress Management, Myofascial Release, and Meridians), Theory and Practice of Hydrotherapy, Florida State Law, and HIV/AIDS.

The 1,125-hour Associate of Science Degree in Natural Health, Advanced Therapeutic Massage Concentration may be completed in fourteen months of day or eighteen months of evening study. Students completing the concentration will become certified in Sports Massage and Neuromuscular Therapy. The program consists of the Therapeutic Massage Training Curriculum plus five general education courses (English, Math, Psychology, Humanities, and Business), and 276 hours of advanced massage courses in Pathology, Advanced Practical Training, Medical Terminology, Medical Documentation, Kinesiology, Athletic Injuries, and Professional Practices.

Admission Requirements

Therapeutic Massage Training applicants must be at least 18 years of age; have a high school diploma or equivalent or demonstrate an ability to benefit from the course; and provide a statement of health from a licensed physician.

Associate of Science Degree applicants must have a high school diploma or equivalent; must provide Scholastic Aptitude Test (SAT) or American College Testing Exam (ACT) results or take FCNH's entrance exam; and provide a statement of health from a licensed physician.

Tuition and Fees

Tuition for the Therapeutic Massage Training program is $5,500, plus an additional $320 for books and supplies.

Tuition for the Associate of Science Degree in Natural Health, Advanced Therapeutic Massage Concentration is $11,580 plus an additional $1,085 for books and supplies.

Financial Assistance

FCNH financing; federal grants, loans, and work-study; and veterans' benefits are available. Acupuncture students are not eligible for Title IV financial aid.

Florida Health Academy

261 9th Street South
Naples, Florida 34102
PHONE: (941) 263-9391
FAX: (941) 263-8680
E-MAIL: Clara@ceuonline.org
WEBSITE: www.ceuonline.org

Florida Health Academy was founded in 1990 by Stanley Hubbard as the Acupuncture Center of Naples. The school was purchased in 1995 by Clara and Dale McElroy. There are seven massage therapy instructors; class sizes average ten students. In addition to the program described below, the academy offers programs in Acupuncture (not ACAOM accredited or candidate) and in Facials and Skin Care.

Accreditation and Approvals

The Florida Health Academy is licensed by the Florida State Board of Independent Postsecondary Vocational, Technical, Trade and Business Schools. Graduates of the massage therapy program are qualified to take the National Certification Examination for Therapeutic Massage and Bodywork (NCETMB).

Program Description

The 540-hour Massage Therapy Program consists of Massage Therapy, Anatomy and Physiology, Hydrotherapy, Allied Modalities, Florida Massage Law, AIDS/HIV Education, and forty hours of Student Clinic.

Continuing Education

The 300-hour Herbology course included in the Acupuncture Program may be taken separately by physicians, chiropractors, or acupuncturists. The course covers Herbal Theory, Herbal Diagnostic Theory, Individual Herbs, Herbal Formulas, Herbal Application, Food Therapy, and Herbal Clinic.

Other continuing education programs are offered to licensed acupuncturists; contact the academy for details.

Admission Requirements

Massage therapy applicants must be at least 18 years of age and have a high school diploma or equivalent.

Tuition and Fees

Tuition for the Massage Therapy Program is $2,500; books are an additional $250. The Herbology course taken independently of the Acupuncture Program is $1,500.

Financial Assistance

A payment plan is available.

Florida Institute of Psychophysical Integration

5837 Mariner Drive
Tampa, Florida 33609
PHONE: (813) 286-2273
FAX: (813) 287-2870
E-MAIL: Dr.Joy@JohnsonMail.com
WEBSITE: www.QuantumBalance.com

The Florida Institute of Psychophysical Integration was founded in 1976 by Joy K. Johnson, Ph.D., a practitioner of gestalt therapy and humanistic psychology who is also trained in craniosacral therapy and is certified as an International Trainer of Postural Integration. There are two instructors, with one to four students per class.

Program Description

The institute offers a 150-hour, fifteen-day residential tutorial program in the field of deep tissue therapy known as postural integration. The training has a maximum of four students, and may be individually tutored and scheduled by mutual agreement. The curriculum includes Theory of Postural Integration, Manipulation, Techniques for the Practitioner, Psychological Testing, Movement, Professional Ethics and Responsibilities, and Setting Up a Postural Integration Practice. Training consists of Phase I: Independent Study, Phase II: Residential Intensive, and Phase III: Work/Study Mastery.

Admission Requirements

Prerequisites are flexible but include completion of ten standard sessions of postural integration or its equivalent; minimum age of 25; a college degree, preferably with a counseling background, and a license to touch; massage experience and knowledge; and knowledge of the muscle system.

Tuition and Fees
Tuition for the entire program is $3,100.

Financial Assistance
Financing is available.

Florida Institute of Traditional Chinese Medicine

5335 66th Street North
St. Petersburg, Florida 33709
PHONE: (727) 546-6565
FAX: (727) 547-0703
E-MAIL: fitcm@gte.net

The Florida Institute of Traditional Chinese Medicine (FITCM) was founded in 1986 by Su Liang Ku, who has served as chairperson of the Florida State Board of Acupuncture, as president of the American Association of Acupuncture and Oriental Medicine (AAAOM), and on the Board of Examiners of the National Commission for the Certification of Acupuncturists (NCCA). There are ten instructors, with ten to twenty students per class. FITCM has two locations in the Tampa Bay area that include classrooms, herbal pharmacies, and on-site treatment clinics.

Accreditation and Approvals
FITCM is accredited by the Accrediting Council for Continuing Education and Training (ACCET) and by the Accreditation Commission for Acupuncture and Oriental Medicine (ACAOM). Graduates of the TCM program are eligible to apply for various state licensing exams and the National Certification Commission for Acupuncture and Oriental Medicine (NCCAOM) exam.

Program Description
FITCM offers a 2,882-hour program in Traditional Chinese Medicine, which includes 2,082 hours of classroom-based study in acupuncture, herbology, and Tui Na massage, and 800 hours in student clinic. The program may be completed in thirty-six months (days) or forty-eight months (evenings and weekends).

Admission Requirements
Applicants must be at least 18 years of age; have completed at least two years of college or postsecondary education (sixty semester credit hours) at an accredited institution; submit two letters of recommendation; submit a statement of health from a TCM or Western physician; have a keen interest in and basic understanding of TCM; and interview with the school director.

Tuition and Fees
Tuition is $7,500 per year for the thirty-six-month program, or $5,700 per year for the forty-eight-month program. Additional expenses include application fee, $25; registration fee, $75; books, approximately $1,500 for the program; and miscellaneous supplies and fees, approximately $1,500.

Financial Assistance
Federal grants, loans and payment plans are available.

Florida School of Massage

6421 SW 13th Street
Gainesville, Florida 32608
PHONE: (352) 378-7891
FAX: (352) 376-7218
E-MAIL: info@massageonline.com
WEBSITE: www.massageonline.com

The Florida School of Massage (FSM) first enrolled students in 1973. In 1979, the American Institute of Natural Health and the Florida School of Massage merged their programs of massage therapy and allied holistic health training. There are twenty-three instructors, with an average of sixty students per class.

Accreditation and Approvals
The Therapeutic Massage and Hydrotherapy Program is accredited by the Commission on Massage Training Accreditation (COMTA), and graduates are qualified to take the National Certification Examination for Therapeutic Massage and Body-

work (NCETMB). FSM is approved as a continuing education provider by the National Certification Board for Therapeutic Massage and Bodywork (NCBTMB) and by the State of Florida, Board of Massage Therapy. FSM is licensed by the Florida State Board of Independent Postsecondary, Vocational, Technical, Trade, and Business Schools.

Program Description

The 705-hour Therapeutic Massage and Hydrotherapy Licensing Program consists of Introduction to Awareness Based Massage/Orientation, Massage Therapy Techniques (including Foundations of Bodywork/Swedish Massage, Connective Tissue Massage, Neuro-Muscular Therapy, Polarity Therapy, Sports Massage, Reflexology, Awareness and Integrated Massage, and Feldenkrais—Awareness Through Movement, Direct Supervision with Feedback, Human Anatomy, Physiology and Kinesiology, Hydrotherapy, Awareness and Communication Skills, Florida Massage Laws and Rules, Business Practices and Ethics, CPR and First Aid, Living with AIDS, Massage Journals, Examination Review/Graduation, and Community Circle.

Students wishing to receive a 1,000-hour diploma must also complete forty-five to fifty hours of electives (which may include such topics as Tai Chi/Chi Kung, Yoga, Meditation, Ayurveda, Infant Massage, Body Image, Choosing Happiness, and others, a 200-hour Directed Independent Study Project, and the fifty-hour Journal Writing elective. Students who wish to take the New York State Massage Examination must take an additional ten-day intensive, Exploring the Art of Shiatsu.

Beginning January 1, 2000, the Directed Independent Study Project will not meet the New York State revised requirements for 1,000 hours. FSM is developing a program that would include the 705-hour program plus a supplementary program designed to comply with the revised New York State requirements; this program will involve additional tuition expense.

Continuing Education

FSM offers a wide variety of advanced trainings and continuing education workshops throughout the year.

A 112-hour Polarity Therapy Certification Program covers Polarity Balancing/Theory, Practical Experience, and Psychophysical Awareness. A phone or personal interview is required.

A 200-hour Sports Massage Program includes Sports Massage Theory and Application, Supervised Field Event Experience, and Supervised Practicum and Independent Study. Topics covered include hydrotherapy protocol, injury evaluation and treatment, strength training and conditioning, and more. The program is open to current massage students or Massage Therapists.

A 200- to 500-hour Teacher's Assistant Program exposes therapists to the theory and techniques necessary to become instructors through observation and experience as classroom assistants. Course work includes Instructional Principles and Procedures and Personal and Video Feedback on Participant Presentations. Applicants must be graduates of a basic massage program plus an awareness oriented advanced training or equivalent.

A 205-hour Therapeutic Hand and Foot Reflexology Program prepares practitioners to offer skilled hand and foot non-diagnostic reflexology sessions within the context of a client-directed holistic health program. Instruction includes Reflexology Theory and Application (which includes history, principles, Oriental and Western allopathic theories, techniques, hydrotherapy, ethics, HIV/AIDS education, and more), as well as Anatomy and Physiology, Supervised Clinical Internship, and Externship. Applicants must be 21 years of age and have a high school diploma or equivalent.

Admission Requirements

Therapeutic Massage and Hydrotherapy applicants must be 19 years of age (this may be waived through a personal interview) and submit written biographical data; an interview with the school administrator may be required. Prerequisite for the Teacher's Assistant program is completion of the basic massage licensing program.

Tuition and Fees

Tuition for the Therapeutic Massage and Hydrotherapy Licensing Program is $5,150. Additional expenses include application fee, $100; massage table, $400 to $600; books, approximately $250; and New York State required shiatsu class, $1,000.

Tuition for the Polarity Therapy Certification Program is $1,275; books cost $75 to $300 (optional).

Tuition for the Sports Massage Program is $1,650; books cost $75 to $100.

Tuition for the Teacher's Assistant Program is $2,500; books are $75 to $100.

Tuition for the Therapeutic Hand and Foot Reflexology Program is $1,500; books are $75 to $100 (optional); and an optional massage table costs $400 to $600.

Financial Assistance
Scholarships, payment plans, work-study, veterans' benefits, and vocational rehabilitation are available, as well as aid from the Bureau of Blind Services.

Florida's Therapeutic Massage School

1300 East Gadsden Street
Pensacola, Florida 32501
PHONE: (850) 433-8212

Florida's Therapeutic Massage School (FTMS) was founded in 1992 by Geraldine Vaurigaud, a licensed massage therapist and teacher. There are twelve instructors and a maximum of twenty-two students per class.

Accreditation and Approvals
FTMS is licensed by the State Board of Independent Postsecondary Vocational, Technical, Trade and Business Schools. Graduates are qualified to take the National Certification Examination for Therapeutic Massage and Bodywork (NCETMB).

Program Description
The 600-hour, six-month Therapeutic Massage and Hydrotherapy Program consists of Therapeutic Massage (which includes Swedish Massage, Reflexology, Neuromuscular Therapy, Connective Tissue Massage, Sports Massage, Polarity, Shiatsu, and Lymphatic Massage), Anatomy and Physiology (which includes Kinesiology and Palpation, and Pathology), Hydrotherapy, History and Massage Laws, Allied Modalities (which includes Awareness and Communication Skills, Ethics, Movement and Body Awareness, Nutrition and Herbology, Business Practices, and introduction to various modalities such as seated chair massage, Trager®, lymph drainage, therapeutic touch, pregnancy, infant and elderly massage), AIDS/HIV Education, and Clinic Internship. Students may elect to complete a Directed Independent Study Project for an additional 100 hours. Students are required to complete First Aid/CPR certification prior to graduation.

Community and Continuing Education
FTMS offers seminars and lectures by experts in the field of massage and natural health care for the benefit of the community, students, and other massage therapists. Topics include Introduction to Massage, Couples Massage, Reflexology, Shiatsu, Polarity, and Using Herbs.

Continuing education provides opportunities for massage therapists to advance their knowledge and techniques. Courses include Advanced Reflexology, Advanced Polarity, Oriental Bodywork, Structural Integration, Advanced Chair Massage, Advanced Neuromuscular Therapy, Communication and Counseling Skills for Massage Therapists, Trager Massage, and Insurance Billing.

Admission Requirements
Applicants must be at least 18 years of age, have a high school diploma or equivalent, and submit an essay and two letters of reference. After enrollment, the student must receive at least one professional massage prior to the first day of school and attend an FTMS Introduction to Massage Workshop.

Tuition and Fees
Tuition is $3,150. Additional expenses include registration fee, $100; books, approximately $300; Introduction to Massage Workshop, $25; American Red Cross First Aid/CPR (if needed), $35; AIDS Awareness Training (if needed), $15; portable massage table (optional), $300 to $500; supplies, $25 to $50; one professional massage, $35 to $45. Fees vary for community and continuing education courses.

Financial Assistance
Payment plans and veterans' benefits are available.

The Humanities Center Institute of Applied Health School of Massage

4045 Park Boulevard
Pinellas Park, Florida 34665
PHONE: (727) 541-5200
FAX: (727) 545-0053

E-MAIL: info@2touch.com
WEBSITE: www.2touch.com

The Humanities Center was founded in 1981 and was purchased by its current owner, Sherry Fears, in 1983. In 1990, the school moved to its current location. There are eight instructors, with an average of sixteen students per class.

Accreditation and Approvals

The school is accredited by the Accrediting Commission of Career Schools and Colleges of Technology (ACCSCT) and approved by the Florida Board of Massage as an approved-curriculum school and as a provider for continuing education units. Graduates are qualified to take the National Certification Examination for Therapeutic Massage and Bodywork (NCETMB).

Program Description

The 625-hour Therapeutic Applications of Massage Program includes Theory and Practice of Massage (which includes Swedish massage, relaxation massage, neuromuscular therapy, and more), Business Practices, Internship, Visiting Professor and Additional Techniques, Massage Law, Hydrotherapy, HIV/AIDS Education, and Anatomy and Physiology. Day and evening programs are available.

Continuing Education

Various continuing education seminars are offered in such areas as lower body sports therapy and cervical dysfunction.

Admission Requirements

Applicants must be at least 20 years old, have a high school diploma or equivalent, be physically able to learn and receive massage, interview with an admissions representative, and observe classes for at least two hours.

Tuition and Fees

There is a $25 application fee; when accepted, candidates pay a $100 registration fee (which is deducted from total charges). Tuition is $5,910, which includes books, supplies, lotion, and five school polo shirts. Linens are additional.

Financial Assistance

Payment plans, federal grants, and loans are available.

International Alliance of Healthcare Educators®

(See Multiple State Locations, pages 396-97)

International Institute of Reflexology

(See Multiple State Locations, page 398)

Loraine's Academy

1012 58th Street North
St. Petersburg, Florida 33710
PHONE: (727) 347-4247
FAX: (727) 347-6491

Loraine's Academy was founded as a cosmetology school in 1966 and began offering a Therapeutic Massage program in 1995. Massage faculty consists of seven full- and part-time members. Class size is limited to twelve.

Accreditation and Approvals

The Academy is accredited by the National Accrediting Commission of Cosmetology Arts and Sciences (NACCAS) and is licensed by the Florida State Department of Education Board of Independent Postsecondary, Vocational, Technical, Trade and Business Schools. The Therapeutic Massage Program is approved by the State of Florida's Board of Massage, and graduates are qualified to take the National Certification Examination for Therapeutic Massage and Bodywork (NCETMB).

Program Description

The 600-hour Therapeutic Massage Program may be completed in twenty weeks of day classes or thirty weeks of evening classes. The program consists of Orientation and Introduction to Therapeutic Massage; Human Anatomy, Physiology and Kinesiology; Pathology and Recognition of Various Conditions (which includes contraindications of massage, medical terminology, HIV/AIDS, CPR/First Aid, and more); Massage/Bodywork Theory and Assessment (which covers client interview and assessment, massage/bodywork for soft tissue, fascia, and energy systems, postural assessment, athletic and sports massage, neuromuscular therapy, Eastern theory, energy techniques, and other allied modalities); Practical Applications of Therapeutic Massage (including safety and sanitary practices, therapist posture and body mechanics, and specialized massage and bodywork application); Related Methods and Techniques; Business Administration/Professional Practices; Florida State Laws and Rules; and Evaluations/ Completion.

Admission Requirements

Applicants must have a high school diploma or equivalent or be at least 18 year of age and have the ability to benefit from the training offered.

Tuition and Fees

Tuition is $4,250. Additional expenses include an administrative fee of $150; lab fee, $275; and books, $300. A professional massage table is highly recommended and available through the school for $584 (Ultra Light).

Financial Assistance

Federal grants and loans, veterans' benefits, and no-interest payment plans are available.

National College of Oriental Medicine

7100 Lake Ellenor Drive
Orlando, Florida 32809
PHONE: (407) 888-8689
FAX: (407) 888-8211
E-MAIL: info@acupunctureschool.com
WEBSITE: www.acupunctureschool.com

National College of Oriental Medicine was founded in 1990; Larry L. Han is the owner. There are nine faculty members and an average of twelve students per class.

Accreditation and Approvals

The professional Masters of Oriental Medicine degree program is accredited by the Accreditation Commission for Acupuncture and Oriental Medicine (ACAOM).

Program Description

The 2,635-hour Master of Oriental Medicine degree program is a four-year academic program accelerated over three years. The program consists of 945 hours of Acupuncture and Basic Oriental Medical Theory; 345 hours of Herbology; 505 hours of Western Medicine; 810 hours of Clinical Training; and thirty hours of Business.

Acupuncture and Oriental Medical Theory courses include Basic Theory and Philosophy of Oriental Medicine, Oriental Medical Diagnostic Skills, General and Clean Needle Technique, Basic General Theory, Acupuncture Point Location, Legal Status of Acupuncture, Identification of Disease Patterns, Oriental Bodywork: Tui Na Therapy, Ear and Scalp Acupuncture, General Principles of Acupuncture Treatment, Acupuncture Case Studies, The Treatment of Common Diseases, and others. Herbology courses include Herbology and Oriental Herbal Diagnostic Methods, Herbal Formulas, Food Therapy, and Integration of Herbal Medicine and Western Science. Western Medicine courses include Anatomy and Physiology, First Aid and CPR, Microbiology, Western Pathology, Western Diagnostics, Radiology, Clinical Psychology, and Western Pharmacology. Clinical Training consists of Clinical Observation, Internship, and Herbal Pharmacy and Dispensary. Business courses are Ethics and Human Service and Practice Management. Classes are held on a day or evening schedule. Postgraduate and senior students may take advantage of a voluntary six-week internship at a hospital in China.

Admission Requirements

Applicants must have a high school diploma and must have completed at least sixty semester hours from an accredited college or university, which must include at least nineteen hours of general education or liberal arts courses. English-language competency is required of all students. Applicants must submit an autobiographical essay, three letters of recommendation, and a physician's health statement, and have a personal interview.

Tuition and Fees

Tuition is $25,200 for the entire program. Additional expenses include a $25 application fee; registration fee, $100; books, approximately $1,000; and graduation fee, $50. Malpractice insurance is optional. The voluntary internship in China is approximately $3,000 including airfare.

Financial Assistance
Federal grants and loans, veterans' benefits, and a monthly payment plan are available.

Reiki Plus® Institute

707 Barcelona Road
Key Largo, Florida 33037
PHONE: (305) 451-9881
FAX: (305) 451-9841
E-MAIL: reikiplu@bellsouth.net
WEBSITE: www.reikiplus.com

The Reiki Plus Institute (RPI) was founded in 1987 by director David G. Jarrell, who became a Reiki Teacher in 1981. RPI is the teaching arm of the Pyramids of Light, a spiritually based church of natural healing. The institute teaches a form of Reiki they call Reiki Plus, an art of natural healing and a unique blending of celestial elements. There are five instructors plus those in training; classes average ten to fifteen students. A home study program is also available; see pages 493-94.

Program Description
The Reiki Plus Practitioner's Program consists of four classes. Reiki Plus First Degree introduces techniques to use with the self and with clients to promote healing, relaxation, and stress reduction through hands-on experience and group treatment. In Reiki Plus Second Degree, students learn how Second Degree is combined with mystical teachings; how to activate, direct and apply energy to self, fellow students and clients; and Distant Healing techniques. Psycho-Therapeutic Reiki Plus identifies psycho-physical, emotional, and mental disorders for which Second Degree is an appropriate intervention and how to remove stored traumas and dis-ease from the chakras and physical body. The Reiki Plus Third Degree Practitioner course increases the depth, intensity and effectiveness of the Practitioner's healing work. Certification as a Reiki Plus Practitioner requires the student to take the Practitioner Examination. A complete Reiki Plus Teachers Training Program is also available.

The Physio-Spiritual Etheric Body (PSEB)® Practitioner's Program consists of seven courses. PSEB is a healing technique that teaches the healer how to unite the physical and Etheric Bodies in order to allow spiritual harmony to flow through them from God. Courses in the program include Physio-Spiritual Etheric Body (PSEB) I, II, and III; Applied Esoteric Psychology and Anatomy; Intuitive Evaluation of Client's Consciousness; Theory of Holographic Energy: Chakra Astrology; and Implementation of Holographic Theory I and II.

Continuing Education
Continuing education classes include Astro-Physiology and Psychology, Astro-Physiology and Healing Techniques, Spinal Attunement Technique, and others.

Tuition and Fees
Tuition is charged separately for each seminar and ranges from $200 to $500 for Reiki Plus and PSEB courses, $30 to $300 for electives.

Financial Assistance
Discounts of $25 to $50 per seminar are offered for early registration.

Sarasota School of Massage Therapy

1970 Main Street
Sarasota, Florida 34236
PHONE: (941) 957-0577
FAX: (941) 957-1049
E-MAIL: massage@bte.net
WEBSITE: www.web-sarasota.com/ssmt/

The Sarasota School of Massage Therapy was founded in 1979, and purchased in 1991 by Michael and Mary Rosen-Pyros. Michael, a chiropractic physician, is the director of the school. There are fifteen instructors, with an average of eighteen to twenty students per class.

Accreditation and Approvals
The school is accredited by the Council on Occupational Education (Atlanta, Georgia). Graduates are qualified to take the

National Certification Examination for Therapeutic Massage and Bodywork (NCETMB).

Program Description

The 600-hour Massage Therapy Program may be taken on either a full-time (thirty weeks, days or evenings) or part-time (sixteen months, evenings) basis. The curriculum includes Anatomy and Physiology, Hydrotherapy, Florida Massage Law, Massage Theory/Practice, Allied Modalities (such as myology and neuromuscular therapy, first aid and CPR, and Massage Cornucopia, which includes a variety of bodywork specialties), AIDS, Oriental Bodywork, Business of Massage, and Student Clinic. Almost every class will include movement and relaxation in such forms as yoga, Feldenkrais®, tai chi, calisthenics, visualization, and meditation.

Admission Requirements

Applicants must be at least 18 years of age, have a high school diploma or equivalent, schedule a pre-enrollment interview, and submit a signed enrollment agreement.

Tuition and Fees

Tuition is $5,000. Additional expenses include application fee, $75; books, $300; First Aid/CPR, $20; optional massage table, approximately $500; and state board exam, $345.

Financial Assistance

An interest-free monthly payment plan and veterans' benefits are available.

Seminar Network International, Inc.

d/b/a SNI School of Massage and Allied Therapies
518 North Federal Highway
Lake Worth, Florida 33460
PHONE: (561) 582-5349 / (800) 882-0903
FAX: (561) 582-0807
E-MAIL: snimassage@mindspring.com
WEBSITE: SNImassage.com

Seminar Network International began in 1985 to provide continuing education for massage professionals. In 1987, the organization acquired the School of Massage Therapy and began to offer training at both the beginning and advanced levels. There are twenty instructors, with ten to twenty students per class. Additional programs offered but not covered here include Facial/Skin Care Specialist, Spa/Hydrotherapy Specialist, Colon Therapy, and SNI Day Spa.

Accreditation and Approvals

The Massage Therapy Program is approved by the Commission on Massage Training Accreditation (COMTA) and exceeds the educational requirement set forth by the Florida State Board of Massage; graduates are qualified to take the National Certification Examination for Therapeutic Massage and Bodywork (NCETMB). The program is also approved by the National Certification Board for Therapeutic Massage and Bodywork (NCBTMB) and by the State of Florida as a continuing education provider.

Program Description

The 600-hour Massage Therapy Program includes Human Anatomy and Physiology, Massage Theory and Practice, Hydrotherapy, Allied Modalities (including introductions to such fields as reflexology, shiatsu, sports massage, nutrition, polarity, infant massage, and others), Statutes/Rules and History of Massage, Practice Building and Business Practice, Basic Psychology, and HIV/AIDS.

Tai Chi and Chi Kung Teacher Training Programs are offered on two levels: a 200-hour Level I and a 250-hour Level II. These programs are open to students who want to learn or teach Tai Chi and Chi Kung to groups or in one-on-one instruction.

Continuing Education

Advanced Training workshops of 100 to 300 hours in length are offered to professional massage therapists in the areas of NISA (Neuromuscular Integration and Structural Alignment), Aromatherapy, Traditional Medical Massage of Thailand, Sports Massage, Clinical Sports Massage, Colon Hydrotherapy, Craniosacral Therapy, Equine Therapies, and Oriental Therapies (including Shiatsu and Thai Massage). As part of these advanced trainings, students receive a total of twenty hours in Advanced Anatomy and Physiology, Advanced Maniken® (nerves and vessels), Advanced Marketing, and Advanced Case Management.

Admission Requirements

Applicants must be at least 18 years of age; have a high school diploma or GED, or demonstrate an ability to benefit by achieving a passing score on the PAR Test (a test of basic skills); complete a personal health inventory; submit a physician's statement; and interview with an admissions representative.

Tuition and Fees

Tuition for the Massage Therapy Program is $5,000; books and fees are $210. Tuition for the Colon Therapy Program is $1,200. There is a $100 registration fee that is applied toward tuition or returned if the student is not accepted.

Tuition for the Tai Chi and Chi Kung Teacher Training programs is $11 per hour.

Financial Assistance

Federal grants and loans are available to qualified applicants; payment plans are also available.

Southeastern School of Neuromuscular and Massage Therapy

(See Multiple State Locations, pages 412–13)

Yogi Hari's Ashram

2216 NW 8th Terrace
Ft. Lauderdale, Florida 33311
PHONE: (800) 964-2553
E-MAIL: yogihari@aol.com
WEBSITE: www.yogihari.com

The Yoga Teachers Training Course at Yogi Hari's ashram was founded in 1989. Sri Yogi Hari and Leela Mata have been disciples of Swami Vishnudevananda since 1975. The Yoga Teacher's Certification course is limited to twenty people.

Program Description

The two-week residential Yoga Teachers Certification Course is personally conducted by Yogi Hari and Leela Mata twice each year. The intensive program permits total immersion in the practice of yoga. The curriculum includes Asanas, Pranayama, Meditation, Vedanta Philosophy, Karma and Reincarnation, Raja Yoga (mys-

teries of the mind), Jnana Yoga (inquiry into the nature of self), Bhakti Yoga (the path of devotion), Nada Yoga (study of sound vibration), Karma Yoga, Bhagavad Gita, Proper Diet, and Yoga Kriyas (cleansing techniques). Two buffet-style vegetarian meals are served daily. Full participation in all activities is required; no meat, fish, eggs, alcohol, tobacco, or narcotics are allowed.

Continuing Education

Continued training is offered through an Advanced Teachers Training Course and Sadhana Week programs.

Admission Requirements

Interest in yoga and self-unfoldment is the only prerequisite. A basic knowledge of asanas and philosophy is helpful, but beginners are welcome.

Tuition and Fees

The Yoga Teachers Training Course costs $1,500, including tuition, accommodations, meals, and course materials.

GEORGIA

Academy of Somatic Healing Arts

7094 Peachtree Industrial Boulevard, Building 4
Norcross, Georgia 30071-1024
PHONE: (404) 315-0394
FAX: (404) 633-1270
E-MAIL: demosthenes@mindspring.com
WEBSITE: www.ashamassage.com

Jim Gabriel's seriously injured elbows led him to seek help from Paul St. John, developer of neuromuscular therapy (NMT). Gabriel's positive response to treatment led him to attend massage therapy school and learn NMT himself. In 1982, he opened the Neuromuscular Center of Atlanta, and in 1991, the Academy of Somatic Healing Arts (ASHA). There are twenty-three instructors, with a maximum of twenty-two students per class.

Accreditation and Approvals

ASHA's Massage Therapy Training Program is authorized by the Nonpublic Postsecondary Education Commission of the

State of Georgia. The curriculum is also approved by the Ohio Medical Board and the boards of massage of the states of Washington and Florida; graduates are qualified to take the National Certification Examination for Therapeutic Massage and Bodywork (NCETMB). ASHA is approved by the National Certification Board for Therapeutic Massage and Bodywork (NCBTMB) and by the Florida State Board of Massage as a continuing education provider.

Program Description

The 775-hour Professional Massage Therapy Program offers graduates a triple certification in massage therapy: Therapeutic Swedish Massage, Clinical Sports Massage/Integrated Restorative Techniques, and Neuromuscular Therapy. The curriculum includes Anatomy and Physiology, Somatic Nutrition, Swedish Massage, Ethical Behavior and Self Care, Clinical Sports Massage, Hygiene/HIV/AIDS Awareness Training, Hydrotherapy and Associated Therapeutic Modalities, Neuromuscular Therapy (NMT), Clinical Practicum and Community Events, and Creating Success. Classes are offered in day, evening, and weekend formats.

Continuing Education

ASHA offers continuing education seminars on such topics as Craniosacral Therapy, Pregnancy Massage, Lymphatic Drainage Massage, and Thai Massage, as well as classes in Aromatherapy and Clinical Assessment and Treatment Planning.

Admission Requirements

Applicants must be at least 18 years of age and of moral character, submit two letters of recommendation, have a personal interview, and submit a physician's report and a massage therapist's verification report.

Tuition and Fees

Tuition is $7,000. Estimated additional expenses include application fee, $25; linens, $40; massage table, $460 to $600; books, $200; clinic shirt and white clothing for class, $100; and CPR certification, $25.

Financial Assistance

An interest-free payment plan is available to all students. A third-party loan program and veterans' benefits are available to those who qualify.

Atlanta School of Massage

2300 Peachford Road, Suite 3200
Atlanta, Georgia 30338
PHONE: (770) 454-7167 / (800) ASM-MASSAGE
FAX: (770) 454-7367
E-MAIL: asmadmit@bellsouth.net [Admissions] asmcraig@bellsouth.net [Continuing Education]
WEBSITE: www.atlantaschoolofmassage.com

The Atlanta School of Massage was established in 1980. There are four full-time and thirty-six adjunct and specialty instructors. The school graduates over 200 massage therapists a year.

Accreditation

The school is accredited by the Accrediting Commission of Career Schools and Colleges of Technology (ACCSCT), the Commission on Massage Training Accreditation (COMTA), and the Integrative Massage and Somatic Therapies Accreditation Council (IMSTAC). Graduates are qualified to take the National Certification Examination for Therapeutic Massage and Bodywork (NCETMB).

Program Description

The school offers three programs: Integrated Massage and Deep Tissue Therapy, Clinical Massage Therapy, and Wellness Massage and Spa Therapies. The four-day-per-week program is 720 hours over seven and a half months. The three-night-per-week evening program is 600 hours over twelve months.

All programs include Foundation Courses: Introduction to Massage, Massage Techniques (including Swedish Massage Comprehensive, Sports, Pregnancy, and Seated Massage, Polarity Therapy, Joint Movements, Body Mechanics, and Energetic Techniques), Human Sciences (Anatomy and Physiology, First Aid/CPR, Illness Care, HIV/AIDS Care, and more), Therapeutic Skills, Practice-Building Skills, Hydrotherapy, and Community Outreach Activities. Also required is a Clinic Practicum, in which students practice massage techniques and interactive skills with the public in a supervised setting at the nearby Student Teaching Clinic.

In addition to the Foundation Courses, each program includes a Specialized Curriculum.

The Integrated Massage and Deep Tissue Therapy Program combines several massage modalities such as Neuromuscular Therapy, Bodyreading, Advanced Therapeutic Skills, Intuitive Massage, and others to prepare graduates to adapt to a variety of work environments.

The Clincal Massage Therapy Program gives students the skills to work in medical and athletic environments. The specialized curriculum includes Thai Massage, Neuromuscular Therapy, Conditions and Assessment, Kinesiology, and more.

The Wellness Massage and Spa Therapies Program prepares students for work in spa and treatment settings as well as private practice. Specialized curriculum includes Shiatsu, Acupressure, Spa Lab Comprehensive, Reflexology (day only), and others.

One-evening introductory classes are scheduled biweekly to explain the school's program and to demonstrate massage techniques.

Admission Requirements

Applicants must be at least 18 years of age, have a high school diploma or equivalent, submit two letters of recommendation from licensed massage therapists or health professionals, submit a physician's examination report, and interview with an admissions representative. Applicants must have received at least one massage from a certified massage therapist; two additional professional massages must be received before graduation.

Tuition and Fees

Tuition is $7,975 for the day programs, $7,695 for evening. Other costs include application fee, $65; books, $300 to $350; massage table, approximately $600; CPR certification, $25; linens, lotion, and supplies, approximately $100; school shirt, $35; and three professional massages, approximately $140.

Financial Assistance

Federal grants and loans, payment plans, and loans are available.

Georgia Institute of Therapeutic Massage

2160 Central Avenue
P.O. Box 3657

Augusta, Georgia 30914-3657
PHONE: (706) 737-9291
FAX: (706) 738-6232
E-MAIL: gitm@MassageOne.com
WEBSITE: www.MassageOne.com

Georgia Institute of Therapeutic Massage (GITM) was founded in 1995 by Vicki N. Platt. There are ten instructors, with an average of fifteen to twenty students per class (maximum twenty-four).

Accreditation and Approvals

GITM is authorized in Georgia by the Nonpublic Postsecondary Education Commission, licensed in South Carolina by the Commission of Higher Education, and approved by the Florida Board of Massage Therapy. Graduates are qualified to take the National Certification Examination for Therapeutic Massage and Bodywork (NCETMB).

Program Description

The 550-hour, forty-week program in Massage Therapy consists of courses in Anatomy and Physiology, Applied Anatomy, Pathology, Introduction to Massage Therapy, Swedish, Deep Tissue, On Site Massage, Neuromuscular, Integration of Technique, Clinical Practice, Business Practices, Ethics and Self Care, Flexibility, Polarity, Shiatsu (Acupressure), Reflexology, Healing Touch, Cranial-Sacral Balancing, Hydrotherapy, Law and History of Massage, and Hygiene. Classes may be taken on a day or evening schedule.

Community and Continuing Education

Introductory classes are offered to the public in such areas as Introduction to Massage, Back and Neck Massage, Shiatsu, Reflexology, Basic Seated Massage, and Acupressure's Potent Points.

Admission Requirements

Applicants must be at least 18 years of age, have a high school diploma or equivalent, submit a physician's report and two letters of recommendation, have received at least one professional massage, and have a personal interview.

Tuition and Fees

Tuition is $5,100, including a $50 application fee. Additional expenses, including books, massage table, linens and oil, school shirt, two professional massages, and First Aid and CPR certification total approximately $950 to $1,250.

Fees for introductory classes are $40 to $75.

Financial Assistance

Tuition may be paid in two installments. Discount for early application, veterans' benefits and Vocational Rehabilitation (Georgia and South Carolina) are available.

Lake Lanier School of Massage

746 Green Street
Gainesville, Georgia 30501
PHONE: (770) 287-0377
FAX: (770) 536-7350
E-MAIL: Rcllsm@bellsouth.com
WEBSITE: www.massageschool.net

The Lake Lanier School of Massage was founded in 1993 and is owned by Sandra K. Easterbrooks, L.M.T. There are four instructors plus guest lecturers; classes average ten to fourteen students.

Accreditation and Approvals

The Lake Lanier School of Massage is accredited by the Integrative Massage and Somatic Therapies Accreditation Council (IMSTAC); authorized by the State of Georgia Nonpublic Postsecondary Education Commission; and approved by the Florida State Board of Massage. Graduates are qualified to take the National Certification Examination for Therapeutic Massage and Bodywork (NCETMB). The school is approved as a continuing education provider by the Florida State Board of Massage and by the National Certification Board for Therapeutic Massage and Bodywork (NCBTMB).

Program Description

The 550-hour Massage Therapy Program consists of Anatomy and Physiology, Massage Theory, Massage Practice (which includes Swedish Massage, Neuromuscular/Trigger Point Therapy, On-Site Seated Massage, Introduction to Russian (a massage system using heat, friction, and specific massage techniques), Myofascial Release Therapy, and Student Clinic/Community Events), Hydrotherapy, AIDS Awareness, History of Massage, Law, Rules and Regulations, and modalities that include Aromatherapy, Nutrition and Prevention, Business Marketing, Stress Management, Applied Kinesiology, Pathology, Craniosacral, CPR, and Assault Prevention. Classes are held days or evenings, with some Fridays and Saturdays required for the student clinic.

Continuing Education

Continuing education courses include Reflexology, Introduction to Shiatsu, Introduction to Infant Massage, Sports Massage 100-Hour Certification Program, and Touch for Health I, II, and III (kinesiology), among others.

Admission Requirements

Applicants must be at least 16 years of age, have a high school diploma or equivalent, be in good physical health and of good moral character, and be sincerely committed to providing quality care. Applicants must submit a physician's statement, two personal references, and a short essay, and interview with an admissions representative.

Tuition and Fees

Tuition is $5,500; books cost approximately $295. Linens and massage table for home practice are additional.

Financial Assistance

Payment plans are available.

Life University School of Chiropractic

1269 Barclay Circle
Marietta, Georgia 30060
PHONE: (770) 426-2884 / (800) 543-3202
FAX: (770) 428-9886
WEBSITE: www.life.edu

Life Chiropractic College was founded in 1974 by Dr. Sid E. Williams and opened in 1975 with twenty-two students; today Life University School of Chiropractic is the largest in the world. In addition to the programs described here, the university offers undergraduate degree programs in Nutrition for Dietetics and Business Administration, and a Master of Science degree in Sport Health Science. There are 312 instructors, with an average of 100 students in lecture, twenty-four in lab.

Accreditation and Approvals

Life University is accredited by the Commission on Colleges of the Southern Association of Colleges and Schools. The School of Chiropractic is accredited by the Council on Chiropractic Education (CCE).

Program Description

The 14-quarter Doctor of Chiropractic (D.C.) Degree Program is provided by seven major organizational components: Division of Chiropractic Sciences (Chiropractic Principles and Philosophy, Clinic Proficiency, and Practice and Professional Relations); Division of Technique and Analysis (Upper Cervical Technique, Full Spine Technique, and Analysis); Division of Clinical Sciences (Diagnosis, Radiologic Clinical Assessment, Psychology, and Public Health); Division of Diagnostic Imaging and Alignment (Radiologic Analysis and Radiologic Technology); Division of Basic Sciences (Anatomy, Chemistry, Microbiology/ Pathology, and Physiology); the Sid E. Williams Research Center; and the Division of Patient Care Facilities (Clinics).

Life University offers a multilevel approach to chiropractic education. Basic and clinical sciences are taught concurrently with chiropractic techniques, and students are taught hands-on techniques beginning in the third quarter. Students are permitted to give chiropractic care to patients during their third academic year.

Students' schedules are "blocked" (that is, they consist of a recommended sequence of courses) to a greater or lesser degree throughout the fourteen quarters of study, although a minimum of eighteen credit hours of electives may be selected beginning with the tenth quarter.

The four-quarter Chiropractic Technician (C.T.) Program covers Chiropractic Philosophy, Chiropractic History, Terminology, Nutrition, Introduction to X-Ray/Physics, Anatomy/ Physiology, Introduction to Clinic, Computer Literacy, CPR/ Basic Life Support, Emergency Procedures, X-Ray Positioning, Clinic/Field Interning, Patient Management/ Office Procedures, Public Relations/Speech, Public Health, Physical Diagnosis, Ra-

diographic Practicum, Office Procedures, Chiropractic Instrumentation, Laboratory Diagnosis, Computerized Office Management, Insurance Management, Spinal Hygiene, and more.

The School of Undergraduate Studies offers a four-year Bachelor of Science in Nutrition for the Chiropractic Sciences which is designed to complement the Doctor of Chiropractic program. In addition to courses in the sciences, humanities, and social sciences, courses offered include Medical Terminology, Introduction to Nutrition, Principles of Meal Preparation, Basic Nutrition, Advanced Nutrition, Nutrition in Health and Disease, Community Nutrition, Pathology, Nutrition Care Practicum, and a choice of Nutrition options (two are required) in such areas as Sports Nutrition, Maternal/Child Nutrition, The Study of Herbs in Health, Geriatric Nutrition, Nutrition and Physical Fitness Assessment, Menu Management, and more.

Continuing Education

The Program of Postgraduate Education offers numerous seminars on and off campus each year to Doctors of Chiropractic; contact the university for schedules and fees of upcoming programs.

Admission Requirements

Doctor of Chiropractic program applicants must have earned a cumulative GPA of 2.25 on a 4.0 scale and must have completed at least sixty semester hours (ninety quarter hours) of prechiropractic, college-level courses, including six semester hours of English, three semester hours of Psychology, fifteen semester hours of Humanities/Social Sciences, six semester hours of Organic Chemistry, six semester hours of Inorganic Chemistry, six semester hours of Physics, and six semester hours of Biological Sciences, in either Animal or Human Biology. Each science course must have a lab and must be passed with a grade of C or better. Students are encouraged to become proficient in written and computer literacy as part of their prechiropractic education. In addition, applicants must submit two letters of recommendation from practicing chiropractors or other professionals who know the applicant.

Chiropractic Technician applicants must be at least 17 years of age, have a high school diploma or equivalent, and submit two letters of recommendation.

Bachelor of Science in Nutrition for the Chiropractic Sciences applicants must have a 2.0 GPA from high school or passing GED score, and minimum recentered SAT score of 860 or a minimum ACT score of 18 (SAT/ACT scores waived for adult/nontraditional students who have been out of school eight years or more).

Tuition and Fees

Tuition for the D.C. program is $3,400 per quarter ($162 per quarter hour) plus a $50 application fee; books, supplies, lab fees, and other fees are additional. Tuition for the C.T. program is $600 per quarter (part-time tuition is $28.57 per quarter hour) plus a $25 application fee; books, supplies, and other fees are additional.

Tuition for the B.S. program is $118 per quarter hour plus a $50 application fee; books, supplies, lab fees, and other fees are additional.

Financial Assistance

Available financial assistance includes federal, state and private grants, scholarships, loans, and work-study.

Living With Herbs Institute

931 Monroe Drive, Suite 102-343
Atlanta, Georgia 30308
PHONE: (404) 607-8222
E-MAIL: LWHerbs@earthlink.net

Instructor Patricia Kyritsi Howell has been a full-time herbal educator for the past eight years; classes have been offered at the Living With Herbs Institute for the last six years. There are three to five instructors per year, with an average of thirty students per class.

Program Description

The ten-month Fundamentals of Herbalism program is designed to give students a solid foundation in the use of herbs for healing, and covers concepts of energetic herbalism rooted in both Eastern and Western traditions. The program of evening and weekend lectures, workshops, and retreats covers Energetic Herbalism, Five Phase Theory and Energetic Healing, Herbs In-Depth, Health Assessment Techniques, Wild Plant Identification and Harvesting, Flower Essences, Aromatherapy, Herbal Therapies in Practice, and Materia Medica.

Community and Continuing Education

The institute offers weekend workshops related to the use of plants as medicines, and a clinical skills training program for practitioners who have successfully completed Fundamentals of Herbalism.

Admission Requirements

No previous herbal experience is required, although students are encouraged to review basic concepts of anatomy and physiology.

Tuition and Fees

The tuition of $2,600 includes lectures, workshops, course materials and two three-day retreats. Books, retreat meals, and medicine-making supplies are additional.

Financial Assistance

Payment plans, an early registration discount ($100), and limited work-exchange options are available.

HAWAII
Aisen Shiatsu School

Interstate Building
1314 South King Street, Suite 601
Honolulu, Hawaii 96814
PHONE: (808) 596-7354
FAX: (808) 593-8282

The Aisen Shiatsu School was founded in 1977 by Fumihiko Indei, a graduate of and former instructor at the Japan Shiatsu College in Tokyo.

Accreditation and Approvals

The Aisen Shiatsu School is licensed by the Hawaii State Department of Education.

Program Description

The 200-hour Shiatsu Therapy Program is designed to produce skilled shiatsu therapists. The curriculum includes eighty hours of anatomy and physiology and 120 hours of theory and practice of shiatsu therapy (therapeutic muscle and nerve shiatsu). Classes are held in the evening.

Admission Requirements

Applicants must have a high school diploma or equivalent, good moral character, and temperate habits; submit a health certificate and three letters of reference; and interview with an admissions representative.

Tuition and Fees

There is a $200 registration fee; tuition is $4,600, including lab fees and books.

American Viniyoga Institute

(See Multiple State Locations, page 385)

Hawai'i College of Traditional Oriental Medicine

3660 Baldwin Avenue
Makawao, Maui, Hawaii
Mailing Address:
P.O. Box 457
Kula, Hawaii 96790
PHONE: (808) 573-0899
FAX: (808) 573-2450
E-MAIL: email@hawaiicollege.com
WEBSITE: www.hawaiicollege.com

The Hawai'i College of Traditional Oriental Medicine, a non-profit corporation, was founded in 1994 by Thomas and Ilene Bellerue. The faculty consists of seventeen full- and part-time members; there are twelve to fifteen students per class.

Accreditation and Approvals

The Hawai'i College of Traditional Oriental Medicine is a candidate for accreditation with the Accreditation Commission for Acupuncture and Oriental Medicine (ACAOM). The college is licensed as a vocational-technical school by the State of Hawaii Department of Education. Graduates are eligible to apply for licensure as an acupuncturist in Hawaii and to sit for the examinations leading to national certification by the National Certification Commission for Acupuncture and Oriental Medicine.

Program Description

The 2,550-hour Master of the Arts of Traditional Oriental Medicine Program may be completed in three years. Year One courses include Classical Chinese Medical Theory, History of Medicine, Acupuncture Points and Meridians, Medical Terminology, Anatomy and Physiology, Qi Gong, Oriental Dietary Principles, Chinese Astrology, Clinical Observation, Herbal Medicine, Oriental Massage Therapy, Five Element Acupuncture, Communication and Counseling Skills, Acupuncture Techniques, and Feng Shui. Year Two courses include Differentiation of Syndromes, Acupuncture Points and Meridians, Herbal Medicine, Pathology, Acupuncture Techniques, Qi Gong, Clinical Observation, Oriental Massage Therapy, and Oriental Massage Therapy Clinic. Year Three courses include Advanced Diagnostic Methods, Herbal Medicine, Clinical Sciences, Clinical Internship, Case History Seminar, Survey of Medical Practices, Physics, Pharmacology, Traditional Pediatrics, Laboratory Test Analysis, Ethics and Practice Management, Qi Gong, and Chinese Astrology.

Admission Requirements

Applicants must have completed at least two years (sixty semester units) of general college education at the baccalaureate level from an accredited institution. Preference is given to applicants who have completed a bachelor's degree. Applicants must also submit two letters of recommendation, an essay, and have a personal interview.

Tuition and Fees

Tuition is $9,000 per year ($9,250 per year for students paying in three payments). Total additional expenses for the three-year program include application fee, $50; books, $1,200; class supplies, $150; clinical supplies, $500; student malpractice insurance, $350.

Financial Assistance

Payment plans and a low-interest student loan program are available.

Hawaiian Islands School of Body Therapies

78-6239 Alii Drive
P.O. Box 390188
Kailua-Kona, Hawaii 96739
PHONE: (808) 322-0048 / (800) 928-9645
FAX: (808) 322-4971
E-MAIL: massages@gte.net

Lynn Wind, former clinical director of the Canadian College of Massage and Hydrotherapy, founded the Hawaiian Islands School of Body Therapies (HIS) in 1988. Unique to the school, the Knight-Wind Method of Restorative Treatment Therapy integrates medical treatment massage with holistic therapies to nurture each student's intuitive abilities. There are seven instructors, with an average of eight to twelve students per class.

Accreditation and Approvals
The program offered by HIS is approved by the Hawaiian State Department of Education. Graduates are eligible to take the Hawaii State Board of Massage licensing exam; graduates of massage therapy programs of 500 or more hours are qualified to take the National Certification Examination for Therapeutic Massage and Bodywork (NCETMB). HIS is approved by the Florida State Board of Massage, as well as by most states with licensing requirements, as a CEU provider.

Program Description
The Knight-Wind Method of Restorative Therapies is a compilation of various bodywork disciplines taught primarily from a series of therapeutic massage manuals written by Lynn Wind.

The 645-hour Professional Massage Therapy Program consists of Levels I through III, three thirteen-week semesters (Level I may be taken alone for 165 hours of training). An extended program—Levels I through IV—offers 1,000 hours (one additional semester) of instruction.

Level I consists of Theory and Practice of Massage (100 hours), Introduction to Anatomy (fifty hours), and Principles of Assessment and Treatment (fifteen hours). Levels II through IV consist of three intensive areas of study (shoulder/thorax/upper extremities; cervical/cranium/TMJ; and low back/pelvis/lower extremities), each in excess of 128 hours. Also included are Anatomy/Physiology/Pathology, Kinesiology,

Clinical Integration, Practical Integration, and Business. Other modalities taught during the course of the program include lomi lomi, hydrotherapy, reflexology, polarity, neuromuscular techniques, aromatherapy, shiatsu, body-mind integration, geriatric massage, lymphatic drainage, brain gym (education kinesiology), subtle body therapies, soft touch, myofascial release, craniosacral, and sports massage.

Students must have completed a Hawaiian Heart Association CPR Course prior to graduation. Classes are held weekday mornings and evenings. Each October, students are part of the world's largest massage team at the annual Ironman Triathlon.

Admission Requirements
Applicants must be at least 18 years of age, have a high school diploma or equivalent, interview with an admissions representative, provide documentation of good health and TB clearance, submit a current résumé, be physically able to perform massage therapy, and be able to finance their education.

Tuition and Fees
There is a $50 application fee that is credited toward tuition upon acceptance. Tuition for Level I is $1,650; books and supplies are approximately $550. Tuition for Levels I to III is $5,676; books and supplies are approximately $950. Tuition for Levels I to IV is $7,800; books and supplies are approximately $1,050.

Financial Assistance
A payment plan is available.

Honolulu School of Massage

1136 12th Avenue, Suite 240
Honolulu, Hawaii 96816
PHONE: (808) 733-0000
FAX: (808) 733-0045
E-MAIL: hsminc@digital-m.com

The Honolulu School of Massage was founded in 1981. There are ten instructors plus guest lecturers, with an average of twenty-five students per Basic Class, thirty to fifty in combined Professional Classes.

Accreditation and Approvals

The Massage Therapy Training Program offered by Honolulu School of Massage meets AMTA standards and exceeds the educational requirements for licensure in Hawaii; graduates of programs of 500 or more hours are qualified to take the National Certification Examination for Therapeutic Massage and Bodywork (NCETMB). The school is approved by the Hawaii Department of Education and by the Hawaii Nursing Association for continuing education.

Program Description

The one-year, 630-hour AMTA Professional Training Program consists of two sections: a 180-hour Basic Massage Therapy Training (which fulfills the minimum academic portion of state of Hawaii licensing requirements) and a 450-hour Professional Massage Therapy Training Program.

The sixteen-week Basic Training consists of eighty hours of anatomy, physiology, and kinesiology, and one hundred hours of theory, demonstration, and practice of massage, including history, basic principles and application of Swedish massage strokes, contraindications, personal hygiene, and client assessment.

The Professional Training consists of 350 hours of classroom study and one hundred hours of supervised student clinic and community service. Topics covered include Foot Reflexology, Pregnancy Massage, Special Population Massage, Hydrotherapy, Professionalism, Lomi Lomi, Shiatsu, Sports Massage, Session Planning, Ethical Issues and the Professional Massage Therapist, HIV and Massage, Craniosacral Technique, Practical Myology, Neuroanatomy, Deep Tissue Massage, Kinesiology, Pathology, CPR/First Aid, and state exam review. Completion takes approximately eight months.

Continuing Education

Individual courses listed under Professional Massage Therapy Training may be taken by students who wish to continue their education after licensing. Advanced workshops for licensed therapists are offered in a variety of techniques and interests beyond the Professional-level training.

Admission Requirements

Applicants must be at least 18 years of age or have the consent of a parent or guardian; have a high school diploma or equiva-

lent and fluent English-language skills; have TB clearance and no diseases or disabilities that would limit physical exertion; interview with an admissions representative; and submit two personal recommendations and a letter of intent.

Tuition and Fees

For all courses, there is a nonrefundable $25 application fee and a $100 registration fee; supplies are approximately $100.

Tuition for the Basic Massage Therapy program (180 hours) is $1,950. Tuition for the Professional Massage Therapy program (450 hours) is $4,600, or $2,300 per semester. Total tuition for the AMTA Professional Massage Therapy Program (630 hours) is $6,550. Tuition includes books, lubricant, taxes, and deposits.

Financial Assistance

Payment plans are available; veterans' benefits are available for the 630-hour program. Various state agencies may approve funding.

Tai Hsuan Foundation College of Acupuncture and Herbal Medicine

Mailing Address:
P.O. Box 11130
Honolulu, Hawaii 96828

STREET ADDRESS:
2600 South King Street, #206
Honolulu, Hawaii 96826
PHONE: (808) 949-1050 / (800) 942-4788
FAX: (808) 947-1152
E-MAIL: 71532.2642@compuserve.com
WEBSITE: acupuncture-hi.com

Tai Hsuan Foundation College was founded in 1970 by Taoist Master Chang Yi Hsiang, Ph.D., the sixty-fourth-generation lineage holder of heavenly Taoist Masters of the Lung He Shan Mountains in China. There are twelve instructors, with an average of twenty students per class.

Accreditation and Approvals

The Master of Acupuncture and Oriental Medicine program is

accredited by the Accreditation Commission for Acupuncture and Oriental Medicine (ACAOM).

Program Description

The college teaches Taoist healing arts through Acupuncture, Chinese Herbology, Qigong, Meditation, Sacred Taoist Magic Arts, Feng Shui, Chinese Astrology, Palmistry, I Ching, Calligraphy, Taoist Charm Language Writing, and Tao of Living Philosophy.

The 2,500-hour Master of Acupuncture and Oriental Medicine Program consists of 1,380 hours of Acupuncture Medical (traditional Chinese medicine, Taoist medicine and treatment, and needle technique) and Clinical Sciences, 500 hours of Herbal Medicine (materia medica, herbs, and herbal formulas) and Clinical Sciences, and 360 hours of Biomedical Sciences (anatomy/physiology, terminology, pathology, disease processes, pharmacology, and lab test/physical exam/clinical process).

Admission Requirements

Applicants must have completed a minimum of two years of college education (sixty college credits) or professional training from an accredited institution, and should have a professional attitude and flexibility in personal relations as evidenced by professional experience, education, life experiences, and letters of recommendation. Applicants must submit a brief essay and professional experience history, two letters of recommendation, and tuberculin skin test or chest X-ray results no more than three months old.

Tuition and Fees

Tuition is $3,450 per semester. Additional expenses include application fee, $50; uniform, $25; and graduation fee, $100.

Financial Assistance

Federal loans and veterans' benefits are available.

Traditional Chinese Medical College of Hawaii

Waimea Office Center/Mamalahoa Highway
P.O. Box 2288
Kamuela, Hawaii 96743
PHONE: (808) 885-9226
FAX: (808) 885-7886
E-MAIL: chinese@ilhawaii.com
WEBSITE: www.ilhawaii.net/~chinese/

The Traditional Chinese Medical College of Hawaii, founded in 1986 by Angela Longo, Ph.D., was the first such college on the Big Island of Hawaii. Dr. Longo apprenticed under Dr. Lam Kong, a two-term chairman of the California Board of Acupuncture. There are six instructors, with an average of seven students per class.

Accreditation and Approvals

The college's Professional Diploma of Oriental Medicine Program is a candidate for accreditation with the Accreditation Commission for Acupuncture and Oriental Medicine (ACAOM). Graduates of the three-year program are qualified to take the Hawaii State Licensing Exam administered by the National Certification Commission for Acupuncture and Oriental Medicine (NCCAOM).

Program Description

The 2,466-hour, three-year program leads to a Diploma in Oriental Medicine. The school year is divided into three fifteen-week trimesters. Courses include Origins of Acupuncture and Fundamental Theory of Oriental Medicine; Comparison of Western and Oriental Medical Models; Traditional Meridian and Point Study; Meridian Theory; Clinical Acupuncture and Moxibustion Procedures; Auriculotherapy; Traditional Diagnosis and Pathology; Chinese Pharmacology; Nutrition and Its Relation to the Disease State; Western Medical Terminology and Lab Analysis; Acupressure Techniques; CPR and Basic Emergency Procedures; Human Anatomy and Physiology; Qigong and Preventive Medicine; Tai Chi; Ethics and Human Services Skills; Chinese Medical Communication Skills; Case Presentations; Neurophysiology and Brain Gym; Clinic Management; Clinical Observation; Clinical Patient Care; Practice Management; and Supervised Clinical Practice.

Admission Requirements

Applicants must be at least 21 years of age; have completed two years (sixty semester credits) of postsecondary education at an accredited college or university; be proficient in English; submit a résumé, an essay, and two letters of recommendation; and interview with an admissions representative.

Tuition and Fees

Tuition is $2,700 per trimester; this includes both classroom and clinical instruction. Other costs include: application fee, $60; new student registration fee, $25; required seminars, $1,080 total; books (annual average), $200 to $300; supplies, $50; needles and moxa (annual average), $50; and annual malpractice insurance, $300.

Financial Assistance

Students are eligible for the MedAchiever educational loan program.

IDAHO

Idaho Institute of Wholistic Studies

1412 West Washington Street
Boise, Idaho 83702
PHONE: (208) 345-2704
FAX: (208) 367-9242
E-MAIL: iiws@micron.net

The Idaho Institute of Wholistic Studies (IIWS) was founded in 1993 by Brandie Redinger, Karen VanDeGrift, and Barbera Bashan.

Accreditation and Approvals

While there is no licensing requirement in Idaho, graduates of massage therapy programs of 500 or more hours are qualified to take the National Certification Examination for Therapeutic Massage and Bodywork (NCETMB).

Program Description

The 350-hour Massage Practitioner Program may be completed in one year of full-time study. The curriculum includes Anatomy, Physiology, Body Work I and II (which includes Swedish, polarity, reflexology, yoga, muscular release, and supervised clinic), Body Work III: Shiatsu, CPR, Chinese Anatomy and Physiology, Emotional Armoring and Trauma, Movement,

Professionalism and Ethics, Self-Healing and Communication, Sports Medicine, and Whole Foods and Health.

The Healing Body/Mind Somatic Therapy Advanced Program adds 250 hours toward the 600 hours required for advanced certification as a body therapist. The curriculum includes Rebirthing, Touching the Trauma of Sexual Abuse, Introduction to Abuse and Recovery, Transference Issues, Interviewing and Screening Clients, Co-Treatment, Treatment from the Victim's Perspective, Post-Traumatic Stress Disorder, Trust and Power Issues, Disassociation, Emotional Healing, Body Image vs. Body Reality, Offender Profile, Assessing Trauma, Keeping Your Balance, Survivor's Spirituality, and Emotional Release Techniques.

IIWS coordinates a 795-hour AMMA Therapy Course with Wellspring, an educational institute dedicated to traditional Eastern medicine. AMMA Therapy integrates bodywork with manipulation of energy channels, diet, herbal and vitamin supplements, detoxification, application of external herbal preparations, and exercise. Completion of this course earns advanced certification as a body therapist and meets qualifications for membership in the American Oriental Bodywork Therapist Association (AOBTA). The curriculum includes Oriental Anatomy and Physiology, AMMA Technique, Applied Technique, Clinic, Food in Treatment of Disharmony, and Oriental Clinical Assessment. Other requirements include sixty hours of tai chi chuan and/or qigong and six private sessions with a senior AMMA therapist; the student must also give a senior therapist one treatment.

Admission Requirements

Applicants must be at least 18 years of age and have a high school diploma. Applicants must also be able to lift fifty pounds, to stand one to two hours at a time, and must see, hear, speak, and move well enough to meet the demands of the work.

Tuition and Fees

There is a $95 registration fee. Tuition for the 350-hour Massage Practitioner Program is $3,770. Tuition for the 600-hour Massage Therapist Program is $6,310. Students transferring in with at least 350 credit hours and taking only the 250 credit hours of the Advanced Program pay $2,750. Contact the Institute for the AMMA Therapy course.

Financial Assistance

A payment plan, Vocational Rehabilitation, and Job Service aid are available.

ILLINOIS

Chicago National College of Naprapathy

3330 North Milwaukee Avenue
Chicago, Illinois 60641
PHONE: (773) 282-2686 / (800) 262-6620
FAX: (773) 282-2688
E-MAIL: cncn@naprapathy.edu
WEBSITE: www.naprapathy.edu

Naprapathic practice is the evaluation of persons with connective tissue disorders through the use of naprapathic case history and palpation or treatment using connective tissue manipulation, postural counseling, nutritional counseling, heat, cold, light, water, radiant energy, electricity, sound, and air. The practice includes the treatment of contractures, lesions, laxity, rigidity, structural imbalance, muscular atrophy, and other disorders. The first chartered school of naprapathy, the Oakley Smith School of Naprapathy, was founded in 1907 in Chicago; it became the Chicago College of Naprapathy. Another school, the National College of Naprapathy, was founded in Chicago in 1949. The two schools merged in 1971 to become the Chicago National College of Naprapathy. There are twenty-two faculty members; the average class size is twenty-five.

Accreditation and Approvals

The Chicago National College of Naprapathy is accredited by the Council of Colleges of the American Naprapathic Association and recognized by the Illinois State Board of Higher Education to grant the degree Doctor of Naprapathy (D.N.). Graduates are eligible to take the examination for licensure as a Doctor of Naprapathy (D.N.) in the State of Illinois.

Program Description

The four-academic-year (three-calendar-year) full-time Doctor of Naprapathy Program (plus qualified part-time four-calendar-year program) consists of sixty-six credit hours in the basic sciences and sixty-four credit hours in the naprapathic

sciences, for a total of 130 credit hours of academic work. An additional sixty credit hours are spent gaining clinical experience. Courses in the basic sciences include Anatomy I, II, and III; Applied Biomechanics; Biochemistry I and II; Embryology/Genetics; Exercise Physiology/Biomechanics; Histology; Connective Tissue Dynamics; Kinesiology; Laboratory Interpretation and Symptomatology; Microbiology and Public Health; Neuroscience I and II; Organic Chemistry; Physiology I, II, and III; Pathology I and II; and Science of Nutrition and Diet I and II. The naprapathic science curriculum covers naprapathic theory and practice; evaluating connective tissue disorders and how they effect neurological control of the connective tissues; how to apply naprapathic therapeutic techniques; the educational, ethical, legal, and psychological issues involved in clinical practice; and courses in therapeutic exercise, biomechanics, and nutrition. The clinical experience phase is supervised by clinic faculty. Courses in this phase include Accessory Technique; Accessory Techniques/Adjunctive Therapies; Clinical Nutrition: Approach to Wellness; Clinical Orthopedic and Neurological Evaluation; Clinical Practice; Clinical Preparation; Ethics and Jurisprudence; Gross Anatomical Examination; Integrational Clinic Seminars; Naprapathic Charting and Clinical Evaluation I, II, and III; Naprapathic History and Philosophy; Naprapathic Technique I and II; Naprapathic Therapeutics; Physiological Therapeutics; Principles of Rehabilitation; Principles of Massage; Spinal Anatomy; Sports and Exercise Injury Assessment; Treatment and Rehabilitation; Therapeutic Exercise; and Clinical Naprapathic Protocol and Evaluation.

Admission Requirements

Degree-seeking candidates must have completed two years of college (sixty semester hours), including a minimum of twenty-four semester hours of general education with a GPA of 2.0 on a 4.0 scale; submit the application form and fees; have a personal interview; and submit two letters of reference. Students-at-large—those undecided about pursuing the degree—should schedule an interview with an admissions counselor.

Tuition and Fees

Tuition is $135 per credit hour. There is a matriculation fee of $50 and an application fee equal to the cost of one class, which is refunded if the student does not enroll. All students pay a registration fee of $25, a student activity fee of $75 per year, and applicable lab fees.

Financial Assistance

Monthly payment plans, veterans' benefits, and vocational rehabilitation benefits are available.

Chicago School of Massage Therapy

2918 North Lincoln Avenue
Chicago, Illinois 60657-4109
PHONE: (773) 477-9444
FAX: (773) 477-7256
E-MAIL: Jeff@csmt.com
WEBSITE: www.csmt.com

The Chicago School of Massage Therapy (CSMT) was founded in 1981. There are over forty faculty members; class sizes average seventy students for lectures, twenty-four for technique classes.

Accreditation and Approvals

CSMT is accredited by the Commission on Massage Training Accreditation (COMTA); graduates are qualified to take the National Certification Examination for Therapeutic Massage and Bodywork (NCETMB). CSMT is approved as a vocational school by the Illinois State Board of Education, and is approved by the National Certification Board for Therapeutic Massage and Bodywork (NCBTMB) as a continuing education provider. CSMT is also approved by the licensing boards of Washington and Ohio.

Program Description

The 662-hour, four-semester Professional Massage Therapy Diploma Program consists of 612 hours of coursework plus fifty hours of community outreach. Courses include Acupressure, Anatomy and Physiology, Business Development, Chair Massage/Outreach Orientation, First Aid and CPR, Kinesiology and Musculo-Skeletal Pathology, Massage Therapy (covering such topics as contemporary Western massage, body mobilization techniques, sports massage, hydrotherapy, trigger points, myofascial techniques, and more), Professional Foundations,

Special Populations, Stress Reduction/Student Clinic Orientation, and Student Clinic. The fifty hours of community outreach includes thirty hours of Special Populations and twenty hours of Special and Sports Events.

Community and Continuing Education

CSMT offers ongoing five- and ten-week Massage Basics classes to acquaint prospective students with the theory and basic skills of massage.

Ongoing continuing education programs and advanced certifications are offered to massage therapy and bodywork professionals. Programs include Advanced Certification Sports Massage, Professional Myofascial Massage Therapy, Post Graduate Certification Course Electives, and Advanced Certification/ Sports Massage/Personal Fitness Training.

Admission Requirements

Applicants must be at least 18 years of age; have a high school diploma or equivalent; have received at least one professional massage; have prior introductory-level training or instruction in massage therapy; be in good health and be physically able to perform massage; submit a completed application including answers to essay questions; and interview with the admissions director.

Tuition and Fees

Tuition is $6,900; an additional $400 book fee covers books, handouts, manuals, lab fees, and professional liability insurance while working as a student. Additional expenses include a massage table, sheets, and oil.

Tuition for the five-week Massage Basics Course is $150; for the ten-week Massage Basics Course, $250.

Integrative Yoga Therapy

(See Multiple State Locations, page 396)

Leidecker Institute

1901 North Roselle Road, Suite 800
Schaumburg, Illinois 60195
PHONE: (847) 844-1933 / (888) 655-6632
FAX: (847) 844-1932

E-MAIL: NGHSchool@aol.com

WEBSITE: www.leideckerinstitute.com

The Leidecker Institute was founded by Arthur A. Leidecker.

Accreditation and Approvals

Leidecker Institute is endorsed by the International Medical and Dental Hypnotherapy Association (IMDHA).

Program Description

The complete program of Hypnotherapy Certification Courses consists of 100 hours of intensive training over three courses.

The Foundational Hypnotherapy Course 101 covers Introduction to Hypnosis, Preliminary Suggestibility Tests, Recognition and Classification of Subjects, How to Hypnotize, Changing Behaviors Using Posthypnotic Suggestions, Depth Stages of Hypnosis, Self-Hypnosis Training, Hypnotic Miscellany, Your Hypnosis Practice, Hypnosis Programs for Smoking Cessation, Weight Management and Stress Reduction, and Business Aspects of Hypnotherapy Practice.

The Advanced Hypnotherapist Certification 102 covers How to Give a Lecture Demonstration, How to Use Modern Advanced Methods of Induction, Hypnotherapy Applications, Use of Tasking, Creating Triggers and Anchors, How to Use Age Regression, and The Law and You.

Graduate Course 103 covers Instantaneous Inductions, Kinesthetic Disorientation, Image Psychology and Hypnosis, Imagination Training, Systematic Desensitization, Color Imagery, Behavioral Therapies, Hypno-Amnesia, Forensic Hypnosis Interviewing, Automatic Writing, Hypnotic Tapes, Electronic Hypnosis, Past Life Regressions, Corporate Marketing, and more.

Community and Continuing Education

Additional programs and workshops are offered in Reiki I, Therapeutic Touch, Child Hypnosis, Medical Hypnotism, NLP Training, and Neuro-subliminal® Communication are offered.

Tuition and Fees

Tuition for Course 101 is $295; for Course 102, $395; and for course 103, $495.

Financial Assistance

Payment plans, spouse or partner discounts, and discounts for enrolling in all three programs are available.

LifePath School of Massage Therapy

7820 North University, Suite 110
Peoria, Illinois 61614
PHONE: (309) 693-7284 / (309) 693-PATH / (888) 2-LIFEPATH
E-MAIL: rwasher@flink.com

The LifePath School of Massage Therapy was founded in 1991 by Rhonda Washer. The school emphasizes the integration of various modalities in order to therapeutically affect body, mind, and spirit. LifePath is in partnership in process with Illinois Community College. There are thirteen instructors, with a maximum of twenty-five students per class.

Accreditation and Approvals

The school is accredited by the Integrative Massage and Somatic Therapies Accreditation Council (IMSTAC), approved by the Illinois State Board of Education as a private vocational school, and a member of the American Massage Therapy Association (AMTA) Council of Schools. Graduates are qualified to take the National Certification Examination for Therapeutic Massage and Bodywork (NCETMB).

Program Description

The ten-month, 700-hour Massage Therapy Program includes Fundamental Massage Techniques, Anatomy and Physiology, Kinesiology, Nutrition, Reflexology, Psychology for the Bodyworker, Wellness Concepts, Massage Technique Variations, Massage Technique Applications, Deep Muscle Therapy, Sports Massage, Joint Mobilization and Stretching, Hydrotherapy, Polarity Therapy, Business Ethics and Professional Practice, Neuromuscular Principles in Deep Tissue Bodywork, and Clinical Experience in Massage Therapy. Classes meet two evenings and one Saturday per week, with one weekend intensive per month.

Admission Requirements

Applicants must be at least 18 years of age; have a high school diploma or equivalent; be proficient in the English language; be in good health and free of communicable disease; submit two letters of recommendation and an autobiographical sketch; and interview with an admissions representative.

Tuition and Fees
Tuition is $7,000 and includes materials and liability insurance. Additional expenses include an application fee, $100, and books and a massage table, $900 to $1,000.

Financial Assistance
Payment plans and veterans benefits are available.

National College of Chiropractic

200 East Roosevelt Road
Lombard, Illinois 60148-4583
PHONE: (630) 629-2000 / (800) 826-NATL
FAX: (630) 889-6554
E-MAIL: juliet@national.chiropractic.edu
WEBSITE: www.national.chiropractic.edu

The National College of Chiropractic (NCC) was established in 1906 in Davenport, Iowa, as the National School of Chiropractic. After years of growth and several moves, the school moved to its current facility in Lombard—the first such facility ever constructed for the exclusive use of chiropractic educators. There are 107 instructors, with approximately 100 students per class.

Accreditation and Approvals
NCC is accredited by the Council on Chiropractic Education (CCE), the Commission on Institutions of Higher Education of the North Central Association of Colleges and Schools, and by registration by the State Education Department of the State of New York.

Program Description
NCC adopted a new curriculum in 1996. The Doctor of Chiropractic Degree Guided Discovery Curriculum allows students to utilize real clinical patient cases as they are developing their basic science knowledge, thereby learning at an early point in the curriculum to integrate basic science knowledge with diagnosis and chiropractic therapies. The curriculum provides

greater focus on the integration of knowledge and skills; all courses are integrated and taught by interdepartmental teams.

The 4,834-hour, ten-trimester Doctor of Chiropractic Degree Program covers, in the first year, Structure and Function of the Spine, Cells/Endocrine, Head and Neck, Molecular Biophysiology, Extremities, and Respiratory System; Clinical Practice including History, Professional Responsibilities, Physical Assessment, Manipulative Therapeutics, and more; and General Education in Ethics, Boundary Training, Community Health, Self-Care, Communication, and Problem Solving. Second-year topics, include Structure and Function of the Viscera, CV, GI, and Life Cycle; Neuromusculoskeletal System topics, including Arthrology/Myology and Spinal/CNS; Clinical Practice including Diagnostic Imaging, Chiropractic Manipulative Therapeutics, and XR Positioning; and General Education topics including Jurisprudence and Research Paper. Third-year courses include Neuromusculoskeletal System: Peripheral Nervous System and Extremities/Arthritides; Viscera; Clinical Practice, including Diagnostic Imaging and Student Clinic; General Education topics, including Risk Management and Doctor-Patient Relationship; and Internship.

Continuing Education
The National-Lincoln School of Postgraduate Education, a division of NCC, offers credit and noncredit courses of instruction taken as residencies or on an extension basis. Programs offered include Diagnostic Imaging, Chiropractic Orthopedics, Clinical Orthopedics, Physiological Therapeutics, Advanced Physiological Therapeutics, Chiropractic Neurology, Chiropractic Clinical Nutrition, Industrial Consulting, Chiropractic Sports Physician, Electrodiagnosis, Clinical Thermography, and Manipulation Under Anesthesia. Contact NCC for additional information about these programs.

In addition, continuing education programs are also offered in Homeopathy and in Acupuncture/Meridian Therapy.

The Homeopathy Program provides a comprehensive summary of the fundamentals of classical homeopathy and consists of twenty-five weekend sessions that meet monthly over a two-year period. Topics covered include homeopathic history and philosophy, homeopathic practice methodology, materia medica, first aid and acute prescribing, chronic case management, practical clinical training, ethics and legal issues, and research.

The Acupuncture/Meridian Therapy Program consists of 120 hours of practical training and an additional 108 hours of advanced acupuncture training. Basic courses include Introduction to Acupuncture, Meridians, Auriculotherapy, Instrumentation and Acupuncture Diagnosis, and Differential Diagnosis; Advanced courses include Five Element Theory, The Eight Principles: Patterns of Disease, Needling Techniques, Pulse Diagnosis, Tongue Diagnosis, Microsystems, Accessory Techniques, Case Studies, and Electrical, Magnetic, and Electromagnetic Forces.

Admission Requirements

Doctor of Chiropractic degree applicants are encouraged to apply for admission at least one year in advance for one of three new classes per year. Applicants are required to have a Bachelor of Science degree prior to entering the college. Specific requirements, completed with a grade of C or better, include a minimum of six semester hours in each of these courses: Human/Cell-related Biological Sciences, General or Inorganic Chemistry I and II, Organic Chemistry I and II, and Physics I and II. All science courses must be completed with the corresponding laboratory. Other requirements include six semester hours of English or Composition, fifteen semester hours of Social Sciences/Humanities, and three semester hours of Introductory or General Psychology.

Tuition and Fees

There is a $55 application fee. Tuition is $225 per credit hour. Books cost $250 to $350 per trimester; lab fees are additional.

Financial Assistance

A payment plan, federal and private scholarships, grants, loans, and work-study programs are available.

Northern Prairie Center for Education and Healing Arts

MAIN SITE:
138 North Fair Street
Sycamore, Illinois 60178
PHONE: (815) 899-3382
FAX: (815) 899-3381
E-MAIL: npschool@earthlink.net

CLASSROOM EXTENSION SITES:
839 North Madison Street
Rockford, Illinois 61107
PHONE: (815) 963-7270
Provena Mercy Center
Aurora, Illinois

The Northern Prairie Center for Education and Healing Arts (a.k.a. the Northern Prairie School of Therapeutic Massage and Bodywork) was founded in 1993. Director/administrator Jeannette Vaupel has been practicing therapeutic massage since 1986. There are nineteen part-time instructors with an average of fifteen (maximum thirty) students per class. Classes are held in Sycamore, Rockford, and Aurora.

Accreditation and Approvals

Northern Prairie School is accredited by the Integrative Massage and Somatic Therapies Accreditation Council (IMSTAC), a member of the American Massage Therapy Association (AMTA) Council of Schools, an institutional member of Associated Bodywork and Massage Professionals (ABMP), and approved by the Illinois State Board of Education as a Private Vocational School.

Program Description

The eleven-month, 600-hour Therapeutic Massage and Bodywork Program consists of 464 hours of in-class instruction, thirty hours of self-study for Anatomy and Physiology (Atlas of Skeletal Muscles, Lab Manual, and Clay Muscle Building), and one hundred practice hours. The curriculum includes Anatomy and Physiology, Anatomy Coloring Book, Fundamental Bodywork Techniques, Guided Imagery, Aromatherapy, Therapeutic Touch, Herbal Remedies, Body Mechanics and Kinesiology, Reflexology, Assessment of Problems and Pathology, Optimal Health Practices, Myofascial Release, Psychology for Bodyworkers, Lymphatic Massage, Shiatsu, Craniosacral: Level 1, RoHun, Special Considerations, Nutrition, and Business Practices. Classes are held in both Sycamore and Rockford.

The nine-month, 200-hour Therapeutic Herbalism Program consists of Herbalism: Gaia in Action, Selection Criteria, Classification of Medicinal Plants, Formulation and Preparation of Herbal Medicines, Digestive System, Cardiovascular System, Respiratory System, Nervous System, Urinary and Reproductive Systems, Musculoskeletal System and Skin, Immunity, Holism and Phytotherapy, Phytotherapy and Children, Phytotherapy and the Elderly, Actions, Aromatherapy, Flower Essences, Materia Medica, Assessment Modalities, Business Practices, and a final exam or project. Labs are held throughout the program to provide hands-on experience with teas, packs, poultices, salves, tinctures, and other forms of treatment.

Admission Requirements

Applicants must be at least 18 years of age; have a high school diploma or equivalent; be proficient in the English language; be in good general health and submit results of TB skin test; and interview with an admissions representative. Therapeutic Massage and Bodywork applicants must be physically able to perform movements and techniques inherent to massage therapy practice.

Tuition and Fees

There is a $35 application fee and a $115 registration fee for all courses.

Total tuition for the Therapeutic Massage and Bodywork Program is $7,800. Additional expenses include books, materials, and liability insurance, approximately $500; massage table, approximately $625; and graduation fee, $45.

Tuition for the Therapeutic Herbalism Program is $2,700; books are $225 and additional optional materials are approximately $200.

Financial Assistance

Payment plans are available.

Redfern Training Systems School of Massage

9 South 531 Wilmette Avenue
Darien, Illinois 60561
PHONE: (630) 960-0844
FAX: (630) 960-3755

The Redfern Training Systems (RTS) School of Massage was founded in 1992 by Rhonda A. Wolski, a certified massage therapist since 1986. There are six instructors, with an average of eight to twelve students per class.

Accreditation and Approvals

RTS was approved in 1992 by the Illinois State Board of Education. Graduates are qualified to take the National Certification Examination for Therapeutic Massage and Bodywork (NCETMB).

Program Description

The 690-hour Massage Certification class meets one day per week for thirty weeks, and includes instruction in the following subject areas: Massage Techniques (including Swedish, French, cranial, and positional release), Theory and History of Massage, Anatomy and Physiology, Benefits and Contraindications, Self-Awareness and the Body-Mind Connection, and practical experience.

Community and Continuing Education

A twenty-four-hour Basic Reflexology class meets one day per week for eight weeks, and includes instruction in the history and basis of reflexology, energy, and the body zones.

An eight-hour class is offered in Day Spa Treatments that includes several different body treatments and wraps.

A twenty-four-hour Sports Massage course is open to certified massage therapists, and meets once a week for eight weeks. Classes are divided into theory and practical sessions, and involve working with the athlete before, during, and after training and competition; theory and history; and preventive, curative, and emergency treatments.

Admission Requirements

Applicants for the Massage Certification, Basic Reflexology, and Day Spa Treatment classes must be at least 18 years of age and have previous exposure to bodywork. Sports Massage applicants must be at least 18 years of age and certified in massage therapy. Applicants are interviewed prior to enrollment.

Tuition and Fees

Tuition for the Massage Certification Course is $5,000, including books and supplies.

Tuition for the Basic Reflexology Course is $400, plus a $100 enrollment fee.

Tuition for the Day Spa Treatments Course is $200, plus a $50 enrollment fee.

Tuition for the Sports Massage Course is $400, plus a $100 enrollment fee.

Financial Assistance
Payment plans are available.

Wellness and Massage Training Institute

1051 Internationale Parkway
Woodridge, Illinois 60517
PHONE: (630) 325-3773
WEBSITE: www.wmti.com

The Wellness and Massage Training Institute (WMTI) enrolled its first students in 1989. The institute moved to a new facility in 1999. There are twenty instructors.

Accreditation and Approvals
The Massage Therapy training program is accredited by the Commission on Massage Training Accreditation (COMTA); graduates are qualified to take the National Certification Examination for Therapeutic Massage and Bodywork (NCETMB). The institute is approved by the National Certification Board for Therapeutic Massage and Bodywork (NCBTMB) as a continuing education provider.

Program Description
The 770-hour Massage Therapy Program consists of 649 hours of required core courses and 121 hours of electives. Core courses include Introduction to Palpation and Anatomy, Introduction to Massage Therapy and Bodywork, Fundamental Massage Techniques, Anatomy and Physiology for Massage and Bodywork, Kinesiology, Introduction to Wellness Concepts, Body/Mind in Perspective, Movement and Energy in Massage, Professional Practice, Deep Tissue Massage, Clinical Experience in Massage Therapy, American Red Cross CPR and First Aid, and Integrative Studies in Massage Therapy. Topics covered in elective courses include Prenatal Massage, Trigger Point, Geriatric Massage, Introduction to Skin Disease, Seated Massage, Positional Release and Massage, Esalen Massage, Sports Massage, Reflexology, Touch for Health, Ortho-Bionomy, Shiatsu, Cranial Sacral, Tai Chi, Nutrition, Boundary Issues, Stress Management, Prescription Medications, and many others. Students may attend full- or part-time; day and evening classes are offered.

The 750-hour Oriental Studies Program consists of 545 hours of required core courses plus fifty-five hours of elective courses and 150 or more hours of declared major track courses. Required core courses include Introduction to Oriental Studies: The Tao of Touch, Oriental Medical Theory I and II, Anatomy and Physiology for Massage and Bodywork, Kinesiology, Introduction to Wellness Concepts, Points and Channels I and II, Professional Practice, Clinical Experience in Oriental Bodywork, and Integrative Studies in Oriental Bodywork: Touch Comes Full Circle. Topics covered in elective courses include Tai Chi, Shiatsu, Jin Shin Do Bodymind Acupressure, Tui Na, Eastern Nutrition, Chinese Herbology, Eastern Philosophy, Feng Shui, Bodymind Awareness, Special Topics in Oriental Studies, and Practicum in Oriental Studies. Students declare a major track in either Shiatsu (151 hours), Jin Shin Do (171 hours), or Tui Na (150 hours). Classes are held day and evening.

Continuing Education
A variety of courses are offered in the continuing education program, including Ortho-Bionomy, Jin Shin Do Acupressure, Aromatherapy, Cranial Sacral, Manual Lymph Drainage, Reflexology, and others.

Admission Requirements
Applicants must be at least 18 years of age, have a high school diploma or equivalent, be in general good health and free of communicable disease, and have received at least one professional massage prior to the start of classes.

Tuition and Fees
Tuition for Massage Therapy required subjects is $5,420; tuition for electives is $60 to $320 per course (total tuition is roughly $7,500); additional expenses include books, depending on electives, $397 to $468; materials, $255; massage table, approximately $500 to $1,000; professional massages, $80 to $100.

Tuition for Oriental Studies required subjects is $4,310, books and materials are an additional $475. Tuition for electives is $100 to $300 per course. Tuition for declared major tracks is $1,595 for Shiatsu, $1,740 for Jin Shin Do, and $1,500 for Tui Na; books are $50 to $131. (Total tuition is roughly $7,500.)

Financial Assistance

Payment plans are available.

INDIANA

Alexandria School of Scientific Therapeutics

P.O. Box 287
809 South Harrison Street
Alexandria, Indiana 46001
PHONE: (765) 724-9152 / (800) 622-8756
FAX: (765) 724-9156
E-MAIL: alexssin@netdirect.net
WEBSITE: www.assti.com
www.pfrimmerii.com

The Alexandria School of Scientific Therapeutics was founded in 1982 by Herbert and Ruthann Hobbs. Ruthann Hobbs is a registered reflexologist, certified iridologist, and certified instructor for the Pfrimmer Technique Deep Muscle Therapist Association. There are fifteen instructors, with an average of thirty students per class.

Accreditation and Approvals

The Massage Therapy program is approved by the Commission on Massage Training Accreditation (COMTA), and licensed and approved by the State of Indiana. Graduates are qualified to take the National Certification Examination for Therapeutic Massage and Bodywork (NCETMB).

Program Description

The 664-hour, forty-two-week, Massage Therapy program includes Anatomy, Physiology, Theory and Practice of Massage, Hydrotherapy, Nutrition, Health and Hygiene, Business Practices, Client Assessment, Polarity Techniques, Muscle Balancing Techniques, Postural Release Techniques, Iridology, Structural Alignment Techniques, Color Therapy, Acupressure, Shiatsu, Craniopathy, Infant Massage, Geriatric Massage, Sports Massage, and Manual Lymph Drainage. Students are also required to take EMR (Emergency Medical Response) training. Weekday and weekend classes are available.

Continuing Education

An eighty-hour postgraduate course in Pfrimmer Deep Muscle Therapy is offered to those with at least 500 hours of anatomy, physiology, hygiene, ethics, and other requirements, and who are willing to abide by the standards imposed by the Therese C. Pfrimmer School and the International Association.

Admission Requirements

Applicants must be at least 18 years of age, have a high school diploma or equivalent, submit two letters of recommendation, interview with an admissions representative, and be in good health.

Tuition and Fees

Tuition for the Massage Therapy program is $5,885 with a $100 registration fee. Tuition for the course in Pfrimmer Deep Muscle Therapy is $3,025.

Financial Assistance

Payment plans are available.

Lewis School and Clinic of Massage Therapy

3400 Michigan Street
Hobart, Indiana 46342
PHONE/FAX: (219) 962-9640

The Lewis School and Clinic of Massage Therapy was founded in 1984 by Rose Marie Lewis, a registered massage therapist who has served on the board of directors of the Indiana Chapter of AMTA.

Accreditation and Approvals

This institution is regulated by the Indiana Commission on Proprietary Education. Graduates are qualified to take the National Certification Examination for Therapeutic Massage and Bodywork (NCETMB).

Program Description

The 550-hour Massage Therapy Program includes Anatomy and Physiology, Craniosacral Concepts, Massage Theory and Hands-On Experience (including a variety of Swedish techniques), Sports Massage, Reflexology, CPR, Hydrotherapy, and Business Ethics and Practices. Classes are held on weekends.

Admission Requirements

Applicants must be at least 18 years of age; have a high school diploma or equivalent; submit three character references, one of which must be from a health care professional; interview with an admissions representative; provide a current photograph; and reveal a sincere interest in the natural health therapies field.

Tuition and Fees

Tuition is $5,000, including books, oils, and linens. There is a $100 registration fee.

Financial Assistance

An interest-free payment plan and veterans' benefits are available.

Midwest Training Institute of Hypnosis

2121 Engle Road, Suite 3A
Fort Wayne, Indiana 46809
PHONE: (219) 747-6774
FAX: (219) 747-6774
E-MAIL: Gzukausky@compuserve.com
WEBSITE: www.mwiofhypnosis.com

The Midwest Training Institute of Hypnosis (a satellite branch of Inner Quest Awareness Center of California) was founded in 1990 by Gisella Zukausky, who has taught internationally and has training in Psychology, Parapsychology, and Clinical and Medical Hypnotherapy, and has a private practice. Zukausky is the only instructor; classes average eight students. Classes 1 and 2 are also offered through correspondence; see description below.

Accreditation and Approvals

Upon completion of Class 1, students are eligible for certification with the International Medical and Dental Hypnotherapy Association, the American Institute of Hypnotherapy, the Hypnotherapy Association of Indiana, and most other hypnother-

apy associations. St. John's University in Louisiana gives credits for MTIH courses; others must be consulted individually.

Program Description

The institute offers a series of classes in hypnotherapy which may be taken in any order without any previous training. Classes 1 and 2 are also offered as correspondence courses.

Class 1: Hypnosis/Hypnotherapy/Regression Therapy consists of eight days of instruction and forty hours of lab and homework for a total of 150 hours. The course covers different depths of hypnosis; motivating clients to stop smoking, control weight, and change other problem behaviors; chronic pain and health; applying hypnosis to regression therapy; and more. Class 1 is also offered as a video correspondence course.

Class 2 is a thirty-hour, three-day course teaching a nonverbal regression technique using only ideomotor yes and no finger signals. In this gentle technique, the client does not have to talk and frequently has no conscious awareness of the incident to which they regressed; this technique uncovers events that may not have been revealed with the verbal approach. Class 2 is also offered as a video correspondence course.

Class 3 is a thirty-hour, three-day course teaching Hypno-Anesthesia, Glove Anesthesia, Pain Control, Improved Health with Imagery, and the use of hypnosis as anesthesia for surgery, childbirth, dental work, and other procedures.

Admission Requirements

MTIH offers training for physical and mental health professionals and those interested in hypnosis for personal growth. Applicants must be at least 18 years of age and have a high school diploma or equivalent.

Tuition and Fees

Tuition for Class 1 is $975 including manual and cassette tapes. Tuition for Class 2 is $365 including manual and cassette tapes. Tuition for Class 3 is $275; cassette tapes included.

Financial Assistance

Full or partial scholarships are given on an individual basis.

IOWA

Capri College

315 2nd Avenue SE
Cedar Rapids, Iowa 52401
PHONE: (319) 364-1541 / (800) 397-0612
FAX: (319) 366-2075
E-MAIL: cradm@mwci.net
WEBSITE: www.capricollege.com

Capri College was founded in 1966 by Charles Fiegen and Edward Bisenius as Capri Cosmetology College. There are four instructors, with an average of twelve students per class. In addition to the program described here, courses are also offered in Cosmetology and Nail Technology.

Accreditation and Approvals

Capri College is accredited by the Accrediting Commission of Career Schools and Colleges of Technology (ACCSCT). Graduates of the Massage Therapy Program are eligible for Iowa state licensing and to take the National Certification Examination for Therapeutic Massage and Bodywork (NCETMB).

Program Description

The 650-hour Massage Therapy Program provides training in Swedish Massage and includes Human Anatomy and Physiology, Pathology, Kinesiology, Massage/Bodywork Theory, Assessment and Practice (which covers Consultation, Draping, Body Mechanics, Contraindications, Swedish Massage Techniques, Athletic/ Sports Massage, Deep Tissue, Specifics, Specialized Massage, Prenatal Massage, Geriatrics, Spa Therapies, Shiatsu, Acupressure and Reflexology), and Adjunct Techniques and Methods (which covers CPR, First Aid, Energy Work, Nutrition, Aromatherapy, Business Practices, Career Planning, Ethics, Iowa Law, and Licensing and Certification).

Admission Requirements

Applicants must have a high school diploma or equivalent, submit two letters of recommendation, have a personal interview, and meet the physical, mental, and communication skill requirements demanded in the workplace.

Tuition and Fees

The application fee is $30. The total cost for tuition, equipment, books, uniform, locker/linen, activity fee, and insurance is $6,200.

Financial Assistance

Scholarships, grants, loans, and payment plans are available.

Carlson College of Massage Therapy

11809 Country Road X28
Anamosa, Iowa 52205-7519
PHONE: (319) 462-3402
FAX: (319) 462-5990
E-MAIL: carlc@inqv.net
WEBSITE: www.carlson-college.com

Carlson College of Massage Therapy was founded in 1985 by Director Ruth A. Carlson. There are seven instructors, with an average of fifty students per year.

Accreditation and Approvals

The Massage Therapy Program at Carlson College is accredited by the Commission on Massage Training Accreditation (COMTA) and by the Integrative Massage and Somatic Therapies Accreditation Council (IMSTAC). The curriculum is approved by the Iowa Board of Examiners for Massage Therapy. Graduates are qualified to take the National Certification Examination for Therapeutic Massage and Bodywork (NCETMB).

The college is also approved by the National Certification Board for Therapeutic Massage and Bodywork (NCBTMB) as a continuing education provider.

Program Description

The 625-hour, five-and-a-half-month Massage Therapy Program consists of Anatomy/Physiology and Massage Theory, Techniques, and Practices (founded on intermediate and advanced Swedish technique), in addition to instruction in therapeutic touch, polarity, stretches, deep and connective tissue massage, reflexology, sports massage, hydrotherapy, musculoskeletal pathology, aromatherapy, shiatsu, myofascial work, herbology, tai chi/body movement, guided imagery, on-site chair massage, CPR, first aid, professional ethics, business practices, and an internship (outreach and clinic). Classes meet during the day.

Admission Requirements
Applicants must have a high school diploma or equivalent, be of high moral character, and be in good health.

Tuition and Fees
Tuition is $5,000, including textbooks and student liability insurance. There is a $25 application fee; linens, uniforms, and massage table are additional.

Financial Assistance
Payment plans are available.

The Foundation for Aromatherapy Education and Research

(See Multiple State Locations, pages 394–95)

Maharishi University of Management

1000 North Fourth Street
Fairfield, Iowa 52557
PHONE: (515) 472-7000 / (515) 472-1110 (admissions office)
FAX: (515) 472-1179
E-MAIL: admissions@mum.edu
WEBSITE: www.mum.edu

Maharishi University of Management (formerly Maharishi International University) was founded in 1971 as Maharishi International University by Maharishi Mahesh Yogi. The university is a leader in research on natural approaches to health and has received research grants from agencies that include the National Institutes of Health.

The university uses a Consciousness-Based® approach to education that incorporates twice-daily group practice of the Maharishi Transcendental Meditation® or TM-Sidhi® program into a more traditional curriculum. The 262-acre campus has over 1.2 million square feet of teaching, research, recreational, and living space; buildings and dorms are nonsmoking and

free of alcohol and other drugs. There are approximately 100 faculty members, with a student:teacher ratio of 10:1.

Accreditation and Approvals
The university is accredited at the doctoral level by the Commission on Institutions of Higher Education of the North Central Association of Colleges and Schools.

Program Description
The university offers doctorate, master's, and bachelor's degrees, certificate, and technical training programs in both the more usual disciplines, such as Computer Science, Business, Chemistry, Literature, Mathematics, and Electronics, and alternative fields including Maharishi Vedic Psychology®, The Science of Creative Intelligence®, Maharishi Vedic Medicine®, Maharishi Gandharva Veda Music®, and Maharishi Ayur-Veda® Technician. Natural health and personal development programs are incorporated into every discipline's curriculum.

The Bachelor of Arts and doctorate degrees in Maharishi Vedic Medicine curriculums cover Vedic anatomy and physiology, study of forty areas of Veda and Vedic Literature applied to individual and collective health; modern medical knowledge relevant to the holistic approach of Maharishi Vedic Medicine; Research in Consciousness through Maharishi Transcendental Meditation and TM-Sidhi programs, including Yogic Flying; and reading the Vedic literature in Sanskrit. Students teach short courses in the Maharishi Vedic Approach to Health to the general public. Courses include Self-Pulse Reading; Maharishi Vedic Science; Vedic Anatomy and Vedic Physiology; Prevention; Diet, Digestion and Nutrition; Maharishi Yoga Asanas; Principles of Physiological Purification; Higher States of Consciousness; and many others.

The Bachelor of Science in Biology qualifies as a premedicine degree with tracks available in Environmental Studies, Sustainable Agriculture (organic farming), and Biology.

The Bachelor of Arts and Bachelor of Science programs in Maharishi's Vedic Psychology include such courses as Maharishi Vedic Psychology; Maharishi Vedic Science; Research Methods; Developmental Psychology; Levels of Mind: Theory and Research; Collective Consciousness; Psychophysiology; Health Psychology; Applied Psychology; Statistics; Seminar in Consciousness, and others.

The Master of Science and doctorate programs in Maharishi Vedic Psychology include advanced courses such as Cognitive Processes; Maharishi Vedic Psychology; Maharishi Vedic Science; Psychophysiology; Theory and Research in Collective Consciousness; Sanskrit; and many others.

Bachelor's, master's, and doctorate degrees are offered in the Science of Creative Intelligence. Courses in this department include Philosophy of Action, Higher States of Consciousness, Creativity, Applications of Maharishi Vedic Science, Scientific Research, Sanskrit, the Unified Field of All Streams of Knowledge, Bhagavad-Gita, Maharishi Vedic Approach to Health, and many others.

Students study one subject at a time through a four-week block system, allowing them to focus deeply on each subject and retain more knowledge without conflicting demands of other classes. The Rotating University program offers courses in India, Italy, France, and other countries.

Community and Continuing Education

The Department of Continuing Education offers noncredit evening and weekend courses in a wide range of subjects, including full-time classes in session.

Continuing medical education for physicians and special degree and nondegree programs for medical students and physicians are planned; contact the university for details.

Distance education programs are also offered in such areas as Maharishi Vedic Science: Sanskrit and Reading the Vedic Literature. Other distance-learning programs, using satellite transmission and the Internet, are planned.

Admission Requirements

Undergraduate applicants must be at least 18 years of age, have a high school diploma or equivalent, and submit standardized test scores, two letters of recommendation, and essays, and have an interview. Students not already practicing the Transcendental Meditation program are instructed in the technique before commencing study.

Tuition and Fees

Undergraduate costs per year are as follows: application fee, $25; tuition and fees, $15,430; single room, $2,720; board, $2,480; and books and supplies, $800.

Graduate costs per year are as follows: application fee, $40; tuition and fees, $16,550; single room, $2,720; board, $2,480; and books and supplies, $800.

Financial Assistance

Federal grants and loans, state grants, university scholarships, and work-study are available. Contact the financial aid office at (515) 472-1156 or by e-mail at finaid@mum.edu.

Palmer College of Chiropractic

1000 Brady Street
Davenport, Iowa 52803-5287
PHONE: (319) 884-5656 / (800) 722-3648
FAX: (319) 884-5414
E-MAIL: pcadmit@palmer.edu
WEBSITE: www.palmer.edu

Palmer College of Chiropractic's founder, D. D. Palmer, performed the first modern chiropractic adjustment in 1895 and held the first classes at the Palmer School and Cure in 1897. The college boasts the profession's largest chiropractic outpatient clinic system, a leading chiropractic research facility, and the most extensive chiropractic library. Today, one of every three chiropractors in the world is a Palmer graduate. There are 141 instructors, with a 1:14 teacher:student ratio.

Accreditation and Approvals

Palmer College of Chiropractic is accredited by the Council of Chiropractic Education (CCE) and the North Central Association of Schools and Colleges.

Program Description

The 4,620-hour Doctor of Chiropractic (D.C.) degree program may be completed in as little as three and one-third consecutive years. Courses are offered in the departments of Anatomy, Chiropractic Protocol, Clinic, Diagnosis, Pathology, Philosophy, Physiology and Biochemistry, Radiology, Research, Special Programs/Electives, and Technique.

Students may also complete a Bachelor of Science degree in general science in addition to the Doctor of Chiropractic degree; this degree must be awarded concurrently with the D.C. degree.

Continuing Education

Advanced studies include the Clinical Teaching Residents program, which prepares graduate doctors of chiropractic to be clinical faculty members. Graduate doctors of chiropractic may also participate in a residency program with the Department of Radiology to qualify for the diplomate exam of the American Chiropractic Board of Radiology.

Admission Requirements

Applicants for admission to the D.C. program must have completed at least sixty semester hours leading to a baccalaureate degree in a college or university program with a minimum GPA of 2.75. Applicants whose GPA falls between 2.5 and 2.74 may be considered after an on-campus interview. Candidates must meet specific course and credit requirements in the sciences, social sciences, and humanities. In addition, applicants must submit letters of recommendation and a personal essay.

Beginning with the November 2001 trimester, the semester credit hours necessary before entering Palmer will increase from sixty to ninety. The minimum GPA will remain the same.

Tuition and Fees

Tuition is $5,235 per trimester full-time, or $200 per credit hour for less than twenty-three hours. Additional expenses include a $50 application fee; activities fee, $150; and liability insurance, $195. Books and equipment costs vary by trimester from approximately $50 to $500. Additional fees for students obtaining a Bachelor of Science degree in conjunction with the Doctor of Chiropractic degree include: application fee, $100; graduation and record fee, $100; and transcript evaluation fee, $50.

Financial Assistance

Scholarships, awards, and federal financial aid are available.

KANSAS

American Academy of Environmental Medicine

(See Multiple State Locations, pages 383–84)

International College of Applied Kinesiology® U.S.A.

(See Professional Associations and Membership Organizations, page 447)

LOUISANA

Blue Cliff School of Therapeutic Massage

(See Multiple State Locations, pages 388–90)

MAINE

Avena Botanicals

P.O. Box 333
West Rockport, Maine 04865
PHONE: (207) 594-0694
FAX: (207) 594-2975
E-MAIL: avena@midcoast.com
WEBSITE: www.avenaherbs.com

Avena Botanicals is a nonprofit educational center founded by Deb Soule, who has been organically growing, wildcrafting, and using medicinal herbs for over twenty years. She is the author of *The Roots of Healing: A Woman's Book of Herbs.* Soule is the primary instructor; classes are limited to twenty-five students.

Program Description

The Women's Medicinal Herb Foundation Course meets for three three-day weekends and is designed for any woman interested in using herbal remedies for nourishment and healing. The course of study includes Hands-On Medicinal Herb Preparation, Nourishing Herbs in Our Daily Life, Tonics Herbs, Herbs for Women's Health, Immune System Herbs, Integrating Herbal Care with Other Modalities, Wild Plant Identification, Biodynamic Gardening Principles, Herb Gardening, Harvesting and Drying Techniques, Tea Ceremony/Earth Ceremony, Plants As Our Allies, Creating Dream Pillows and Medicine Bundles, and more.

The Women's Intermediate Medicinal Herb Course meets for three three-day weekends. The course of study includes Materia Medica, Energetics of Herbs, Understanding the Energetics of the Five Seasons, Herbal Tonics and Foods for the Five Seasons, Homeopathic and Herbal First Aid, Homeopathy and Herbs for Children, Respiratory Complaints, Medicinal Mushrooms, Doctrine of Signatures, Using Herbs and Flower Essences Together, and Women's Herbs.

Matthew Wood, clinical herbalist, offers a year-long advanced herbal course at Avena; contact Avena for details.

Tuition and Fees

Tuition for the Foundation Course in $615 to $675 (depending on payment plan), and includes lab materials, camping, and six vegetarian meals each weekend. Tuition for the Intermediate Course is $675 to $750, and includes camping and six vegetarian meals each weekend.

Financial Assistance

Payment plans are available.

Birthwise Midwifery School

66 South High Street
Bridgton, Maine 04009
PHONE: (207) 647-5968
E-MAIL: birthwise@ime.net
WEBSITE: www.birthwisemidwifery.org

Birthwise was founded in 1994 by Heidi Fillmore-Patrick. Enrollment is limited to fifteen students; there are nine faculty members.

Accreditation and Approvals

Birthwise is accredited by the Midwifery Education Accreditation Council (MEAC). Graduates are eligible to become certified nationally through the North American Registry of Midwives (NARM) as Certified Professional Midwives (CPMs).

Program Description

The curriculum encompasses both theoretical and practical aspects of midwifery care. The program is divided into three sessions and may be completed in fifteen months; classes are pass/fail and meet one to two days per week. Courses include

Orientation, Anatomy and Physiology for Midwives, Physical Assessment, Normal Prenatal, Normal Labor and Birth, Postpartum, Prenatal Complications, Complications of Labor and Birth, The Art of Traditional Midwifery, Newborn, Hospital Birth, Lab Work, Pharmacology, Well Woman Care, Homeopathy, Mind/Body Connection, Business of Midwifery, Counseling Techniques, Integration Days, and Seminar Days. Students are offered to local hospitals as doulas, are paired with local midwives to observe clinic days, and are invited to attend a limited number of home births with local midwives when possible.

Only those students who successfully complete the academic program at Birthwise are eligible to enroll in the clinical component. Length of preceptorships is determined by the period of time needed to fulfill the following requirements: attendance at twenty births as active participant; attendance at twenty births as primary midwife; performing seventy-five prenatal exams; performing forty postpartum exams; performing twenty newborn exams; and performing twenty well-woman exams. Students may have to travel to complete this portion of their studies.

Continuing Education

Continuing education workshops are offered to practicing midwives, student/apprentice midwives, aspiring midwives, doulas, birth assistants, and childbirth educators. These workshops have included Labwork Skills and Interpretation for Midwives; Normal Labor and Birth; Pharmacology for Midwives; Counseling for Health Professionals; Introduction to the Heart, Mind and Skill of a Midwife; and Well Woman Care and Physical Exam Skills Workshop.

Admission Requirements

Applicants must have a high school diploma; have a strong interest in women's health issues and birth at home; have a strong motivation to learn; and have completed training as a doula (may be obtained at Birthwise prior to enrollment or during the first semester of the program); submit two letters of reference; and have a phone or in-person interview.

Tuition and Fees

Tuition is $6,000. Additional expenses include books and materials; approximately $550; clinical session fees, $500; additional fees up to $2,000 may be required by the preceptor of choice.

Tuition for continuing education workshops ranges from $80 to $575.

Financial Assistance

Tuition is paid in four installments. Work-study (four hours per week) is available for two students per class for a 20 percent tuition reduction.

Downeast School of Massage

P.O. Box 24
99 Moose Meadow Lane
Waldoboro, Maine 04572-0024
PHONE: (207) 832-5531
FAX: (207) 832-0504
E-MAIL: admissionsdsm@midcoast.com
WEBSITE: www.midcoast.com/~dsm

The Downeast School of Massage (DSM) was established in 1981 by Nancy Dail and moved to its current location in 1993. The faculty consists of twenty-two instructors, with a maximum class size of thirty.

Accreditation and Approvals

Downeast School of Massage is accredited by the Commission on Massage Training Accreditation (COMTA) and a member of the American Massage Therapy Association (AMTA) Council of Schools; graduates are qualified to take the National Certification Examination for Therapeutic Massage and Bodywork (NCETMB). Downeast is approved by the National Certification Board for Therapeutic Massage and Bodywork (NCBTMB) as a continuing education provider.

Program Description

DSM offers three programs which may be completed over ten months or over two ten-month periods; programs start in January and September. The primary focus of each program is Swedish Massage technique; in addition, students must choose one of three areas of concentration: Sports Massage (Program I; 609 hours), Shiatsu (Program II; 708 hours), or Body/Mind (Program III; 605 hours).

Required courses include Business Design, Business Panel, Ethics, Integrating Business, IRS, Seated Massage Presentation,

Children's Massage Clinic, Clinic, Geriatric Massage, Hydrotherapy, Intro to Shiatsu, Neuromuscular Therapy, Postural Assessment, Pregnancy Massage, Reflexology, Swedish Massage, Video Mechanics, Kinesiology, Maniken Muscles, Anatomy, HIV/AIDS, Nutrition, Pathology, Physiology, Chronic Pain, First Aid/CPR, Introduction, Intro to Homeopathy, Intro to the Impact of Trauma, Movement Analysis, and Tai Chi.

As a commitment to good physical health, students are required to perform and log any form of exercise during the school year.

Continuing Education

Separate from any of the three programs, electives and special guest workshops are offered to students, graduates, and professional Massage Therapists.

Admission Requirements

Applicants must be at least 18 years of age, have a high school diploma or equivalent, be of good physical and mental health, and have high moral character.

Tuition and Fees

Tuition for Program I: Swedish and Sports Massage is $5,625. Tuition for Program II: Swedish and Shiatsu is $6,519. Tuition for Program III: Swedish and Body/ Mind is $5,500. Additional expenses for each program include application fee, $50; registration fee, $100; deposit, $200; books and manuals, $480; four professional massages, $140; massage table and accessories, approximately $700 to $800; lotion and oil, $150; linen, $75; thermophore (optional), $65; BP cuff, $30; stethoscope, $15; AMTA student membership, $169; and shiatsu mat (Program II only), $85.

Tuition for electives and special guest workshops ranges from $65 to $400 each.

Financial Assistance

Payment plans and veterans' benefits are available.

Footloose

Box 112, Egypt Road
Alna, Maine 04535
PHONE: (207) 586-6751
FAX: (207) 586-6702

Footloose was founded in 1989 by Janet E. Stetser, a Certified Reflexologist who has been teaching reflexology since 1984. There is one instructor; classes sizes range from two to ten students.

Accreditation and Approvals

Footloose one-day courses are approved for continuing education credit by the Maine Council of Reflexologists. The Reflexology for Certification Course meets and surpasses all current national standards set by the American Reflexology Certification Board (ARCB). Graduates are eligible to sit for National Certification.

Program Description

The 300-hour Reflexology for Certification Program consists of nine three-day weekends covering Anatomy and Physiology and Reflexology; a practicum consisting of seventy different pairs of feet, one person five times, and one person ten times; and a paper on an allied field to be written and presented. Major areas covered are Foot/Hand Reflexology with an Introduction to Ear Reflexology; Joint Mobility; Dr. Wickler's Foot Assessment: Theory and Practical Use; Business Practices; Standards and Ethics; State, National, and International Organizations of Reflexology; National Testing Standards and Procedures; Meridian Theory, History of Reflexology; Techniques and Methods for Sessions; Introduction to Iridology; Bio Mechanics of the Foot; General Foot Care; Special Considerations for Chronically Ill Clients; Universal Procedures; and Record Keeping.

Community and Continuing Education

One-day workshops open to the public include Iridology, Self-Hypnosis for Personal Growth, Personal Numerology, Beginning Dowsing, and Simple Ear Reflexology.

Admission Requirements

Applicants must have a high school diploma or equivalent.

Tuition and Fees

Tuition for the Reflexology Program is $3,500. Tuition for one-day workshops is $93.

Financial Assistance

There is a discount for payment two weeks in advance.

New England School of Clinical Hypnotherapy

700 Atlantic Highway
Northport, Maine 04849
PHONE: (207) 338-9774 / (888) 338-9774

The New England School of Clinical Hypnotherapy was founded by Harold and Jane Nealy, who are the primary instructors.

Accreditation and Approvals

New England School of Clinical Hypnotherapy is endorsed by the International Medical and Dental Hypnotherapy Association (IMDHA). Accreditation is being pursued.

Program Description

The 100-hour Clinical Hypnotherapy Program consists of two parts. Part I: Basic Hypnosis consists of Preliminary Suggestibility Test, Recognition and Classification of Subjects, Favorable and Unfavorable Influences and Dangers of Hypnosis, How to Hypnotize, Method of Awaking, Depth Stages of Hypnosis, Self-Hypnosis Training, Hypnosis Miscellany, Advanced Induction Techniques, Your Hypnosis Practice, Group Leadership, and Private Training. Part II: Advanced Hypnotherapy consists of What Is Hypnosis?; The First Session With a Client; Behavior Assessment, Goal Setting, and Reinforcement; Image Psychology and Hypnosis; Sessions Two, Three, and Four with a Client; Designing and Teaching a Six-Hour Self-Hypnosis Course; A Successful Hypnosis Practice; Age Regression; and The Modern Group Hypnotherapy Experience. All students are required to schedule one private hypnotherapy session with instructor prior to graduation at no additional cost.

Admission Requirements

Applicants must be at least 18 years of age; have a high school diploma or equivalent or demonstrate comparable education through life or work experience; and have a personal interview.

Tuition and Fees
Tuition is $1,995 and includes training manuals, and audio- and videotapes. There is a $25 application fee.

New Hampshire Institute for Therapeutic Arts

(See Multiple State Locations, pages 403-4)

Polarity Realization Institute

(See Multiple State Locations, pages 408-9)

MARYLAND
Baltimore School of Massage

6401 Dogwood Road
Baltimore, Maryland 21207
PHONE: (410) 944-8855
FAX: (410) 944-8859
E-MAIL: registrar@bhhc.com
WEBSITE: www.bsom.com

The Baltimore School of Massage (BSM) was founded in 1981 by Jerry Toporovsky, past chairman of the American Massage Therapy Association (AMTA) Council of Schools and chairman of the Zero Balancing Association. There are nineteen instructors for the 510-hour CMTP, twenty-five for the 610-hour PMTP, and eighteen for the Shiatsu program; class sizes average twenty-four students.

Accreditation and Approvals
BSM is accredited by the Accrediting Commission of Career Schools and Colleges of Technology (ACCSCT) and approved by the Maryland Higher Education Commission (MHEC).

BSM is currently seeking accreditation with the Commission on Massage Training Accreditation (COMTA), and is a member of the AMTA Council of Schools. Graduates of the PMTP and CMTP are eligible to take the National Certification Examination for Therapeutic Massage and Bodywork (NCETMB).

Graduates of the Shiatsu Program are eligible to take the

National Certification Commission for Acupuncture and Oriental Medicine's (NCCAOM) National Certification in Oriental Bodywork Therapy exam.

BSM is also approved by the National Certification Board for Therapeutic Massage and Bodywork (NCBTMB) as a continuing education provider.

Program Description
The 510-hour Professional Massage Training Program consists of three terms, a series of elective trainings, First Aid training, and CPR certification. The twenty-week First Term Basic Massage teaches how to give a full body massage and includes such topics as Swedish massage, energy work, seated massage, body mechanics, anatomy, and physiology. The twenty-week Second Term Intermediate Massage covers such topics as deep tissue work, energy concepts, body-type analysis, progressive relaxation techniques, stress management, massage for pregnant women, communication skills, elective trainings in such areas as reflexology and sports massage, and participation as practitioners in the Student Clinic. The twenty-week Third Term Advanced Massage teaches myofascial release techniques, living anatomy, physiology, deep massage, body mechanics, body awareness and movement education, the development of essential touch and sensitivity training, elective trainings in such areas as marketing massage and small business accounting, and extensive work in the Student Clinic. Day or evening classes are offered on a part-time basis.

A 610-hour Professional Program in Comprehensive Massage Therapy for a Medical or Clinical Setting offers education in relaxation, therapeutic and medical massage, and related subjects. The first 510 hours of training are the three terms of the Professional Massage Training Program (above), including the supervised lab, elective trainings, CPR/First Aid trainings, and Student Clinic. The medical massage component of the CMTP includes pathophysiology, medical conditions and contraindications, communication skills for the health professional, introduction to working in a medical setting, safe practice protocol, and Therapeutic Touch. Students may take the program on a full- or part-time basis.

The 620-hour Professional Program in Shiatsu and Asian Bodywork, first offered in April 1999, meets one weekend per month for seventeen months. The curriculum consists of Foundation: Basic Massage, Beginning Shiatsu and Acupressure, Intermediate: Zen Shiatsu, and Advanced Eclectic Shiatsu. Topics covered in these courses include essential Shiatsu techniques; five elements and twelve meridians; vital acu-points, locations, and traditional treatments; abdominal hara assessment; beginning moxibustion; acupressure, tuina, and other Asian bodywork techniques; tai chi; and business and communication skills.

Community and Continuing Education

An evening Introduction to Massage workshop gives participants an enjoyable and informative introduction to massage.

The 120-hour, twenty-week Basic Avocational Massage Training Program teaches how to give a full body massage and covers such topics as Swedish massage, seated massage, and energy work techniques.

BSM also offers seminars to professional massage therapists and bodyworkers for continuing education. Such seminars have included Zero Balancing®, Chakra Energy Workshop, Medical Massage Therapy, Muscle Energy Techniques, Fundamentals of Acupressure, Bach Flower Remedies for the Healer and the Home, Aromatherapy, Gentle Massage for the Frail, Sports Massage, and others.

Admission Requirements

Applicants must be at least 18 years of age, have a high school diploma or equivalent, be physically capable of performing massage manipulations, interview with a school representative, and complete a biographical sketch.

Tuition and Fees

Tuition for the 510-hour Professional Massage program is $4,750. Other expenses include a $100 application fee and $300 for books and supplies; linens are additional.

Tuition for the 610-hour CMTP Program and for the Professional Program in Shiatsu and Asian Bodywork is $5,850. (For graduates of an approved 500-hour program, advanced standing tuition for the Shiatsu program is $4,450.) Other expenses for these programs include a $100 application fee and $400 for books and supplies; linens are additional.

The fee for the Introduction to Massage workshop is $10. Tuition for the 120-hour Basic Avocational Massage Training Program is $775. Continuing education seminars range from $100 to $495.

Financial Assistance

Payment plans, veterans' benefits, and financial aid are available.

Maryland Institute of Traditional Chinese Medicine

4641 Montgomery Avenue, Suite 415
Bethesda, Maryland 20814
PHONE: (301) 718-7373 / (301) 907-8986 / (800) 892-1209
FAX: (301) 718-0735
E-MAIL: martindell@aol.com
WEBSITE: www.MITCM.org

The Maryland Institute of Traditional Chinese Medicine (MITCM) was founded in 1987 and held its first classes in 1992. In 1996, MITCM moved to its current site. There are seventeen instructors, with a maximum of thirty students per class.

Accreditation and Approvals

The master's degree–level acupuncture program is accredited by the Accreditation Commission for Acupuncture and Oriental Medicine (ACAOM).

Graduates are eligible to be licensed as professional acupuncturists in Maryland and other states, and to sit for the National Certification Commission for Acupuncture and Oriental Medicine (NCCAOM) exam.

Program Description

The three-year, 1,890-hour master's degree–level program in Traditional Chinese Medicine consists of 900 hours of academic instruction and 900 hours of clinical training. Course work includes History and Theory of TCM, Channel Theory, Clinical Anatomy and Pathophysiology, Clean Needle Technique, Research Project Planning, Diagnostic Theory of TCM, Acupuncture Points, Introduction to Clinical Western Medicine, Acupuncture Techniques, Acupuncture Treatment, Western Medicine Diagnostic Methods, Chinese Tui Na, Advanced Therapeutics, Clinical Observation, Clinical Treatment of Patients, and Business Management.

Community Education

Tai Chi and Qi Gong are offered to the public as well as to currently enrolled students.

Admission Requirements

Applicants must have completed at least sixty semester hours of undergraduate study (including six college credits of anatomy and physiology, which must be completed before entering the second year of study) from an accredited college or university, and must interview with one or more members of the admissions committee.

Tuition and Fees

Tuition is $21,390 for the entire program. Additional expenses include books, approximately $300, and acupuncture needles, approximately $200.

For medical doctors and those not required to take the Western medicine curriculum, tuition is $18,330 for the entire program.

The Tai Chi and Qi Gong Courses are $80 for students, $100 standard.

Financial Assistance

Payment plans, loans, and veterans' benefits are available. MITCM is also in the process of establishing a federal and state loan program.

Traditional Acupuncture Institute

American City Building
10227 Wincopin Circle, Suite 100
Columbia, Maryland 21044-3422
PHONE: (301) 596-6006 / (410) 997-4888
FAX: (410) 964-3544
E-MAIL: bklaits@tai.edu
WEBSITE: www.tai.edu

The concept for the Traditional Acupuncture Institute was formed in 1973 by a group of American acupuncturists completing their clinical residence in England. There are forty-three faculty members plus thirty-five assistants, with an average of twenty students per class.

Accreditation and Approvals

The Master of Acupuncture Program is accredited by the Accreditation Commission for Acupuncture and Oriental Medicine (ACAOM) and conforms to the licensing requirements of most states, including Maryland and California. Those seeking California licensing must meet specific course requirements, including the Chinese Herbs class.

Program Description

The Master of Acupuncture Degree Program may be taken in either a twenty-nine-month or a forty-month track. The curriculum consists of three levels of study.

Level I courses include a ten-day SOPHIA (School of Philosophy and Healing in Action) Theory Intensive that introduces basic laws, language, and diagnostic skills of traditional acupuncture; Clinical Observation and Diagnosis; Embodying Qigong; Acupuncture Theory/Elements; Basic Acupuncture Anatomy; Touching the Energy; Zero Balancing®; Partnership with Nature; Mentor Groups; and more.

Level II courses focus on the development of diagnostic skills and include Introduction to Traditional Diagnosis: The Patient Examination and Physical Diagnosis; Introduction to Treatment Planning; Principles of Treatment; Introduction to Classical Chinese Medical Literature; Tai Chi/Breathing/Meditation; Spirit of the Points; Acupuncture Anatomy Lecture and Lab; Acupuncture Theory; Zang Fu; Patterns of Disharmony; History of Chinese Medicine and Philosophy; Diagnostic Interaction; Introduction to Western Medicine: Clinical Science and Pathology; Professional Project: Research/Communication; Treatment of Addiction and Community Health; and others.

Level III courses focus on clinical work and begin with a four-day student retreat. Courses continue to build on the foundations of Acupuncture Anatomy, Theory, and Diagnosis, and also include Distinct Traditions; Business, Ethics, and Legal Issues; Treatment Planning and Case Presentation; Patterns of Disharmony Lab; Being Practitioner: Observation; Mentor Groups; Professional Project: Research/Communication; and others.

Community and Continuing Education

The ten-day SOPHIA Theory Intensive, two-day Five Element Approach to Redefining Health workshop, evening Introduction to Traditional Acupuncture, and other programs are open to the public as a community service.

Admission Requirements

Applicants must have a bachelor's degree from an accredited institution with a minimum GPA of C; at least fifteen semester credits in the biosciences, which include anatomy, physiology, and nutrition; and fifteen semester credits in the social sciences, which include introductory-level Psychology and Sociology. In addition, applicants must have at least 130 hours of clinical work as follows: a minimum of 80 hours/maximum of 105 hours in a Western medical setting, such as a hospital, mental health facility, hospice, doctor's office, or similar situation; and a minimum of twenty-five hours/maximum of 50 hours in hands-on bodywork, such as massage, acupressure, or reiki. Applicants must also have completed or plan to complete a CPR course from the Red Cross or American Heart Association. Also, applicants must submit a letter from a practitioner documenting that they have received Five-Element treatment; and interview with two faculty members, graduates, or administrators.

Tuition and Fees

There is a $65 application fee. A tuition deposit of $800 is required; the tuition balance is $27,000. Books and materials cost approximately $500.

Financial Assistance

A payment plan and federal loans are available.

The Yoga Center

8950 Route 108, Suite 114
Columbia, Maryland 21045
PHONE: (410) 720-4340

The Yoga Center was founded in 1992. Director Bob Glickstein is a certified Iyengar yoga teacher and holistic body worker who has taught yoga for twenty years.

Program Description

A six-month Teacher Training Course for Level I classes trains participants in the instruction and modification of asanas for Level I Hatha yoga classes based on the Iyengar method. Instruction includes effectively communicating step-by-step instruction for each Level I asana, recognizing and making adjustments for common problems, using props effectively, teaching relaxation and restorative poses, and identifying body types according to structural alignment. Topics include Standing Poses, Seated Poses, Forward Bends, Twists, Hip Openers, Arm Work, Simple Backbends, Restorative Poses, Savasana and Philosophy, and review and evaluation. Participants meet one weekend per month for six months, and assist during Level I yoga classes once a month.

Admission Requirements

To participate in the Teacher Training Course and receive maximum benefit, applicants must have a regular daily practice, have completed a Level I class and be enrolled in at least a Level II class, and be committed to studying and developing the skills necessary to teach a Level I class.

Tuition and Fees

Total tuition is $995.

MASSACHUSETTS

American School for Energy Therapies

17 Spring Street
Watertown, Massachusetts 02472
PHONE: (617) 924-9150
FAX: (617) 924-2828
E-MAIL: energydj@ix.netcom.com

The American School for Energy Therapies was founded in 1990 by director Douglas Janssen, a polarity and craniosacral practitioner and teacher since 1981. There are ten instructors, with ten to sixteen students per class.

Accreditation and Approvals

Both the Level 1 and Level 2 Programs are approved by the American Polarity Therapy Association (APTA). The American School for Energy Therapies is licensed by the Department of Education of the Commonwealth of Massachusetts.

Program Description

The American School for Energy Therapies offers both Level 1 (A.P.P.) and Level 2 (R.P.P.) certification programs.

The Level 1 Registered Polarity Practitioner Training, Part 1 (also A.P.P.) consists of 170 hours of instruction divided into five classes: Theory and Practice of Polarity, Energetic Nutrition and Exercises, Introduction to Anatomy and Physiology, Energetic Evaluation and Integration and Building Your Polarity Practice, and Basic Communications and Clinical Supervision. To graduate, students must successfully complete all classes; give thirty documented one-hour polarity sessions; receive ten one-hour polarity sessions from three Registered Polarity Practitioners; pass three out of four competency examinations; comply with all rules and regulations of the school; have valid CPR/First Aid certification; have all tuition and fees paid in full; and select an approved R.P.P. to serve as a postgraduate supervisor for private practice for a period of one year after graduation.

The Level 2 Registered Polarity Practitioner Training, Part 2 consists of 530 hours in addition to Level 1. Classes include Integrating Theory and Practice of Polarity; Polarity Body Systems and Structural Alignment; Orthodox Anatomy and Physiology; Energetic Theory and Evaluation Skills; Polarity Communication and Facilitation Skills; Energetic Nutrition and Exercises; Practice Management, Promotion, Ethics, and Law; Clinical Supervision and Internship; and Energetic Components of Personality. To graduate, students must successfully complete all classes; give seventy documented one-hour polarity sessions; receive twenty one-hour polarity sessions from three Registered Polarity Practitioners; pass three out of four competency evaluations; comply with all rules and regulations of the school; have valid CPR/First Aid certification; have all tuition and fees paid in full; and select an approved R.P.P. to serve as a postgraduate supervisor for private practice for a period of one year after graduation.

Admission Requirements

Level 1 applicants must be at least 18 years of age; have a high school diploma or equivalent; agree to not use drugs, alcohol, or cigarettes during the training weekends; provide a list of all medications and dosages at time of application and throughout the program; and if under the care of a physician, psychiatrist, or counselor at the time of application, a letter from that health care provider stating the applicant's ability to participate in the program. Applicants must also submit two letters of recommendation and answers to essay questions. Level 2 applicants must also have completed the Level 1 training (or the equivalent from another school).

Tuition and Fees

Tuition for Level 1 is $1,350. Other costs include: application fee, $50; student liability insurance, $40; ten sessions received, approximately $400; and books and handouts, approximately $40 to $165.

Tuition for Level 2 is $4,840. Other costs include: application fee, $50; student liability insurance, $50; twenty sessions received, approximately $800; and books and handouts, approximately $185.

Financial Assistance

Work-study positions are available.

Bancroft School of Massage Therapy

333 Shrewsbury Street
Worcester, Massachusetts 01604
PHONE: (508) 757-7923
FAX: (508) 791-5930
E-MAIL: BSMTTank@aol.com
WEBSITE: www.bancroftsmt.com

Henry LaFleur established the Bancroft School of Massage Therapy in 1950. There are twenty-five instructors, and an average of twenty-four students per class.

Accreditation and Approvals

Bancroft is accredited by the Accrediting Commission of Career Schools and Colleges of Technology (ACCSCT). The Certificate Program in Massage Therapy is approved by the Florida Massage Board; graduates are qualified to take the National Certification Examination for Therapeutic Massage and Bodywork (NCETMB). By taking the additional Florida Statutes and Laws course, graduates may seek licensure in Florida.

Program Description

The 940-hour Certificate Program in Massage Therapy includes classes in Massage Techniques and Theory, Movement and Palpation, Reflexology, Anatomy and Physiology, Sports Massage, Oriental Massage Applications, Internship Program, Clinical Massage Applications, Hydrotherapy, Health (CPR/First Aid), Business Practices/Life Skills, Student Clinic, and Seated/On-Site Massage. Classes meet two days or one weeknight and one Saturday per week.

Continuing Education
Additional courses that are not part of the certificate program are available for students who wish to further their education. These include Myology, Neurology, and Florida Statutes and Laws.

Admission Requirements
Applicants must be at least 20 years of age (exceptions may be made for those 18 to 20), have a high school diploma or equivalent, submit personal references and a medical history form, have received a professional massage, and interview with the director of the school.

Tuition and Fees
Tuition for the entire program is $11,750, although some courses may also be taken individually. Other costs total approximately $1,500 and include application fee, books and anatomy equipment, uniform, portable massage table, and supplies.

Financial Assistance
A payment plan and federal loans are available.

Blazing Star Herbal School

P.O. Box 6
Shelburne Falls, Massachusetts 01370
PHONE: (413) 625-6875
FAX: (413) 625-6972
E-MAIL: bshschool@aol.com

Gail Ulrich, founder and director of the Blazing Star Herbal School, has been an herbalist for over twenty-five years and has organized the New England Annual Women's Herbal Conference for the past twelve years. She is an author, vice president of the Northeast Herbal Association, and a plant spirit medicine practitioner. Blazing Star Herbal School was founded in 1983. There are eight instructors, with ten to twenty students per class.

Program Description
The Weekday Apprenticeship Program for beginner and intermediate students meets one day per week for ten months. Instruction is given in Herbal Preparation, Herb Gardening, Ethical Wildcrafting, Herbs for Children, Flower Essences, Study of the Organ Systems, Developing Diagnostic Skills, Chronic Ailments, Herbal First Aid, Natural Cosmetics and Skin Care, Plant Culture and Cultivation, Herbal Business Practices, and more.

The Weekend Apprenticeship Program in Therapeutic Herbalism meets one weekend per month for seven months and is designed for those who are traveling some distance to attend. Course work includes Integration of Traditional and Western Medicine, Classification of Medicinal Plants, Formulation and Preparation of Herbal Medicines, Botanical Terminology, Plant Pharmacology, Sources of Herbal Information, Body Systems and Therapeutics, Herbal Actions, Materia Medica, and Selection Criteria.

A five-day Apprenticeship Intensive is offered to beginning and intermediate students. The course includes Herb Walks and Identification, History of Western Herbalism, Herb Gardening, Herbal Pharmacy, Herbal Preparation, Wildcrafting, Kitchen Cosmetics, Wild Foods Cooking, Herbal First Aid, and Flower Essences.

A Flower Essence Practicum is offered one Saturday per month from June through September.

Community and Continuing Education
A variety of one-day and longer workshops are offered throughout New England. These include Aromatherapy, Diagnostic Skills for Herbalists, The Business of Herbs, and many others.

Admission Requirements
There are no minimum age or educational requirements.

Tuition and Fees
The Weekday Apprenticeship Program costs $1,500. The Weekend Apprenticeship Program in Therapeutic Herbalism costs

$1,050, including text. The five-day Apprenticeship Intensive costs $400, including camping. The Flower Essence Practicum is $250. Fees for all programs include written materials.

Financial Assistance
A payment plan is available.

Boston Shiatsu School

(See East West Institute of Alternative Medicine, below)

Centre of the Web

Jade Hill Farmstead
Box 175
Manchaug, Massachusetts 01526-0175
PHONE/FAX: (508) 476-7081
E-MAIL: jadehill@telegram.infi.net

The Centre of the Web was founded in 1987 by Jane I. LaForce, a wise woman herbalist. The number of instructors varies; classes range from five to thirteen participants.

Program Description
The Basic Apprentice Program consists of a minimum of sixty hours of instruction and a unifying project. The program combines hands-on practical experience of the natural world with scientific information. Topics covered include medical herbology, plant identification, wild foods, wildcrafting, wise woman ways, herbal preparations, development of intuition, cooking with herbs, basic anatomy and physiology, spirit healing, earth awareness and ceremony, plant culture, personal care, women's health, and more. Classes meet in day-long sessions on either Saturdays or Tuesdays; weekends or continuous residency are also offered.

Admission Requirements
Applicants must have a command of the English language, ability to be out-of-doors, and a willing heart and mind.

Community and Continuing Education
Weed walks, workshops, and presentations are offered throughout the year and by appointment. Courses recently of-

fered include Changing Woman, Herbs for Women's Health, Deep Roots, Kitchen Kosmetics, and others.

Work/playshops are hands-on and can be designed to meet a group's needs; minimum $25 per hour. Inquire for a complete description.

Tuition and Fees
Tuition for the Basic Apprentice is $750 to $900 per year. Weed walks and workshops are $30 to $70.

Financial Assistance
Some barter and work exchange is available.

DoveStar Institute

(See Multiple State Locations, pages 391–93)

East West Institute of Alternative Medicine

1972 Massachusetts Avenue
Cambridge, Massachusetts 02140
PHONE: (617) 876-4048
FAX: (617) 497-4892
E-MAIL: eastwestinst@mindspring.com
WEBSITE: www.eastwestinstitute.com

The East West Institute of Alternative Medicine (formerly the Boston Shiatsu School) was founded in 1988 as the Boston School of Ki. There are five faculty members; all technique classes are limited to eighteen students per instructor.

Accreditation and Approvals
The East West Institute is a member of the American Massage Therapy Association (AMTA) Council of Schools and of the American Oriental Bodywork Therapy Association (AOBTA). Graduates of the Shiatsu Certification program are eligible to become AOBTA certified practitioners.

Program Description
The twelfth-month, 720-hour Shiatsu Certification Program may also be taken on a part-time basis over twenty-four months. Courses include Basic Form, Side Position, Supervised

Practice, Anatomy, Zen Shiatsu, Sotai, Chi Development, Physiology, Advanced Techniques/Traditional Chinese Medicine, Business and Ethics, Clinic, Pathology, Advanced Zen Shiatsu, Skills and Dynamics/Elective Introductory Classes, Case Histories/Integration of Techniques/TCM Lab, and electives. Students are required to perform at least fifty treatments in the student clinic.

The 400-hour, three-semester Integrative-Ayurvedic Therapist Certification Program consists of 234 classroom hours with 166 hours of guided studies in clinic and lab work. Courses include Foundation/Theory (covering theory, elements, doshas, physical and mental attributes, Ayurvedic psychology, anatomy and physiology, nutrition and herbology, Ayurvedic pulse diagnosis, and evaluation and management of doshas); Subtle and Physical Therapies (covering herbal medicine, aromatherapy, bodywork, marma points, energy, and vibrational healing); and Advanced Ayurvedic Practices—Pancha Karma (covering five levels of Pancha Karma, Jyotish "Ayurvedic astrology," Ayurvedic numerology, Ayurvedic yoga and Tantric yoga, and clinic). Classes are held over three-day weekends.

A nine-day Basics of Eastern Aromatherapy training is held over three weekends. Topics covered include herbal healing history, olfactory and dermal application processes, home care and treatment room applications, botanical distillations and quality of plant substances, contraindications and safety, Eastern/Ayurvedic energetics and therapeutics, and nine blending labs.

Other programs under development include Comprehensive Nutrition Training, Chinese Herbal Formulas Training, Cranial Sacral Workshop, and TouchPro Chair Massage; contact the Institute for details.

Admission Requirements
Applicants must be at least 18 years of age, have a high school diploma or equivalent, submit an essay and a letter of reference, and be in good health. It is strongly recommended that applicants receive at least one professional shiatsu treatment prior to beginning the program.

Tuition and Fees
Tuition for the Shiatsu Certification Program is $7,200. Additional expenses include a $25 application fee and approximately $250 for books.

Tuition for the Integrative-Ayurvedic Therapist Program is $4,775, including supplies and equipment charges.

Tuition for Basics of Eastern Aromatherapy is $1,095 including supplies; books and essential oils are additional.

Financial Assistance
Payment plans are available.

Ellen Evert Hopman

P.O. Box 219
Amherst, Massachusetts 01004
E-MAIL: saille333@mindspring.com
WEBSITE: www.neopagan.net/WillowsGrove/

Ellen Evert Hopman, M.Ed., is a psychotherapist, master herbalist, lay homeopath, and international coordinator of Keltria, the International Druid Fellowship. She has written several books on the spiritual and healing aspects of plants and has been teaching classes in herbalism since 1983. Classes are held near Amherst, though Ms. Hopman also travels to conduct workshops. Ms. Hopman is the primary instructor; classes are limited to twenty students. (See pages 472–73 for videos.)

Program Description
Ms. Hopman offers a six-month Introduction to Herbal Healing and Self-Care Program that meets one night per week. The course includes an introduction to Chinese Five Element theory and basic diagnostics, the art of formula making, Bach and FES flower essences, herbal therapeutics, and preparation of tinctures, salves, infusions, decoctions, poultices, and more. Classes include 400 pages of printed material, slides, case-taking techniques, and hands-on herbalism.

Herb walks are offered in the summer; write or e-mail for details.

Admission Requirements
Students should be able to read college-level material.

Tuition and Fees
Tuition is $800.

Hands of Light

28 Green Street
Leominster, Massachusetts 01453
PHONE: (978) 466-1249

Hands of Light (formerly Holistic Training) was founded in 1987. There are six instructors; classes are limited to fourteen students. In addition to the programs described here, Hands of Light offers programs in Holistic Labor Assistant and Traditional Midwifery.

Program Description

The one-year Clinical Herbal Program consists of thirteen classes that meet roughly once a month. Topics covered include Spiritual and Psychological Aspects of Healing, Taking a History, Herbal Preparations, Laws of Cure and Disease, Oriental Philosophies, Formula Making, Dosages, Botanical Identification, Diagnosing Imbalances, Intro to Iridology, Nutrition and Allergies, Digestive Problems, Breath: The Life Force, Fatigue, Immune System, Stress and Healing, Toxicity in the Body, Urogenital System, and Harmonizing the Circulation, among others.

The Midwife's Herbal consists of four classes covering Fundamentals of Healing, Formula Making, Counter-indications, Herbs in Pregnancy and Birth, Gynecological Herbal Treatments, Well Woman Care, and Herbs for the Childbearing Year; students will make tinctures, salves, syrups, pills, and suppositories. Each student will make an herbal kit to take home.

Tuition and Fees

Tuition for the Clinical Herbal program is $1,000. Tuition for The Midwife's Herbal is $220 plus $25 for materials.

Financial Assistance

Payment plans, early payment discounts, and a limited number of work-study positions are available.

International Ayurvedic Institute

(See Multiple State Locations, pages 397-98)

Kripalu Center for Yoga and Health

Box 793
Lenox, Massachusetts 01240-0793
PHONE: (413) 448-3152 / (800) 741-7353
FAX: (413) 448-3384
WEBSITE: www.kripalu.org

The Kripalu Center was founded as an ashram in 1972 by Yogi Amrit Desai, and moved from Pennsylvania to Lenox, Massachusetts, in 1983. The current president is Richard Faulds. More than 15,000 people come to Kripalu each year. The faculty consists of several Kripalu teachers as well as nationally known presenters; classes range from ten to ninety-five students and conferences average around 300.

Accreditation and Approvals

Kripalu is approved by the National Board of Certified Counselors and by the National Certification Board for Therapeutic Massage and Bodywork (NCBTMB) as a continuing education provider. Some programs are eligible for continuing education credit for nurses and social workers.

Program Description

Kripalu offers a wide variety of seminars and workshops in such areas as yoga, self-discovery, health and well-being, and bodywork. Introductory workshops include Kripalu Yoga for Beginners, Welcome Weekend, Kripalu Meditation Retreats, Introduction to Kripalu Bodywork, and others.

Certificate programs include Kripalu Yoga Teacher Training, Holistic Health Teacher Training, and the Kripalu Bodywork Training month-long certification program.

The month-long Kripalu Yoga Teacher Training: Basic Certification includes learning how to teach postures with clarity and to lead students into a heightened sense of body awareness. Topics covered include warm-ups, basic postures and their benefits and contraindications, and anatomy and physiology as applied to yoga, pranayama, relaxation, meditation, and yogic philosophy. It is recommended that students practice yoga regularly for at least six months prior to attending. This program is also offered in a three-segment option for those unable to participate in a month-long training.

The month-long Holistic Health Teacher Training Program

prepares participants to teach a wide range of workshops in wellness and stress management, including communication and self-expression; body awareness through yoga and movement; relaxation; meditation; learning to play; transforming attitudes about work; conscious eating; and creating a supportive environment and lifestyle.

The 200-hour, month-long Kripalu Bodywork Training Certification Program offers an in-depth experience of Kripalu's unique approach to bodywork, grounded in the conscious awareness and use of energy. In-depth stroke instruction blends Swedish massage with energy balancing and "tissue listening." Daily yoga and a strong emphasis on body dynamics provide the foundation for bodywork practice that includes grounding and centering as central components. The program is beneficial for both beginning and experienced bodywork practitioners, yoga teachers, holistic health practitioners, and others in health-related fields.

Continuing Education
Programs eligible for continuing education credits change three times per year. Please contact the center for additional information.

Admission Requirements
Programs are generally open to guests 18 years of age and older. Special programs are available to children and youths.

Tuition and Fees
Tuition for Kripalu Yoga Teacher Training: Basic Certification is $1,485 plus twenty-seven or twenty-eight nights' room and meals. Tuition for Holistic Health Teacher Training is $1,190 plus twenty-eight nights' room and meals. Tuition for the Kripalu Bodywork Training Certification Program is $1,190 plus twenty-eight nights room and meals.

Room and meals for twenty-seven-night programs range from $1,026 to $3,645 per person depending on accommodations; room and meals for twenty-eight-night programs range from $1,008 to $3,640 per person depending on accommodations.

Financial Assistance
Partial scholarships and group and senior discounts are available.

Kushi Institute

P.O. Box 7
Becket, Massachusetts 01223-0007
PHONE: (413) 623-5741 / (800) 975-8744
FAX: (413) 623-8827
E-MAIL: kushi@macrobiotics.org
WEBSITE: www.macrobiotics.org

The Kushi Institute was founded in 1979 by Michio and Aveline Kushi. In 1994, the Institute and the University of Minnesota were the recipients of a grant from the National Institutes of Health (NIH) for research on the macrobiotic approach to cancer therapy. Mr. Kushi is also the founder of the One Peaceful World society (see page 459) and the author of several dozen books. The institute sells a variety of books, tapes, and other products (see pages 489–90). The faculty includes sixteen full- and part-time members; classes average twenty students.

Program Description
The Macrobiotic Career Training Program consists of three month-long levels that include comprehensive instruction in the macrobiotic diet and lifestyle, gaining proficiency in macrobiotic diagnosis, macrobiotic cooking classes and participatory workshops, macrobiotic shiatsu, and how to set up a macrobiotic center, run educational programs, and access resources on the Internet. After successful completion of all three levels with an additional one hundred documented treatments, students are eligible to apply for the Associate Degree in Shiatsu through the American Oriental Bodywork Therapy Association (AOBTA).

A five-day Teachers' Seminar conducted by Michio and Aveline Kushi is offered to all macrobiotic teachers who have been practicing for at least one year. The seminar includes presentations by selected teachers, discussions, and classes with Michio Kushi.

The Macrobiotic Educators Association (MEA) is a membership organization of teachers and counselors. Successfully passing a testing program, offered twice yearly at the Kushi Institute, is a prerequisite to becoming a member; for more information, contact Mirea Pencke at the institute or see page 443.

Community Education

A week-long introductory program, The Way to Health, is offered an average of three times per month and offers instruction in such areas as choosing foods for health, basic ingredients of the macrobiotic diet, macrobiotic Oriental diagnosis, daily cooking classes, menu planning, natural home remedies, shiatsu massage workshop, and more.

Tuition and Fees

There is a $100 application fee for week-long programs and a $300 fee for month-long programs. Tuition for the Macrobiotic Career Training Program is $4,200. Tuition for the Teacher's Seminar is $500. Tuition for The Way to Health is $1,745. All prices include accommodations and macrobiotic meals.

Financial Assistance

Financial assistance is available only for the Way to Health program. Prepayment discounts are available for all programs.

Massage Institute of New England

22 McGrath Highway, Suite 11
Somerville, Massachusetts 02143
PHONE: (617) 666-3700
FAX: (617) 666-0109

The Massage Institute of New England (MINE) was established in 1982.

Accreditation and Approvals

Graduates are qualified to take the National Certification Examination for Therapeutic Massage and Bodywork (NCETMB).

Program Description

The 750-hour Massage Therapist Certification Program may be completed in nine months of full-time or seventeen months of part-time evening study. The program consists of Core Classes (Anatomy, Physiology, and Theory and Technique), Clinical Practicum, and eighty-five hours of electives.

Admission Requirements

Prospective students must have a high school diploma or equivalent; be physically, emotionally, and academically quali-

fied to practice massage; interview with a school representative; and attend the Introduction to Swedish Massage workshop.

Tuition and Fees

Tuition is $7,500.

Financial Assistance

Payment plans are available.

Muscular Therapy Institute

122 Rindge Avenue
Cambridge, Massachusetts 02140
PHONE: (617) 576-1300
FAX: (617) 864-8283
E-MAIL: info@mtinstitute.com
WEBSITE: www.mtinstitute.com

The Muscular Therapy Institute (MTI) was founded in 1974 by Dr. Ben E. Benjamin, who developed muscular therapy from a synthesis of approaches. The Benjamin System of muscular therapy is a unique combination of treatment, education, and exercise designed to promote health and reduce muscle tension. There are forty instructors, with an average of twenty-seven students per class.

Accreditation and Approvals

MTI is accredited by the Accrediting Council for Continuing Education and Training (ACCET) and licensed by the Commonwealth of Massachusetts Department of Education. Graduates are qualified to take the National Certification Examination for Therapeutic Massage and Bodywork (NCETMB).

Program Description

The 51.6-credit-hour Intensive Professional Training in Muscular Therapy program may be completed in either a three-semester/fifteen-month format meeting two days per week, or a four-semester/twenty-month format meeting one and a half days per week. One classroom day in the first semester will be held at a retreat center. Courses include Skills and Dynamics of Therapeutic Relationships, Anatomy and Kinesiology, Physiology, Clinical Considerations and Pathology,

Muscular Therapy Technique, Sports Massage, Approaches to Holistic Therapy, Practice Development, Professional Development, Perspectives on Bodywork, Business Practice for Massage Professionals, and fifteen private lessons with a faculty member.

Students interested in applying are required to attend a one-day introductory workshop, held about once a month. These workshops include classes in Muscular Therapy Technique, Alignment in Movement, Tension Analysis and Communication Skills. Participants have the opportunity to interact with faculty, students, and graduates to obtain firsthand information about the program.

Career Nights are free evenings at which prospective students may learn more about the school and about massage as a career.

Admission Requirements
Applicants must be at least twenty years of age, have a high school diploma or equivalent, be in good health and free of communicable diseases, and attend the introductory workshop. In addition, applicants are interviewed and evaluated for their aptitude for working with their hands, working with people in a professional fashion, and for motivation and self-directedness.

Tuition and Fees
Tuition is $12,890. Additional expenses include the introductory workshop, $25; application fee, $100; books, approximately $295; massage table, $525; Student Therapy Center uniform, $75; CPR/First Aid certification, $125; and massage treatment, $500. Linens are additional.

Financial Assistance
Federal grants and loans, alternative loans, no-interest payment plans, and veterans' benefits are available; MTI is approved for training under the Massachusetts Rehabilitation Commission.

New England School of Acupuncture

40 Belmont Street
Watertown, Massachusetts 02472
PHONE: (617) 926-1788

FAX: (617) 924-4167
E-MAIL: info@nesa.edu
WEBSITE: www.nesa.edu

The New England School of Acupuncture (NESA), the oldest acupuncture school in the United States, was founded in 1975 by master acupuncturist James Tin Yau So. There are seventy faculty members, with an average of forty students per class.

Accreditation and Approvals
NESA is accredited by the Accreditation Commission for Acupuncture and Oriental Medicine (ACAOM) and approved by the Massachusetts Board of Higher Education to grant a Master of Acupuncture degree.

Program Description
The three-year Master of Acupuncture degree program includes more than 1,000 hours of hands-on clinical instruction and a full year of clinical internship in acupuncture and herbal medicine. NESA offers two options as part of its master's degree: an Oriental Medicine Program (2,722.5 hours) and an Acupuncture program (2,392 hours). Electives offer students exposure to diverse acupuncture techniques such as Japanese styles, Five Element, and other approaches. In addition, students gain a solid grounding in Western science and medicine, nutrition, Tui Na, and qi gong. Students may choose day or evening options.

During the clinical experience, students progress from observing and assisting acupuncture practitioners to treating patients under the supervision of clinical faculty during a year-long internship. Students have opportunities for assistantship and internship in the NESA Clinic, a thirty-patient treatment room facility, and at off-campus clinical sites, including a hospital-affiliated clinic and at the AIDS Care Project.

Continuing Education
NESA's Continuing Education Department offers an extensive program of courses and seminars throughout the year on acupuncture, herbal medicine, wellness, and other related topics.

Graduates have the opportunity to do advanced clinical training at the Zhejiang College of Traditional Chinese Medicine in Hangzhou, China, through programs arranged by the Continuing Education Department.

Admission Requirements

Applicants must have a bachelor's degree from an accredited institution and have an admission interview. All required science courses may be taken as corequisites; however, it is recommended that students complete anatomy and physiology before starting the program.

Tuition and Fees

Full-time tuition for 2000–2001 is $9,750 for the first year (three semesters) of the program; tuition may vary based on the number of credits taken; the per-credit tuition for full-time students is $250 ($275 for part-time). Books and supplies are approximately $1,250 to $1,500 for the three years of study. Other costs include malpractice insurance coverage.

Financial Assistance

Federal financial aid in the form of loans is available.

New England School of Homeopathy

(See Multiple State Locations, pages 402–3)

Phoenix Rising Yoga Therapy

See Multiple State Locations, page 407)

Polarity Realization Institute

(See Multiple State Locations, pages 408–9)

The School for Body-Mind Centering

(See Multiple State Locations, page 411)

The Stillpoint Program at Greenfield Community College

270 Main Street
Greenfield, Massachusetts 10301
PHONE: (413) 775-1620
FAX: (413) 774-2285
E-MAIL: nursing@gcc.mass.edu
WEBSITE: www.gcc.mass.edu

The Stillpoint Program at Greenfield Community College was founded in 1981 in Hatfield, Massachusetts, as the Stillpoint Center School of Massage. Stillpoint recently brought its comprehensive massage therapy training program to Greenfield Community College, thereby combining the highly qualified Stillpoint faculty with the resources of higher education in a joint certificate program. There are ten instructors in the massage therapy program; average class sizes are sixteen in technique and applied sciences, thirty-two in professional development classes.

Accreditation and Approvals

Stillpoint's Massage Therapy Certification Program operates as a department within the Division of Nursing and Health Occupations at the College. Graduates are qualified to take the National Certification Examination for Therapeutic Massage and Bodywork (NCETMB).

Program Description

The 700-hour/twenty-five-credit Massage Therapy Certification Program is guided by three interrelated principles: Holism, Massage with Awareness, and Compassionate Action. The curriculum includes courses in Anatomy, Physiology, Myology, Swedish Massage, Professional Development, Pathology, Kinesiology, Hydrotherapy, Professional Worklife, on-site massage clinics, and a service learning project.

Advanced certification courses include Hydrotherapy, Sports Massage, Healing Modalities, and Therapeutic Techniques.

Full-time day and evening programs are offered.

Community and Continuing Education

Workshops are offered on a variety of topics, including basic massage, craniosacral therapy, reflexology, and others through the college's community services program.

Admission Requirements

Applicants must be at least 18 years of age, have a high school diploma or equivalent, and attend an informational meeting.

Tuition and Fees

Tuition is $4,300. Additional expenses include a $25 application fee; books, supplies, and massage table are approximately $1,400.

Financial Assistance

Full financial aid services are available through the College.

MICHIGAN

Ann Arbor Institute of Massage Therapy

2835 Carpenter Road
Ann Arbor, Michigan 48108-1123
PHONE: (734) 677-4430
FAX: (734) 677-4520

Ann Arbor Institute of Massage Therapy (AAIMT) was founded in 1993 by Jocelyn Granger and Jane Anderson. AAIMT is affiliated with the Chicago School of Massage Therapy, with a portion of the AAIMT program being taught by the Chicago School core faculty. There are thirteen instructors, with an average class size of sixteen to twenty-six students and a teacher:student ratio of 1:12 for technique classes.

Accreditation and Approvals

AAIMT is licensed by the Michigan Department of Education. Graduates are qualified to take the National Certification Examination for Therapeutic Massage and Bodywork (NCETMB). AAIMT is approved by the National Certification Board for Therapeutic Massage and Bodywork (NCBTMB) as a continuing education provider.

Program Description

The 650-hour Massage Therapy Professional Training Program consists of two semesters that include Anatomy and Physiology, Therapeutic Massage and Related Approaches, Myofascial Therapy, Neuromuscular Therapy, Sports Massage, Shiatsu, Seated Massage, Business Management and Professionalism, Student Clinic: Internship, and Student Outreach Program: Externship. Students must receive at least three professional massages during the class year.

Continuing Education

Weekend workshops in advanced therapies are open to practicing massage therapists for continuing education credits. Topics typically covered include Seated Massage, Pathology, Shiatsu, Myofascial Therapies, Sports Massage, Refinement, and Neuromuscular Therapy.

Admission Requirements

Applicants must be at least 18 years of age, have a high school diploma or equivalent, and be of sound mind and body.

Tuition and Fees

Tuition for the 650-hour program is $5,900. Additional expenses include application fee, $25; registration fee, $50; books, approximately $160; lab fee, $185; massage table, $450 to $750; and sheets and massage oil.

Financial Assistance

A payment plan is available.

Discovery Institute of Clinical Hypnotherapy

6470 Belding Avenue
Fenwick, Michigan 48834
PHONE: (616) 761-3453
E-MAIL: Discovery@Ionip-mi.net

Discovery Institute of Clinical Hypnotherapy was founded in 1996 by Charles Kinney. There are two primary instructors; classes are limited to thirty students.

Accreditation and Approvals

The Discovery Institute of Clinical Hypnotherapy is endorsed by the International Medical and Dental Hypnotherapy Association (IMDHA).

Program Description

The forty-four-hour Basic Hypnosis Program covers History of Hypnosis, Suggestibility Testing, Group Participation and Practice, Principles of Suggestion, Psychology of Hypnosis, Pre-Induction Talk, Relaxation Stress Management, Guided Mental Imagery, Group Hypnosis, Weight Loss, Stop Smoking, Formulating Suggestions, Self Hypnosis, Setting Up a Practice, Induction Methods, and more.

The forty-four-hour Advanced Hypnosis Program covers Advanced Methods, Rapid Inductions, Age Regression, Hypnotherapy, Dreams and Meaning, Visual Hallucination, Medical/Dental Hypnosis, Introduction to NLP, Waking Hypnosis, Hickman Method, Amnesia and Surgery, Post Hypnotic Suggestion, Glove Anesthesia and Dentistry, Stage Hypnosis, the Elman Method, and more.

The forty-eight-hour Hypnoanalysis Program consists of Fundamentals of Hypnosis, Basic Communication Type, Initial Comprehensive Intake, Word Association in Hypnosis, Dream Analysis in Hypnosis, Hypnoanalysis Goals in Therapy, Spiritual Cleansing/Healing, Subconscious Motivation of Health and Disease, Client Time Line, The Five "R"s of Hypnotherapy, Sexual Disorders, Theology in Hypnoanalysis, Techniques for Release of Negative Energy, Regression Therapy, and more.

Admission Requirements

Applicants must be at least 18 years of age and have a high school diploma or equivalent.

Tuition and Fees

Tuition for Basic Hypnosis is $495; for Advanced, $495; and for Hypnoanalysis, $495.

Financial Assistance

Scholarships in the form of reduced tuition, discounts for spouse or assistant, and discounts for full payment fourteen days prior to class are available.

Health Enrichment Center

1820 North Lapeer Road
Lapeer, Michigan 48446-7771
PHONE: (810) 667-9453
FAX: (810) 667-4095
E-MAIL: hec@tir.com
WEBSITE: www.healthenrichment.com

Health Enrichment Center (HEC) was founded in 1985 and is owned and operated by Sandy Fritz. Decentralized facilities for the Therapeutic Massage program are offered regionally throughout Michigan. There are twenty-five instructors with a maximum of twenty students in a primary class.

Accreditation and Approvals

HEC is accredited by the Accrediting Commission of Career Schools and Colleges of Technology (ACCSCT). HEC has an articulation agreement with Siena Heights College in Adrian, Michigan, where graduates may transfer some credits toward an associate's or bachelor's degree. Graduates of the Therapeutic Massage program are qualified to take the National Certification Examination for Therapeutic Massage and Bodywork (NCETMB). HEC is approved by the National Certification Board of Therapeutic Massage and Bodywork (NCBTMB) as a continuing education provider. HEC has program approval in Ontario, Canada.

Program Description

The 1,000-hour, thirty-three-credit Therapeutic Massage Program consists of 500 classroom hours and 500 directed-study hours. Topics covered in the classroom include Anatomy and Physiology, Biology of Health and Wellness, Muscle Stress Reduction Techniques, Movement Reeducation, Muscle Energy Techniques, Therapeutic Massage Techniques, Sports Massage, Clinical Experience Lab, and Ethics and Business Practices. Directed-study hours require a massage log, written essay exams, research paper, presentation, and a business project. Classes are held days, evenings and weekends.

The 244-hour, fifteen-credit Clinical Approaches Course is open to graduates of any 500-hour massage therapy program from a state-licensed school. The program focuses on the application of therapeutic massage in more complex situations, with courses in Joint Anatomy and Physiology, Functional Assessment, Manual Therapies, Chronic Health Problems, Professional Interactions, Craniosacral Therapies, and Myofascial Techniques. Students attend classes for thirteen weekends.

A 256-hour, fifteen-credit Subtle Energy Therapies course is open to graduates of any 500-hour massage therapy program from a state-licensed school. The core curriculum consists of Advanced Craniosacral; Anatomy and Physiology of Energy; Essence, Aromatherapy, and Homeopathy; One Brain; Power of Word Intention; Somato Positional Release; Supervised Practice Time; Triune Polarity Energy; Movement and Yoga; Tools of the Trade; Reiki I and II; and review and testing.

Continuing Education

Graduates are eligible to take the 2,000-hour, sixty-six-credit Advanced Practitioner and 5,000-hour, 156-credit Master Bodywork Therapist advanced diploma programs. These programs are continuations of the Therapeutic Massage Program. See the catalog for details.

Individual workshops ranging from four hours to six days are offered in various fields of bodywork, including Therapeutic Seated Massage, Precision Muscle Skeletal Anatomy, Shiatsu, Manual Medicine, and many others.

Admission Requirements

Applicants must be at least 18 years of age, have a high school diploma or equivalent, be physically capable of performing massage, be of good moral character, and be able to read, write, and speak in the English language.

Tuition and Fees

There is a $25 application fee. Tuition for the Therapeutic Massage Program is $4,500; books are approximately $350. Tuition for the Clinical Approaches Course is $2,650; books are approximately $360. Tuition for the Subtle Energy Therapies course is $2,650; books are approximately $300. Tuition for the Advanced Practitioner and the Master Bodywork Therapist Programs varies depending on choices.

Financial Assistance

Limited scholarships and a payment plan are available. A two-year loan is available at a local bank.

Infinity Institute International

4110 Edgeland, Suite 800
Royal Oak, Michigan 48073-2285
PHONE: (248) 549-5594
WEBSITE: www.infinityinst.com

Anne H. Spencer, Ph.D., founded both the Infinity Institute International (in 1980) and the International Medical and Dental Hypnotherapy Association (in 1987), a referral service for certified hypnotherapists to health care providers and the general public.

Accreditation and Approvals

Infinity Institute International has been granted course approval by the State of Michigan Board of Higher Education, and is approved by the International Medical and Dental Hypnotherapy Association (IMDHA).

Program Description

Courses are offered in Basic Hypnosis, Advanced Hypnosis, and Hypnoanalysis. Courses are given on two weekends and include directed independent study as well as classroom instruction and practice.

The forty-hour Basic Hypnosis Course covers the History of Hypnosis, Suggestibility Testing, Group Participation and Practice, Principles of Suggestion, Relaxation/Stress Management, Induction Methods, Guided Mental Imagery, Group Hypnosis, Weight Loss, Stop Smoking, Self-Hypnosis, Setting Up a Practice, and more.

The forty-hour Advanced Hypnosis Course includes Advanced Methods, Rapid Inductions, Age Regression, Hypnotherapy, Dreams and Meaning, Visual Hallucination, Medical/Dental Hypnosis, Group Participation and Practice, Waking Hypnosis, Hickman Method, Amnesia and Surgery, Somnambulism, Post-Hypnotic Suggestion, and more.

In the forty-hour Hypnoanalysis Course, topics covered include Fundamentals of Hypnoanalysis, Basic Communication Type, Initial Comprehensive Intake, Word Association and Dream Analysis in Hypnosis, Spiritual Cleansing/Healing, Techniques for Release of Negative Energy, Regression Therapy, and more.

Admission Requirements

Applicants must be at least 18 years of age and have a high school diploma.

Tuition and Fees

Tuition for the Basic Hypnosis program is $575; for the Advanced Hypnosis program, $575; and for the Hypnoanalysis program, $575.

Financial Assistance

Limited scholarships are available and a discount is given for prepayment.

Institute of Natural Health Sciences

20270 Middlebelt Road, Suite 4
Livonia, Michigan 48152
PHONE: (248) 473-5458
FAX: (248) 473-8141

The Institute of Natural Health Sciences (INHS) was founded in 1986. There are nine faculty members, with an average of fifteen (maximum eigtheen) students per class. In addition to the programs described here, an additional 200-hour certificate program is offered in Acupuncture Training.

Accreditation and Approvals

INHS is in the process of applying for accreditation with the Council on Homeopathic Education (CHE).

Program Description

The 334-hour Diploma in Homeotherapeutics and the Natural Health Sciences requires completion of the 234 resident class hours in Basic Body Balancing, Early Family Health Enhancement, Homeotherapeutics, Hypnotherapy, Nutrition, Othamo Somatic Analysis, Homeopathy and Psychosocial Development, and Pharmacognosy; eighty hours of independent Homeotherapeutic Case Study Research; twenty hours of Community Service Enrichment; demonstration of the ability to take, repertorize and solve a case; and satisfactory completion of written assignments and exams.

The 768-hour Diploma in Bio-Energetics and the Natural Health Sciences requires completion of the Diploma in Homeotherapeutics and Natural Health Sciences above, plus 234 additional resident class hours in Acupuncture, Bio-Energetics, Electrodermal Analysis, Homeotherapeutics, Pharmacognosy, and Clinical Practicum; eighty hours of independent EAV Case Study Research; twenty hours of independent Community Service Enrichment; demonstration of the ability to take, repertorize and solve a case; 100 hours of Clinical Internship; certification in First Aid and CPR; and satisfactory completion of written assignments and exams.

Resident classes meet on the third weekend of each month for fifteen months.

Admission Requirements

Applicants must have completed a bachelor's degree or equivalent in the liberal arts or physical sciences, and must have completed courses in anatomy, biology, chemistry, and physiology with a GPA of 2.0 or better. Applicants not meeting these requirements may be admitted under special circumstances.

Tuition and Fees

Tuition is $4,680 for fifteen weekends of resident classes; books are additional. There is a $25 application fee.

Financial Assistance

Payment plans are available.

Institute of Natural Therapies

P.O. Box 222
Hancock, Michigan 49930
PHONE: (906) 482-2222

The Institute of Natural Therapies (INT) was founded in 1994 by Harold Roy Rudnianin, who is the primary instructor; from time to time, guest lecturers present special techniques. Classes are limited to twenty students.

Accreditation and Approvals

INT is licensed by the Michigan Board of Education. Graduates are qualified to take the National Certification Examination for Therapeutic Massage and Bodywork (NCETMB).

Program Description

The Professional Massage Therapist Training consists of 500 in-class hours, 100 hours of outside massage practice, 200 hours of workbook and practice, and six hours of public presentation for a total of 806 hours. Coursework includes Traditional Swedish Massage, Anatomy and Physiology, Yoga and Stretch Kinesiology, Hydrotherapy and Living Foods, CPR, Deep Tissue Massage, Muscular Anatomy and Physiology, Orthobionomy Kinesiology, Neuro-Muscular Therapy, Neuro-Anatomy and Physiology, Somatic Movement Kinesiology, Traditional Chinese Techniques, Traditional Chinese Theory and Culture, Qi Gong and Tai Chi Kinesiology, Healing Touch,

Myofascial Release/Connective Tissue, Fascial Anatomy/Somatic, Postural Analysis Kinesiology, Business Ethics, Supervised Clinic Experience, Final and Review, and Review of Personal Professional Growth.

Community and Continuing Education

A Free Massage Lecture and Open House offers prospective students an introduction to the school. The twelve-hour Weekend Family Massage Class is open to the public.

Admission Requirements

Applicants must be at least 18 years of age, have a high school diploma or equivalent, be physically and emotionally able to perform massage, submit two letters of recommendation, and have a personal interview, where literacy and basic science knowledge will be assessed by a written test.

Tuition and Fees

Tuition is $4,400; there is a $25 application fee.

Financial Assistance

Payment plans are available.

International Center for Reiki Training

21421 Hilltop Street, # 28
Southfield, Michigan 48034
PHONE: (248) 948-8112 / (800) 332-8112
FAX: (248) 948-9534
E-MAIL: center@reiki.org
WEBSITE: www.reiki.org

The International Center for Reiki Training was founded in 1988 by William L. Rand. There are twenty instructors, with an average of eight to ten students per class. See page 493 for a catalog of products.

Accreditation and Approvals

Continuing education units (CEUs) are available for nurses, athletic trainers, and massage therapists.

Program Description

The Licensed Teacher Certification Program is an advanced course for Reiki Masters who wish to teach the programs offered by the International Center for Reiki Training and to become Center Licensed Teachers.

The program is self-paced; at least one year is suggested for completion. Requirements include sending a letter of intent to the certification office; trusting the reiki energy to provide the perfect healing result; actively working on one's own healing; working to fully express the reiki principles and the center's philosophy and purpose; agreeing to teach the minimum subjects required for each class and using the center manuals; taking Reiki I and II, ART, and Reiki III from a Center Licensed Teacher twice; practicing reiki for one year or more before enrolling in the program; providing proof of doing fifty or more complete reiki treatments; passing a written test; writing a paper on the reiki subject of your choice; co-teaching a Reiki I and II class with another Center Licensed Teacher; and paying an annual membership fee of $100 to the Center.

Reiki I and II are taught together during a weekend intensive. Topics covered include reiki hand positions and giving a complete reiki treatment, the Reiki II symbols and how to use them, using reiki for specific conditions, and distant healing, scanning, and beaming.

Advanced Reiki Training (ART) is a one-day intensive that includes the Usui Master attunement, the Usui Master symbol, reiki meditation, advanced techniques to achieve goals, using reiki to protect yourself and others, using crystals and stones with reiki, reiki psychic surgery, guided meditation, and more.

Reiki III/Master is a two-day intensive that includes the complete Reiki III Usui/Tibetan Master attunement, instruction in giving all attunements, the healing attunement, two Tibetan symbols, advanced reiki meditation, and the values and spiritual orientation of a Reiki Master.

A three-day, weekend Karuna Reiki Class is offered to those who have completed Reiki Master Training. Reiki, guided meditation, NLP, past life regression, and other techniques are used to heal blocks to developing a thriving reiki practice. Connections are strengthened to guides, angels, ascended masters, and higher self. The class is complete with two levels, two attunements, three master symbols, and nine treatment symbols. Those completing the course will be able to teach all four levels of Karuna Reiki (two practitioner levels and two master levels).

Continuing Education

An Advanced Teacher Licensing Program is offered to those who have completed Reiki I and II, ART, and Reiki III/ Master; contact the center for details.

Tuition and Fees

The Reiki I and II courses cost $310. The Advanced Reiki Training (ART) course costs $205. The Reiki III/Master course costs $620. The Karuna Reiki course costs $825. Prices may vary with the instructor.

Financial Assistance

Financial assistance may be possible in some cases.

Irene's Myomassology Institute

18911 Ten Mile
Southfield, Michigan 48075
PHONE: (248) 569-HAND
FAX: (248) 569-4261
WEBSITE: www.myomassology.com

Irene's Myomassology Institute was founded by Irene Gauthier in 1992. "Myomassology" is a term used to describe a massage that includes therapeutic techniques beyond basic Swedish massage, such as reflexology, energy balancing, craniology, muscle testing, Polarity, Shiatsu, and others. There are fourteen instructors for core classes and thirty-five elective instructors. Classes average twenty students.

Accreditation and Approvals

Irene's Myomassology Institute is a state-licensed school approved by the International Myomassethics Federation (IMF). Graduates are qualified to take the National Certification Examination for Therapeutic Massage and Bodywork (NCETMB).

Program Description

The 500-hour, forty-eight-week Myomassology Program consists of 216 hours of core classes, forty-five documented Clinical Massage hours, and 140 hours of electives. The core curriculum includes Basic Myomassology, Therapeutic Myomassology, Anatomy, Physiology, Pathology, Sanitary Practices, Posture, Ethics, Business Procedures, and Review/Exams.

Electives may be chosen from a variety of topics in bodywork and related studies, which include Myofascial Release, Sports Massage, Craniology, Shiatsu, Polarity, Touch for Health, Chair Massage, Trigger Points, Reiki, Prenatal Massage, Labor Massage, Infant Massage, Therapeutic Touch, Reflexology, Pet Massage, Lymphatic Health, Herbology, Nutrition, Macrobiotics, Applied Iridology, Biomagnetics, Crystal Healing, Bach Flower Essences, Yoga for Therapists, Colon Health, and others.

Community and Continuing Education

A variety of classes (including the elective classes listed above and others) are open to members of the community; some require a minimum of twelve weeks' prior massage training.

Admission Requirements

Applicants must be at least 18 years of age, have a high school diploma or equivalent, attend an entrance interview, and demonstrate emotional maturity and a genuine desire to serve the public.

Tuition and Fees

Tuition is $4,550 full-time, $4,760 part time. Additional fees required for some elective classes range from $5 to $25. Additional expenses include registration fee, $50, and books, $225.

Tuition for electives for those not enrolled in the 500-hour program ranges from $70 to $175 plus a registration fee of $40 to $75; material fees are an additional $5 to $25.

Financial Assistance

Payment plans are available.

Kalamazoo Center for the Healing Arts

3715 West Main Street, Suite 3
Kalamazoo, Michigan 49006-2842
PHONE: (616) 373-0910
FAX: (616) 373-0271
E-MAIL: kchands@aol.com
WEBSITE: www.kcha.com

Kalamazoo Center for the Healing Arts (KCHA) was founded in 1986; the school's program was started and state-licensed in 1993. KCHA is also a health care center offering private bodywork sessions, a store, and a variety of other services and classes. There are four instructors, with an average of twenty-two students per class.

Accreditation and Approvals

KCHA is accredited by the Integrative Massage and Somatic Therapies Accreditation Council (IMSTAC). Graduates are qualified to take the National Certification Examination for Therapeutic Massage and Bodywork (NCETMB).

Program Description

The 520-hour Professional Training Program begins with a 120-hour Basic Massage class followed by 400 hours of professional-level classes. Basic Massage covers anatomy (including names, locations, and functions of organs; the digestive, circulatory, lymphatic, skeletal, and nervous systems; and muscles); range of motion; introduction to acupressure; and specific techniques for hips, pelvic region, shoulders, legs, head, arms, and diaphragm release. The Professional Training classes cover Integrated Bodywork Therapies (including myofascial release, craniosacral therapy, polarity, and related concepts), Acupressure, Advanced Anatomy, The Business of Being a Bodyworker, and 100 hours of Practicum (forty lab hours, thirty on-site hours, and thirty hours of elective seminars).

Community and Continuing Education

A free Introduction to KCHA's Massage Programs, held monthly, introduces students to KCHA, accreditation and certification, state licensing, course descriptions, and more. In addition, a two-evening Massage as a Profession workshop provides a sampling of hands-on massage experience and information from instructors, students, and graduates.

Admission Requirements

Applicants must be at least 18 years of age (or have the consent of the director of services); submit two letters of recommendation, a completed application and enrollment agreement; and interview with the enrollment director.

Tuition and Fees

Tuition for the 520-hour Professional Training Program is $4,720; there is a $100 application fee.

Transportation to on-site and/or field trip locations, books,

pillow, towel, colored markers, and massage table are additional.

Tuition for the two-day Massage as a Profession workshop is $75; $25 will be applied to tuition if the student is accepted into the program.

Financial Assistance

Payment plans and student loan programs are available.

Kirtland Community College

10775 North St. Helen Road
Roscommon, Michigan 48653-9981
PHONE: (517) 275-5121
FAX: (517) 275-6710
E-MAIL: pavelekn@kirtland.cc.mi.us
WEBSITE: www.kirtland.cc.mi.us

Kirtland Community College was founded in 1966 and offers fifty vocational certificate and degree programs and five transfer degree programs. In the Massage Therapy Program, there are seven instructors and a maximum of sixteen students per class.

Accreditation and Approvals

Kirtland Community College is accredited by the Michigan Commission on College Accreditation and the North Central Association of Colleges and Secondary Schools. Students completing either the Associate Degree or the Certificate program will be qualified to take the National Certification Examination for Therapeutic Massage and Bodywork (NCETMB).

Program Description

The sixty-three-credit hour Associate in Applied Science in Massage Therapy may be completed in four semesters (two years). Courses required for the Massage Therapy Major include Introduction to Massage Therapy, Swedish Massage, Introduction to Clinic Operations, Structural Based Bodywork Systems, Energy Based Bodywork Systems, Massage Therapy Clinic I and II, Topics in Massage Therapy, Internship, and Directed Study—Massage Therapy I and II. General Education requirements for graduation include Standard First Aid, Essentials of Anatomy and Physiology, Business Seminar, Writing

Lab, English Composition I, Technical Writing, Medical Terminology, Finite Math, Conditioning Activities—Blueprint for a Healthy Back, Lifetime Fitness and Wellness, Introduction to American Government, Introduction to Psychology, Introduction to Sociology, Introduction to Interpersonal and Public Communication, and a Humanities elective.

A thirty-eight-credit hour, 640-contact hour Certificate in Massage Therapy includes all of the courses listed under the Massage Therapy Major (above), plus Medical Terminology, Standard First Aid, Essentials of Anatomy and Physiology, Business Seminar, Conditioning Activities, and Lifetime Wellness and Fitness. Students must also demonstrate proficiency in English, reading, and mathematics based on test scores or completion of recommended classes. Students may complete the program in less than two years by attending summer session or completing hours on an accelerated basis.

Admission Requirements

Applicants must be at least 18 years of age, have a high school diploma or equivalent, be physically able to perform the massage techniques, and must complete a physical examination verifying the applicant is free of communicable diseases.

Tuition and Fees

Tuition for in-district residents is $48.65 per credit hour; for out-of-district residents, $66.70 per credit hour. Additional expenses include registration fee ($3 per credit hour), student activity fee ($1 per credit hour), course lab fees, books, and supplies.

Financial Assistance

Numerous scholarships, grants, loans, work study, tuition deferral, and veterans' benefits are available.

Lansing Community College

400–600 North Washington Square
P.O. Box 40010
Lansing, Michigan 48901-7210
PHONE: (517) 483-1410 / (517) 483-1200
FAX: (517) 483-1508
E-MAIL: rdisbrow@lansing.cc.mi.us
WEBSITE: www.lansing.cc.mi.us/index2html

Lansing Community College (LCC), founded in 1957, is one of the largest community colleges in the country and offers over 150 degree and certificate programs, including a certificate program in Massage Therapy. The Massage Therapy classes average twenty-four students; there are eight faculty members.

Accreditation and Approvals

LCC is accredited by the North Central Association of Schools and Colleges. Graduates are qualified to take the National Certification Examination for Therapeutic Massage and Bodywork (NCETMB).

Program Description

The Massage Therapy Certificate of Completion Program consists of twenty-five credits of required courses and two credits of limited choice requirements. Required courses include Introductory Anatomy and Physiology, Massage Therapy: Beginning, Massage Therapy: Intermediate, Independent Study Massage Practicum (consisting of ninety-six hours of massage work, reading, and a report), Human Structural Dynamics for Massage Therapy, Touch for Health, Polarity Therapy I, Business Applications for Massage Therapists, Clinical Approaches to Therapeutic Massage, Sports Massage Techniques, Healthy Lifestyles, and Stress Management. Students must complete two credits chosen from Polarity Therapy II, Self-Awareness: Key to Wellness, Medical Alternatives in Health and Wellness or Yoga and Therapeutic Touch.

Admission Requirements

Applicants must be at least 18 years of age and have a high school diploma. Those who are under 18, enrolled in high school, and working to fulfill high school requirements may be admitted under the Dual Enrollment or Special Admission Programs.

Tuition and Fees

Tuition per credit hour is $48 for residents, $77 for nonresidents, and $106 for out-of-state or international students. Additional expenses include a $10 application fee, a registration fee of $20 per semester, and an activity fee based on the number of credits.

Financial Assistance

Financial assistance is available in the forms of scholarships, grants, loans, employment, and special situation funds.

Michigan School of Myomassology

School of Basic and Therapeutic Bodywork
3270 Greenfield Road
Berkley, Michigan 48072-1161
PHONE: (248) 542-7228
FAX: (248) 542-5830
E-MAIL: touch@concentric.net
WEBSITE: www.therapeutic-touch.com

The Michigan School of Myomassology (MSM) changed owners and locations in May 1997. Owner/director Marilyn A. Rotko is a practicing Myomassologist and Clinical Hypnotherapist. There are four core class instructors, and sixteen methods class instructors; the maximum class size is twenty students.

Accreditation and Approvals

MSM is state licensed, and approved by the National Certification Board for Therapeutic Massage and Bodywork (NCBTMB) as a continuing education provider. Graduates are qualified to take the National Certification Examination for Therapeutic Massage and Bodywork (NCETMB).

Program Description

The 650-hour, forty-six-week Myomassology Program consists of Core Classes, Methods Classes, and Practical Hours. Core Classes cover such topics as Basic and Therapeutic Myomassology Techniques, Anatomy, Craniology, Proprio-neuro Receptor Facilitation, Reflexology, Body Mechanics, Myofascial Release, Paraffin Therapy, Hydrotherapy, Heliotherapy, Modified Massage, Energy Balancing, Business Procedures, Sanitary Practice, and Massage Ethics. Methods Classes (some of which are required for graduation) may include Sports Massage, Shiatsu, Polarity, Touch for Health, One Brain, Prenatal and Infant Massage, Myofascial Release, Herbs, Nutrition, Iridology, CPR, Aromatherapy, Neurolinguistic Programming, Clinical Approaches to Carpal Tunnel, Clinical Approaches to Headaches, Clinical Approaches to Low Back Pain, Nuat Thai, and others. In addi-

tion, students must complete eighty Practical Hours either at the facility or under preapproved supervision.

Admission Requirements

Generally, applicants must be at least seventeen years of age and have a high school diploma or equivalent; however, some exceptions may be made.

Tuition and Fees

Total tuition of $4,090 includes instruction manual, coloring book, handouts, and oils. Books, supplies, and massage table are additional.

Financial Assistance

Payment plans are available.

Wellspring School of Therapeutic Bodywork

20312 Chalon
St. Clair Shores, Michigan 48080
PHONE: (810) 772-8520

The Wellspring School of Therapeutic Bodywork has seven instructors and a maximum class size of twenty-five students. In addition to the program described here, Wellspring offers a 300-hour program in Therapeutic Massage and in Advanced Therapeutic Bodywork.

Accreditation and Approvals

Wellspring is licensed by the Michigan State Board of Education. Graduates of massage therapy programs of 500 or more hours are qualified to take the National Certification Examination for Therapeutic Massage and Bodywork (NCETMB).

Program Description

Wellspring offers 500-hour programs in Therapeutic Massage and in Advanced Therapeutic Bodywork.

The 500-hour Therapeutic Massage Program consists of their 300-hour Therapeutic Massage and Basic Bodywork Education Program (which covers Basic Massage, Acupressure or Shiatsu, Therapeutic Touch, Emotional Self-Influencing, Reflexology, Practice Management, Sports Massage, Massaging the Elderly, plus additional elective workshops if needed), plus

Advanced Massage Practicum, Elective Workshop Hours, Anatomy Coloring Book, Reading Study Program, and Special Credit.

The 500-hour Advanced Therapeutic Bodywork Professional Development Program consists of the 300-hour Advanced Therapeutic Bodywork Professional Development Program (which covers Advanced Massage Practicum, Practical Anatomy, Modern Medical Massage, Clinical Practice, and Independent Study Project), plus additional elective class hours and clinical practice.

Electives include such courses as Introduction to Trust Level (TORI) Theory, Communication Skills Workshop, Applied Compassion, Relieving Osseous Calcification in Feet, Stress Management for Bodyworkers, Jin Shin Acupressure Facial, Trigger Point Therapy, Massaging the Disabled, Hot Herbal Wraps, Polarity Therapy, and others.

Admission Requirements

Applicants must be at least 18 years of age (or have consent of the director); be physically, mentally, and emotionally able to perform massage; be of good moral character; and be free of any major communicable disease.

Tuition and Fees

Tuition for either of the 500-hour programs is $3,650 to $4,749 depending on electives chosen and payment plans).

Financial Assistance

Payment plans are available.

MINNESOTA

Center for a Balanced Life

1535 Livington Avenue, Suite 105
West St. Paul, Minnesota 55118
PHONE: (651) 455-0473
WEBSITE: www.saintpaul.com/bodywork.htm

Center for a Balanced Life was founded in 1987 by Sister M. Janine Rajkowski, who is the primary instructor; the center also uses guest lecturers and contracted faculty for specific courses. The maximum class size is twelve students (minimum four).

Accreditation and Approvals

Center for a Balanced Life is registered with the Minnesota Higher Education Services Office. Graduates are qualified to take the National Certification Examination for Therapeutic Massage and Bodywork (NCETMB). Courses may be taken by massage therapists for continuing education credit.

Program Description

The 650-hour Professional Massage Training Program consists of three 200-hour modules plus a fifty-hour internship. Classroom work covers Swedish Massage, Deep Muscle Therapy, Acupressure, Reflexology, Polarity/Energy Work, Sports Massage, Anatomy and Physiology, CPR and First Aid, Charting and Terminology, Communication Skills, Professional Ethics, and Business Skills. The program requires fifteen to twenty-four months to complete. Classes meet one or two evenings per week and some Saturdays.

Admission Requirements

Applicants must be at least 18 years of age, have a high school diploma or equivalent, be in good physical condition and physically able to perform massage, submit a physician's statement, be emotionally stable and of good moral character, be able to handle college level work, and interview with the director. It is recommended that applicants receive at least one professional massage prior to enrollment.

Tuition and Fees

Tuition is $1,700 per module (total $5,100). Additional expenses include a $50 application fee; books, $250 to $350; massage table, $500 to $800; optional massage chair, $550; and professional massage treatments, $120 to $150.

Financial Assistance

Tuition may be paid in three installments over three months.

Minneapolis School of Massage and Bodywork

85 22nd Avenue NE
Minneapolis, Minnesota 55418
PHONE/FAX: (612) 788-8907

E-MAIL: MSMB@mplsschoolofmassage.org
WEBSITE: www.mplsschoolofmassage.org

Minneapolis School of Massage and Bodywork (MSMB) was founded in 1975. There are sixteen instructors, with an average of sixteen students in hands-on classes.

Accreditation and Approvals
MSMB is accredited by the Accrediting Commission of Career Schools and Colleges of Technology (ACCSCT) and by the Integrative Massage and Somatic Therapies Accreditation Council (IMSTAC). The 626-hour Therapeutic Bodywellness Massage Training Program is approved by the Wisconsin Educational Approval Board. Graduates are qualified to take the National Certification Examination for Therapeutic Massage and Bodywork (NCETMB).

Program Description
A 202-hour Massage Practitioner Training Program is offered to students who are unsure about career in massage therapy. Upon completion of the program, students may transfer into the 626-hour program described below. Courses in the 202-hour program include Basic Therapeutic Massage, Pressure and Release Points, Communications and Boundaries, Massage Related Business, Massage Related Ethics, Anatomy/ Physiology, and CPR.

The 626-hour Therapeutic Bodywellness Massage Training Program consists of the 202-hour program described above with the addition of Pre- and Post-natal Massage, Infant Massage, Connective Tissue and Physiology, Swedish Massage Techniques, and First Aid.

Community and Continuing Education
Workshops previously offered include Aromatherapy Blending, Infant Massage Instructor Certification, Myofascial, CPR, First Aid, and others.

Admission Requirements
Applicants must be at least 18 years of age, have a high school diploma or equivalent, and have an on-site interview.

Tuition and Fees
Tuition for the 626-hour Therapeutic Bodywellness Massage program is $5,340; additional expenses include application fee, $25; registration fee, $75; and books, $189.

Financial Assistance
Minnesota State Grants, veterans' benefits, and payment plans are available.

The Minnesota Center for Shiatsu Study

1313 Fifth Street SE, Suite 336
Minneapolis, Minnesota 55414
PHONE: (612) 379-3565
FAX: (612) 379-3568
E-MAIL: shiatsumn@aol.com

The Minnesota Center for Shiatsu Study (MCSS) was founded in 1992 by Cari Johnson Pelava. There are twenty-six instructors, with an average of twenty-two students in practical classes, twenty-eight in lectures.

Accreditation and Approvals
MCSS is licensed as a private career school by the Minnesota Higher Education Services Office, and is a member of the AOBTA Council of Schools and Programs. Graduates are eligible to take the National Certification Commission for Acupuncture and Oriental Medicine (NCCAOM) certification exam in Oriental Bodywork. Nurses and acupuncturists may earn CEUs at MCSS continuing education workshops.

Program Description
The 560-hour Professional Shiatsu Training Program consists of four levels of study and is offered as a one-year day program or a one-and-one-half- to two-year evening program. Level I courses include Anatomy, Physiology, and Introduction to Shiatsu and Development of the Healer. Level II courses include Traditional Chinese Medicine, Shiatsu Anma, Supervised Clinical Practice, Qi Gong, and Adult CPR and First Aid. Level III courses are Eastern Pathology, Shiatsu Anma Application, Supervised Clinical Practice, Western Pathology, Business Essentials, Professional and Legal Considerations, Ethics and Boundaries, and Personal Financial Preparedness. Level IV consists of Supervised Clinical Practice and Summary Session. In addition to course work, students must complete at least one externship.

A Special Accelerated Studies program is offered to currently certified/licensed bodywork professionals (i.e., massage therapists, physical therapists, chiropractors, osteopaths) and acupuncturists. Qualified students may enter directly into Level II and may transfer out of most of the Level III business-related seminars, the electives/externships, and all but 12.5 hours of Supervised Student Clinic.

Community and Continuing Education

A 123-hour graduate-level Zen Shiatsu program is offered to MCSS graduates and/or AOBTA-certified Oriental bodywork therapists. Students attend class one evening per week for nine months, completing 108 hours of class time plus fifteen hours of Student Clinic.

Community and continuing education workshops are offered on a variety of topics including Extraordinary Vessels, Tui Na Chinese Medical Massage, Shiatsu Basics, Foot Reflexology, and Sooji Korean Hand Therapy.

Admission Requirements

Applicants must be at least 18 years of age, have a high school diploma or equivalent, submit at least two letters of recommendation, and have a personal interview. MCSS encourages all applicants to attend an Information Session and to experience a Shiatsu in their professional clinic prior to starting the program.

Tuition and Fees

Tuition and fees for the day Shiatsu Program is $5,380. Additional expenses include CPR and First Aid class, approximately $45; AOBTA Student Membership, $40; student liability insurance, $76; electives and externships, up to $250; and books, approximately $330. Optional expenses include Shiatsu futon, $148 to $210; Shiatsu table, $485 to $885; and body support cushions, $290 to $570.

Tuition for courses in the evening studies Program are paid before the start of each level of study. Tuition and fees for Level I is $1,700; for Level II, $1,650; for Level III, $1,510; and for Level IV, $520. Additional expenses are similar to those listed for the day program.

Tuition and fees for the graduate-level Zen Shiatsu program are $1,065 to $1,115. Additional expenses include books and supplies, approximately $80. Optional expenses include Shiatsu futon, $148 to $210, and recommended books and supplies, $95.

Financial Assistance

Grants, loans, dislocated workers benefits, rehabilitation benefits, veterans' benefits, and MCSS payment plans are available.

Minnesota Institute of Acupuncture and Herbal Studies

1821 University Avenue, 278-S
St. Paul, Minnesota 55104
PHONE: (651) 603-0994
FAX: (651) 603-0995
E-MAIL: miahs@millcomm.com

The Minnesota Institute of Acupuncture and Herbal Studies was founded in 1990.

Accreditation and Approvals

MIAHS has been granted candidate status with the Accreditation Commission for Acupuncture and Oriental Medicine (ACAOM).

Program Description

The 2,645-hour Oriental Medical Program may be completed in four years. The program requires a minimum of 1,889 classroom hours, 606 clinical hours, and 150 hours of observation, and provides comprehensive education and training in Traditional Oriental Medical Concepts (physiology, pathology, diagnostics, energetics, and treatment principles); Acupuncture Principles and Skills; Tui Na; Traditional Chinese Herbalism; Western Medical Concepts; Chinese Culture and Philosophical Foundations of Oriental Medicine; Related Chinese Studies (tai chi chuan, qigong, and introductory language skills); and Holistic Skills (counseling, nutrition, communication skills, bodywork, touch, and subtle energy therapies).

The 2,129-hour Professional Acupuncture Program is similar to the Oriental Medicine Program but does not include herbal studies. The program may be completed in three years plus one quarter; clinical requirements are 510 hours of supervised practice and 150 hours of observation.

Admission Requirements

Applicants must have completed at least two years of college-level education at an accredited school, submit two letters of recommendation and a personal essay, and interview with an admissions representative.

Tuition and Fees

Tuition is $11 per contact hour. Other costs include: application fee, $60; registration fee, $10 per course; and books, approximately $200 to $300 per year; tuition, books, and other fees can be estimated at about $7,500 for the first year for full-time students. Total costs vary based on the number of hours for which a student registers.

Financial Assistance

State of Minnesota loans are available. Students who do not hold a bachelor's degree may be eligible for state grants based on financial need.

Northern Lights School of Massage Therapy

1313 SE Fifth Street, Suite 209
Minneapolis, Minnesota 55414
PHONE: (612) 379-3822
FAX: (612) 379-5971
E-MAIL: nlsmt@pro-ns.net

Northern Lights School of Massage Therapy (NLSMT) was founded in 1985. There are eight instructors, with a maximum class size of forty students for lectures and a functional teacher:student ratio of 1:8 for techniques classes.

Accreditation and Approvals

Northern Lights is a member of the American Massage Therapy Association (AMTA) Council of Schools, and is in the process of applying for accreditation with the Commission on Massage Training Accreditation (COMTA). Graduates are qualified to take the National Certification Examination for Therapeutic Massage and Bodywork (NCETMB).

Program Description

The 600-hour Massage Therapy Training Program may be completed in ten months of full-time study; part-time options

are also available. The program consists of a 550-hour core curriculum and fifty hours of electives. The Core Curriculum consists of Science (covering Anatomy, Physiology, Pathology, and Kinesiology), Massage Therapy Techniques (covering Swedish, Integrative, and Deep Tissue Massage), Professional Development, and Clinic. Electives are offered on a rotating basis and may include Reflexology, Aromatherapy, Positional Release, Hospice Massage Therapy, Self-Care, and Body Mobilization and Tune-Up. Students must complete a CPR/First Aid course prior to the first day of class.

Community and Continuing Education

A varied selection of continuing education workshops and classes are offered throughout the year.

A two-day weekend Introductory Massage Therapy Techniques workshop provides an introduction to massage for interested laypersons or potential students.

Admission Requirements

Students must be at least 18 years of age, have a high school diploma or equivalent, be physically able to perform the manipulations of massage therapy, have a personal interview, and have received at least one verified professional massage.

Tuition and Fees

Tuition is $5,600. Other costs include application fee, $50; linen service, $120; books, $300 to $500; professional massage treatments, $120 to $160; and AMTA student membership, $95 to $105.

The Introductory Massage Therapy Techniques workshop costs $125; $100 is credited toward tuition when the student enrolls within one year of taking the workshop.

Financial Assistance

Payment plans are available.

Northwestern Academy of Homeopathy

10700 Old County Road #15, Suite 300
Plymouth, Minnesota 55441
PHONE: (612) 794-6445
FAX: (612) 525-9518
E-MAIL: info@homeopathicschool.org
WEBSITE: www.homeopathicschool.org

The Northwestern Academy of Homeopathy was founded in 1994 by Eric Sommermann and Valerie Ohanian. The academy's three core faculty members have years of clinical practice and teaching experience; they are all registered with the North American Society of Homeopaths (NASH). There is a maximum class size of thirty-five students.

Accreditation and Approvals
The school is currently applying for both state and federal accreditation and expects to receive it in 2001.

Program Description
The Northwestern Academy of Homeopathy provides a four-year, 1,440-hour course of professional training designed to meet the guidelines of the International Council of Homeopathy. The curriculum in Year One provides a basic foundation in homeopathic philosophy, an introduction to the repertory, case taking, case analysis, materia medica or major homeopathic remedies, and lectures on constitutional treatment. Year Two continues with advanced training in materia medica, case management, and computer software, and begins clinical training with observation of live cases. Year Three continues with didactic subjects with one-half the time spent in a supervised Student Clinic. Year Four is a full-time Student Clinic which develops progressively toward a more advanced clinical experience.

Admission Requirements
The course is open to all dedicated students with a variety of backgrounds. Some course work may be required; a five-week Pathology course is offered by the school. Contact the school for further admission details.

Tuition and Fees
Tuition is $5,200 per year.

Financial Assistance
Payment plans are available.

Northwestern College of Chiropractic

2501 West 84th Street
Minneapolis, Minnesota 55431

PHONE: (612) 888-4777
FAX: (612) 888-6713
E-MAIL: admit@nwchiro.edu
WEBSITE: www.nwchiro.edu

Northwestern College of Chiropractic was founded in 1941. It was among the first colleges to adopt the six-year academic program, several years before it was required by the Council on Chiropractic Education (CCE). The teacher:student ratio is 1:11; each incoming class is divided into sections of 28.

Accreditation and Approvals
Northwestern is accredited by the Council on Chiropractic Education (CCE) and by the Commission on Institutions of Higher Education of the North Central Association of Colleges and Schools.

Program Description
The Doctor of Chiropractic (D.C.) curriculum consists of five academic years of chiropractic college instruction; each academic year is composed of two fifteen-week trimesters (Northwestern offers three trimesters: fall, winter, and summer). A twelve-month public clinic internship and preceptorship constitutes the last three trimesters.

The required curriculum for the D.C. degree consists of 4,380 contact hours of study, exclusive of electives. A Bachelor of Science degree in human biology is granted to candidates who have completed the equivalent of 133½ trimester credits by fulfilling specific requirements; see the catalog for more information.

First-year courses include Gross Anatomy, Biochemistry, Embryology, Histology, Skeletal Radiology, Professional Issues, Infection Control, Principles and Philosophy, Introduction to Chiropractic, Spine and Pelvis, Physiology, Peripheral Nervous System, and Chiropractic Methods.

Second-year courses include Physiology, Biochemistry, Central Nervous System, Pathology, Skeletal Radiology, Physical Diagnosis, Critical Thinking, Chiropractic Methods, Neuromusculoskeletal, Principles and Philosophy, Microbiology, Neurodiagnosis, and Critical Appraisal of Scientific Literature.

Third-year courses include Skeletal Radiology, EENT, Clinical Pathology, Infectious Diseases, Community Health, Chiropractic Methods, Physiological Therapeutics, Clinical Nutrition,

Neuromusculoskeletal, Patient Interviewing, Introduction to Clinical Chiropractic, Radiation Physics and Safety, Radiology of the Abdomen and Chest, Respiratory System, Cardiovascular System, Gastrointestinal System, Clinical Pathology, Clinic Internship, and Principles and Philosophy.

Fourth-year courses include Radiographic Technology and Positioning, Gynecology, Endocrinology, Dermatology, Obstetrics, Emergency Procedures, Pharmacology and Toxicology, Mental Health, Chiropractic Methods, Physiological Therapeutics, Clinical Nutrition, Pediatrics, Clinic Internship, Clinical Case Studies, and Northwestern Clinical Practice.

The fifth year consists of Clinic Internship, Clinical Case Studies, The Business of Clinical Practice, and Legal Aspects of Chiropractic Practice.

Continuing Education

The postgraduate department sponsors more than 150 continuing education seminars each academic year, including topics in radiology, orthopedics, neurology, sports injuries, family practice, rehabilitation, and occupational health. These courses may also fulfill relicensure requirements set by the State Board of Chiropractic Examiners.

Admission Requirements

Applicants must have completed at least two academic years (sixty semester hours) of college credit acceptable toward a bachelor's degree. Prechiropractic courses must be completed at a regionally accredited institution. Specific course requirements include biology and/or zoology with lab (six semester hours), general or inorganic chemistry with lab (six semester hours), organic chemistry with lab (six semester hours), physics with lab (six semester hours), psychology (three semester hours), English or communication skills (six semester hours), humanities or social sciences (fifteen semester hours), and electives (twelve semester hours). All of these courses must have been passed with a grade of C or better. Applicants must have earned a cumulative GPA of at least 2.5 and a science GPA of at least 2.0. Applicants must also possess the strength, coordination, manual dexterity, and visual, hearing, and tactile senses (compensated, if necessary) to perform all required aspects of diagnosis and treatment, and must submit three character references or letters of recommendation.

Tuition and Fees

Tuition for the Doctor of Chiropractic Program is $5,165 per semester. Other costs include: application fee, $50; lab fee, $50 per lab; elective courses, $220 per credit hour; activity fee, $40 per trimester; health service fee, $10 per trimester (trimesters one through seven); graduation fee, $135; split schedule/part-time schedule fee, $300; B.S. degree diploma and registration fee, $200; and books and supplies, approximately $3,300 for the four-year period.

Financial Assistance

Available financial assistance includes federal grants, loans, and work-study; state grants; Chiroloans; Worldwide Grants; scholarships; and private loans.

MISSISSIPPI
Blue Cliff School of Therapeutic Massage

(See Multiple State Locations, pages 388-90)

MISSOURI
Cleveland Chiropractic College

Kansas City Campus
6401 Rockhill Road
Kansas City, Missouri 64131-1181
PHONE: (816) 501-0100/ (800) 467-CCKC
FAX: (816) 361-0272
E-MAIL: pub@cleveland.edu
WEBSITE: www.clevelandchiropractic.edu

Cleveland Chiropractic College of Kansas City was founded in 1922 by Dr. C. S. Cleveland Sr., Dr. Ruth R. Cleveland, and Dr. Perl B. Griffin. In 1992, the college joined with its sister school, Cleveland Chiropractic College of Los Angeles (see pages 77-78), to form a multicampus system. There are forty instructors, with an average of fifty students per class.

Accreditation and Approvals

Cleveland Chiropractic College is accredited by the Council on Chiropractic Education (CCE) and the North Central Association of Colleges and Schools.

Program Description

The 4,410-clock-hour, twelve-trimester (forty-eight-month) Doctor of Chiropractic (DC) degree may be completed in as little as nine trimesters (thirty-six months). The core program is divided among the departments of Basic Sciences, Diagnostic Sciences, Chiropractic Sciences, and Clinical Sciences.

Students may earn a bachelor's degree in human biology independently of the Doctor of Chiropractic degree or as they work toward completion of the D.C. degree.

The Preprofessional Health Science Program offers required prerequisite courses that meet requirements for both the bachelor's and Doctor of Chiropractic degrees. Courses are offered in eight-week modules and include General Chemistry I and II, Organic Chemistry I and II, General Physics I and II, Anatomy and Physiology, General Biology, and Mathematics.

Continuing Education

The Postgraduate and Related Professional Education Program provides the practicing Doctor of Chiropractic with continuing education in areas of special interest.

Admission Requirements

Applicants for the Doctor of Chiropractic Degree Program must have completed at least two academic years (sixty semester hours) of undergraduate work leading to a baccalaureate degree at an accredited college or university, and must have earned a minimum GPA of 2.50. Specific hours of course work in such subjects as biology, inorganic chemistry, organic chemistry, physics, English composition/communication, psychology, and humanities/social sciences are also required. Applicants must submit two letters of recommendation (one from a health care professional).

Applicants for the upper division of the bachelor's degree in human biology must first complete sixty credit hours from an accredited postsecondary institution, including six hours each in biology, inorganic chemistry, organic chemistry, and physics. (These courses may be taken on campus in the Preprofessional Health Science Program.)

Tuition and Fees

Tuition is $165 per weekly clock hour (for example, tuition for the first trimester on the twelve-trimester program is $3,690; for the first trimester on the nine-trimester program, $4,950).

Other costs include: application fee, $50; student activity fee, $67 per trimester; and books and supplies, approximately $400 per trimester. Dormitory rooms for single students are available at University of Missouri–Kansas City.

Financial Assistance

Federal and private scholarships, grants, loans, and work-study are available.

Logan College of Chiropractic

1851 Schoettler Road
P.O. Box 1065
Chesterfield, Missouri 63006-1065
PHONE: (636) 227-2100 / (800) 782-3344 / (800) 533-9210 (admissions)
FAX: (636) 207-2425
E-MAIL: loganadm@logan.edu
WEBSITE: www.logan.edu

Logan College of Chiropractic, named for founder Hugh B. Logan, D.C., enrolled its first class in 1935. There are eighty-six instructors; class sizes range from fifty to 110 students.

Accreditation and Approvals

Logan College is accredited by the Commission on Accreditation of the Council on Chiropractic Education (CCE) and the Commission of Institutions of Higher Education of the North Central Association of Colleges and Schools.

Program Description

The 5,265-hour, ten-trimester Doctor of Chiropractic degree program includes courses in the Basic Science division such as Gross and Spinal Anatomy, Physiology, Biochemistry, Pathology, Microbiology, and Embryology; in the Chiropractic Division, such courses as Adjusting Technique, Orthopedics, Biomechanics, Jurisprudence, and Practice and Office Management; in the Clinical Science division, such courses as Physical Diagnosis, Radiographic Diagnosis and Fundamentals, GI/UG, OB/Gyn, Pediatrics, Geriatrics, and others; in the Health Center division, educational programs, student patient and outpatient clinical rotations; and student research projects.

Logan also offers a Bachelor of Science degree in Human

Biology (133 hours minimum). Students may matriculate to Logan for the B.S. degree without continuing to study for the Doctor of Chiropractic degree. Required coursework in biology, general chemistry, organic chemistry, and physics is offered in the Accelerated Science Program (ASP) or may be transferred into Logan from an accredited institution.

The Chiropractic Paraprofessional Program consists of 214 classroom hours that include six modules: Anatomy and Physiology, Basic X-Ray Proficiency, Clinical Training, General Office Procedures, Laboratory Procedures, and Physiological Therapeutics.

Continuing Education

Postdoctoral educational programs include Residency Programs in Chiropractic Diagnostic Imaging (three years) and Chiropractic Family Practice (two years); Diplomate Programs in Chiropractic Neurology (DACNB), Chiropractic Orthopedics (DABCO), and Sports Injuries and Physical Fitness (DABCSP); and Certification Programs in Acupuncture/Acupressure/ Meridian Therapy, Certified Chiropractic Sports Physician (CCSP), Chiropractic Utilization Review/Quality Assessment Consultant, Impairment Rating, Manipulation Under Anesthesia (MUA), Physiologic Therapeutics, and Skeletal Radiology.

Other continuing education seminars are also offered to Doctors of Chiropractic, including special event seminars such as the Spring Training Baseball Specific Seminar, Chiropractic Management of Women's Health, Pediatrics for the Chiropractor, and Nutrition for the Chiropractor.

Admission Requirements

Doctor of Chiropractic program applicants must have completed sixty semester hours leading to a bachelor's degree at an accredited college or university with a cumulative GPA of 2.5 or better; specific hours in language and/or communications, psychology, social sciences or humanities, biological science, general and organic chemistry, and physics are required. Applicants must submit a recommendation from a licensed Doctor of Chiropractic, three references, and a personal essay, and have a personal interview.

Prerequisites for the Bachelor of Science program include twenty-seven hours specifically defined as psychology, communication skills, social sciences, and math, which must be

transferred into Logan from an accredited institution. Required coursework in biology, general chemistry, organic chemistry, and physics is offered in the Accelerated Science Program (ASP) or may be transferred into Logan from an accredited institution.

Tuition and Fees

Tuition for the D.C. degree program is $4,595 per trimester. Additional expenses include application fee, $50; activity fee, $25 per trimester; technology fee, $60 per trimester; and books, approximately $600 per year.

Tuition for the B.S. degree program is contingent upon the number of credit hours taken per trimester; contact the school for details. The application fee for the BS program is $15.

Financial Assistance

Scholarships, grants, loans, and employment (including federal grants, loans, and work-study; state grant programs; and Chiroloan and Canadian Chiroloan) are available.

Massage Therapy Training Institute LLC

9140 Ward Parkway, Suite 100
Kansas City, Missouri 64114
PHONE: (816) 523-9140
FAX: (816) 523-0741
WEBSITE: www.mtti.net

The Massage Therapy Training Institute (MTTI) was founded in 1988 and is Missouri's first and Kansas City's only massage school certified to operate by the Missouri Coordinating Board for Higher Education. There are twenty-five instructors, with an average of sixteen students in technique classes.

Accreditation and Approvals

MTTI is accredited by the Integrative Massage and Somatic Therapies Accreditation Council (IMSTAC). Graduates of the 500-hour program are eligible to take the National Certification Examination for Therapeutic Massage and Bodywork (NCETMB). MTTI is approved by the National Certification Board for Therapeutic Massage and Bodywork (NCBTMB) as a continuing education provider.

The State of Missouri requires 500 hours for licensure; licensing requirements in Kansas vary by city. There are no licensing requirements for personal trainers or energy therapy practitioners.

Program Description

The 500-hour Massage Therapy Practitioner Program includes courses in Basic Swedish Massage, Anatomy and Physiology, Sports Massage, Reflexology, Shiatsu or Chinese Meridian Therapy, Creating a Successful Practice, Creating Clarity in Bodywork: Defining Sexuality and Ethical Issues, Integrating Bodywork Techniques, Therapeutic Touch, Myofascial Release Massage, CPR/First Aid, Exploring Touch for Bodyworkers, Introduction to Vibrational Healing, Pathophysiology, Tai Chi, and approximately one hundred hours of electives. On average, students complete the program in eighteen months by attending classes two evenings per week and one weekend per month; a more accelerated or extended pace is possible.

The 300-hour Wellness Consultant Program combines counseling skills with competency in nutritional consulting, stress management facilitation, environmental awareness, and lifestyle assessment skills. Courses include Anatomy and Physiology, Basic Counseling Skills for Wellness Consultants, Creating a Successful Practice, Environmental Influences on Wellness, Gender Specific Issues and Wellness, Nutrition and Wellness Consulting, Practicum for Wellness Consultants, Stress Management Facilitation, and Stress Management Workshop.

A 200-hour Energy Therapy Program includes Introduction to Vibrational Healing, Energy Therapy, Aromatherapy, Craniosacral Balancing, Therapeutic Touch, Flower Essence Therapy, Color Therapy, Polarity Therapy, Music and Healing, Creating Clarity in Bodywork: Defining Sexuality and Ethical Issues, and Creating a Successful Practice.

All courses may be taken individually providing the student meets the prerequisites for the course.

Continuing Education

Many MTTI courses are eligible for continuing education credit for massage therapists, nurses, licensed counselors, and other health professionals.

Admission Requirements

Applicants must be at least 18 years of age, have a high school diploma or equivalent, and be physically, mentally, and emotionally capable of performing the work. Applicants must submit two letters of recommendation and have a personal interview.

Tuition and Fees

Tuition for the Massage Therapy Practitioner Program is $5,800 plus approximately $300 for books. Tuition for the Wellness Consultant program is $3,500 plus approximately $150 for books. Tuition for the Energy Therapy program is $2,300 plus approximately $80 for books.

Additional expenses include a $75 application fee; massage table, $400 to $600; and oil and linens.

Financial Assistance

Payment plans and early-payment discounts are available.

St. Charles School of Massage Therapy

Corporate Parc 94
2440 Executive Drive, Suite 100
St. Charles, Missouri 63303
PHONE: (314) 949-0448
FAX: (314) 949-7896
E-MAIL: Oasis@anet-stl.com
WEBSITE: webusers.anet-stl.com/~oasis/com

St. Charles School of Massage Therapy was founded in 1987. There are six instructors; classes are limited to twenty students.

Accreditation and Approvals

St. Charles School of Massage Therapy is certified to operate by the Coordinating Board for Higher Education of the State of Missouri and the City of St. Charles. Graduates are qualified to take the National Certification Examination for Therapeutic Massage and Bodywork (NCETMB).

Program Description

Beginning September 1999, the Massage Therapy Program will

be expanded to 600 hours; contact the school for information on the new program.

The 520-hour Massage Therapy Program may be completed in as little as seven months (ten months maximum). The course of study covers Swedish Massage; Anatomy and Physiology; Specialized Bodywork Training, which includes Foot Reflexology, Hydrotherapy, Trigger Point Therapy, Shiatsu, Polarity, Acupressure, CPR and First Aid, Tai Chi, Sports Massage, Aromatherapy, Chair Massage, Lymph Drainage, and Myofascial Techniques; and Clinical Practice. Classes are held days and evenings; some weekend classes will be required.

Admission Requirements

Applicants must be at least 18 years of age, have a high school diploma or equivalent, attend an Open House, have received at least one professional massage, and interview with the director.

Tuition and Fees

The total cost of $5,245 includes tuition, registration fee, books and supplies, and liability insurance. Additional expenses include sheets, approximately $15, and oil, $25.

Financial Assistance

Payment plans are available.

MONTANA

Asten Center of Natural Therapeutics

(See Multiple State Locations, page 386)

Rocky Mountain Herbal Institute

P.O. Box 579
Hot Springs, Montana 59845
PHONE: (406) 741-3811
E-MAIL: rmhi@rmhiherbal.org
WEBSITE: www.rmhiherbal.org

Rocky Mountain Herbal Institute (RMHI) was founded in 1987 by Roger W. Wicke, Ph.D. The school began as the Colorado Herbal Institute and moved to Montana in 1991. Forty graduates have completed the program; the majority of these were li-

censed health professionals. There are three instructors, with five to a maximum of twelve students per class.

Accreditation and Approvals

RMHI is accredited by the American Association of Drugless Practitioners.

Program Description

The two-year Chinese Herbal Sciences training program qualifies the student to develop herbal formulas tailored to individual needs. The program is offered to professionals and serious students unable to relocate for full-time study, and consists of three six-day residential intensives in Hot Springs, each preceded by reading and homework assignments completed through correspondence. Study and homework time is estimated at fifteen to twenty hours per week. Topics covered include Traditional Chinese Health Assessment Methods (tongue inspection, pulse palpation, abdominal palpation, and body characteristics); TCM Herbal Pharmacopoeia; Tailoring Herbal Formulas to Individual Circumstances; Ordering Herbs and Inspecting Quality; Establishing a Practice; Legal and Ethical Issues; Alternative Perspectives in Epidemiology; Overcoming Environmental Pollution; Electromagnetic Fields and Human Health; Food Sensitivities and Intolerance; and much more.

Community and Continuing Education

Courses for nonprofessionals are occasionally offered on such topics as family health, environmental health, immunity and epidemics, herbal principles, and diet.

Courses in Advanced TCM Herbal Training are open to all herbalists with basic training in TCM assessment, materia medica, and herbal formulation. Each year, RMHI sponsors courses in various specialties of TCM that may include problems of the immune system, endocrine system, gastrointestinal tract; menopause; epidemic illnesses; and others.

Admission Requirements

Admission requirements include high-level literacy, common sense, the ability to think and reason clearly, and prior training in anatomy and physiology. A sample homework assignment and textbook order is sent once the application is accepted; final admission to the program is contingent upon receiving a grade of 70 percent or above on the homework assignment.

Tuition and Fees

Tuition for the Chinese Herbal Sciences training program is $4,635. Other costs include an admission fee of $90; books, herb kits, and materials are approximately $850. Meals and lodging are additional.

Tuition for the Advanced TCM Herbal training program is $525 per six-day seminar.

Financial Assistance

A payment plan is available.

NEBRASKA

Gateway College of Massage Therapy

2607 Dakota Avenue
South Sioux City, Nebraska 68776
PHONE: (402) 494-8390
FAX: (402) 494-4561
E-MAIL: gcmass1@aol.com

In 1995, Darrell J. Peck, Joan Knott, and Donald Knott purchased the Sioux City Branch of Dr. Welbes's College of Massage Therapy. There are five instructors; typically, eight to twelve students enter the program each quarter.

Accreditation and Approvals

Gateway College of Massage Therapy is accredited by the Nebraska Department of Education and the Nebraska Department of Health and Human Services, and approved by the Iowa Department of Health. Graduates are eligible to apply for licensure in Nebraska or Iowa, and are qualified to take the National Certification Examination for Therapeutic Massage and Bodywork (NCETMB).

Program Description

Two Massage Therapy Programs are offered. The twelve-month program consists of 1,000 hours of lecture, lab, and internship over four quarters; the nine-month program consists of 500 in-class hours over three quarters. Courses in both programs include Basic Anatomy and Physiology, Basic Massage Technique, Clinical Practice Subjects (Professional Issues, Human Relationships), Advanced Anatomy and Physiology, Pathology, Advanced Massage Technique (Deep Tissue, Acupressure, Sports, Pregnancy, Executive), Clinic, Public Service, Health Service Management (Business Ethics, Laws, Licensing, Administrative, Résumés, Marketing), Hydrotherapy, CPR/First Aid, and Advanced Massage Techniques (Myofascial Therapy, Trigger Point Therapy, Infant, Reflexology). The fourth quarter of the 1,000-hour program includes Advanced Massage Techniques, Senior Seminar, and an off-campus Clinical Internship.

Admission Requirements

Applicants must be at least 18 years of age; have a high school diploma or equivalent; and submit an autobiographical letter of intent, two personal references, and a statement indicating that the applicant has no felony record.

Tuition and Fees

Tuition for the 12-month program is $5,950; tuition for the nine-month program is $4,950. There is a $50 application fee; books, equipment, and supplies are additional.

Financial Assistance

Payment plans are available.

Omaha School of Massage Therapy

9748 Park Drive
Omaha, Nebraska 68127
PHONE: (402) 331-3694 / (800) 399-3694
FAX: (402) 331-0280
E-MAIL: OSMTSCHOOL@aol.com
WEBSITE: www.OSMT.com

Ann Reuck founded the Omaha School of Massage Therapy in 1991; the school moved to its current location in 1995. There are twelve instructors with an average of fifteen students per class.

Accreditation and Approvals

The program is accredited by the Accrediting Commission of Career Schools and Colleges of Technology (ACCSCT) and is approved by the Nebraska State Board of Health upon the recommendation of the Nebraska State Board of Examiners of Massage Therapy and the Nebraska State Board of Education.

Graduates are qualified to take the National Certification Examination for Therapeutic Massage and Bodywork (NCETMB).

Program Description

The 804-hour, nine-month Massage Therapy Program consists of Massage Theory and Practice, Community Service, Physiology, Anatomy/Kinesiology, Hydrotherapy, Exercise Training, Business and Health Service Management, Wellness, Professional Issues, Pathology, CPR and First Aid Training and Certification, and 190 hours of Student Massage Clinic.

Admission Requirements

Applicants must submit a completed application packet and high school and college transcripts.

Tuition and Fees

The total cost of the Massage Therapy Program is $7,605, which includes tuition, application fee, books, equipment, CPR/First Aid, gym fee, school shirt, linen, and hydrotherapy lab. Additional expenses include marketing supplies, massage oil and cream, and two reams of copy paper.

Financial Assistance

Qualified individuals may apply for federal grants and loans or veterans' benefits. Payment plans are also available.

NEVADA

Aston-Patterning®

P.O. Box 3568
Incline Village, Nevada 89450
PHONE: (775) 831-8228
FAX: (775) 831-8955
E-MAIL: AstonPat@aol.com
WEBSITE: www.aston-patterning.com

Aston-Patterning® is an educational system developed by Judith Aston based on nearly forty years of teaching experience. The process includes a combination of bodywork, movement coaching, ergonomics, and fitness training. Although the work can be helpful to those in acute and chronic pain and those wishing to improve their body's posture, efficiency, and effec-

tiveness, it is also useful for athletic performance and personal growth. There are five senior faculty and seven faculty in training; class size averages twenty students.

Accreditation and Approvals

Certification as an Aston-Patterning Practitioner, open only to already trained practicing health professionals, is dependent on completion of the Level III clinical evaluation, signing the licensing agreement, and paying an annual licensing fee. Practitioners may then use the Aston-Patterning trademarks and logos and be included in the directory of practitioners. Applicants should check with their home state to determine specific licensing requirements.

Program Description

To become a certified Aston-Patterning Practitioner, a student must complete approximately fifteen weeks of training (eighty-four days) over a period of one and a half to two years. Training includes movement education (neurokinetics), soft tissue work (myokinetics), advanced massage, and ergonomics. The courses meet in three-week segments, followed by blocks of time for the application of skills in work situations.

Prior to beginning the Aston-Patterning Practitioner Program, students must complete the prerequisite courses Aston Therapeutics I (three days), Aston Therapeutics II (three days), Aston Therapeutics: Bodyworks I (four days), and Aston Therapeutics: Bodyworks II (four days).

Continuing Education

The Aston-Patterning corporation offers continuing education courses for already licensed/registered health professionals. Continuing education of three days every four years is encouraged following certification. Continuing education courses are offered in Aston Fitness, Arthro-Kinetics, Facial Toning, and small group tutorials for specialized interests.

Admission Requirements

The Aston-Patterning corporation offers continuing education courses for already licensed/registered health professionals. Applicants must be at least 21 years of age; submit a letter of endorsement from an Aston-Patterning practitioner and a statement of purpose; have completed the prerequisite courses;

have a bachelor's degree or academic training in education, health care, or a related field or demonstrated career success; have knowledge of anatomy and physiology equal to one semester of college work; have a diploma from or be currently enrolled in an accredited school of massage, or have a comparable license as a health professional. Students are encouraged to have six private Aston-Patterning sessions with certified practitioners.

Tuition and Fees

There is a $25 application fee for the Aston-Patterning Practitioner Program. The Aston Practitioner Program course fees may be determined by multiplying the number of days in the program by approximately $125 per day. There is a four-day evaluation following the program at approximately $350.

Financial Assistance

Payment plans and discounts for advance payment are available.

Utah College of Massage Therapy

(See Multiple State Locations, pages 417-18)

NEW HAMPSHIRE

DoveStar Institute

(See Multiple State Locations, pages 391-93)

New Hampshire Institute for Therapeutic Arts

(See Multiple State Locations, pages 403-4)

North Eastern Institute of Whole Health

22 Bridge Street
Manchester, New Hampshire 03101
PHONE: (603) 623-5018
FAX: (603) 623-4689
E-MAIL: lionman@xtdl.com
WEBSITE: www.neiwh.com

The North Eastern Institute of Whole Health was founded in 1993 by Gabrielle Grigore, M.D., N.D., D.O.M., L.M.T., and shiatsu master, and Douglas H. DuVerger. It is the largest school of massage therapy in New England. There are thirty-two faculty members; each program is limited to thirty students.

Accreditation and Approvals

The institute and its curriculum are approved by the State of New Hampshire Department of Education. Graduates are qualified to take the National Certification Examination for Therapeutic Massage and Bodywork (NCETMB).

Program Description

The 750-hour Massage Therapy Program consists of Anatomy and Physiology, Hydrotherapy, CPR/First Aid, Health Service: Management, Ethics and Professionalism, Chair Massage, Health and Hygiene for Bodyworkers, Introduction to Craniosacral Therapy, Eastern Traditional Medicine and Its Philosophies, Introduction to Touch Therapies, Massage Practicum, Neuromuscular Technique, Reflexology, Shiatsu, Sports Massage, and Swedish Massage, plus electives in Acupressure, Advanced Neuromuscular Massage, Aromatherapy, Craniosacral Therapy Level I, Equine Massage, Esalen Massage, Feng Shui, Geriatric Massage, Hawaiian Lomi Lomi Massage, Hypnotic Techniques for Bodyworkers, Lymphatic Drainage Massage, Marketing for Results, Pregnancy Massage, Polarity Therapy, Russian Massage, and Trigger Point Therapy. Students may attend full- or part-time; eight different program choices are offered, with morning and evening programs available.

Admission Requirements

Applicants must be at least 18 years of age, have a high school diploma or equivalent by the end of the program, and submit a physician's note of good health and a completed Whole Health medical form.

Tuition and Fees

Tuition is $5,550; the application fee is $50. Allow an additional $400 for books, handouts, body wrap, school T-shirt, diploma fee, graduation fee, and other expenses.

Financial Assistance

Payment plans, veterans' benefits, and vocational rehabilitation are available.

NEW JERSEY
Academy of Massage Therapy

401 South Van Brunt Street, 2nd Floor
Englewood, New Jersey 07631
PHONE: (201) 568-3220
FAX: (201) 568-5181
E-MAIL: massageschool@mindspring.com

The Academy of Massage Therapy was founded in 1991 by Joanna Sechuck. There are ten instructors, with a maximum of fourteen students in hands-on classes, eighteen students for lecture classes.

Accreditation and Approvals

The Academy of Massage Therapy is accredited by the Accrediting Commission of Career Schools and Colleges of Technology (ACCSCT) and by the Commission on Massage Therapy Accreditation (COMTA). Graduates are qualified to take the National Certification Examination for Therapeutic Massage and Bodywork (NCETMB). The academy is approved by the National Certification Board for Therapeutic Massage and Bodywork (NCBTMB) as a continuing education provider.

Program Description

The 554-hour Massage Therapy Certificate Program (Program 1) consists of Anatomy and Physiology (including Myology and Neurology); Massage Therapy (including Swedish Massage Theory and Practice, Body Mechanics, Swedish Massage Clinic, Hydrotherapy, Medical Massage and Pathology, Sports Massage and Related Injuries, HIV/AIDS Education, Pre-natal Massage, Chair Massage, and Medical and Sports Massage Clinic); Electives, chosen from Anma: Japanese Medical Massage, Body Wisdom: Energetic Healing, or Reflexology; Business and Marketing; and Community Service.

The 559-hour Shiatsu Therapy Certificate Program (Program 2) consists of Anatomy and Physiology (including Myology and Neurology); Shiatsu Theory and Practice (including Shiatsu Theory and Technique, Practice and Clinic, Anma, and Tai Chi); Electives, chosen from Body Wisdom: Energetic Healing or Reflexology; Business and Marketing; Survey of Western Massage; and Community Service.

Admission Requirements

Applicants must be at least 18 years of age; have a high school diploma or equivalent; be of sound physical and mental health; be able to read, write and speak English; and have a personal interview.

Tuition and Fees

Tuition for Program 1 is $5,000, plus a $100 registration fee and approximately $300 for books and supplies. Tuition for Program 2 is $5,000, plus a $100 registration fee and approximately $350 for books and supplies. Students may purchase a massage table for $400 to $600.

Financial Assistance

Title IV financial aid, payment plans, and veterans' benefits are available to those who qualify; the academy is also approved by the New Jersey Department of Vocational Rehabilitation and various workforce agencies.

The Chrysalis Center

442 Route 31 N
Lambertville, New Jersey 08530
PHONE: (609) 466-7410
FAX: (609) 466-7442
E-MAIL: ChrysalisC@aol.com / Pakajomi@aol.com

Patricia Chichon, an herbalist and nurse practitioner, has been teaching herbal classes since 1986. Chichon is the primary instructor with occasional special guests; classes average fifteen students.

Program Description

A Year with the Plants is a year-long series of thirteen classes plus three intensives held on Saturdays, Sundays, and Thursday evenings. The classes may be taken as a series or individually. The Spring Series: Beginning/Developing (classes 1 through 3 plus intensive) covers such topics as Spring Tonics (including surviving allergy season, Lyme disease, chronic fatigue, candida, and more), Spring Nourishing (taking in and letting go; the skin, hair, and nails; gastrointestinal tract; respiratory system); Women Through the Life Cycle (infancy, puberty, pregnancy, menopause, wise woman); and Spring Pharmacy (harvesting with nature and storing for the winter). The Summer Series: Building/Growing (classes 4 though 8 plus intensive) covers such topics as Summer Tonics (alternatives), Musculoskeletal (toning and supporting), The Brain and the Nerves (attune with the world), Hormones and Glands (balance and adaptation), and Summer Pharmacy. The Fall Series: Harvest/Stability (classes 9 through 13 plus intensive) covers Fall Tonics (alternatives, immunity), The Fluids of Life (the blood and heart, kidneys, and lymphatics), Winters Ills, and Fall/Winter Pharmacy.

A second year of classes, requiring clinical time and homework, is currently under development.

Community and Continuing Education
Two-hour, Thursday evening classes are offered in Summer Ills (skin things; working with rashes) and Packing a First Aid Kit.

Admission Requirements
Classes are open to all, at the beginner level.

Tuition and Fees
Tuition for the entire series is $800 ($600 without intensives) or taken individually, $30 to $90 per class. There is a $10 materials charge for intensives. Two-hour Summer Ills and Packing a First Aid Kit classes are $30 each.

Financial Assistance
Sliding scale or work-study available.

Five Elements Center

115 Route 46 West
Building D, Suite 49
Mountain Lakes, New Jersey 07046
PHONE: (973) 402-8510
FAX: (973) 402-8510

Five Elements Center was founded in 1992 by Jane Cicchetti, who has been practicing homeopathy since 1981 and has had extensive training in Five Elements Chinese medicine. There are three instructors; classes average fifteen students (maximum thirty).

Program Description
Five Elements Center offers a three-year course in Essentials of Constitutional Homeopathy. Classes meet eight weekends (150 hours) per year. The first year includes an in-depth study of twenty-eight polycrest remedies; topics include How to Study Materia Medica, Introduction to Organon, History of Vitalist Medicine, Structure of Repertory, Case Taking, Theory of Miasms, Remedy Antidotes, Obstacles to Cure, and more. Second-year topics include an in-depth study of twenty-eight lesser-known polycrest remedies, as well as Acute Illness During Chronic Treatment, Case Analysis, Analysis and Use of Nosodes, Vaccinations, Diet and Detoxification, Selection of Potency (Advanced), Practice Management/Licensing, and more. In the third year, students learn many small and rarely used remedies, as well as Small Plant Remedies, Herbology and Mother Tinctures, Analysis of Difficult Cases, Homeopathy and Computer Technology, Student Cases, Failed Cases, and more.

An introductory Homeopathy Workshop is available as a weekend course or on audiocassettes for home study. It includes acute treatment for first aid, flu, colds, and headaches, as well as basic principles.

Admission Requirements
There are no prerequisites for the first year. For the second year, students must have completed the first-year program or a minimum of 140 hours of study in classical homeopathy. Third-year applicants must have completed the second year or a minimum of 250 hours of study in classical homeopathy.

Tuition and Fees
Tuition for the three-year homeopathy course is $1,800 (or $1,690 for early registration); books are additional. The Homeopathy Workshop weekend course costs $195; the home study course costs $89.

Financial Assistance
A payment plan is available.

Garden State Center for Holistic Health Care

1195–1203 Route 70 West and Airport Road
Lakewood, New Jersey 08701
PHONE: (732) 364-0882
FAX: (732) 364-7096
WEBSITE: www.bodywork4u.com

Garden State Center for Holistic Health Care was founded in 1992 by Gloria Coppola. There are eight instructors and teacher assistants, with an average of twelve to eighteen students per class.

Accreditation and Approvals
The center is approved by the New Jersey Department of Education. Graduates are qualified to take the National Certification Examination for Therapeutic Massage and Bodywork (NCETMB). The center is approved by the National Certification Board for Therapeutic Massage and Bodywork (NCBTMB) as a continuing education provider.

Program Description
The 700-hour Holistic Health Massage Certification Training may be taken over six or twelve months and consists of three semesters. Semester I: Building Your Foundation includes Anatomy/Physiology/Myology, Neurology, Pathology, Swedish Theory and Practice of Massage, On-Site Seated Massage, Foot Reflexology, and Stress Management/Meditation. Semester II: Development of a Healer consists of Anatomy and Physiology, Pathology, Medical Massage/Myology, Clinical Hours, Yoga, Cranio-Sacral/Energy Therapy, and Stress Management. Semester III: Fine Tuning Your Skills covers Business Management, Medical Massage/Clinic Hours, CPR, Oriental/Vedic, Allied Modalities, and Externship.

Continuing Education
Students who already have a background in bodywork but need additional hours to qualify for the national certification exam, or students who would like to specialize in a particular area, may take trainings in such areas as Nuat Thailand Massage (Level I and II), Energy Anatomy (150 hours), Reiki (all levels), Medical Massage Treatments (200 hours), Cranio

Sacral Therapy Level I, and Neuromuscular Therapy I, II, or III. Prerequisites and/or pretesting may be required for some trainings.

Admission Requirements
Applicants must be at least 18 years of age, have a high school diploma or equivalent, submit a photo and physician's statement, and interview with the director.

Tuition and Fees
Tuition is $5,500. Additional expenses include application fee, $25; registration fee, $100; books, approximately $190; a massage table (optional), $350 to $700; plus sheets and oil.

Financial Assistance
Payment plans are available.

Healing Hands Institute for Massage Therapy

41 Bergenline Avenue
Westwood, New Jersey 07675
PHONE: (201) 722-0099
FAX: (201) 722-0690
E-MAIL: HHI@aol.com
WEBSITE: www.HealingHandsInstitute.com

Healing Hands Institute was founded in 1990 by sisters Olga Kubicek and Alice Feuerstein. There are twenty-six instructors, with twelve to twenty-five students per class; the teacher:student ratio is 1:8 or less.

Accreditation and Approvals
Healing Hands Institute is accredited by the Commission on Massage Training Accreditation (COMTA), approved by the State of New Jersey Department of Education, and a member school of the American Massage Therapy Association (AMTA) Council of Schools. Graduates are qualified to take the National Certification Examination for Therapeutic Massage and Bodywork (NCETMB). The Institute is approved by the National Certification Board for Therapeutic Massage and Bodywork (NCBTMB) as a continuing education provider.

Program Description

The 600-hour Therapeutic Massage Program includes courses in Anatomy and Physiology, Pathology, Introduction to Massage, Art of Touch and Biomechanics, Principles of Massage Therapy, Palpation Skills, HIV/AIDS Awareness, Deep Tissue Massage, Sports Massage, Pre- and Post-Natal Massage, Hydrotherapy, Business Management, Kinesiology, Neuroanatomy and Neuromuscular Application, Reflexology, Shiatsu, On-Site Chair Massage, National Certification and License Review, and CPR/First Aid. Students may elect a six-month day program or a year-long evening program.

Students enrolled in the program have the option of extending the curriculum to 1,000 hours with electives in Advanced Shiatsu Massage, Herbology, and a 300-hour Medical Massage Certification.

Continuing Education

A variety of seminars and workshops are offered throughout the year. Courses offered include Cancer/HIV Certification, Geriatric Massage, Chinese Massage, Aromatherapy, Tai Chi, Post-Mastectomy Massage, Holistic Bodywork Certification, Medical Massage Certification, Baby's First Massage, and others.

Admission Requirements

Applicants must be at least 18 years of age; have a high school diploma or GED; be in good health and free of communicable diseases or any medical problems which would interfere with training and the practice of massage therapy; provide evidence of emotional maturity, domestic and economic stability, and the necessary motivation; and interview with a member of the administration.

Tuition and Fees

The total cost for the program is $5,945 which includes application and registration fees, books, and tuition; a massage table is recommended and will cost $500 to $750. Tuition varies for continuing education courses.

Financial Assistance

Payment plans, veterans' benefits, and State Retraining Programs are available.

Healing Hands School of Massage

515 White Horse Pike
Haddon Heights, New Jersey 08035
PHONE: (609) 546-7471 / (215) 676-9891
FAX: (609) 546-7491

Healing Hands School of Massage was founded in 1978; Kristina Shaw has been the director since 1994. There are five instructors plus guest lecturers; classes are limited to fourteen students.

Accreditation and Approvals

Graduates are qualified to take the National Certification Examination for Therapeutic Massage and Bodywork (NCETMB).

Program Description

The 550-hour, thirteen-month Professional Massage Therapy Program includes both American and Oriental massage styles. Courses include Introduction to Massage, Swedish Massage, Lymphatic Massage, Anatomy and Physiology, Professionalism and Self-Development, Business Practices and Ethics, Shiatsu and Oriental Health Assessment, Polarity Massage, Abdominal Massage and Nutrition, Pathology and Physiology, Oriental Massage Styles, Deep Tissue and Medical Massage, Business and Promotion, Hydrotherapy and Liniments, Body Psychology, Women's Health Issues, National Massage Exam Tutoring, Student Clinics, Tutorials, and Clinic Supervision. Classes meet evenings and weekends.

Admission Requirements

Applicants must be at least 21 years of age; have attended a New Student Orientation Evening at the School; have a professional massage from a staff member before classes begin; submit two letters of recommendation; be physically able to perform the manipulations of massage therapy; and have a personal interview.

Tuition and Fees

Tuition is $5,600. Additional expenses include books ($250 for required texts, $90 for optional Anatomy texts); massage table, $400 to $700; and liability insurance, $95.

Financial Assistance

Payment plans are available.

Health Choices

170 Township Line Road, Building B
Belle Mead, New Jersey 08502
PHONE: (908) 359-3995
FAX: (908) 359-3902
E-MAIL: hc@health-choices.com
WEBSITE: www.health-choices.com

Health Choices was founded in 1977 and is owned by Renate Novak. There are fifteen instructors, with a maximum of twenty-four students per class and forty-eight students per enrollment period.

Accreditation and Approvals

Health Choices is approved as a private vocational school by the Department of Education of the State of New Jersey. Graduates are qualified to take the National Certification Examination for Therapeutic Massage and Bodywork (NCETMB). Health Choices is approved as a continuing education provider by the National Certification Board for Therapeutic Massage and Bodywork (NCBTMB).

Program Description

Health Choices offers a 630-hour, one-year Holistic Massage Practitioner training. Courses include Swedish Massage, Shiatsu, Polarity, Deep Tissue, Anatomy and Physiology, Clinical Application, Field Work, Self-Development, Business Skills, Associated Studies, electives, and student clinic. Other associated studies include yoga, relaxation and breathing skills, and guest lectures in nutrition, chiropractic, and other topics. Classes are held days and evenings.

Community and Continuing Education

Courses with no prerequisites include Reiki I, Newborn Massage, Infant Massage, and Introduction to Hakomi.

Continuing education workshops offered to those who have completed basic massage training include Sports Massage, the Totally Effortless Massage, and On-Site Massage.

Advanced training in shiatsu, aromatherapy, pregnancy massage, post-mastectomy, cancer/HIV/hepatitis, geriatric massage, reflexology, reiki, and polarity is offered to those with prior training.

Admission Requirements

Applicants must attend one of the school's free introductory afternoons; it is recommended that they receive a full-body massage from one of the graduates or from the student clinic.

Tuition and Fees

Tuition is $6,185. Additional expenses include a $25 application fee and approximately $380 for books.

Financial Assistance

A payment plan is available.

Helma Institute of Massage Therapy

853 Garrison Avenue
Teaneck, New Jersey 07666
PHONE: (201) 836-8176
FAX: (201) 836-8767
CLASSROOMS:
101 Route 46 West
Saddle Brook, New Jersey 07663
PHONE: (201) 226-0056 / (201) 226-0057

Helma Institute of Massage Therapy was founded in 1981 by Kitty Leer. There are eight instructors, with an average of sixteen students per class.

Accreditation and Approvals

Helma Institute is approved by the State Education Department of New Jersey. Graduates are qualified to take the National Certification Examination for Therapeutic Massage and Bodywork (NCETMB). Helma Institute is approved by the National Certification Board for Therapeutic Massage and Bodywork (NCBTMB) as a continuing education provider. The institute is authorized under federal law to enroll non-immigrant alien students.

Program Description

The Helma Institute offers a 550-hour Massage Therapy Program I which may be combined with the 450-hour Massage Therapy Program II for a 1,000-hour program.

The 550-hour, thirty-week Program I includes Swedish Massage, Anatomy and Physiology, Clinical Internship, Body Mechanics, Trager® Technique, Business and Marketing, Ethics, Hygiene, Hydrotherapy, Sportsmassage, Shiatsu, Lymph Drainage, On Site Massage, Prenatal Massage, CPR, Reflexology, and Geriatric Massage.

The 450-hour, thirty-week Program II covers Applied Topics in Anatomy and Physiology, Neurology, Pathology, Myology, Shiatsu, Hygiene and Professionalism, and Kinesiology.

Admission Requirements

Applicants must be at least 18 years of age, have a high school diploma or equivalent, submit a health statement, and have a personal interview.

Tuition and Fees

Tuition for Program I is $3,995 and includes liability insurance. Tuition for Program II is $3,500. The application fee is $25; books and massage table are additional.

Financial Assistance

A payment plan and veterans' benefits are available.

Herbal Therapeutics School of Botanical Medicine

P.O. Box 553
Broadway, New Jersey 08808
PHONE: (908) 835-0822
FAX: (908) 835-0824
E-MAIL: dwherbal@nac.net

CLASSROOM LOCATION:
51 S. Wandling Avenue
Washington, New Jersey 07882

The Herbal Therapeutics School of Botanical Medicine was founded by David Winston, a founding member of the American Herbalists' Guild, herbal consultant to physicians and industry, and noted lecturer at American and Canadian universities, medical and herbal school, and symposia. The faculty consists of three members. Class size is limited to twenty-eight.

Program Description

The two-year Herbalist's Training Program meets one evening per week, forty-five weeks per year. (The 2000–2002 Tuesday class is scheduled to start September 2000.) The curriculum includes Introduction to Healing, Field Botany, Wildcrafting, Introduction to the Phytochemistry of Medicinal Plants, Introduction to Chinese Medicinal Concepts, Introduction to Cherokee Medicine and Culture, Herbal Pharmacy, Diagnostics, Materia Medica, Therapeutics Protocols, Constitutional Therapy, Case Histories and Clinic, and History of Western Herbal Medicine. In addition to lecture, demonstration and discussion, students take monthly herb walks and submit one class project each year (40- to 60-page reports, demonstrations, videos, slides, lecture, etc.).

Admission Requirements

Applicants who have not completed a college-level Anatomy and Physiology course will be required to take Introduction to Anatomy and Physiology offered by Michael Anthonavage at the same location. Applicants must also submit an application form and have a personal interview.

Tuition and Fees

Total tuition for the two-year program is $3,200 to $3,600, depending on payment method.

Financial Assistance

Payment plans are available.

Institute of Aromatherapy

3108 Route 10 West
Denville, New Jersey 07834
PHONE: (973) 989-1999
FAX: (973) 989-0770
E-MAIL: essence@aromatherapy4u.com
WEBSITE: www.aromatherapy4u.com

The Institute of Aromatherapy was founded in 1997 by Mercedes Hnizdo, Clinical Aromatherapist, and Vincent Iuppo, Naturopath. The faculty consists of four members; class sizes are limited to twenty-five. The institute also offers an Internet-based Aromatherapy Consultant Program, which covers the same material as the in-class program.

Accreditation and Approvals

The Institute of Aromatherapy is approved by the New Jersey Department of Education and the South Carolina Commission on Higher Education.

Program Description

The 200-hour Aromatherapy Consultant Program is forty days in length. Subjects covered include Aromatherapy (definition, history, and modern-day practices); The Sense of Smell; Essential Oils (definition and general characteristics); Methods of Essential Oil Extraction and Yields; Essential Oil Adulteration, Quality and Testing; Toxicity and Contraindications; Methods of Application, Dilutions and Dosages; Hydrosols; Carriers for Essential Oils; Lab Work (including general blending, perfume blending, consultation practice and blending, and case discussions); Essential Oils in Relation to the Body Systems, Aromatic Materia Medica, Aromachemistry, Botanical Families, Consultation Guidelines and Procedures, and Business Practices and Ethics. Students are also required to complete written and oral tests, fifteen case studies, and a 2500- to 3000-word research paper.

The institute also offers an Internet-based Aromatherapy Consultant Program, which covers the same material as the in-class program.

Admission Requirements

Applicants must be at least 18 years of age, have a high school diploma or equivalent, and submit a doctor's note (no allergic reactions or sensitivity to scents or essential oils).

Tuition and Fees

Tuition for either the in-class or Internet-based program is $2,995. Additional expenses for either program include application fee, $50; textbook, $17; essential oil kit, $300; and lab coat (required but not supplied by the institute).

Financial Assistance

A payment plan and bank loans are available.

Light Lines Wholistic Center

4 Leigh Street
Clinton, New Jersey 08809
PHONE: (908) 735-7403
FAX: (908) 735-4949
E-MAIL: light@webspan.net
WEBSITE: www.light-lines.com

The Light Lines Wholistic Center was founded in 1992. The Integrated Hypnotherapy course is the first of its kind, based on the twenty-five years' experience of Light Lines owner Carol Gill in helping others overcoming self-sabotage on the road to mental, physical, and spiritual health. There are two instructors, with an average of four students per class.

Accreditation and Approvals

Students completing the Healing Awareness—Integrated Hypnotherapy course are eligible for certification through the International Association of Counselors and Therapists as a certified hypnotherapist.

Program Description

The four-day Healing Awareness—Integrated Hypnotherapy Course teaches a wholistic, cocreative healing process. The curriculum consists of separate courses in Hypnotherapy, Kinesiology, and Yoga Therapy.

Admission Requirements

Applicants must complete an application form.

Tuition and Fees

Total tuition for the Healing Awareness—Integrated Hypnotherapy course is $400.

Financial Assistance

A payment plan is available.

Morris Institute of Natural Therapeutics

The Mareen Building
3108 Route 10 West
Denville, New Jersey 07834

PHONE: (973) 989-8939
FAX: (973) 989-5554
E-MAIL: essence@aromatherapy4u.com
WEBSITE: www.aromatherapy4u.com

The Morris Institute of Natural Therapeutics (MINT) was founded in 1963 and offers certification and continuing education in a wide variety of holistic health modalities. There are six instructors, with an average of ten students per class.

Accreditation and Approvals

Graduates are qualified to take the National Certification Examination for Therapeutic Massage and Bodywork (NCETMB). Hands-on courses, workshops, and seminars meet American Massage Therapy Association (AMTA) and Associated Bodywork and Massage Professionals (ABMP) continuing education requirements.

Program Description

The 500-hour Therapeutic Massage Course covers Principles of Massage, Terminology, Practical Techniques, Complete Body Massage and Body Movements, Indications/Contraindications, Preparation/Draping, Sanitation/Attire/Oils, Massage-Related Anatomy and Physiology (including an Introduction to Spatial Relationships and Systems of the Body) Professional Ethics, Legislation/Insurance, and How to Become Established. Classes are held days and evenings.

Continuing Education

A two-day workshop in applied kinesiology and muscle balancing enables the student to put the body in balance to improve posture and increase energy, use muscle-balancing techniques, and test for allergies. Topics include Chinese Concepts of Medicine, Cross Crawl Exercise, Pain Relief, Visual Inhibition, Auricular Exercise, Balancing with Food, Forty-Two Major Muscle Testing, Surrogate Testing, Emotional Stress Release, Massage Reflexes, Holding Points, Meridians and Meridian Massage, Alarm Points, Muscle Origin/Insertion Technique, Pulse Testing, and Body Balancing.

A three-day workshop in reflexology covers such topics as Theory and Origin, Thumb and Finger Movements, Location of Reflex Points, Basic Anatomy, Breathing and Relaxation, Practice of Complete Pressure Massage, Work with Oil, Special Health Problems, and more.

A two-day workshop in sports massage covers specialized techniques, such as Neuromuscular Therapy, Neuroproprioceptive Therapy, Pre- and Post-Event Sports Massage (including Theory of Sports Massage, Proper Pre- and Post-Event Strokes, Muscle Problems, and Preventing and Improving Sports Injuries), and more.

A two-day shiatsu workshop covers Theory and Practice, Yin/Yang Meridians, Points of the Meridians, Adjunctive Techniques (including moxa, cupping, infant massage, seated shiatsu, and more), Emergency/Quick Fix Shiatsu Techniques (for headaches, fainting, hiccoughs, insomnia, relaxation, and others), and more.

Reiki training (Traditional Usui Method), taught by a Reiki Master, is offered in three sessions: Reiki I, Reiki II, and Reiki Master certification.

Additional seminars are offered in Touch for Health, RejuvenEssence facial massage, neuromuscular therapy (NMT), craniosacral therapy, lymph drainage therapy, herbology, nutrition, and other areas.

Admission Requirements

Applicants must be at least 18 years of age and have a high school diploma or equivalent. Other prerequisites vary depending on the program chosen.

Tuition and Fees

Tuition for the Therapeutic Massage course is $3,295; for the Applied Kinesiology course, $325; for the Reflexology course, $325; for the Sports Massage course, $325; and for the Shiatsu workshop, $325. Reiki sessions vary in cost; contact the institute for additional information.

Our Lady of Lourdes Institute of Wholistic Studies

900 Haddon Avenue, Suite 100
Collingswood, New Jersey 08108
PHONE: (609) 869-3134
FAX: (609) 869-3129
WEBSITE: www.lourdesnet.org

Our Lady of Lourdes Institute of Wholistic Studies was founded in 1993 by Sr. Helen Owens, Dean and Vice President of Mission. There are ten to twelve instructors, with an average of twenty to twenty-four students per class.

Accreditation and Approvals

Graduates of the 500-hour Wholistic Massage program receive thirty-three credit hours toward an Associate's Degree in Applied Science at Camden County College, and are qualified to take the National Certification Examination for Therapeutic Massage and Bodywork (NCETMB). Lourdes Institute is approved by the National Certification Board for Therapeutic Massage and Bodywork (NCBTMB) as a continuing education provider. Graduates of the Foot Reflexology program are eligible to take the National Reflexology Certification Exam. The Foundations of Aromatherapy program follows the National Association for Holistic Aromatherapy guidelines for Level I certification.

Program Description

The 550-hour Wholistic Massage Certification Program consists of 500 instructional hours and fifty hours of independent practice. Students are encouraged to choose their own curriculum provided they stay within the guidelines of the National Certification Exam; that is, students must take 100 hours of Anatomy and Physiology, a minimum of 200 hours of Massage and Bodywork, and a maximum of 200 hours in Related Education. Courses offered include Wholistic Massage Foundational Course, Anatomy and Physiology, Wholistic Living, Independent Practice Hours, Kinesiology: Tai Chi Chuan and Qi Gong, Clinical Pathology, Infectious Diseases, Reiki, Professional Ethics for the Bodyworker, Kinesiology: The Study of Human Movement, Massage for the Elderly, Pregnancy and Massage, Infant Massage, Introduction to Deep Tissue Massage, Traditional Chinese Medicine, Foot Reflexology, Seated Chair Massage, Introduction to Shiatsu, Introduction to CranioSacral Therapy, Guided Imagery, Vibrational Healing, Introduction to Ayurveda, Word Becomes Flesh, CPR/First Aid, Therapeutic Touch, Medical Massage, Sports Massage, and others. Classes are offered days, evenings, and weekends.

The 150-hour Wholistic Yoga Teacher Training Program consists of seventy instructional hours and eighty hours of practice and application; applicants should have some prior Yoga experience. Students learn new ways to access energy through breath and body awareness, effective warm-ups, basic postures, meditation, prayer, and deep relaxation.

An eight-hour Christian Yoga Teacher Training Certification Program may be taken as an adjunct to the Wholistic Yoga Teacher Training Program or as an individual certification. Students learn how to use yoga as a sacred encounter with God, as an experience of the body at prayer.

The 110-hour Foot Reflexology Certification is conducted by the Laura Norman School of Reflexology (NY). The program is composed of four levels of training: Beginner Level I, an in-depth study of the principles of reflexology covering the location of reflex areas and points; Intermediate Level II, which adds additional therapeutic techniques and explores anatomy and physiology; Advanced Level III, which begins with a comprehensive examination of the foot and lower leg and the role of biomechanics, gait analysis, foot function, and shoe assessment; and Certification Level IV, which focuses on pathologies, professional ethics, and working with special populations. Students must also complete 100 hours of documented practical work. A thirty-six-hour Foundations of Aromatherapy Certification Program introduces the therapeutic properties and uses of aromatherapy oils, blending, basic chemistry of essential oils, and more.

Continuing Education

All of the courses at Lourdes Institute are offered as continuing education courses, including those listed as part of the 500-hour curriculum.

An advanced level seventy-five-hour Shiatsu Certification Program is offered in which students learn the art of Shiatsu acupressure massage and advanced energy balancing techniques.

Other certification courses offered beginning in summer 1999 are Palpation Skills for Massage Therapists, Introduction to CranialSacral Therapy, and Shiatsu Seated Chair Massage.

Admission Requirements

Applicants must be at least 18 years of age, submit three letters of recommendation and a physician's statement, and have a personal interview.

Tuition and Fees

Tuition is $4,910 plus a $25 application fee; books are additional. Tuition for the Wholistic Yoga Teacher Training Program is $1,100. Tuition for Christian Yoga Teacher Training is $150. Tuition for the Foot Reflexology program is $500 per level (total $2,000). Tuition for Foundations of Aromatherapy is $375.

Tuition for the Shiatsu Certification Program is $800.

Financial Assistance

Financial assistance is available in the form of student loans, a two-installment payment plan, and one work-study scholarship per session.

School of Asian Healing Arts

1930 East Marlton Pike, G-38
Cherry Hill, New Jersey 08003
PHONE: (609) 424-7501
FAX: (609) 424-7379
E-MAIL: acwsaha@bellatlantic.net
WEBSITE: members.bellatlantic.net/~acwsaha

The School of Asian Healing Arts was founded in 1986. Ruth Dalphin, one of the cofounders, serves as director. There are five instructors, with three to fifteen students per class.

Accreditation and Approvals

The School of Asian Healing Arts is a member of the American Oriental Bodywork Therapy Association (AOBTA) Council of Schools and Programs, and is approved by the State of New Jersey Department of Education as a private vocational school.

Program Description

The school offers day or evening Shiatsu Certification Programs from 150 to 500-plus hours. Each semester includes seventy to seventy-five hours of instruction. A Basic Level (150-hour) certificate in shiatsu is awarded after completion of Levels IA and IB, 100 treatment reports, and receiving three treatments from a certified instructor or practitioner.

Level IA includes Meridian Theory, Fourteen Major Meridians, Chinese Anatomy and Physiology, the Four Examinations, Qi, Yin/Yang, Shiatsu in Relation to Other Healing Arts, Basic Full-Body Treatment, Use of Yu/Shu Points, Shiatsu Self-Care, Energetics of Food/Lifestyle, and Introduction to Western Anatomy and Physiology.

Level IB covers Principles of Assessment (Hara and Pulses), Law of Five Elements, Special Points, Ampaku, Traditional and Masunaga Bo Points, Side Shiatsu, Special Stretches, Balancing Yin and Yang in Diet, Whole Foods, and more.

Level IIA instruction includes Element Points, Eight Principles, Six Evils, Assessment, Home Remedies, Transitional Cooking, Application of Assessment Skills, Psychological/Emotional Bodywork, and more.

In Level IIB, students are exposed to Source/Luo Points, Review of Zang Fu Functions, Detailed Study of Pathologies with Signs and Symptoms, Assessment and Treatment Plan, Case Studies, and more.

Level IIIA includes Review of 100 Major Points, Five Elements: Pathologies and Personal Relationships, Muscle Channels, Extraordinary Vessels, and a continuation of Level IIB shiatsu work.

Level IIIB consists of seventy hours of clinic, in which students give full shiatsu treatments under supervision.

For Level III certification, in addition to class requirements, students must also take two semesters of Western anatomy and physiology, complete CPR training, and receive ten shiatsu treatments.

A 200-hour Yoga Teacher Training Course includes fifty hours of yoga classes, taken over one to two years; fifty hours (one semester) of anatomy and physiology; and 100 of postures, history, and philosophy (in four twenty-five-hour segments).

Community and Continuing Education

Additional classes and workshops are offered in a variety of subjects, including Meditation, Thai Massage, Yoga, Tai Chi, Do-in, Acupressure, and others.

Admission Requirements

For the Shiatsu Certification program, applicants must have a high school diploma or equivalent. For Yoga Teacher Training, applicants must be in good physical and mental condition; prior completion of at least one six-session series of yoga classes is recommended. No experience is necessary for introductory workshops

Tuition and Fees

Tuition is $750 per semester for all shiatsu classes. There is a one-time $100 registration fee; books and supplies average $60 per semester.

Tuition for the anatomy and physiology course is $780 ($390 per semester).

Tuition for the Yoga Teacher Training course is $2,000; books, mats, and optional equipment are additional.

Financial Assistance

A payment plan is available.

Somerset School of Massage Therapy

E-MAIL: ssmt@massagecareer.com
WEBSITE: www.ssmt.org

SOMERSET LOCATION:
7 Cedar Grove Lane
Somerset, New Jersey 08873
PHONE: (732) 356-0787
FAX: (732) 469-3494

WALL CIRCLE PARK LOCATION:
1985 Highway 34
Wall Circle Park at Allaire Road
Wall Township, New Jersey 07719
PHONE: (732) 282-0100
FAX: (732) 282-1108

Somerset School of Massage Therapy was founded in 1987. There are twenty-five instructors; the teacher:student ratio is no higher than 1:12 (actual ratio in 1999 was 1:9).

Accreditation and Approvals

The massage therapy program is accredited by the Commission on Massage Training Accreditation (COMTA) and approved by the New Jersey Department of Education, the Florida Board of Massage, and the Iowa Massage Therapy Board. Graduates are qualified to take the National Certification Examination for Therapeutic Massage and Bodywork (NCETMB). Somerset School of Massage Therapy is approved for recommendation for college credit by the American Council on Education (ACE).

Program Description

Somerset offers three massage therapy programs:

The 550-hour Professional Track Program includes required courses in Anatomy and Physiology, Therapeutic Massage and Related Modalities, Myofascial and Deep Tissue Techniques, Reflexology, Sports Massage, Prenatal Massage, Student Clinic, Business Management and Professional Ethics, CPR/First Aid, Hydrotherapy, HIV/AIDS Awareness, and Tai Chi. Students may complete the program in twelve months on either a morning or evening schedule, or in six months in the accelerated program, which meets two full days per week plus one evening or Saturday.

The 670-hour Eastern Track Program consists of the Professional Track program plus an additional 120 hours of Shiatsu.

The 670-hour Western Track Program consists of the Professional Track Program plus an additional 120 hours of Neuromuscular Therapy (NMT).

Continuing Education

Elective courses are open to both practicing massage therapists and enrolled students. Some classes have no prerequisites and are open to the general public.

The school invites top professional presenters from across the country. Courses include Beyond the Routine (required for Florida licensing), Myofascial Massage Therapy—An Advanced Certification Training Program, Neuromuscular Therapy (NMT), Shiatsu, Reiki, Acupressure for Headaches, and Pathology. New courses are continually being added.

Admission Requirements

Applicants must be 18 years of age or older, have a high school diploma or equivalent, be of sound mind and body, and interview with an admissions representative.

Tuition and Fees

Tuition for the Professional Track program is $5,400. Tuition for the Eastern or Western Track programs is $6,400.

Additional expenses include application fee, $25; registration fee, $100; books, approximately $350; recommended massage table, $400 to $600; two school shirts, $35 to $45; and linens, $25 to $50.

Financial Assistance

A monthly payment plan, Sallie Mae student loans, and veterans' benefits are available.

Studio Yoga

P.O. Box 99
Chatham, New Jersey 07928
PHONE: (973) 966-5311
FAX: (800) 310-9833
E-MAIL: studioyoga@yoga.com
Teacher Workshops:
Studio Yoga Madison
2 Green Village Road, Room 301
Madison, New Jersey

Studio Yoga was founded in 1979 by Theresa Rowland. There are seventeen instructors, with an average of twenty-five students in the First Degree Teacher Workshop Certification classes.

Program Description

The Teacher Preparation Workshop meets one Saturday a month for three hours over six months, and was created to better prepare students for the Teacher Certification Workshop (below). The program is centered around asana, with at least three poses assigned each month to study and practice. Principles of Yoga and other aspects of teaching and practice may also be covered, but will not be the focus of the course.

The First Degree Yoga Teacher Certification Workshop meets one Saturday a month for six hours over twenty-four months. Participants learn and experience how to conduct a class (themes, goals, rhythm, and sequencing); how to observe the students; how to demonstrate; Vedanta (yoga philosophy); Principles of Yoga; Principles of Yoga Teaching; Peer Teaching; Sitting and Chanting practice; and, through study of asana and pranayama homework assignments, Basic Instructions for the raw beginner, Instructions for the continuing student, Form and actions of the ultimate pose, Ways to modify pose (including use of props), Relevant anatomy and physiology, Timings/Repetitions/Sequencing, Effects, and Basic Therapeutics.

Community and Continuing Education

Advanced Degree Certification Workshops are ongoing at the Studio. In addition, several times a year visiting teachers present special workshops for the continuing education of yoga teachers.

Other regularly scheduled yoga workshops are Yoga for Teens and Children, Prenatal Yoga, Yoga for Golf and Tennis, Yoga and Scoliosis, Introduction to Meditation, Vedanta Seminars, Yoga for a Healthy Heart, and Yoga for Hypertension.

Supporting programs at the Studio include Experiential Anatomy, Kinetic Awareness, Eye Workshops, Tai Chi, Qi Gong, and African Drum and Dance.

Admission Requirements

Applicants should have a minimum of one year attending classes (at least once per week) with a certified Iyengar yoga instructor. For the Teacher Certification Workshop, students are expected to either have a background in or to pursue a course in anatomy and physiology.

Tuition and Fees

Tuition is $1,360 per year or $378 per quarter.

Financial Assistance

Out-of-state students have individualized payment plans; work-study is available.

Unlimited Potential Institute

623 Eagle Rock Avenue
West Orange, New Jersey 07052
PHONE: (973) 325-0900
FAX: (973) 403-9789

Unlimited Potential Institute was founded in 1989 by Roxanne Louise, a Certified Hypnotherapist and Reiki Master. Louise is the primary instructor; class sizes average four to five students.

Accreditation and Approvals

Unlimited Potential Institute is approved by the International Medical and Dental Hypnotherapy Association (IMDHA).

Program Description

The 150-hour Basic Hypnosis Training consists of seventy-five classroom and seventy-five outside hours. Four weekend modules include: Introduction to Hypnosis (healing visualizations, stress management, goal setting, formulating suggestions, and more); Inductions and Script Writing (trance principles, extensive practice, hypnotic language, recognizing levels of trance); Hypnotic Problem Solving (creative problem solving; hypnotic interventions such as anchoring, secondary gain, and crystal ball; age regression/progression); and Practice Supervision (work with clients in class, case supervision, support and practical help, new techniques, case studies). These four classes may also be taken as a nine-day summer intensive.

Reiki I, Reiki II, Reiki III, and Reiki Master Apprenticeships are also offered. In the twelve-hour Reiki I class, students learn hands-on treatment for self and others. In the twelve-hour Reiki II class, students learn emotional/mental/distant healing, how to amplify Reiki healing energy, and how to integrate hypnosis and Reiki for a synergistic effect. In the twelve-hour Reiki III class for mind-body healing, students learn to enhance their ability to channel healing energy, several advanced Reiki techniques, emotional healing visualizations, interface more fully with hypnotic techniques, use symbols to clear negativity and bless a space, and more. The Reiki Master Apprenticeship takes three to four months to complete and involves four additional class days, assisting with Reiki classes, mind/body healing, and working with private clients.

Community and Continuing Education

Workshops and self-help classes are offered to the public, covering such topics as goal setting, self-hypnosis, understanding and changing our patterns, prosperity, therapeutic dowsing and telepathic healing, and others. A healing prayer group is planned.

Admission Requirements

Adult applicants of good character are welcome to apply; an interview is required for all programs.

Tuition and Fees

Tuition for Basic Hypnosis Training is $285 per weekend or all four weekends for $1,000; books are additional.

Tuition for Reiki I is $150; for Reiki II, $225; for Reiki III, $225; and for the Reiki Master Apprenticeship, $775.

Financial Assistance

A payment plan, prepayment discounts, and discounts for additional family members are available.

NEW MEXICO
The Ayurvedic Institute

11311 Menaul NE
Albuquerque, New Mexico 87112
PHONE: (505) 291-9698
FAX: (505) 294-7572
E-MAIL: registrar@ayurveda.com
WEBSITE: www.ayurveda.com

MAILING ADDRESS:
P.O. Box 23445
Albuquerque, New Mexico 87192-1445

The Ayurvedic Institute was founded in 1984 in Santa Fe, New Mexico. Dr. Vasant Lad, president, and Dr. Robert Svoboda, both well-known authors in the field of Ayurveda, are board and faculty members. The institute offers educational programs in Ayurvedic studies both in the classroom and through correspondence (see page 470), as well as a membership organization (see page 448). There are three faculty members, four full-time instructors, and four part-time instructors. The average class size for the Ayurvedic and Jyotish classes is forty; for Gurukula classes, twelve.

Accreditation and Approvals

The Ayurvedic Institute is recognized and licensed by the State of New Mexico's Commission on Higher Education as a private postsecondary institution. Dr. Vasant Lad's seminars and weeklong intensives are approved for continuing education hours in collaboration with the University of New Mexico Division of Continuing Education Nursing and Allied Health Professional Development Programs.

Program Description

The 700-hour, three-trimester Ayurvedic Studies Program is an introduction to the medical science of Ayurveda for laypersons and medical professionals. The first trimester covers basic principles and concepts; the second trimester covers client assessment and the causes and progress of imbalance and disease; and the third trimester covers treatment and rejuvenation. First-year students will learn how to read, write, and pronounce the Devanagari script through working with Ayurvedic and yogic vocabulary and memorizing several chants that are regularly recited in institute classes. Classes are held afternoons and evenings.

The Gurukula Certificate Program offers continuing education to individually selected students dedicated to learn, present, and practice Ayurveda in a manner consistent with the principles and practices of Dr. Lad and the institute. In the traditional form of this relationship, the student is expected to trust the teacher as to what, when, and how to teach the subjects the teacher feels are appropriate. The program includes several components: attendance at Dr. Lad's morning classes, attendance at two Sanskrit classes per week, attendance at two yoga classes per week, and completion of a self-study anatomy and physiology class. Students will work with traditional Ayurvedic texts.

Jyotish is a Sanskrit term that translates to "the study of Light"—a systematized knowledge of the astronomical principles that govern our solar system and of their effect on our existence. The Jyotisha Program consists of three six-week modular segments: the Jyotish Foundation Course, the Intermediate Jyotish Course, and the Advanced Jyotish Course. Successful completion requires reading, active listening, completion of review assignments, and focused commitment. Classes meet in the afternoon.

Admission Requirements

Applicants to the Ayurvedic Studies Program must have a high school diploma or equivalent. Some understanding of Ayurveda, anatomy and physiology, Sanskrit, and other Vedic traditions will greatly enhance comprehension of the program material.

Applicants to the Gurukula Certificate Program must have a thorough understanding of the material in the Ayurvedic Studies Program and of human anatomy and physiology, and an ability to pronounce Sanskrit in the Devanagari script. Each prospective student is individually considered.

Community and Continuing Education

Weekend seminars and intensives are open to anyone who is interested in learning more about Ayurveda. Topics have included Spirituality, Psychology and Healing; Ayurveda and Modern Health Care; and Pregnancy, Childcare, and Parenting.

Tuition and Fees

Tuition for the Ayurvedic Studies Program totals $5,500 plus a $200 registration fee. Tuition for the Gurukula Program is $2,800 plus a $200 registration fee. Tuition for the Jyotish Programs is $900. Weekend seminars are $210; week-long intensives are $450.

Financial Assistance

Veterans benefits and a limited number of work-study positions are available.

Body Dynamics School of Massage Therapy

3901 Georgia Street NE, Suite B-4
Albuquerque, New Mexico 87110
PHONE: (505) 881-1314 / (505) 889-3736
FAX: (505) 830-0542
E-MAIL: bdmassage@aol.com

Body Dynamics School of Massage Therapy was founded in 1998 by Darlene Stone. There are twelve to fifteen instructors, with an average of twelve students per class.

Accreditation and Approvals

The state-registered certification course meets the State of New Mexico requirements for certification and licensure. Graduates are qualified to take the National Certification Examination for Therapeutic Massage and Bodywork (NCETMB).

Program Description

The 675-hour Massage Therapy curriculum includes a 450-hour core curriculum of Anatomy and Physiology, Structural Kinesiology, Pathology, Massage Therapy, Business and Professional Ethics, CPR and First Aid for Health-Care Providers, Marketing Strategies for Success, Hydrotherapy Techniques, and Clinical/Practical Internship. Students choose an additional 225 hours of electives from Concepts of Reflexology, Reflexology Techniques, Aromatherapy and Aroma-therapeutic Massage, Introduction to Oriental Therapies, Psychology of Touch, Stretching Techniques, Introduction to Geriatric Massage, Special Techniques for Geriatric Massage, Principles of Homeopathy, Injury Prevention and Exercises for the Therapist, Corporate Chair Massage, Sports Massage, Trigger Point/Myofascial Therapy, Advanced Palpation Techniques, Medical Massage and Bodywork, Reiki, Introduction to Herbology, Introduction to Ayurveda, Tincturing, Body Mechanics for the Massage Therapist Using the Feldenkrais Method, Special Techniques for Specific Pathologies, Shiatsu/Acupressure, and Craniosacral Therapy.

Admission Requirements

Applicants must be at least 18 years of age, have a high school diploma or equivalent, submit a health statement, and interview with a school administrator.

Tuition and Fees

Tuition is $3,000 and includes books, manuals, and five individual bodywork sessions; additional expenses include linens, oils, personal massage table, and supplies.

Financial Assistance

Payment plans, work-study, and limited scholarships are available.

Crystal Mountain Apprenticeship in the Healing Arts

118 Dartmouth SE
Albuquerque, New Mexico 87106-2218
PHONE: (505) 268-4411 / (800) 967-5678
FAX: (505) 268-4007
E-MAIL: crystalm@rt66.com

Crystal Mountain first opened its massage therapy clinic in 1980 and began offering classes through the University of New Mexico's continuing education program in 1982. In 1992, the program was expanded to its current 700 hours. There are sixteen instructors, with an average of twenty-four students per class.

Accreditation and Approvals

Crystal Mountain is registered with the New Mexico State Board of Massage and is a member of the Associated Bodywork and Massage Professionals (ABMP). Graduates are qualified to take the National Certification Examination for Therapeutic Massage and Bodywork (NCETMB).

Program Description

Crystal Mountain's 700-hour Massage Therapy Licensure Program includes Therapeutic Massage; Anatomy, Physiology, Pathology, and Kinesiology; Sports Massage and Therapeutic Exercise; Shiatsu; Esalen Massage; Polarity Therapy; Reflexology; Polar Reflexology; Aromatherapy; Chair/Seated Massage; Neuromuscular Therapy; Deep Tissue Massage; Postural Analysis; Craniosacral Therapy; Body Centered Healing; Movement Reeducation; Pregnancy Massage; Hydrotherapy; Business Skills; Ethics; Herbology; Nutrition; Clinical Internship Forum; and Internship Program. Programs are offered both days and evenings.

Admission Requirements

Applicants must be at least 18 years of age and have a high school diploma or equivalent. The academy looks for motivated students.

Tuition and Fees

Tuition is $5,000, including books, manual, and a minimum of five private training sessions.

Financial Assistance

Payment plans and work-study are available.

Hypnosis Career Institute

10701 Lomas NE, Suite 216
Albuquerque, New Mexico 87112
PHONE: (505) 292-0370
FAX: (505) 292-4580

The Hypnosis Career Institute was founded in 1984. All course are taught by Joseph P. Reel, Ph.D; classes consist of approximately six students.

Accreditation and Approvals

The Hypnosis Career Institute is licensed by the New Mexico Commission on Higher Education to issue a Diploma in Hypnotherapy. All courses are approved by the New Mexico Counseling and Therapy Practice Board and by the New Mexico Board of Social Work Examiners.

Program Description

The Hypnotherapy Certification Program is scheduled in four five-day modules held over four months. Basic Professional Hypnosis 101 covers History of Hypnosis, Nature of Hypnosis, Nature of Suggestion, Suggestibility Testing, Induction Techniques, Deepening Techniques, Termination Techniques, Handling Resistance, Waking Hypnosis, Group Hypnosis, Indirect Methods, Self-Hypnosis Training, Supervised Practice, and more. Advanced Professional Hypnosis 201 covers such topics as Rapid Hypnosis Methods, Age Regression, Developing Rapport, Establishing Realistic Goals, Explanation and Utilization of Basic and Advanced Techniques, Meditative Approaches, Left/Right Brain Approaches, Supervised Practice, and others. Hypnotherapy 301 covers Ericksonian Approaches plus Responsibility as Practitioner, Competence, Client Welfare, Interprofessional Relations, The Process of Self-Scrutiny, Applications of Hypnotherapy, and Supervised Practice. Hypnotherapy 401 covers NLP, Video Case Histories, Developing a Successful Practice, and Supervised Practice.

Admission Requirements

Courses are open to all who are over 21 years of age and who wish to learn hypnosis theory and application for personal or professional growth; a personal interview may be required.

Tuition and Fees

Tuition for each course is $445 ($395 with early registration discount).

Financial Assistance

There is a discount for early registration.

International Institute of Chinese Medicine

P.O. Box 29988
Santa Fe, New Mexico 87952-9988

PHONE: (505) 473-5233 / (800) 377-4561
FAX: (505) 473-9279
E-MAIL: 102152.3463@compuserve.com
WEBSITE: www.thuntek.net/iicm

The International Institute of Chinese Medicine was founded in 1984 by Dr. Michael Zeng, who brought his extensive knowledge of acupuncture and traditional Chinese medicine from the People's Republic of China. There are fifty instructors, with a teacher:student ratio of 1:12.

Accreditation and Approvals

The Master of Oriental Medicine degree program is accredited by the Accreditation Commission for Acupuncture and Oriental Medicine (ACAOM). IICM is approved by the New Mexico State Board of Acupuncture and by the Medical Board of California Acupuncture Committee.

Program Description

The 2,400-hour, eight-semester Master of Oriental Medicine degree program includes 915 hours spent in observation, hands-on experience, and actual treatment. Graduates of the program are qualified to take licensing examinations in New Mexico, California, and other states, and the diplomate exam of the National Certification Commission for Acupuncture and Oriental Medicine (NCCAOM). New Mexico legislation awards the title Doctor of Oriental Medicine (DOM) upon completion of this program and passage of the New Mexico licensing exam.

First-year courses include Traditional Chinese Medicine, Five Element Theory and Application, Theory of Meridians, Chinese Medicine Etiology and Pathology, Meridian and Acupoint Energetics, Acupuncture Practicum, Human Anatomy, Surface Anatomy, Western Approaches to Illness and Medical Terminology, Tai Chi Chuan, Human Physiology, Chinese Herbology, Acupuncture and Moxibustion Therapy, and others.

Second-year classes include Chinese Medicine Diagnosis, Chinese Patent Medicine, Treatment of Disease, Clinical Diagnosis by Lab Data, Qigong, CPR, Chinese Medicine Prescriptionology, and others.

Third-year classes include Chinese Acupressure and Tui Na Techniques, Chinese Medicine Diet and Food Therapy, Nutrition and Vitamins, General Psychology, Advanced Student Clinic, Ethics and Human Service Skills, Basic Chemistry, Organic and Biochemistry, and others.

Fourth-year courses include Chinese Medicine Internship, Advanced Student Clinic, Western Pharmacology, Clinical Aspects of Western Medicine, General Physics, and others.

Classes are usually held three days per week. An evening/weekend schedule is available at the Albuquerque campus.

Continuing Education

A forty-credit Continuing Education Certificate Program is open to licensed acupuncturists, graduates of Master of Acupuncture or Oriental Medicine degree programs, current students of IICM's degree program, and other qualified healing arts practitioners. Courses in Chinese herbology and Chinese medicine prescriptionology are prerequisites. These courses will eventually develop into the academic Doctor of Oriental Medicine (D.O.M.) degree program, which is currently awaiting approval by ACAOM on a national basis.

Students in the Continuing Education Certificate Program must complete forty credits. Courses offered include Advanced Student Clinic, Extraordinary Acupuncture Points, Chinese Internal Medicine, Chinese Medicine Longevity, Chinese Medicine Gynecology, Chinese Sports Medicine, Animal Acupuncture, Chinese Medicine Surgery, Laser Acupuncture, Basic Chinese Language, Chinese Medicine Ophthalmology, Herb Cultivation and Preparation, and others.

Admission Requirements

Applicants to the Master of Oriental Medicine degree program must have completed sixty credit hours of general education at the college level from an accredited institution, supply official transcripts, complete an autobiographical sketch, submit two letters of recommendation and a letter from a licensed health care practitioner regarding the applicant's physical condition, and interview with an admissions representative.

Tuition and Fees

Tuition is $150 per credit for fifteen credits or more, or $165 per credit for fourteen credits or fewer. Other costs include: application fee, $50; registration fee, $30 per semester; graduation fee, $150; student activity fee, $20 per semester; clinic fee, $20 per semester; and books and supplies, approximately $300 per semester.

Financial Assistance

A payment plan, work-study, and federal loans are available.

The Medicine Wheel—A School of Holistic Therapies

1243 West Apache
Farmington, New Mexico 87401
PHONE: (505) 327-1914 / (888) 327-1914
FAX: (505) 327-2234
E-MAIL: medicinewheel@arcnet.com
WEBSITE: www.acrnet.com/medicinewheel

The Medicine Wheel is the educational branch of Wholistic Innerworks Foundation, Inc., a nonprofit corporation founded by Randy and Susan Barnes. Wholistic Innerworks began offering a complete certification program in 1992. There are six instructors, with an average of twelve students per class.

Accreditation and Approvals

The Medicine Wheel is accredited by the Integrative Massage and Somatic Therapies Accreditation Council (IMSTAC), approved by the National Certification Board for Therapeutic Massage and Bodywork (NCBTMB) as a continuing education provider, and registered with the State of New Mexico Board of Massage Therapy for the 750-hour program and the 1,200-hour Associate of Occupational Studies degree. Graduates are qualified to take the National Certification Examination for Therapeutic Massage and Bodywork (NCETMB).

Program Description

The 750-hour Basic Massage Training Program consists of 360 hours of related classes in Anatomy and Physiology, Business, Client Relationships and Stress Management, Diet and Nutrition, Ethical Issues, First Aid and CPR, Herbology, Hydrotherapy, Legal Guidelines, Traditional Chinese Medical Theory, and the Mind-Body Connection, plus an additional 390 hours of training in Chinese Massage (Tui Na), Cranio-Sacral, Lymphatic Massage, Neuromuscular Therapy, Polarity, Swedish Massage and Body Mechanics, and TMJ Work.

The 840-hour Oriental Studies Program adds ninety hours of Traditional Chinese Medical Theory to the 750-hour program above.

The 1,200-hour Associate of Occupational Studies Holistic Health Practitioner Program offers an in-depth study of holistic practices by combining the Basic Massage Training program with advanced training in Advanced Anatomy and Physiology, Advanced Mind-Body Connection, Advanced Chinese Massage, Aromatherapy, Neuromuscular Therapy, Pathology, Muscle Checking, Medical Qi Gong, Traditional Chinese Medical Theory II, Yoga for Specifics, and 105 hours of research and a written report of this research.

Community and Continuing Education
Most electives and several massage classes are open to the public; these may also be taken for continuing education by health care professionals.

Admission Requirements
Applicants must be at least 18 years of age, have a high school diploma or equivalent, and be emotionally stable and physically able to perform massage manipulations taught in the program.

Tuition and Fees
Tuition for the 750-hour program is $6,500; additional expenses include liability insurance, $75, books, $350, and oil and supplies, $80.

Tuition for the 840-hour program is $7,280.

Tuition for the 1,200-hour program is $11,000, plus books, approximately $500, and oil and supplies, $100.

Other expenses for either program include: application fee, $100; ten required professional massages, $350; and portable massage table, approximately $780.

Tuition for elective courses taken by non-enrolled students is $15 per hour if received two weeks before scheduled class; $15 is added to the total after that time.

Financial Assistance
A payment plan and veterans' benefits are available.

National College of Phytotherapy

3030 Isleta Boulevard SW
Albuquerque, New Mexico 87105
PHONE: (505) 873-8107
FAX: (505) 873-4530
E-MAIL: phyto@swcp.com
WEBSITE: www.MotherGAIA.com/phyto

The National College of Phytotherapy was founded in 1996 by Amanda McQuade Crawford. There are ten part-time instructors, with an average of fifteen to twenty students per class.

Accreditation and Approvals
The college is licensed with the Commission of Higher Education in New Mexico, and is pursuing accreditation.

Program Description
The college offers a three-year diploma program leading to a Bachelor of Science degree in Phytotherapy (herbal medicine). Year One courses include Philosophy of Healing I: A Western Constitutional Perspective, Philosophy of Healing II: The Practitioner in Health, Illness, and Healing—Personal Progressions, Study Habits, Botany, Materia Medica, The History of Western Herbal Medicine, Philosophy of Herbal Medicine, Herbal Traditions and Culture of New Mexico, Biochemistry, Ecology and Ethics of Harvesting, Herbal Pharmacy, Cellular Physiology, Histology, Philosophy of Western Medicine, Anatomy and Physiology, Pharmacology/Pharmacokinetics, Western Energetics, and English (composition). Year Two courses include Materia Medica, Introduction to Pathophysiology, Pathophysiology, Therapeutic Ethics, Nutrition, Computer Skills, Stress Management, Pharmacognosy, Botanical Field Work, Introduction to the Client, The Physical Exam, Diagnostic Skills, Diagnostic Tests, Drugs and Herbal Medicine, Integrated Phytotherapy, Behavioral Medicine, Medical Microbiology, and Applied Materia Medica. Year Three courses include Orientation to the Clinic, Clinical Practicum, Ballant Group (discussion group), Round Table, Business Skills for the Phytotherapist, Practice Management, Introduction to Western Drugs, Working with the Pregnant Woman, Herbal Pediatrics, Herbal Geriatrics, Traditional Chinese Medicine, TCM Materia Medica, Advanced First Aid, CPR, Nutrition, Psychology, Thera-

peutic Counseling, Introduction to Research, Toxicology, Massage, Introduction to Homeopathy, Ayurvedic Medicine, Ayurvedic Materia Medica, Public Health Issues, Environmental Health, Hospice, Basic Orthopedics, and Networking.

The Foundations of Herbalism Program is an introductory course meeting one weekend per month for nine months. Topics include Introduction to Herbalism: Philosophy and History, Introduction to Herbal Preparation, Anatomy and Physiology (of the respiratory system, digestive system, women's health, and immune system), Materia Medica, Healing and Ritual, Herbal Pediatrics, Herbs for Elders, Gaia: Lectures/Discussion, Herbal Protocols for Men's Health, Herb Walks, and more.

Admission Requirements

Bachelor of Science degree applicants must be at least 18 years of age, fluent in English, have a high school diploma or equivalent, submit two letters of recommendation, and have a personal interview. Applicants should have completed one year of college or advanced placement high school English and biology and one semester of college or advanced placement high school Chemistry.

There are no prerequisites for the Foundations of Herbalism program.

Tuition and Fees

Tuition for the Bachelor of Science degree program is $5,000 per year; books, fees, and supplies are additional. Tuition for the Foundations of Herbalism program is $1,095.

Financial Assistance

Payment plans and work study are available.

New Mexico Academy of Healing Arts

501 Franklin Avenue
P.O. Box 932
Santa Fe, New Mexico 87504-0932
PHONE: (505) 982-6271
FAX: (505) 988-2621
E-MAIL: nmaha@trail.com
WEBSITE: www.nmhealingarts.org

The New Mexico Academy of Healing Arts was founded in 1979.

There are thirty instructors with an average class size of twenty-four to twenty-six students.

Accreditation and Approvals

The academy's massage therapy certification programs are approved by the New Mexico Board of Massage Therapy; graduates are qualified to take the National Certification Examination for Therapeutic Massage and Bodywork (NCETMB). The polarity certification programs are approved by the American Polarity Therapy Association (APTA).

Program Description

The 1,000-hour daytime Massage Program includes, in the first semester, Anatomy, Physiology, Anatomy with Maniken®, Massage, Body Mechanics, Communication Skills, Professional Development and Ethics, and Student Intern Clinic. The second semester includes Anatomy, Physiology, First Aid, CPR, Professional Development, Medical Massage, Student Intern Clinic, Orthobionomy, and Aromatherapy.

The 650-hour day or evening programs are designed for very directed students who want a solid foundation in massage therapy in the shortest possible time. Instruction includes Massage, Anatomy, Physiology, Body Mechanics, Communication Skills, Clinical Exposure, and Professional Development and Ethics.

The six-week, 155-hour Associate Polarity Practitioner (A.P.P.) Program provides an overview of polarity theory and bodywork techniques. Graduates are eligible to apply to APTA for an A.P.P. certificate.

The six-month, 650-hour Registered Polarity Practitioner (R.P.P.) Program provides an immersion in polarity theory, bodywork, nutrition, and counseling. The curriculum includes Polarity Stretching Postures; Business Management, Promotion, Professional Ethics, and Law; Communication and Facilitation: Didactic Study and Guided Personal Exposure; Anatomy and Physiology; Polarity Theory and Principles; Energetic Nutrition; Polarity Bodywork; Evaluation and Integration Skills; electives; and clinical supervision. Graduates are eligible to apply for membership in APTA as a Registered Polarity Practitioner.

Continuing Education

A variety of introductory courses and weekend workshops are offered for continuing education credit. These may include

Massage Sampler, Polarity Sampler, Introduction to Hydrotherapy, Aromatherapy, Ayurvedic Massage, Traditional Amma Shiatsu, Sports Massage, Cranial-Sacral and Cranial-Structural, Thai Medical Massage, Soft Tissue Injuries, and Massage Teacher's Training.

Admission Requirements
Applicants must be at least 18 years of age, have a high school diploma or equivalent, and interview with an admissions representative. It is recommended that prospective students view the academy's Healing Touch video and observe classes.

Tuition and Fees
There is a $35 application fee. Massage students must have access to massage tables before the sixth week of the semester.

Tuition for the 1,000-hour massage program is $8,000; books and supplies cost $450 to $625.

Tuition for the 650-hour massage program is $6,000; books and supplies cost $360 to $500.

Tuition for the Associate Polarity Practitioner (A.P.P.) Program is $1,550; books and supplies cost approximately $145.

Tuition for the Registered Polarity Practitioner (R.P.P.) Program is $5,000; books and supplies cost $560 to $860; professional bodywork costs $750 to $1,050.

Financial Assistance
"Pay as you study," partial deferred payment plans, and limited scholarships (generally limited to ten percent of total tuition) are available.

New Mexico College of Natural Healing

P.O. Box 211
Silver City, New Mexico 88062
PHONE: (505) 538-0050 / (888) 813-8311
WEBSITE: www.zianet.com/nmcnh

New Mexico College of Natural Healing, Inc., was founded in 1996 by codirectors Gwynne Unruh and John Deckebach. There are ten instructors plus guest lecturers. Class sizes are limited to fourteen students in Massage Therapy, eighteen in Herbal Medicine; several lecture classes are scheduled with the combined student body of thirty-two students.

Accreditation and Approvals
The Massage Therapy Program is approved by the State of New Mexico; graduates have the certified hours necessary to take the National Certification Examination for Therapeutic Massage and Bodywork (NCETMB).

Program Description
The 800-hour Massage Therapy Program consists of Anatomy and Physiology; Kinesiology; Clinical Pathology; History of Massage and Bodywork; Getting Ready to Touch; Massage Manipulations and Techniques; Designing the Massage or Bodywork Session; Advanced Massage Techniques; Lymph Massage; Reflexology; Trigger Point Therapy; Connective Tissue Approaches; Face and Scalp Massage; Shiatsu; Intuitive Bodywork; Spinal Release; Effects, Benefits, Indications and Contraindications; Hydrotherapy; Business and Professional Practice Management; Confidentiality; Hygiene, Sanitation and Safety; Professional and Legal Issues; Body Movement; Special Populations; Authentic Movement; Intern Program; Voice Therapy; Wellness Education; Range of Motion; Therapeutic Exercise Methods and Techniques; Structural Integration; Herbology; Theory of Field/Contact in Gestalt Therapy; Theory of Feedback and Interruption of Contact in Gestalt Therapy; Reichian Theory of Segments in Bioenergetics; Bioenergetic Exercises; Nutrition East; and Traditional Chinese Medicine. Tuition includes ten Rolfing® Structural Integration sessions.

The 500-hour Herbal Medicine Program consists of 370 or more hours of Standard Classes, thirty or more hours of Herb Store Internship/Classes, and 100 or more hours of Field Classes. The curriculum includes Anatomy and Physiology; Materia Medica; Internship in a Unique and Professional Herb Store; Plant Pharmacy; Wild Edibles; Nutrition; Field Pharmacy and Field First Aid; Herbal First Aid; Hygiene, Sanitation and Safety; Herbal Traditions and Culture of the Southwest; Self-Sufficiency and Survival Techniques; Herbal Intuition; Professional and Legal Issues; Hydrotherapy; Communication and Healing Across Cultures; The Power of Talismans; Holistic Herbal Medicine; Business and Professional Practice Management; Natural Healing; Energetic Healing; The Emotional Body; Botany and Plant Identification; Ethical Wildcrafting;

Constitutional Herbal Medicine; Client Interview and Assessment; Case Studies Review; Shamanism and the Ritual Use of Plants; Reflexology; Spinal Release; Intern Massage Participation; Pathophysiology; Clinical Evaluation; Confidentiality; and The New Ethnobotany.

Admission Requirements

Applicants must be at least 18 years of age, have a high school diploma or equivalent, complete a personal interview and essays, and submit two character references.

Tuition and Fees

Tuition for the Massage Therapy program is $5,500. Additional expenses include books, $379; two required massages, $60; optional massage table, $350 to $550; supplies, $100; and insurance, $49. Tuition for the Herbal Medicine program is $3,600. Additional expenses include books, $200; insurance, $49; and travel expenses for field trips, $800 to $1,000.

Financial Assistance

Work-study positions, discounts for early payment, and individualized payment plans are available.

The New Mexico Herb Center

3030 Isleta Boulevard SW
Albuquerque, New Mexico 87105
PHONE/FAX: (505) 452-3468

Founded in 199, the New Mexico Herb Center is a not-for-profit educational facility and herbal clinic. Located at the same address and under the same directorship is the National College of Phytotherapy (see pages 247-48).

Program Description

The Clinical Practicum is an intensive, advanced training program for herbalists with a working knowledge of herbal therapeutics and an understanding of physiology. Herbalists see clients in the NMHC clinic under the supervision of a professional herbalist, prepare plant medicines in the apothecary, and discuss cases several times a month at Round Tables with a physician advisor. Classes include Applied Materia Medica, Herbal Pharmacology, Herbal Pharmacy and Formulations,

Understanding Herbal Constituents, Interactions of Western Drugs and Earth Medicine, Toxicology, Introduction to Clinical Skills, Introduction to the Client, the Physical Examination, Taking a Health History, and Accessing Medline and the Net.

Tuition and Fees

Tuition for the Clinical Practicum is $1,600, plus a $15 application fee.

Financial Assistance

Payment plans are available.

New Mexico School of Natural Therapeutics

202 Morningside SE
Albuquerque, New Mexico 87108
PHONE: (505) 268-6870 / (800) 654-1675
FAX: (505) 268-0818
E-MAIL: jpendry@swcp.com
WEBSITE: www.nmsnt.org/nathealth

The New Mexico School of Natural Therapeutics (NMSNT) was founded in 1974 and moved to its present Nob Hill location in 1997. The school emphasizes an integration of many different systems of healing, including Bach flower remedies, homeopathy, herbology, and others, and offers more polarity therapy than any other basic massage course in the country. There are eighteen faculty members; the average class size is thirty to forty day students, twenty evening students.

Accreditation and Approvals

NMSNT is registered with the New Mexico Board of Massage Therapy, is a member of the AMTA Council of Schools, and is currently seeking accreditation through Integrative Massage and Somatic Therapies Accreditation Council (IMSTAC). Graduates are qualified to take the National Certification Examination for Therapeutic Massage and Bodywork (NCETMB).

Program Description

The 750-hour massage therapy curriculum consists of Massage Techniques (including Swedish, sports massage, Swedish gymnastics, neuromuscular therapy, tai chi/table posture, pregnancy and infant massage, and postural analysis), Polarity

Therapy (including body/mind counseling skills and reflexology), Anatomy and Physiology, Internship/Clinical Practice, Shiatsu, Herbology (including traditional Chinese medicine diagnostics and mountain herb walk), Business Procedures and Professional Ethics, Flower Remedies/Homeopathy, Philosophy of Nature Cure, Hydrotherapy, Nutrition, AIDS Education, and First Aid, CPR, and Hygiene. A six-month day program and a one-year evening program are offered.

Continuing Education

An ongoing continuing education program includes such courses as craniosacral therapy, colonic irrigation, advanced polarity, myofascial release, Thai massage, chair massage, and others. A thirty-hour sports massage course is offered annually that fulfills AMTA sports massage certification requirements.

Admission Requirements

Applicants must be at least 18 years of age and have a high school diploma or equivalent. Applicants must submit an application form, including a personal statement and a completed health evaluation form, show evidence of financial readiness, interview with an admissions representative, and provide character references. Prospective students should submit applications two to six months prior to the program starting date.

Tuition and Fees

Tuition is $5,700. An application and supply fee of $600 includes books and linens. Optional expenses include a portable massage table, $450 to $600; Bach flower kit, $200; anatomical and treatment charts, $100; and products and remedies from the dispensary, approximately $40 per month.

Financial Assistance

Tuition may be paid in two installments; prepayment discounts and veterans' benefits are available. Students receive 100 percent of all donations for treatments given at student clinics; students may earn back approximately 15 percent of their tuition in four weeks of clinical internship practice.

Scherer Institute of Natural Healing

935 Alto Street
Santa Fe, New Mexico 87501

PHONE: (505) 982-8398 / (505) 751-3143 (In Taos)
FAX: (505) 982-1825
E-MAIL: tsi@rt66.com
WEBSITE: www.newmexiconet.com/scher.htm

The Scherer Institute of Natural Healing first enrolled students in 1979, and in 1984 became a nonprofit 501-c-3 educational organization. There are twenty instructors, with an average of twenty-four students per class.

Accreditation and Approvals

The institute is a registered school with the State of New Mexico Board of Massage Therapy. Graduates are qualified to take the National Certification Examination for Therapeutic Massage and Bodywork (NCETMB). The institute is approved as a continuing education provider by the National Certification Board for Therapeutic Massage and Bodywork (NCBTMB).

Program Description

The 750-hour, six-month Massage Therapy Training Program includes the Healing Quality of Touch and Professional Development; Nurturing and Therapeutic Massage, in which students learn to give a complete Swedish massage; Connective Tissue Bodywork; Human Anatomy, Physiology, and Pathology; the Principles of Natural Therapeutics Using Herbal Medicine and Hydrotherapy; Shiatsu; Naturopathic Principles and Techniques; Energy Work Modalities; Business; Movement; and Clinical Internship.

A 650-hour, nine-month Massage Therapy training program meets evenings and weekends at the Santa Fe location.

Continuing Education

Additional courses for both beginning and advanced students are offered throughout the year. These include Life Impressions Bodywork, Shiatsu, Trigger Point Therapy, Massage for the Child-Bearing Year, Basic Herbology and Herb Walks, Hakomi for Bodyworkers, Orthobionomy, Process Work (based on the work of Dr. Arny Mindell), Deep Tissue–Specific Ailment Work, Trigger Point Intensive, Exploring Boundaries, and Cranio-Sacral.

Admission Requirements

Applicants must be 18 years of age and have a high school

diploma or equivalent. Students are screened for health, character, financial preparation, stability, and sincerity.

Tuition and Fees

Tuition for the Massage Therapy training program is $6,000. Other costs include: application fee, $50; books, $300; massage table, $500 (optional); linens, $50; and massage oil, $30.

Continuing education courses cost $160 to $350 each.

Financial Assistance

Payment plans and some scholarships and work-study are available.

Southwest Acupuncture College

(See Multiple State Locations, pages 413–14).

Taos School of Massage

5112 NDCBU
Taos, New Mexico 87571
PHONE/FAX: (505) 758-2725
E-MAIL: tsm@newmex.com

The Taos School of Massage was founded in 1994 by J. Frederick Ritchie, whose focus is on working with people in a transformational bodymind context. Ritchie is trained in aikido and Feldenkrais®, has done graduate work in family therapy, and has trained with Lar Short in BodyMind Clearing®. There are ten instructors, with an average of eight students per class.

Accreditation and Approvals

The 650-hour Massage Therapy Course is registered with the New Mexico Board of Massage Therapy; graduates are eligible to take the New Mexico State licensing exam and/or the National Certification Examination for Therapeutic Massage and Bodywork (NCETMB).

Program Description

The 650-hour Massage Therapy Course consists of Therapeutic Massage (interviewing clients, contraindications, basic massage, Swedish massage, draping, corrective exercises, and reflexology), Advanced Sports Massage, Anatomy and Physiol-

ogy, Hydrotherapy, Business Skills, Professional Ethics, CPR Certification/First Aid, Iridology, Aromatherapy, and Shiatsu, for a total of 450 hours. The remaining 200 hours consist of BodyMind Clearing (a system of transformational deep-tissue massage), applied kinesiology, and body-centered facilitation skills, as well as meditation.

Admission Requirements

Applicants must be at least 18 years of age, have a high school diploma, and interview with an admissions representative.

Tuition and Fees

Tuition is $4,400; a summer intensive from mid-July through August costs $350 per week.

Financial Assistance

A payment plan and work-study are available.

3HO International Kundalini Yoga Teachers Association

(See Multiple State Locations, page 415)

Universal Therapeutic Massage Institute

3410 Aztec Road NE
Albuquerque, New Mexico 87107-4403
PHONE: (505) 888-0020 / (800) 557-0020
FAX: (505) 881-0749
E-MAIL: info@utmi.com
WEBSITE: www.albshoppingmall.com/massage

Universal Therapeutic Massage Institute was founded by Mary Jo Jones in 1993. There are eight instructors; classes are limited to twenty-six students .

Accreditation and Approvals

Universal Therapeutic Massage Institute is registered with the New Mexico Board of Massage Therapy. Graduates are qualified to take the National Certification Examination for Therapeutic Massage and Bodywork (NCETMB).

Program Description

The 670-hour Massage Therapy Program consists of 520 hours of classroom instruction and 150 hours of clinical internship. Courses include Anatomy and Physiology, Kinesiology and Pathology, Business and Ethics, Hydrotherapy, First Aid/CPR, Basic Massage Techniques, Myotherapy, Traditional Chinese Medicine, Tui Na, Shiatsu, Cranio-Sacral Techniques, Sports Massage, Techniques for Disabled Clients or Clients with Terminal or Chronic Pathologies, Trigger Point Techniques, Bach Flowers/Polarity/Ayurveda, and Internship. The full-time morning program may be completed in six months; the evening classes meet three nights per week and one Saturday each month for nine months.

Admission Requirements

Applicants must be at least 18 years of age, have a high school diploma or equivalent (students who are age 17 and seniors in high school may enroll with parental permission), adhere to student codes of conduct and ethics, and have a personal interview.

Tuition and Fees

Tuition is $3,850 and includes all required textbooks, handouts, oil, additional learning aids, and the CPR/First Aid certification course. Students must supply one set of twin sheets.

Financial Assistance

Payment plans and limited work-study are available.

NEW YORK

Academy of Natural Healing

40 West 72 Street #117
New York, New York 10023
PHONE: (212) 724-8782
FAX: (212) 724-2535
E-MAIL: chihealer@mindspring.com
WEBSITE: www.chihealer.com

The Academy of Natural Healing was founded in 1974 by Lewis Harrison. There are ten instructors, with an average of fifteen students per class.

Accreditation and Approvals

The Academy of Natural Healing is approved by the American Polarity Therapy Association (APTA) for both Associate Polarity Practitioner (A.P.P.) and Registered Polarity Practitioner (R.P.P.) training.

Program Description

The Academy of Natural Healing is an educational and transformational networking and support community of over 1,600 students, coaches, healers, Shamanic practitioners, bodyworkers, physicians, massage therapists, philosophers, herbalists, caregivers, and teachers guided by the mentoring system developed by Lewis Harrison. The academy offers individualized educational programs; mentoring and personal effectiveness coaching; the self-healing program; community service projects and training; over 400 classes and workshops; and forty-five certification programs, including Polarity, Stress Management, Ayurveda, Flower Remedies, Acupressure, On-Site Chair Massage, Hands-On Healing, Taoist Studies, Energetic Bodywork, Spiritual Mythology, Yoga Studies, Natural Healing, Bodywork, Asian Healing Studies, Native American Studies, Herbology, and others. Each certification program consists of over 255 hours of training, plus use of the academy's extensive library of videotapes, audiotapes, and books.

Tuition and Fees

Tuition ranges from $40 for single classes to $4,900 for full accredited degree programs.

Financial Assistance

Payment plans are available.

The American Institute for Aromatherapy and Herbal Studies

9 Gerry Lane
Huntington, New York 11743
PHONE/FAX: (516) 271-4246
E-MAIL: info@aromatherapyinst.com
WEBSITE: www.aromatherapyinst.com

In 1990, Mynou de Mey, Regional Director for the National Association for Holistic Aromatherapy (NAHA), opened Les

Herbes, Ltd., which offers aromatherapy products to professionals and retail establishments (see page 466). She created The American Institute for Aromatherapy and Herbal Studies (AIAHS) in 1990 and is the primary instructor. Classes are limited to fifteen students, and held in Great Neck and Cold Spring Harbor, New York. The Aromatherapy Certification Course described here is also offered through correspondence.

Program Description

The three-day Aromatherapy Certification Course covers History, The Olfactory Sense, Essential Oils and the Mind, Essential Oils and the Body, Extraction Process, The Chemistry of Essential Oils, Blending Essential Oils, The Essential Oils from A to Z, and Recipes.

Tuition and Fees

Tuition for the classroom-based program is $450. Tuition for the correspondence course is $415, including essential oils.

Financial Assistance

There is a $25 discount for early registration.

Atlantic Academy of Classical Homeopathy

Lawrence Galante, Ph.D., C.C.H., Director
365 West 28 Street, Suite 9J
New York, New York 10001
PHONE: (212) 414-1266
FAX: (212) 414-1793
WEBSITE: www.holistic-arts.com

The Atlantic Academy of Classical Homeopathy (AACH) was founded in 1989. AACH offers a multifaceted approach to homeopathic study that includes introductory seminars, a professional training program, and advanced seminars. There are six instructors, with an average of thirty students per class. Classes are held in Manhattan.

Accreditation and Approvals

Graduates of the 500-hour program are eligible to take the national examination given by the Council for Homeopathic Certification (CHC).

Program Description

The 500-hour professional program culminates in a Certificate in Homeopathy (CHom.). The program consists of a one-year foundation module and two years of advanced studies, plus advanced seminars that may be taken at the student's own pace. The Foundation Year may be taken on its own as a complete course in acute homeopathic therapeutics; more advanced students may enter at the second level.

The Foundation Year is designed to give the student a comprehensive overview of classical homeopathy and a strong foundation in homeopathic history, principles, and philosophy; other topics covered include case taking, analysis, principles of health and disease, materia medica (including comparative materia medica), and acute prescribing (with an introduction to treatment of chronic disease).

The Second Year focuses on a deeper understanding of homeopathic philosophy, in-depth analysis of chronic disease, enlarged materia medica, clinical case analysis and management, the archetypal/symbolic dimension of selected remedies and their specific symptomatology, and a variety of approaches to case analysis.

The Third Year consists of the application of advanced philosophy to clinical situations, expanded materia medica including important but underprescribed remedies, the utilization of homeopathy in advanced pathological states, clinical analysis and management of complex cases, and obtaining a better understanding of the subtle processes of the human psyche and the outer expression of these processes as symptoms.

Classes meet one weekend per month for ten months, for a total of 140 credit hours per year. Students must take additional hours of study through optional AACH advanced seminars or at affiliated homeopathic schools in order to complete the 500 hours. Anyone may attend individual weekends without matriculating.

Admission Requirements

Either previous to or concurrent with classroom studies, students must complete college-level Anatomy/Physiology and Pathology, CPR, and Red Cross First Aid.

Tuition and Fees

Annual tuition is $3,500; there is a $200 application fee. The Advanced Class qualifying exam is $100.

Financial Assistance

Payment plans are available.

Ayurveda Holistic Center

82A Bayville Avenue
Bayville, New York 11709
PHONE: (516) 628-8200
E-MAIL: mail@ayurvedahc.com [Distance learning] lotus fair@aol.com [Classroom-based program]
WEBSITE: ayurvedahc.com/aycertif.htm

The Ayurveda Holistic Center was founded in 1988 by Swami Sada Shiva Tirtha; certification courses began in 1991. The center offers instruction both on-site and via correspondence.

The Ayurveda Holistic Center is an affiliate member of Westbrook University (distance learning). There is one instructor; maximum ten students per class.

Program Description

The two-year, 750-hour Certification Program consists of 300 hours of classroom and internship plus 450 hours of a guided study program. Year One includes Ayurvedic anatomy and physiology, herbology, nutrition, lifestyle and food plans for each dosha, aromatherapy, Ayurvedic hatha yoga, sound therapy, seasons, exercise, Vedic psychology, and music, color, and gem therapy; Year Two covers the various systems of the body and corresponding disorders, as well as Feng Shui, Vedic architecture, scientific research, setting up an Ayurvedic business, and a final.

Each semester lasts for five months; classes meet one evening per week plus five Sundays per semester.

Certification is granted when students are properly practicing and understanding their own Ayurvedic routine, display adequate knowledge through homework, exams and internships, and integrate spirituality, ethics, humility, and respect with classroom knowledge.

Admission Requirements

The program is designed for health care professionals or those who plan to practice. Prior to beginning either the on-site or correspondence program, students must receive an Ayurvedic consultation and follow the suggestions for some months; read required texts; and interview (in person or by phone, mail, or e-mail) with a center representative.

Tuition and Fees

Tuition is $2,500 per year; books $75.

Financial Assistance

Payment plans are available ($1,000 per semester or $200 per month). A $100 discount is given for full payment in advance.

Biofeedback Instrument Corporation

(See Multiple State Locations, pages 386-87)

Finger Lakes School of Massage

1251 Trumansburg Road
Ithaca, New York 14850
PHONE: (607) 272-9024
FAX: (607) 272-4271
E-MAIL: admissions@flsm.com
WEBSITE: www.flsm.com

The Finger Lakes School of Massage was founded in 1993 by Andrea Butje, who originally ran it as a branch of the Florida School of Massage. In December 1995, Andrea Butje and Cindy Black purchased the school. There are eighteen instructors, with an average of thirty-two students per class; the teacher:student ratio is 1:18.

Accreditation and Approvals

The Therapeutic Massage and Hydrotherapy Licensing Program is approved by the New York State Board of Education and by the National Certification Board for Therapeutic Massage and Bodywork (NCBTMB) as a continuing education provider. Graduates may take the New York or Florida state licensing exams and/or the National Certification Examination for Therapeutic Massage and Bodywork (NCETMB).

Program Description

The 1,000-hour Therapeutic Massage and Hydrotherapy Licensing Program may be completed in five and a half months of full-time study. The curriculum consists of Massage Therapy (including techniques of Swedish massage, neuromuscular therapy, sports massage, energy palpation, shiatsu, and connective tissue massage), Allied Modalities (including New York State massage law and business practices, pregnancy massage, infant massage, elderly massage, and others), Oriental Theory and Introduction to Practical Shiatsu, Massage Practicum: Clinic Internship, Hygiene and Hydrotherapy, Human Anatomy and Physiology and Kinesiology, CPR and First Aid, and a directed independent study project.

Community and Continuing Education

Weekend continuing education workshops and advanced trainings are offered throughout the year. Introductory courses open to those with little or no experience include Introduction to Massage, Reflexology, and Polarity. Classes open to practicing massage therapists include Advanced Shiatsu, Polarity, Pregnancy Massage, Present Centered Awareness, Reflexology, and many others.

Admission Requirements

Applicants must be at least 18 years of age, have a high school diploma or equivalent, submit a completed application and two letters of reference from health care professionals, interview with an admissions representative, and have received massage. A tour of the school or attendance at an introductory workshop may, at the discretion of the staff, be substituted for the personal interview.

Tuition and Fees

Tuition is $9,500 to $9,700. Additional expenses include an application fee, $50; books, approximately $350; supplies, approximately $200; and optional massage table, $500 to $700.

Financial Assistance

Veterans benefits are available, as well as aid through Vocational Education Services for Individuals with Disabilities (VESID) and the Job Training Program Administration (JTPA).

Flynn's School of Herbology

60 East 4th Street
New York, New York 10003
PHONE: (212) 677-8140

Flynn's School of Herbology (formerly the Meadowsweet School of Herbology) was founded in 1980. Founder and primary instructor Arcus Flynn has been teaching herbal medicine for sixteen years; class sizes average ten students. Flynn's also has a medicine and gift shoppe, and offers colonics by appointment.

Program Description

The Herbal Beginner/Intermediate Course meets once a week for five weeks. Topics covered include the medical actions of herbs, guidelines for administration of herbal medicines, therapeutic groupings, Chinese herbs and patent medicines, herbal formulas in capsule and tincture form, a discussion of colon therapy, and preparation of herbal tinctures, poultices, and embrocations.

The Advanced Treatment Course covers all the systems of the body and the most common problems and diseases for each system, as well as foods to eat and to avoid, vitamin and mineral supplements, and herbal supplements.

Admission Requirements

Applicants must be over 16 years of age.

Tuition and Fees

Tuition for the Beginner/Intermediate Course is $250 and includes books and notes.

Financial Assistance

Work exchange is possible.

Gulliver's Institute for Integrative Nutrition

120 West 41st Street
New York, New York 10036
PHONE: (212) 730-5433
E-MAIL: iiin@earthlink.net

Gulliver's Institute for Integrative Nutrition (formerly Gulliver's Living and Learning Center) was founded in 1993. Each year, 120 new students enroll in the Professional Training Program.

Accreditation and Approvals

Graduate of the program are Certified Health Counselors accredited by the American Association of Drugless Practitioners.

Program Description

The Professional Training Program focuses on holistic nutrition and prepares students for careers in such fields as health counselor, whole foods chef, wellness counselor, cooking class instructor, dietary and lifestyle counselor, and others. The curriculum covers The Basics (food selection, seasonal cooking, menu planning, etc.), Nutrition as Therapy, Modern Health Concerns and Treatments, Walk Your Talk, Philosophy of Living, Intuitive Massage, Counseling/Teaching, Creating a Professional Practice, and Communication/Community. Classes meet one weekend per month from October to May. In addition to class time, students participate in a six-month program in which they meet individually with a certified health counselor for further support in their own health and personal growth. Students also attend monthly cooking classes and meetings.

Free Thursday night orientations provide prospective students an opportunity to meet teachers and other students and learn about the curriculum in greater detail.

Continuing Education

In the Graduate Program, an additional year of ongoing studies is offered to those who want to work professionally in this field. Emphasis is on personal health, integration, counseling skills, and creating a successful practice.

Tuition and Fees

Annual tuition is $4,400.

Financial Assistance

Discounts are available for early registration, payment in full before the start of class, enrolling friends and family members, and for young people. Student loans are also available.

International Woodstock Retreat Center

Bio Sonic Enterprises
P.O. Box 487
High Falls, New York 12440
PHONE: (914) 687-4767/ (800) 925-0159
FAX: (914) 687-0205
E-MAIL: JohnB310@aol.com
WEBSITE: BioSonic Enterprises.com

Founded in 1982 by John Beaulieu, the International Polarity Wellness Network curriculum as taught at the International Woodstock Retreat Center has been used to train hundreds of polarity practitioners worldwide. There are two instructors, with twenty to thirty students per class.

Accreditation and Approvals

The Polarity Wellness programs at the International Woodstock Retreat Center are approved by the American Polarity Therapy Association (APTA).

Program Description

A 450-hour Polarity Wellness Educator program is offered to Associate Polarity Practitioners (A.P.P.s) who wish to expand upon their learning; completion leads to certification by the International Polarity Wellness Network and fulfills eligibility requirements for status as a Registered Polarity Practitioner (R.P.P.). Requirements include Basic Craniosacral Balancing, Cranial Rhythms and Cerebrospinal Fluid, Advanced Craniosacral Balancing, Nervous System and Five Star Balancing, Energetic Nutrition, Cleansing and Bodywork, Spinal Energy Balancing, Polarity Counseling II or Body/Trance Counseling, Advanced Polarity Exercise Seminar, Professional Speaking, Practice Building and Business, Ethics and Law, clinic, supervision, electives, polarity evaluation and internship, ten receiving sessions, and fifty giving sessions. The recommended time frame for completion is twenty-one months.

The 160-hour Polarity Structural Balancing Program and the 300-hour Polarity Counseling program are designed for bodyworkers and other health professionals who would like to incorporate aspects of polarity into established practices.

Completion of the Polarity Structural Balancing Program leads to certification through the International Polarity Wellness Network in polarity structural balancing. Requirements include Basic Craniosacral Balancing, Cranial Rhythms and Cerebrospinal Fluid, Advanced Craniosacral Balancing, Nervous System and Five Star Balancing, Spinal Energy Balancing, Anatomy Home Study, twenty receiving sessions, and thirty giving sessions. The program may be taken over one to two years.

Completion of the Polarity Counseling program leads to certification through the International Polarity Wellness Network in polarity counseling. Requirements include Basic Polarity Counseling, Polarity Counseling II, Body/Trance Counseling, Relationship Counseling, Dream Counseling, Counseling Supervision/Study Groups/Clinic, receiving session, and giving sessions/apprenticeship. The program may be taken over two or more years.

Community and Continuing Education

A four-day retreat is offered in BioSonic Repatterning®, which uses music, sounds, color, and movement therapies to tune in to, enhance, and balance life energy. The program integrates diverse forms of vibrational healing into a practical approach for self-healing as well as clinical applications, which may be with modalities such as polarity therapy, massage, chiropractic, energy medicine, and others. Topics covered include Tuning Forks, Touch Toning, Environmental Toning, Color Toning, Voice Energetics, Mantras, Chanting, Sacred Geometry, Music Healing, Five Element Movement, Sonic Anatomy, and others. A set of four home study videos are sent upon registration for viewing prior to the retreat.

Admission Requirements

Applicants to the Polarity Wellness Educator Program must be graduates of an A.P.P.-level program.

Tuition and Fees

Tuition for the Polarity Wellness Educator program is $4,500, not including electives, supervision, study groups, and personal polarity sessions received.

Tuition for the Polarity Structural Balancing program is $1,650, not including sessions received.

Tuition for the Polarity Counseling program is $2,400.

Tuition for the BioSonic Repatterning program is $695 and includes videos; board and lodging are available for an average of $150 for four days.

Financial Assistance

Payment plans are available.

The Linden Tree Center for Wholistic Health

8 Noxon Road
Poughkeepsie, New York 12603
PHONE: (914) 471-8000

The Linden Tree Center, founded in 1991 by Regina and Gary Siegel, was designed to provide wholistic care and educational experiences in such areas as herbs, nutrition, personal development, and alternative health practices.

Accreditation and Approvals

The Polarity Therapy Training professional certification program is approved by the American Polarity Therapy Association (APTA).

Program Description

In addition to seminars in such areas as Yoga, Tai Chi, and Health Building, the Linden Tree Center offers certificate programs in Polarity Therapy, Reiki, and Foot Reflexology.

The 175-hour Polarity Therapy Training professional certification program offers Level I training in polarity therapy; graduates are eligible to apply for national certification as an A.P.P. (Associate Polarity Practitioner). The course is divided into four independent courses that altogether take about a year to complete: Roots, a twenty-hour foundation course that teaches basic skills; Elements, a thirty-hour course in which students learn how Earth, Water, Fire, and Air manifest in the body through the chakras and in other ways; Systems, a thirty-hour course that offers an understanding of the nervous system and its functions from an energy perspective; and Clinical, a final thirty-hour course that explores the human body as a series of energetic systems and provides clinical practitioners training and more refined skills. Roots and Clinical are weekend intensives; Elements and Systems each consist of three ten-hour weekends.

Reiki I is an introduction to reiki that teaches the students to channel healing energy for themselves or loved ones for the relief of stress and disease and for personal growth. In Reiki II, students receive one attunement and three symbols used for increasing the flow of energy, accessing the subconscious mind, and distance healing. Reiki III is available on an individual basis.

Tuition and Fees

Reiki I costs from $100 to $150 on a sliding scale. Reiki II costs from $225 to $300 on a sliding scale.

Tuition for the polarity therapy courses is as follows: Roots, $300; Elements, $300; Systems, $300; and Clinical, $400.

Mercy College

Graduate Program in Acupuncture and Oriental Medicine
555 Broadway
Dobbs Ferry, New York 10522
PHONE: (914) 674-7401
FAX: (914) 674-7374
E-MAIL: acu@mercynet.edu
WEBSITE: mercy2.mercynet.edu/programs/graduate/
acupuncture

Mercy College was founded in 1950 as a junior college by the Sisters of Mercy. The college offered its first graduate program in 1981 and was authorized to offer the Master of Professional Studies in Acupuncture and Oriental Medicine in 1996. Mercy College enrolls more than 7,000 students in undergraduate and graduate programs; the Acupuncture and Oriental Medicine department has seventeen instructors.

Accreditation and Approvals

The Acupuncture and Oriental Medicine Program is a candidate for accreditation with the Accreditation Commission for Acupuncture and Oriental Medicine (ACAOM). Graduates are eligible to sit for the examination of the National Certification Commission for Acupuncture and Oriental Medicine (NC-CAOM) and, after successful completion of the exam, for state licensure in New York as a Licensed Acupuncturist.

Mercy College is accredited by the Middle States Association of Colleges and Secondary Schools, and registered with the Board of Regents of the University of the State of New York to award associate's degrees, bachelor's degrees, and master's degrees.

Program Description

The Acupuncture and Oriental Medicine Program leads to a simultaneous Bachelor of Science in Health Science and Master of Professional Studies in Acupuncture and Oriental Medicine. It is a full-time program designed to be completed in three calendar years taken in nine consecutive semesters (including summer semesters). Enrollment is limited to one class of thirty-five students to be admitted annually.

First-year courses include Human Anatomy with Cadaver, Oriental Medicine, Acupuncture Points, Medical Terminology, Chinese Herbal Medicine, Chinese Massage Therapy, Introduction to Clinical Skills, and Elements of Biochemistry.

Second-year courses include Pathophysiology, Oriental Medicine, Acupuncture Points, Chinese Herbal Medicine, Research Methods and Concepts, CPR, Clean Needle Technique, Clinical Diagnosis and Assessment, Diet and Nutrition: East and West, Clinical Counseling, Clinical Observation, Pharmacology and Toxicology, and Clinical Assistantship.

The third year consists of Diagnostic Skills and Treatment Planning, Clinical Internship, Survey of Clinical Sciences, Microbiology, Neuroscience, Advanced Topics, History of Medicine: East and West, Clinical Practicum, Professional Issues, a master's thesis, and an elective.

Admission Requirements

Applicants must have completed at least sixty semester credits at Mercy College or another accredited degree-granting college or university or junior or community college prior to admission. Undergraduate prerequisites include three semesters of biology, including a two-semester introductory Biology course with lab and one additional bioscience course acceptable to the program; General Introductory Chemistry I and II with lab; and Developmental Psychology. In addition to transcripts, applicants must also submit three letters of reference and an essay.

Tuition and Fees

Tuition for the Acupuncture and Oriental Medicine program is $13,050 per year; Clean Needle Technique and CPR are provided by outside institutions and have additional tuition and fees. Other fees include a graduate application fee, $60; graduation fee, $85; and books and supplies, approximately $900 per year.

Financial Assistance

Federal, state, and private scholarships, grants, loans, work-study, and veterans' benefits are available.

The Natural Gourmet Cookery School

48 West 21st Street, Second Floor
New York, New York 10010
PHONE: (212) 645-5170
FAX: (212) 989-1493
E-MAIL: info@naturalgourmetschool.com
WEBSITE: www.naturalgourmetschool.com

The Natural Gourmet Cookery School was founded in 1977 by Annemarie Colbin, author of the best-selling books *Food and Healing, The Natural Gourmet,* and *The Book of Whole Meals.* The Chef's Training Program was instituted in 1985. There are twenty-three instructors.

Accreditation

The school is licensed by the State of New York as a proprietary school.

Program Description

The 600-hour Chef's Training Program emphasizes whole-grain baking techniques, converting recipes from traditional to natural and vegan ingredients, and understanding the fundamentals of human nutrition and the connection between food and healing. The focus of the program is mostly vegetarian, though it also provides instruction in fish and organic poultry; meals are high in fiber and complex carbohydrates, and contain no white sugar and minimal amounts of dairy products. Instruction is given through lectures, workshops, demonstrations, and hands-on cooking classes in knives and knife skills, selection and identification of quality ingredients, culinary techniques, equipment and sanitation, cost control and pricing, special diet cookery, theoretical approaches to diet and health, opportunities in the food business, and more. Students prepare four-course gourmet meals offered to the public at Friday Night Dinners; internships are available at professional food establishments. The program is offered on a full-time (four months) or part-time (ten to fifteen months) basis.

Community Education

Public classes are offered in a variety of topics:

The Core Program provides a complete introduction to the theory and techniques of whole-foods cooking. The program consists of four courses: Basics of Healthy Cooking (two sessions); Vegetarian Cooking Techniques (four sessions); Principles of Balance (four sessions); and Basic Knife Skills (one session).

An annual Two-Week Basic Intensive covers Menu Planning, Knife Skills, Herbs and Spices, Grain and Bean Cookery, Soups, Salads and Dressings, Sea Vegetables, Medicinal Cooking, Tofu and Tempeh, Seitan, Fish, Desserts, and more.

One-session courses are offered in other areas of natural cookery.

Admission Requirements

Applicants must have a high school diploma or equivalent, submit two letters of recommendation, and answer essay questions.

Tuition and Fees

Tuition for the Chef's Training Program is $11,550. Tuition for the Core Program is as follows: Basics 1, $110; Basics 2, $240; Basics 3, $175; and Basics 4, $65. Tuition for the Two-Week Basic Intensive is $1,195.

Financial Assistance

Payment plans, long-term financing, and discounts for students over 65 are available.

New York Chiropractic College

2360 Route 89
Seneca Falls, New York 13148-0800
PHONE: (315) 568-3040 / (800) 234-6922
FAX: (315) 568-3015
E-MAIL: enrolnow@nycc.edu
WEBSITE: www.nycc.edu

New York Chiropractic College (NYCC) was founded in 1919 by Dr. Frank E. Dean as Columbia Institute of Chiropractic. It is the oldest chiropractic college in the Northeast. There are ninety-six instructors (forty-six full-time and fifty part-time); class sizes vary from sixty to 120 students.

Accreditation and Approvals

NYCC is accredited by the Commission on Accreditation of the Council on Chiropractic Education (CCE) to award the Doctor of Chiropractic (D.C.) degree. NYCC holds an Absolute Charter from the New York State Board of Regents and is regionally accredited by the Commission on Higher Education, Middle States Association of Colleges and Schools.

Program Description

The 4,905-hour Doctor of Chiropractic (D.C.) degree may be completed in ten trimesters. Course hours are divided into three areas: Center for Preclinical Studies (1,365 hours) includes anatomy, biochemistry, physiopathology, and microbiology and public health; Center for Clinical Studies (1,995 hours) includes diagnosis, diagnostic imaging, clinical laboratory, associated studies, chiropractic principles, chiropractic procedures, and ancillary therapeutic procedures; and Center for Clinical and Outpatient Services (1,545 hours) includes clinical conferences and seminars, and clinical services.

Continuing Education

NYCC offers a wide variety of seminars enabling practicing doctors of chiropractic to keep abreast of new techniques and advances in the profession.

Programs leading to the diplomate status include Neurology, Clinical Nutrition, Orthopedics, Chiropractic Pediatrics, Rehabilitation, and Sports Injuries.

Programs leading to certification include Acupuncture, Certified Chiropractic Sports Physician, Electrodiagnostic Testing, Homeopathy, and Independent Medical Examination.

License renewal/certification programs include Applied Kinesiology, Autoimmune Deficiency Syndrome (AIDS), Chiropractic Adjunctive Therapy, Chiropractic Assistant Training, Flexion-Distraction Technique, Chiropractic Risk Management and Practice Liability, Chiropractic Management of Headache, Chiropractic Subluxation Complex, Diagnostic Imaging, Extremity Adjusting, Impairment Rating, Managed Care/Utilization Review, Meridian Therapy, Myofascial Techniques, Topics in Nutrition, and Whiplash-Diagnostic, Treatment and Legal Consideration.

Admission Requirements

Applicants must have completed at least seventy-five hours of credit toward a baccalaureate degree from an accredited degree-granting institution. Specific courses in the sciences, social sciences, and humanities are required. A high percentage of candidates selected for admission have completed baccalaureate degrees and have an average cumulative GPA of 3.0 (on a 4.00 scale) and a 2.5 or higher GPA in the science as prerequisites. Applicants must submit three letters of recommendation (one from a Doctor of Chiropractic) and interview with an admissions representative.

Special prechiropractic programs of study are available, some leading to joint B.S./D.C. degrees, in conjunction with other institutions. Articulation agreements with selected institutions lead to the assurance of admission to NYCC for students completing the programs with a specified GPA and meeting all other admission criteria. These programs are designed to provide the exact preparation needed by students planning to enroll at NYCC. Contact the admissions office for more information.

Tuition and Fees

Tuition is $5,650 per trimester for twenty to twenty-eight credit hours, and $224 per credit hour above or below this range. Other expenses include an application fee of $60 and a general fee of $145; books and supplies are additional.

Financial Assistance

Federal grants, loans, and work-study; NYCC and New York State scholarships; and additional student loans, including ChiroLoan and Canadian ChiroLoan are available.

New York College for Wholistic Health Education and Research

6801 Jericho Turnpike, Suite 300
Syosset, New York 11791
PHONE: (516) 364-0808
FAX: (516) 364-0989
E-MAIL: NYCinfo@nycollege.edu
WEBSITE: www.nycollege.edu

The New York College for Wholistic Health Education and Research was founded in 1981 by Robert and Tina Sohn as the New Center for Wholistic Health Education and Research. There are sixty-two faculty members, with maximum class sizes of forty-five students in lectures, twenty in technique classes, and nine in clinic.

Accreditation and Approvals

New York College is registered by the New York State Education Department and chartered by the Board of Regents of the University of the State of New York.

The Acupuncture and Oriental Medicine Programs are accredited by the Accrediting Commission for Acupuncture and Oriental Medicine (ACAOM). Graduates of the Acupuncture program are eligible to sit for the New York State Licensing Exam in Acupuncture and for the National Certification Commission for Acupuncture and Oriental Medicine (NCCAOM) Acupuncture certification exam. Graduates of the Oriental Medicine Program are eligible to sit for the New York State Licensing Exam and for the NCCAOM certification exams in both Acupuncture and Herbal Medicine. Graduates of the Chinese Herbal Medicine Program are eligible to sit for the NCCAOM certification exam in Chinese Herbal Medicine.

Graduates of the Massage Therapy program are eligible to take the New York State licensing exam and the National Certification Exam for Oriental Bodywork Therapy given by the NCCAOM.

Graduates of the AMMA Therapy® Program are eligible for certification as AMMA Therapists through the AMMA Therapy Association.

Graduates of the Wholistic Nursing Program receive a certificate in Wholistic Nursing with AMMA Therapy and are eligible to sit for the NCCAOM Oriental Bodywork certification exam.

New York College is approved as a continuing education provider by the New York State Nurses Associations Council on Continuing Education and by the National Certification Board for Therapeutic Massage and Bodywork (NCBTMB).

Program Description

The 144-credit Bachelor of Professional Studies/Master of Science degree program in Health Sciences/Acupuncture integrates methodologies of the East and West and may be completed in three years (nine semesters). Year One of the Acupuncture program includes courses in Palpatory Assessment, Health Psychology and Clinical Counseling, Introduction to TCM Philosophy and Wholistic Health, Oriental Physiology, Anatomy of Energy, Point Location Lab, AMMA Therapy for OM Practitioners, Tai Chi Chuan for OM Practitioners, Biochemistry, TCM Pathogenesis, Introduction to Chinese Herbal Medicine, Western Pathophysiology, Diagnostic Methods, Acupuncture Techniques and Clean Needle Technique, and Introduction to Clinic. Year Two courses include Western Nutrition, Clinical Neuroscience, Syndrome Analysis and Differential Diagnosis, Acupuncture Points Review, Clinic Grand Rounds, Professional and Medical Ethics, Tai Chi Chuan for OM Practitioners, Medical Microbiology and Immunology, Western Medical Diagnosis, Treatment Principles, Acupuncture Techniques and New Methods, Eastern Nutrition, Western Medical Treatment Principles, Western Pharmacology, Internal Medicine, Clinical Skills Review, Clinical Application of Wholistic Medicine, Clinic Assistantship, and Electives. Year Three includes Current OM Research Data and Methodology, Internal Medicine, Acupuncture Clinic, Clinical Analysis and Case Histories, Professional Business and Practice Management, Master's Thesis, and Electives.

The 170-credit Bachelor of Professional Studies/Master of Science degree program in Health Sciences/Oriental Medicine integrates the study of Acupuncture and Herbal Medicine and may be completed in forty months (ten semesters). Years One and Two of the Oriental Medicine Program are identical to Years One and Two of the Acupuncture Program with the addition of Chinese Materia Medica and Chinese Herbal Formulas in place of Electives. Year Three consists of Current OM Research Data and Methodology, Internal Medicine, Chinese Herbal Formulas, Oriental Medicine Clinic, Clinical Analysis and Case Histories, Patent Herbs, Clinic Application of Herbal Medicine, Pharmacognosy and Toxicology of Herbs, and Han Dynasty Classics. The tenth semester (Year Four) consists of Master's Thesis, Oriental Medicine Clinic, Clinical Analysis and Case Histories, Professional Business and Practice Management, and Electives.

The 143-credit, 2,730-hour diploma program in Chinese Herbal Medicine focuses on Oriental Medicine without Acupuncture and may be completed in three years (nine semesters). Year One courses include Palpatory Assessment, Introduction to TCM Philosophy and Wholistic Health, Oriental Pathophysiology, Introduction to Chinese Herbal Medicine, Chinese Materia Medica, Health Psychology and Clinical Counseling, Clinic Observation, Tai Chi Chuan for OM Practitioners, Biochemistry, AMMA Therapy for OM Practitioners, Eastern Nutrition, Diagnostic Methods, Western Nutrition, Western Pathophysiology, Syndrome Analysis and Differential Diagnosis, and Patent Herbs. Year Two consists of Western Pharmacology, Medical Microbiology and Immunology, Chinese Herbal Formulas, Internal Medicine, Treatment Principles, Clinic Grand Rounds, Tai Chi Chuan for OM Practitioners, Western Medical Diagnosis, Current OM Research Data and Method, Professional and Medical Ethics, Clinical Application of Wholistic Medicine, Western Medical Treatment Principles, Clinical Neuroscience, Classics: Shang Han Lun and Wen Bing, Clinical Skills Review, and Clinic Assistantship. Year Three consists of Pharmacology and Toxicology, Internal Medicine, Herbal Medicine Clinic, Clinical Analysis and Case Histories, and Professional Business Practice and Management.

Elective courses offered in the Oriental Medicine Programs include such topics as Basic Chinese Language, Needling Practice Class, TCM Traumatology and Orthopedics, Introduction to Zazen, Hatha Yoga, Introduction to Qi Gong, Introduction to Shiatsu, Introduction to Tui Na, Pharmacy Assistantship, and others.

All students in the Acupuncture, Oriental Medicine, and Chinese Herbal Medicine Programs are required to pass a CPR and First Aid Course prior to entry into the final academic year of clinic.

The Massage Therapy Program is a sixty-eight-credit Associate of Occupational Studies degree program that may be completed in sixteen months (four semesters) of full-time study, or may be taken on a part-time basis. First-year courses include Anatomy and Physiology, Myology, AMMA Therapy Basic Technique, European Technique, Oriental Anatomy and Physiology, Public Health, Tai Chi Chuan, Ethics and Professional Development, and Bodywork Modalities. Second-year courses include Neurology, Pathology, AMMA Therapy Applied Technique, European Applied Technique, Business Management and Massage Practice, Massage Therapy Clinic, Tai Chi Chuan, Oriental Clinic Assessment, and Kinesiology. Students are required to complete a CPR and First Aid course outside of the school prior to graduation.

The AMMA Therapy Program is a sixty-six-credit Bachelor of Professional Studies degree program requiring 16 months (four semesters) of diagnostic and practical skill beyond the sixty-eight-credit Massage Therapy program. First Year courses include Advanced AMMA therapy Technique, TCM Pathogenesis, Eastern Nutrition, Biochemistry, Introduction to Chinese Herbal Medicine, AMMA Therapy Clinic, Clinic Observation, Patient Management and Case History, Tai Chi Chuan for OM Practitioners, Diagnostic Methods, Medical Microbiology and Immunology, and Western Medical Diagnosis. Year Two courses includes Advanced AMMA Therapy Technique, Syndrome Analysis and Differential Diagnosis, Western Nutrition, Western Medical Treatment Principles, AMMA Therapy Clinic, Clinic Observation, Patient Management and Case History, Point Location, Patent Herbs, Western Pharmacology, Health Psychology and Clinical Counseling, and Electives.

The 804-hour Wholistic Nursing program is open to Registered Nurses and may be completed in thirty months (five semesters). First Year courses include Oriental Anatomy and Physiology, Conceptual and Theoretical Frameworks for Wholistic Nursing Practice, Basic AMMA Therapy Technique, Wholistic Nursing Lab, Stress Management, and Tai Chi Chuan. Second Year courses include Oriental Clinical Assessment, Stress Management, Applied AMMA Therapy Technique, Clinical Nutrition, Clinical Observation, Tai Chi Chuan, Eastern Nutrition, Applied Wholistic Nursing, and Clinical Practice. Third Year (fifth semester) courses include Oriental Diagnosis, Advanced AMMA Therapy, Eastern Nutrition, Professional Development, Clinical Observation and Practice, and Tai Chi Chuan. Supervised clinical experience is done on-site at the Wholistic Health Center or at one of the college's affiliated hospitals.

Community and Continuing Education

A variety of community and continuing education courses are offered to meet the needs of health professionals, students in the healing arts, and the general public.

Admission Requirements

All applicants must be at least 18 years of age; have a high school diploma or equivalent; be a U.S. citizen or an alien lawfully admitted for permanent residence, or hold a valid visa; submit two recommendations; have a personal interview; and complete an entrance exam and brief essay.

In addition, applicants to any of the Oriental Medicine programs must have completed at least sixty undergraduate semester credits in an accredited college or university program with a minimum GPA of 2.5.

AMMA Therapy applicants must furnish verification of licensure or a New York State Limited Permit and transcripts from the Massage Therapy school from which they graduated. Applicants must have either graduated from the New York College's Massage Therapy Program or have satisfactorily completed the prerequisite requirements for a Certificate in AMMA Therapy (460 hours).

Wholistic Nursing applicants must be Registered Nurses. Applicants must submit a copy of their current Registered Nursing License, current CPR certification, and proof of malpractice insurance.

Tuition and Fees

Tuition for the Acupuncture, Oriental Medicine, and Chinese Herbal Medicine Programs is $275 per credit. Additional expenses for these programs include an application fee of $85; registration fee, $25 per semester; liability insurance fee, $15–30 per semester; clinic entrance exam fee, $50; graduation fee, $100; and books and supplies, approximately $2,000.

Tuition for the Massage Therapy Program is $275 per credit; additional expenses include an application fee of $50; registration fee, $25 per semester; clinic entrance exam fee, $50; insurance liability fee, $15–30 per semester; Anatomy and Physiology I and II lab fees, $60 total; graduation fee, $100; books and supplies, approximately $1,300; massage table, $400–500.

Tuition for the AMMA Therapy Program is $275 per credit. Additional expenses include an application fee $65; registration fee, $25 per semester; liability insurance fee, $15 to $30 per semester; graduation fee, $100; and books and supplies, approximately $400.

Tuition for the Wholistic Nursing Program totals $9,648, based on a rate of $12 per clock hour. Additional expenses include an application fee of $50; registration fee, $35 per year; insurance liability fee, $35 per year; graduation fee, $50; and books and supplies, approximately $400.

Financial Assistance

Federal grants and loans, payment plans, and veterans' benefits are available.

New York Institute of Massage

MAILING:
P.O. Box 645
Buffalo, New York 14231
LOCATION:
4701 Transit Road
Williamsville, New York
PHONE: (716) 633-0355 / (800) 884-NYIM
FAX: (716) 633-0213
E-MAIL: NYIM@compuserve.com
WEBSITE: www.nyinstituteofmassage.com

The New York Institute of Massage (NYIM) was founded in 1994. Director David Kasprzyk has been a practicing massage therapist for over fourteen years and has served as President of the Florida State Massage Therapy Association (FSMTA). There are twenty part-time instructors, with a maximum of forty-five students per class.

Accreditation and Approvals

NYIM is accredited by the Accrediting Commission of Career Schools and Colleges of Technology (ACCSCT), approved by the New York State Board of Regents, and registered with the Department of Education. Graduates are eligible to sit for the New York State licensing exam, and/or the National Certification Examination for Therapeutic Massage and Bodywork (NCETMB).

Program Description

The 1,104-hour Massage Therapy Program may be completed in fifty-one weeks of full-time study (four terms) or 103 weeks of part-time study (eight terms); students may attend mornings, afternoons, or evenings. The program includes courses in Anatomy, Business Management, Health and Hygiene, Hydrotherapy, Law, Massage (covering such topics as Swedish massage history and theory, ethics, postural analysis, trigger point and neuromuscular therapy, therapeutic sports massage, and more), Myology, Neurology, Oriental Massage, Pathology,

Physical Assessment, and Physiology. Students are required to complete sixty therapies in the Student Clinic and to complete twenty hours of community service at NYIM-sponsored events.

Admission Requirements

Applicants must be at least 17 years of age; have a high school diploma or equivalent; interview with an admissions representative; submit a completed application, two letters of recommendation, a medical release form and a background check form; and be of good moral character. Prospective applicants should schedule an admissions appointment and tour as part of the admissions process.

Tuition and Fees

Tuition for the 1,104-hour program is $9,500; additional expenses include a $25 application fee and a $525 book and supply package.

Financial Assistance

Financing programs and veterans' benefits are available; financial aid will be available in 2000.

New York Open Center

83 Spring Street
New York, New York 10012
PHONE: (212) 219-2527
FAX: (212) 226-4056
E-MAIL: nyoc@micro-net.com
WEBSITE: www.opencenter.org

The New York Open Center was founded in 1984 by Walter Beebe and Ralph White as a nonprofit organization and emphasized one-day or weekend workshops covering a variety of holistic practices. The center is now moving toward longer-term, in-depth programs. There are over 100 instructors; class sizes vary from ten to 200.

Accreditation and Approvals

The Reflexology program prepares students for the national certification exam given by the American Reflexology Certifi-

cation Board. The A.P.P.-level Polarity Therapy Training Program is approved by the American Polarity Therapy Association (APTA).

Program Description

The one-year Aromatherapy diploma course is held over ten weekends and focuses on the safe and practical application of over 140 essential oils, twenty perfume absolutes, and over twenty carriers. Topics include Introductory Weekend; Chemistry; Botany; Blending, Customizing, and Perfumery; Aromatherapy Massage and Reflexology; Skin and Hair Care; Consultation and Designing Treatments; Pregnancy, Children, and First Aid; Subtle Aromatherapy and Aroma Fitness; and Psycho-Aromatherapy and the Business of Aromatherapy. The first weekend may be taken separately without registering for the year-long program; space permitting, some weekends may be taken separately.

Green Medicine: An Eight-Month Training in Herbalism offers a comprehensive overview of the medicinal and nutritional uses of Western herbs. Topics covered include A Brief History of Western Herbalism, Preparations and Dosages, Herbal Pharmacy: Making Herbal Products, The Digestive System and Liver, The Respiratory System, The Nervous System and Brain, The Endocrine System/Immune System, The Circulatory System: Blood and Lymph/Immune Systems, The Skin, Herbal Energetics, Women's Reproductive System, Men's Reproductive System, Seasonal Cleansing/Spring Tonics, Musculoskeletal System, Urinary Tract and Kidneys, Traditional Herbal Diagnosis, Materia Medica/Herbal Medicine Chest, Wild Edibles Field Trip, and Case Taking I and II. Sessions are held on Monday evenings and occasional weekends.

A 200-hour training program in reflexology prepares students for the national certification exam given by the American Reflexology Certification Board. The curriculum includes forty-two hours of hands-on practice, twenty-eight hours of lectures and demonstrations, seventeen hours of anatomy and physiology, ninety one-hour documented sessions, three hands-on tutorial refinement sessions, and one reflexology treatment from the instructor. Instruction is divided into three sections (Basic, Advanced, and Masters) held on Saturdays and Sundays; there is a weekday Basic in the spring. The thirty-hour Basic course may be taken independently.

The 185-hour Polarity Therapy Training Program prepares students to become an Associate Polarity Practitioner (A.P.P.). Courses include Basic Polarity I and II, Basic Polarity Counseling, Polarity Reflexology, Polarity Clinic, Supervision, and Evaluation and Preparation for Practice. Courses are held Tuesday evenings or on weekends, and may be taken separately.

Tuition and Fees
Tuition for the Aromatherapy diploma course is $2,200 to $2,700; the introductory weekend may be taken separately for $170 to $190. Fees include all materials, workbooks, and a complete aromatherapy kit.

Tuition for the Green Medicine Course is $990 to $1,020.

Tuition for the Training Program in Reflexology is $1,400 to $1,500. The Basic course is $600 plus one $50 tutorial; Advanced is $500 plus one $50 tutorial; Masters is $400 plus one $50 tutorial.

Tuition for the Polarity Therapy Training Program is $1,800 to $2,000; workbook and personal polarity sessions received are additional.

Financial Assistance
Discounts are given to members and for full payment in advance; payment plans and need-based full and partial scholarships are available.

Northeast School of Botanical Medicine

P.O. Box 6626
Ithaca, New York 14851
PHONE: (607) 564-1023

Northeast School of Botanical Medicine was founded in 1994. Director and primary instructor 7Song has been studying and teaching herbology for over fifteen years. 7Song has a clinical practice in Ithaca specializing in men's health, first aid skills, and constitutional care, and teaches throughout the United States. There is a maximum of sixteen students per class.

Program Description
Two programs are offered in Western Clinical Herbalism: the six-month program meets three days per week; the seven-week program meets one weekend per month. These two programs offer similar classes, though they are more condensed in the weekend format. Classes include Anatomy and Physiology, Business Practicum, Clinical Evaluation/Diagnostic Skills, Counseling Skills, First Aid, Herbal Formulation, Herbal Pharmacy/Medicine Making, Herbalist as Educator, Materia Medica, Networking and Resources, Plant Identification/Field Botany, Wild Edibles, Wildcrafting, and Student Clinic. In addition, field trips, guest speakers, and other events are scheduled.

Three positions are offered for apprentices. The Apprenticeship Program is a demanding, active apprenticeship working closely with 7Song from April through December for those interested in training as herbalists.

Continuing Education
An Advanced Western Clinical Herbal Intensive meets for seven days. This program is designed for practicing clinical herbalists to refine and intensify their clinical skills.

Admission Requirements
A personal interview is required.

Tuition and Fees
Tuition for the six-month Western Clinical Herbalism program is $1,850; tuition for the seven-month weekend program is $875. There is no tuition for apprentices, though they must provide their own housing, tools, books, and other supplies.

The Advanced Western Clinical Herbal Intensive is $650. Additional expenses for all of these programs include those for tools, books, and herbal supplies.

Ohashi Institute

(See Multiple State Locations, pages 404-5)

Omega Institute

260 Lake Drive
Rhinebeck, New York 12572
PHONE: (914) 266-4444 / (800) 944-1001
WEBSITE: omega-inst.org

Founded in 1977, Omega Institute offers over 250 workshops, retreats, professional trainings, conferences and wellness vacations, including programs taught by internationally known figures such as Deepak Chopra, Susan Powter, David Carradine, Jack Kornfield, Phil Jackson, and others. The institute's lakeside campus is set on eighty acres in the Hudson River Valley.

Accreditation and Approvals

Many programs may be taken for continuing education credit; contact the institute for specific information.

Program Description

Omega Institute offers programs in many areas of alternative health care for personal benefit, career preparation, and continuing education credit; consult the catalog or website for a complete listing. Programs offered may change from year to year.

The month-long Interdisciplinary Yoga Teacher Training covers yoga postures and breathing techniques, including Astanga, Hatha, Iyengar, and Kripalu yoga; anatomy and kinesiology; how to teach a posture and design lesson plans; yoga philosophy and the chakra system; integrating Western psychospiritual principles with yoga philosophy; and the practicalities of establishing a yoga class, marketing, and networking.

Shorter Yoga Teacher Training Programs of three to five days are also offered; consult the catalog for details.

A seven-day Reflexology Training Program covers the fundamentals of reflexology; classical Western techniques; Ayurvedic and Chinese energy pathways; basic anatomy and physiology; which reflexes to use for specific imbalances and ailments; and using the Alexander Technique.

The four-day Integrative Medicine: A Use-Friendly Approach to Healing Program is open to all but designed for physicians and other health care professionals. Topics covered include the history and impact of integrative medicine; merging Western, Chinese, body-mind, functional, nutritional, and herbal medicine; combining nutrition, herbs, and supplements with conventional medications; holistic detoxification; meditation, yoga, and other body-mind approaches; and incorporating integrative medicine into your health practice.

A four-day course is offered in Developing a Holistic Learning Center, taught by two of the founding members of Omega Institute. Topics covered include financial viability within not-for-profit or profit status; developing programs that speak to your constituency; identifying and reaching your market; creating an organizational structure; choosing faculty; and developing a board of directors and advisors.

Admission Requirements

Interdisciplinary Yoga Teacher Training applicants should have some previous yoga experience. Integrative Medicine: A Use-Friendly Approach to Healing program is open to all but designed for physicians and other health care professionals.

Tuition and Fees

Tuition for the described programs is as follows: for the month-long Interdisciplinary Yoga Teacher Training, $1,850; for the Reflexology program, $395; for the Integrative Medicine program, $210; and for Developing a Holistic Learning Center, $350.

Financial Assistance

Omega Institute members receive tuition discounts.

Pacific College of Oriental Medicine

(See Multiple State Locations, pages 405-6)

R.J. Buckle Associates, LLC

(See Multiple State Locations, page 409)

The Rubenfeld Synergy Center

(See Multiple State Locations, pages 409-10)

The School of Homoeopathy, New York

964 Third Avenue, 8th Floor
New York, New York 10155-0003
PHONE: (212) 570-2576
FAX: (212) 758-4079
E-MAIL: kathy@homeopathyschool.com
WEBSITE: www.homeopathyschool.com

The School of Homoeopathy, New York was founded in 1998 and incorporates the curriculum and senior faculty of the twenty-year-old School of Homeopathy, Devon, England. There are seven instructors, with an average class size of twenty students. Classes are held at the College of Insurance in lower Manhattan.

Accreditation and Approvals

The School of Homoeopathy, New York is seeking accreditation with the Council on Homeopathic Education (CHE).

Program Description

The four-year Professional Homeopathy program is the classical homeopathy of Samuel Hahnemann as set out in The Organon. The first two years concentrate on philosophy, case taking, and in-depth study of materia medica. In the second half of the course, an emphasis is given to clinical practice, case analysis and management skills, pathology, disease, and homeotherapeutics. Classes meet one weekend per month for ten months each year; home research and written assignments extend the study time to more than 500 hours per year.

Admission Requirements

Applicants must complete an application with personal statement; applicants within 200 miles must have a personal interview (others may substitute a phone interview). Applicants must complete an Anatomy and Physiology course by the end of Year One. Advanced students and practitioners may apply for second-year advanced entry.

Tuition and Fees

Tuition is $3,050.

Swedish Institute

School of Massage Therapy
School of Acupuncture and Oriental Studies
226 West 26th Street, 5th Floor
New York, New York 10001
PHONE: (212) 924-5900
FAX: (212) 924-7600

Founded in 1916, the Swedish Institute is the oldest school of massage therapy in the United States. The institute started its Acupuncture program in 1996.

Accreditation and Approvals

The Swedish Institute is accredited by the Accrediting Commission of Career Schools and Colleges of Technology (ACC-SCT). The massage curriculum at the Swedish Institute is approved by the Council of Schools and Programs of the American Oriental Bodywork Therapy Association (AOBTA); graduates are qualified to take the National Certification Examination for Therapeutic Massage and Bodywork (NCETMB). The Institute is approved by the National Certification Board for Therapeutic Massage and Bodywork (NCBTMB) as a continuing education provider. The Acupuncture Program is registered with the New York Education Department and has candidacy status with the Accreditation Commission for Acupuncture and Oriental Medicine (ACAOM).

Program Description

The 1,226-hour Massage Therapy program may be completed in sixteen months of full-time (day or evening/Saturday) or thirty-two months of part-time (evening) study. Courses include Orientation, Anatomy and Physiology, Myology and Kinesiology, Palpation, Swedish Massage, Introduction to Eastern Bodywork and Theory, Professional Development and Ethics, Neurology, Sports Massage and Kinesiology, Shiatsu, Clinical Internship, Off-Site Internship, Pathology for the Massage Therapist, Applied Topics in Anatomy and Physiology, Assessment and Treatment of Soft Tissue Conditions, Trigger Point and Myofascial Technique, Eastern Evaluation and Treatment Strategy, Clinical Strategies: East and West, Complementary Techniques (including Self Care, Reflexology, and Tui Na), plus electives in either the Western Modalities Sequence (Lymphatic Drainage Massage, Craniosacral Therapy, and Polarity Therapy) or the Eastern Modalities Sequence (Thai Massage, Sotai, and Introduction to Pulse, Moxa, and Other Advanced Topics). CPR and First Aid training is included in the Clinical Internship course.

The 2,713-hour Acupuncture and Oriental Studies Program may be completed in three years of full-time or six years of part-time study. Year One courses include Oriental Medicine, Acupuncture Energetics, Point Location and Energetics, Anatomy and Physiology, Myology and Kinesiology, Palpation, Oriental Medical Energetics, Neurology, Diagnostic Skills, Biomedical Nutrition, Biomedical Pathology, and CPR and First Aid. Year Two courses include Oriental Medical Energetics, Diagnostic and Clinical Skills of Acupuncture, Biomedical Pathology, Clinical Observation, Clinical Assistantship, Tui Na, Tai Chi Chuan, Practice Management, and Western Medicine Appreciation. Year Three includes Clinical Internship, Grand Rounds,

Clinical Case Review, and The Classics. Most classes are held Monday through Friday evenings, with required weekend intensive scheduled throughout.

Continuing Education

The Swedish Institute offers a comprehensive program of professional continuing education.

Admission Requirements

Massage Therapy applicants must be at least 18 years of age; have a high school diploma or equivalent; take an entrance exam; be a U.S. citizen or lawfully admitted for permanent residence in the United States; submit a personal essay, three recommendations, and proof of immunization; be in good physical health; be of good moral character; and have a personal interview.

Acupuncture applicants must be at least 18 years of age; have a high school diploma or equivalent; have completed at least sixty semester hours from a college or university; have at least nine semester hours in the biosciences; be of good moral character; be professional in attitude and appearance; be in good physical health and submit a health certificate; and submit three letters of recommendation and a personal statement.

Tuition and Fees

Tuition for the Massage Therapy Program is $13,900. Other expenses include a $45 application fee plus approximately $1,600 for books, supplies, massage table, and uniforms.

Tuition for the Acupuncture and Oriental Studies Program is $26,700 for the full-time three-year program. Additional expenses include application fee, $50; clinic (third-year students), $150; malpractice insurance (third-year students), $300; and books and uniforms, $900 for the three-year program.

Financial Assistance

Payment plans, federal grants and loans, veterans' benefits, and other forms of aid are available.

Teleosis School of Homeopathy

61 W. 62nd Street, #18E
New York, New York 10023

PHONE/FAX: (212) 707-8481
E-MAIL: teleosis@igc.org
WEBSITE: www.Teleosis.com

The Teleosis School of Homeopathy began its educational programs in 1997 under the direction of Dr. Joel Kreisberg, a Doctor of Chiropractic (D.C.) with a degree in classical homeopathy. Dr. Kreisberg completed his advanced clinical training at a homeopathic hospital in Calcutta, India, and serves as the president of the Council on Homeopathic Education (CHE). There are seven instructors, with an average of twenty students per class.

Accreditation and Approvals

The Teleosis School of Homeopathy is in the process of seeking accreditation by the Council on Homeopathic Education (CHE). Upon completion of the practitioner program, graduates will be eligible to take examinations from the Council on Homeopathic Certification, ABHT, and the HAWP.

Program Description

The practitioner program is divided into two self-contained modules, each of which takes two years to complete. Ideally, the student will complete both modules in order to be a fully trained practitioner.

The 300-hour Professional Program begins in the fall and meets one weekend per month, ten months a year, for two years. The program will cover homeopathic philosophy; materia medica; seventy of the most common polycrests; differentials for the twenty most common diseases treated by homeopathy; homeopathic practice methodology, including case taking, case analysis, case management, and repertory; and personal and practitioner development.

The 350-hour Clinical Program begins in the fall and will meet one weekend per month, ten months a year, for two years. The program includes 175 hours of classroom training and 175 hours of clinical supervision. Topics include long-term case management; advanced topics in philosophy; materia medica of the smaller remedies; materia medica differentials of extreme pathologies; clinical case management; practice management; and supervision.

Continuing Education

Homeopathy's Garden is a five-day intensive seminar offering an integrated, systematic approach to studying the plant kingdom in homeopathy. The program consists of five interlinked learning modules in Wildcrafting, Proving, Studying, Practicing, and Reflecting.

Admission Requirements

It is recommended that Professional and Clinical Program applicants hold a license in a healing profession; equivalent experience is considered.

Homeopathy's Garden is open to those with two years or 250 hours of homeopathic classroom experience.

Tuition and Fees

There is a $50 application fee. Tuition for the Professional Program is $3,000 per year. Tuition for the Clinical Program is $3,000 per year. Tuition for Homeopathy's Garden is $575 ($525 with early enrollment).

Financial Assistance

A payment plan is available.

Tri-State College of Acupuncture

P.O. Box 890
Planetarium Station
New York, New York 10024-0890
PHONE: (212) 496-7869
FAX: (212) 496-0648

MAIN CAMPUS AND CLINIC:
80 8th Avenue (4th Floor)
New York, New York 10011

BRANCH CLINIC:
16 East 16th Street
New York, New York 10003

The Tri-State Institute of Traditional Chinese Medicine is one of the oldest acupuncture schools in the United States; it was founded in 1979 as an affiliate of the Institute of Traditional Chinese Medicine of Montreal. There are twenty-two instructors, with an average of fifty students per class.

Accreditation and Approvals

The College is accredited by the Accreditation Commission for Acupuncture and Oriental Medicine (ACAOM).

Program Description

Tri-State College of Acupuncture offers a three-year combined Bachelor of Professional Studies, Master of Science Degree Program in acupuncture designed to train acupuncture therapists to work in clinics, hospitals, medical offices, or private practice. Students must complete 1,914 hours of work at the institute, plus 290 hours of corequisites.

Year One includes Philosophical Bases, Pathways of Qi, Surface Energetics and Primal Reserves, Treatment Planning and Basic Techniques, American Acupuncture, Acupuncture Electives, Acupuncture Human Service Skills, Acupuncture Skills Review, Western Clinical Pathophysiology, Acupuncture Clinical Observation/Personal Treatment (students must receive ten acupuncture treatments), and Independent Study Project.

Year Two includes Energetic Pathogenesis and TCM Patterns of Disharmony, Western Medical Disorders and Traditional Chinese Medical Pathology, Acupuncture Energetics, Reaction Patterns and Advanced Zang Fu Differentiation, American Acupuncture, Acupuncture Electives, Acupuncture Human Service Skills, Acupuncture Skills Review, Western Clinical Pathophysiology, Clinical Observation/ Personal Treatment, Clinical Grand Rounds, and Independent Study Project.

Year Three includes Clinical Field Seminars, Acupuncture Electives, Acupuncture Skills Review, Clinical Practicum, Optional Clinical Externship, Supervision, Clinical Grand Rounds, Personal Acupuncture Treatment, Independent Study Project, and Case Presentation.

In addition to regular class work, students must complete the following outside classes: bodywork, anatomy and physiology, 100 hours of direct patient contact, and CPR certification.

Continuing Education

The Postgraduate Institute offers a four-module, 450-hour program in Chinese herbal medicine, designed to meet or exceed the standards for eligibility for the NCCAOM certification examination in Chinese Herbology. Courses focus on materia medica, theoretical models for organizing Chinese herbal formulas, clinical specialties and their commonly used formulas, and clinical practice. Classes are held on weekends.

Admission Requirements

Applicants must have completed sixty credits at an accredited college or university, including nine credits in the biosciences and eight credits of anatomy and physiology, which must be completed before Year Three. Applicants must submit copies of professional licenses or certificates in health care (if applicable), a completed five-page essay, two letters of recommendation from health professionals, and official transcripts.

Those applying for the Acupuncture Certification Program for physicians must submit an application form along with proof of a current license in medicine, osteopathy, or dentistry.

Those applying for the program in Chinese herbal medicine must be second-year students or graduates of an accredited or candidate school of acupuncture and Oriental medicine recognized by the ACAOM. Applicants trained outside the United States must also be Diplomates in Acupuncture of the National Certification Commission for Acupuncture and Oriental Medicine (NCCAOM).

Tuition and Fees

Tuition for the Acupuncture Therapy Institute is $5,500 per semester. Additional expenses include application fee, $50; books and materials, approximately $500 to $700 for three years; and Clinical Pathophysiology fee, $100 to $200.

Tuition for the program in Chinese herbal medicine is as follows: Module 1 (first year), $1,750; Modules 2 through 4 (second year), $1,950.

Financial Assistance

Payment plans and federal loans are available.

Susun S. Weed

Wise Woman Center
P.O. Box 64
Woodstock, New York 12498
PHONE/FAX: (914) 246-8081
E-MAIL: [checked infrequently] weedwise@webjogger.net or
   ashtree@webjogger.net

Susun S. Weed, founder of the Wise Woman Center, editor-in-chief of Ash Tree Publications, and a high priestess of Dianic Wicca, offers workshops, intensives, and apprenticeships in herbal medicine and shamanic healing, as well as correspondence courses (see page 477) and books and videos (see page 473). The Wise Woman Center was founded in 1982. There are ten instructors, with ten to twenty students per class.

Program Description

Shamanic Apprenticeships (for women only) are full-time, live-in learning apprenticeships. The curriculum includes organic gardening, weed walks, hands-on herbal medicine, anatomy, herbal pharmacy, nutrition, herbal animal care, tarot readings, shamanic trances, moonlodges, workshops, field trips, and visiting teachers.

Weed Wise Apprenticeships are part-time, live-out apprenticeships that include sixty hours of instruction, field trips and classes, tarot readings, consultations, and more.

Community and Continuing Education

Three-day herbal medicine intensives and one-day workshops are offered spring through fall. Courses include Green Witch Intensive, Using Herbs Simply and Safely, Herbal Medicine Chest, Chronic Problems, Magical Plants, Herbs for Women, Breast Health, Spirit Healing Skills, Talking with Plants, and many others.

Admission Requirements

Beginners and advanced students are welcome; no prior experience or education is required.

Tuition and Fees

Shamanic Apprenticeships are $3,650 for eight weeks, $350 per week thereafter; includes meals and lodging. Weed Wise Apprenticeships are $900 to $1,000 (including all books and materials). Three-day intensives range from $195 to $450. One-day workshops cost $45 to $65.

Financial Assistance

Financial assistance in the form of 50 percent work/barter is available to all students; full and half scholarships are available to women of color and Native American women.

NORTH CAROLINA

Body Therapy Institute

South Wind Farm
300 South Wind Road
Siler City, North Carolina 27344
PHONE: (919) 663-3111
FAX: (919) 663-0369
E-MAIL: rick@bti.edu
WEBSITE: www.bti.edu

The Body Therapy Institute (BTI) is owned by Rick Rosen and Carey Smith. BTI was founded in Chapel Hill, North Carolina, in 1983, and moved to its present location in 1995. There are twelve instructors, with thirty-two students per class.

Accreditation and Approvals

BTI is licensed by the North Carolina Community College System, Division of Proprietary School Services. The massage therapy program is approved by the Florida State Board of Massage. Graduates are qualified to take the National Certification Examination for Therapeutic Massage and Bodywork (NCETMB). BTI is approved as a continuing education provider by the National Certification Board for Therapeutic Massage and Bodywork (NCBTMB).

Program Description

The 650-hour Massage Therapy Certification Program is a synthesis of Eastern and Western bodywork systems. Courses include Fundamentals of Massage Theory and Practice, Myofascial Massage, Polarity Therapy, Introduction to Oriental Massage Theory, Synthesis of Clinical Skills, Anatomy, Physiology and Kinesiology, Business and Marketing Practices, Professional Ethics, Massage Laws and Organizations, Personal Integration, Group Dynamics, Somatic Psychology, Hydrotherapy and Allied Modalities, Supervised Clinical Practicum, Community Service Project/Externship, and HIV/AIDS Awareness. Students must also complete an American Red Cross module in First Aid/CPR, and are required to receive at least four professional bodywork sessions during the training. The daytime program is eight months in length; the evening/weekend program runs twelve months.

Community and Continuing Education

Two-day introductory massage workshops are periodically offered to the public, featuring an introduction to Swedish massage. Additionally, a thirty-hour, ten-week Introduction to Massage Therapy series is also offered to the public.

BTI offers a range of continuing education workshops and advanced training programs to the professional practitioner.

Admission Requirements

Applicants must be at least 21 years old, have a high school diploma or equivalent, be free of communicable disease, be physically and emotionally capable of practicing massage, and have a personal interview. Additionally, applicants must have received at least two massage therapy/bodywork sessions and must have taken an introductory massage class or workshop before they enroll.

Tuition and Fees

Tuition is $7,500. Additional expenses include a $25 application fee; books, approximately $400; Maniken® model, $150; massage table, $500 to $700; school shirt, $40; First Aid/CPR, $35; and four professional bodywork sessions, $40 to $60 each.

Tuition for the Introductory Massage Workshop is $95. Tuition for the ten-week Introduction to Massage Therapy Course is $250.

Financial Assistance

Payment plans and work-study are available.

Carolina School of Massage Therapy

1000 Corporate Drive, Suite 101
Hillsborough, North Carolina 27278
PHONE: (919) 732-3390
FAX: (919) 732-3772

The Carolina School of Massage Therapy (CSMT) is a program of the Community Wholistic Health Center, a not-for-profit membership organization that has provided educational and health care services since 1978. The Carolina School of Massage Therapy was founded in 1987.

Accreditation and Approvals

Graduates are qualified to take the National Certification Examination for Therapeutic Massage and Bodywork (NCETMB).

Program Description

The 650-hour Massage Therapy Program includes classes in Anatomy and Physiology, Communications and Somatics, Swedish Massage/Clinic, Sports Massage/Clinic, Deep Muscle Massage/Clinic, Joint Mobilization, Polarity, Oriental Bodywork, Business Practices, Case Studies, Hydrotherapy, and Integrative Seminars. Weekday and weekend scheduling options are available.

Community and Continuing Education

Faculty members offer additional classes outside the curriculum throughout the year that can enhance the learning experience of the student. These classes include Body Centered Therapy, Tai Chi, Experiential Anatomy, Reflexology, Polarity, Acupressure, Pregnancy Massage, and related topics.

Community education workshops are offered throughout the year. Recent topics have included Introduction to Massage, Pregnancy Massage, and Reflexology.

Admission Requirements

Applicants must be 18 years old by the first day of class; have a high school diploma or equivalent; be emotionally and physically capable of performing the required activities; have some experience giving and receiving massage; and satisfy all requirements described in the application.

Tuition and Fees

There is a $50 application fee. Tuition is $6,275; books are approximately $300; a massage table costs $400 to $800, or a rental table costs $32 per month.

Financial Assistance

An extended payment plan and scholarships are available.

North Carolina School of Natural Healing

20 Battery Park Avenue, Room 510
Asheville, North Carolina 28801
PHONE: (828) 252-7096

North Carolina School of Natural Healing was founded in 1991 by Craig Ellis. There are ten instructors, with a maximum class size of twenty-two students.

Accreditation and Approvals

Graduates of the massage therapy program are qualified to take the National Certification Examination for Therapeutic Massage and Bodywork (NCETMB).

Program Description

The 625-hour Massage Therapy Certification Program consists of Massage/Bodywork, covering Assessment and Body Awareness, Movement Awareness/Reeducation and Corrective Exercise, Neuromuscular Therapy, Structural Balancing/Connective Tissue Massage, Joint Mobilization, and Holistic, Energetic and Bodymind Studies; Anatomy and Physiology; Clinical Pathology/Recognition of Various Conditions/Injury Assessment and Treatment; Business Practices and Professionalism; and CPR Certification and Standard First Aid.

The 250-hour Meditation Instructor and Energy Healing Program consists of Meditation Methods and Energy Activation Methods: Sacred Technologies for Inner Power and Mastery; Theory and Practice of Energy Healing; Energy Anatomy; Psychology of Inner Being; and Healing as a Profession.

Two programs are offered in Herbal Studies:

The sixty-five-hour, twelve-week Fundamentals of Herbs and Plant Energetics Program covers Plant Identification, Wild Crafting and Herb Walks, Earth Ceremony, Herbal Medicine Making, Spiritual Properties of Plants, Communication with Plant Devas, Blood and Liver Cleansing, Herbal Home Medicine Chests, Flower Essences and Aromatherapy, and more. Classes are held one evening per week and every other Saturday.

The nine-month Apprenticeship Program is an experiential study of the plants that develops the fundamental skills introduced in the twelve-week program. Topics covered include organizing material for public presentation, field trips in a variety of ecosystems, and supervised independent study. Classes meet one weekend per month from March to November.

Admission Requirements

Those applying for the Massage Therapy and Meditation Instructor Programs must be at least 18 years of age, have a high school diploma or equivalent, be in good physical and mental health, and interview with the director.

Admission to the Herbal Studies program is decided by the director of that program; an interview is required for the Apprenticeship.

Tuition and Fees

There is a $50 application fee. Tuition for the Massage Therapy program is $5,200. Tuition for the Meditation Instructor Program is $2,200. Tuition for the Fundamentals of Herbs Program is $425. Tuition for the Apprenticeship is $1,000.

Financial Assistance

Payment plans are available.

Nurturing the Mother

(See Multiple State Locations, page 404)

Southeastern School of Neuromuscular and Massage Therapy

(See Multiple State Locations, pages 412–13)

Therapeutic Massage Training Institute

726 East Boulevard
Charlotte, North Carolina 28203
PHONE: (704) 338-9660
FAX: (704) 523-4389
E-MAIL: AskTMTI@aol.com
WEBSITE: www.massagetraining.com

The Therapeutic Massage Training Institute (TMTI) was founded in 1987. There are twelve instructors plus guest faculty. Classes are limited to sixteen students; the teacher:student ratio for hands-on classes is generally 1:4.

Accreditation and Approvals

TMTI is licensed by the North Carolina State Board of Community Colleges. Graduates are qualified to take the National Certification Examination for Therapeutic Massage and Bodywork (NCETMB).

Program Description

The 600-hour Professional Certification Program is divided into three 200-hour units of study. Unit I courses include Swedish Massage, Anatomy and Physiology, Business Practices, and Practical Anatomy. Unit II covers Deep Tissue Massage, Anatomy and Physiology, Movement Therapy, Evaluation and Treatment, Kinesiology, Introductory Sports Massage, and Evaluation Standards. Unit III courses include Polarity Therapy/General Energetics, Anatomy and Physiology, Clinical Research, Practical Application, Seated Massage, Nutrition, CPR/First Aid, Evaluation Standards, and forty-five hours of Bodywork Electives. These electives may include Acupressure, Deep Holding Remedies, Integrative Therapeutic Movement, Medical Massage, Neuromuscular Re-Education, Reflexology, Seated Massage Level II, Self-Care, Somatic Psychology, or workshops offered elsewhere if approved in advance. Classes are held evenings and weekends.

Community and Continuing Education

Many of the elective classes listed above are open to the community and may be taken for continuing education credit.

Admission Requirements

Applicants must be at least 18 years of age, have a high school diploma or equivalent, be in good health and physically capable of performing hands-on techniques, be emotionally stable and committed to completing the training, and interview with the director.

Tuition and Fees

Tuition is $5,135 based on 555 hours of required curriculum; the cost of forty-five hours of electives will range from $590 to $685. Additional expenses include a $25 application fee; registration fee, $300; books, $200; massage table, approximately $600; oils and other supplies are additional.

Financial Assistance

Payment plans are available.

The Wellness Training Center

Suite A, P.O. Box 599
Leicester, North Carolina 28748
PHONE: (704) 683-3369

The Wellness Training Center was founded in 1997 by Robert M. Luka, a Registered Nurse and Certified Hypnotherapist. Luka is the primary instructor with occasional guest speakers; class sizes are limited to twenty students.

Accreditation and Approvals

The Wellness Training Center is endorsed by the International Medical and Dental Hypnotherapy Association (IMDHA) and approved as a continuing education provider by the North Carolina Nurses Association.

Program Description

The eighty-hour Hypnosis Training and Certification for the Health Care Professional Program meets for three three-day weekends.

Weekend 1: Basics of Hypnosis covers History and Nature of Hypnosis, Classifications of Hypnosis, Roles of Conscious/Subconscious Mind, Laws of Suggestion, Suggestibility Testing, Directive/Non-Directive Suggestions, Post-Hypnotic Suggestion, Rules for Successful Programming, Pre-Induction Interview, Breathing Techniques, Various Induction Techniques, Induction/Emerging Procedures, Trance Deepening, Trance Management, Obtaining Somnambulism, and Ethical/Legal Issues.

Weekend 2: Comprehensive Hypnosis covers Recognizing Levels of Trance, Self-Hypnosis Conditioning, Medical Applications, Acute Pain Management, Chronic Pain Management, Emergency Hypnosis, Working with Children, Managing and Using Fear, Developing Hypnotic Rapport, Dangers of Hypnosis, Handling Resistance, Developing Refined Semantics, Removing Phobias, Waking Hypnosis, Advanced Induction Techniques, and Handling Abreactive States.

Weekend 3: Advanced Hypnotherapy includes Age Regression Process, Initial Interview, History Taking, Identifying Core Issue/Key Phrase, Regression Techniques, Processing Regression Experience, Integration and Closure Issues, Managing Stress, Hypnotherapy Overview, Hypnoanalysis Overview, Tapping Creativity, Resourceful States, Empowering Behavior, Re-framing/Rescripting, Integrating NLP, and Hypnosis and Meditation.

Admission Requirements

The program is designed for physicians, dentists, nurses, mental health counselors, social workers, psychologists, and other health care workers.

Tuition and Fees

Tuition is $250 per weekend.

The Whole You School of Massage and Bodywork

143 Woodview Drive
Rutherfordton, North Carolina 28139
PHONE: (828) 287-0955
FAX: (828) 287-0067
E-MAIL: institute@blueridge.net
WEBSITE: www.wholeyou.com

The Whole You School of Massage and Bodywork was founded in 1990 by Cheryl Shew. There are six instructors; classes are limited to twenty-four students.

Accreditation and Approvals

The Whole You is licensed by the North Carolina Community College System for Proprietary Schools. Graduates are qualified to take the National Certification Examination for Therapeutic Massage and Bodywork (NCETMB).

Program Description

The 525-hour Massage and Bodywork Program consists of three units. Unit I covers Swedish; Hydrotherapy; Maternity; Introductions to Sports, Oriental Therapies, and Deep Tissue; and certification in Reiki I. Unit II includes Medical, Neuromuscular, Visceral-Somatic Reflex, Structural Rebalancing, TMJ Sequence, Lymph Drainage, Nutrition, and Psyche/Soma Techniques. Unit III consists of Shiatsu, Polarity, Cranial Sacral, certification in Foot Reflexology and Touch for Health, as well as Missing Link in Communication and "Creating." Anatomy and Physiology, Business and Marketing, and Professional Ethics are presented in all units. Classes meet on nineteen weekends over seventeen months. Unit III classes may be taken concurrently with Unit I or II, allowing students to graduate in eleven months.

Admission Requirements

Applicants must be at least 18 years of age (age requirement may be waived through personal interview) and have a high school diploma or equivalent.

Tuition and Fees

Tuition is $3,900 for the entire program. Additional expenses include application fee, $30, and books, approximately $300. Massage table and supplies are additional.

Financial Assistance

Payment plans are available; approved for NC Vocational Rehabilitation.

OHIO

Central Ohio School of Massage

1120 Morse Road, Suite 250
Columbus, Ohio 43229
PHONE: (614) 841-1122 / (800) 466-5676
FAX: (614) 841-0387

The Central Ohio School of Massage (COSM) was founded in 1964.

Accreditation

The COSM Massage Therapy Program is approved by the State Medical Board of Ohio. Graduates are eligible to take the Ohio State Medical Board exam for massage therapist licensure as well as the National Certification Examination for Therapeutic Massage and Bodywork (NCETMB).

Program Description

The 670-hour, eighteen-month Basic Swedish Massage Course includes Anatomy and Physiology (including cytology, osteology, myology, neurology, and angiology); Massage (including theoretical and practical study of techniques, uses, indications, contraindications, use of heat and cold, restorative exercises, and physiological effects); and additional studies including Ethics, Business Practices, Patient Approach, and others. Students are required to complete a course in Basic Life Support and First Aid. Classes may be taken on a day or evening schedule.

Continuing Education

The 170-hour, twenty-week Myofascial Therapy Course is an advanced studies program that combines advanced Swedish massage techniques with trigger point techniques, somatic fascial releases, post-isometric muscle relaxation, and other deep tissue therapies.

The eighty-one-hour Foot Reflexology Course consists of fifty-one classroom hours plus thirty hours of patient documentation. The course covers history, theory, and a wide range of techniques for optimum positive benefits.

Admission Requirements

Basic Swedish Massage applicants must have a high school diploma or GED; complete and submit a Massage Preliminary Education Form (with a $35 fee) to the State Medical Board of Ohio; and submit two character references, an essay, and a completed health certificate.

The Myofascial Therapy Course is open to massage therapists licensed in the State of Ohio, to other health professionals by special arrangement, and to those who have completed the first nine months of the Basic Course.

Tuition and Fees

Tuition for the Basic Swedish Massage Course is $6,300. There is an application fee of $60; books cost approximately $350; and a massage table is additional. Tuition for the Myofascial Therapy Course is $2,150, including books and supplies. Tuition for the Reflexology Course is $750.

Financial Assistance

An interest-free payment plan is available.

Healing Heart Herbals

32654 McCumber Road
Rutland, Ohio 45775
PHONE: (740) 742-8901

E-MAIL: cindyp@eurekanet.com

WEBSITE: www.eurekanet.com/~jimp

Healing Heart Herbals was founded in 1988 by Cindy Parker. It is a folkloric school, primarily focusing on wise woman tradition. There are two primary instructors and nine guest instructors; foundation classes are limited to thirteen, grassroots gatherings to forty.

Program Description

The Foundations of Herbalism Program meets one weekend per month from March to October; students must attend at least six weekends to receive a certificate of completion. Topics covered include History of Herbalism, Spring Tonics, Herb Gardening, Stress Management, Nervine Herbs, Infusions and Decoctions, Medicine Making, Creating First Aid Kits, Working with Creative Energy, Herbs During Pregnancy, Natural Remedies for Children, Diet, Culinary and Flower Cooking, Flower Essences, Aromatherapy, Grassroots Gathering, Cold Care, Hydrotherapy, Legal and Ethical Issues, and more.

A 250-credit hour Herbal Apprenticeship Program is offered to those students wishing to study herbs in depth, and includes the courses in the Foundations of Herbalism Program, Herbal Intensives, and Rosemary Gladstar's Science and Art of Herbology correspondence course. Other activities such as retreats, classes, and conferences as well as work experience may be applied as credit hours. Options are discussed on an individual basis.

Community and Continuing Education

Herbal Intensives, day-long sessions focusing on specific aspects of herbalism, are offered in such areas as Field Botany and Medicine Making, The Healing Flowers, and Business of Herbs.

Admission Requirements

Applicants must be at least 18 years of age.

Tuition and Fees

Tuition for Foundations of Herbalism is $1,250 prepaid ($1,600 on the payment plan).

Tuition for the Science and Art of Herbology Correspondence Course is $375 for the ten-lesson Course; students may try Lesson One for $35.

Tuition for Herbal Intensives is $100.

Financial Assistance

Work exchanges and a payment plan are available.

Integrated Touch Therapy for Animals

7041 Zane Trail Road
Circleville, Ohio 43113
PHONE: (740) 474-6436 / (800) 251-0007
FAX: (740) 474-2625
E-MAIL: wshaw1@bright.net

Integrated Touch Therapy, Inc., was established in 1998 by Patricia Whalen-Shaw, a nationally certified and licensed massage therapist. As a cofounder of the previous Optissage program, she has been teaching animal massage since 1992. Whalen-Shaw is the primary instructor with two assistant instructors; the teacher:student ratio is 1:6 or less. Instructional videos are also available; see page 494.

Accreditation and Approvals

ITT is approved by the National Certification Board for Therapeutic Massage and Bodywork (NCBTMB) as a continuing education provider.

Program Description

Courses are offered in equine, feline, and canine massage. Each class covers Animal Anatomy and Physiology, Massage Theory, Massage Clinical Practical, and Application.

Equine Level I is a six-day introductory massage course that emphasizes Swedish and sports massage techniques of pre- and post-event massage theory and practice. Call the school for information on bringing your horse to the clinic. The Equine Level II course includes more in-depth anatomy and physiology and massage technique.

Canine Level I is a three-day introductory course emphasizing general relaxation massage and sports massage. Participants are encouraged (but not required) to bring a canine friend. Canine Level II teaches more in-depth anatomy and massage applications.

Feline Level I is a two-day class using Swedish and sports massage techniques and exploring anatomy, physiology, and personality traits. Participants are encouraged (but not required) to bring a feline companion.

Admission Requirements

There are no minimum age or educational requirements for the Level I courses. Although not required, it is helpful if the participant is familiar with the animal's skeletal musculature and behavior and/or has studied massage therapy.

Canine Level I is a prerequisite course for Canine Level II. Equine Level I or individual therapist training and experience is a prerequisite for Equine Level II.

Tuition and Fees

There is a nonrefundable deposit of $150. Tuition for the Equine courses ranges from $780 to $899. Tuition for the Canine courses ranges from $300 to $399. Tuition for the Feline Level I course is $299.

Financial Assistance

Assistance may be offered on individual case request. Prepayment may be made in installments; credit cards accepted.

International Academy for Reflexology Studies

4759 Cornell Road, Suite D
Cincinnati, Ohio 45241-2432
PHONE: (513) 489-9328
FAX: (513) 489-9354
E-MAIL: nmd007@aol.com
WEBSITE: nmd007.com

The International Academy for Reflexology Studies (IARS) was founded in 1992 by Marcia L. Aschendorf, N.M.D., D.R. There are ten instructors and an average of eight students per class.

Accreditation and Approvals

IARS is approved by the Ohio State Board of Proprietary Schools.

Program Description

The 1,500-hour, eighteen-month Reflexology Practitioner Diploma Program consists of 1,200 hours of classroom study and 300 hours of Internship. Courses include Anatomy and Physiology; Terminology and Pathology; Reflexology History and Theory; Foot, Hand and Ear Reflexology; Basic and Advanced Therapies; Zone and Meridian Theory; Charts and Mapping; Communication Skills; Documentation Skills; Assessment Skills; Business Practices; Ethics; HIV/AIDS Training; Reflexology Clinical Lab; Adult, Child and Infant CPR; and Advanced First Aid.

Admission Requirements

Applicants must be at least 18 years of age, have a high school diploma or equivalent with a 2.5 GPA, attend an orientation interview, and submit referrals.

Tuition and Fees

Tuition is $1,000 per term for six terms. Additional expenses include a $100 application fee; special weekend seminar, $150; book and lab fees, $550; and LaFuma chair or massage table, $500 and up.

Financial Assistance

State financial aid and Loans are available.

National Institute of Massotherapy

2110 Copley Road
Akron, Ohio 44320
PHONE: (330) 867-1996
FAX: (330) 869-6422

ADDITIONAL LOCATION:
12684 Rockside Road
Garfield Heights, Ohio 44125
PHONE: (216) 662-6955
FAX: (216) 662-6980

The National Institute of Massotherapy (NIM) was founded in Akron in 1991 and continues under the direction of Stephen Perkinson. The faculty includes twenty-one full- and part-time members; class sizes average twelve students, with a maximum of twenty-four.

Accreditation and Approvals

NIM is approved by the State Medical Board of Ohio. Graduates are qualified to take the National Certification Examination for Therapeutic Massage and Bodywork (NCETMB).

Program Description

The 740-hour Massotherapy Program may be completed in one year of full-time study or two years of part-time study. The program consists of Basic Sciences (261 hours); Massage (314 hours); Integrated Classes and Weekend Seminars (135 hours); and Electives (thirty hours). Courses include Anatomy, Physiology, Massage Theory, Massage Practicum, Polarity Seminar, Shiatsu Seminar, Clinic, Neuromuscular Therapy Seminars, OrthoBionomy Seminar, and Business Seminars. Additional electives beyond thirty hours may be taken for additional fees. Electives offered include such topics as Polarity Certification, Shiatsu Certification, OrthoBionomy Certification, Reflexology Certification, Spinal Orthopathic Syndesmobilization (SOS) Certification, Spinal Touch Certification, Touch for Health, Sports Massage, Chair Massage Certification, Infant Massage, Manual Lymph Drainage, Craniosacral Therapy, Geriatric Massage, Reiki, and Massage for the Childbearing Years.

Continuing Education

Students, practicing massage therapists, and other health care workers may take any of the continuing education courses offered by NIM (listed as Electives under Program Description).

Admission Requirements

Applicants must have a high school diploma or equivalent, attend an Information Session at the school, and submit an application package which includes a physician's health certificate.

Tuition and Fees

Tuition is $7,450. Additional expenses include a $50 application fee and approximately $600 for books.

Financial Assistance

Payment plans, low-interest loans, veterans' benefits, and other government funding through retraining programs are available.

Ohio Academy of Holistic Health

3033 Dayton-Xenia Road
Dayton, Ohio 45434
PHONE: (937) 427-0506 / (800) 833-8122
FAX: (937) 426-8883
E-MAIL: oah@earthlink.net

The Ohio Academy of Holistic Health (OAH) was founded in 1987 by Patti McCormick, Ph.D., and offers a variety of educational programs in the holistic health professions.

Accreditation and Approvals

OAH is registered by the Ohio Board of Proprietary School Registration. Contact hours awarded by OAH have been approved by the American Board of Hypnotherapy, American Board of NLP, American Osteopathic Association, National Board of Hypnotherapy and Hypnotic Anesthesiology, State of Ohio Counselor and Social Worker Board, Ohio Nurses Association, and the American Massage Therapy Association.

Program Description

Vocational programs are offered in Clinical Hypnotherapy and Reflexology.

The 225-hour Clinical Hypnotherapy Certification Program consists of courses in Basic Hypnotherapy, Psychology for Hypnotherapists, Advanced Hypnotherapy, Hypnotherapy Preceptorship, Community First Aid/CPR, Medical Terminology, Anatomy and Physiology: A Holistic Model, and Therapeutic Communications.

The 202-hour Reflexology Certification Program includes Basic Reflexology, Advanced Reflexology, Reflexology Preceptorship, Community First Aid/CPR, Medical Terminology, Anatomy and Physiology: A Holistic Model, and Therapeutic Communications.

Students must maintain a cumulative grade of 80 percent or higher.

Continuing Education

Continuing education certification programs are offered in Aromatherapy, Botanical Health, Holistic Nutrition, Iridology, Neurolinguistic Programming (NLP), Non-Directive Imagery, Reiki, and Touch for Health.

The 130-hour Aromatherapy Certification Program consists of Aromatherapy Levels I through IV (covering such topics as specific indications and contraindicaitons; method of delivery of specific essential and carrier oils; basic biochemistry in relation to aromatherapy; blending; basic hand, foot and body reflexology techniques; legal and ethical office operations; and development of health products), Community First Aid/CPR, Medical Terminology, Anatomy and Physiology: A Holistic Model, and Therapeutic Communications. Case studies, client assessment, research material, and a written and practical exam are required for the certification process.

The 120-hour Botanical Health—Herbal Certification Program consists of Botanical Health Levels I through IV (covering such topics as herbs for health, basic precautions, legal and ethical aspects, wildcrafting, indications and contraindications, materia medica index study, assessment techniques, and creation of herbal formulas and compounds), Medical Terminology, Anatomy and Physiology: A Holistic Model, and Therapeutic Communications.

The seventy-seven-hour Holistic Nutrition Certification Program consists of Holistic Nutrition Levels I through III (covering such topics as basic nutrition guidelines; emotional relationships with food; eating according to blood type; food combining; overview of vitamins, antioxidants, herbs and personal supplementation; Ayurvedic theories and dosha balance; macrobiotic theories; assessing clients' nutritional needs; creating personal eating plans; and legal and ethical aspects) and Anatomy and Physiology: A Holistic Model.

The 129-hour Iridology Certification Program consists of Iridology Levels I through III (covering such topics as history of iridology, assessing hereditary weaknesses and strengths, interpreting iris topography, sclerology, metabolic pigments, protocols for reading the live eye and for iris photography, lighting techniques, and techniques for building a practice) and Anatomy and Physiology: A Holistic Model. The certification process involves written exams at each level plus an oral and practical exam in Level III.

The forty-two-hour Neurolinguistic Programming (NLP)—Practitioner Certification Program is an accelerated seven-day program in which participants will study and achieve the art of Human Excellence. Topics covered include developing rapport and a positive self-image, negotiating skills, conflict resolution, achievement of goals, nonverbal communication, and more.

Participants must review a library of twenty-four tapes by Dr. Tad James twice and successfully pass the pre-admission exam prior to the beginning of classes.

The forty-five-hour Non-Directive Imagery (NDI) Certification Program offers instruction in NDI, a therapeutic process utilized during trance work. Topics covered include Communication with Inner Advisor (Inner Guide), Dealing with Resistance, Polarities, Conflict Resolution, Search for Purpose, Death and Dying, Regression, Inner Child Work, and more.

The forty-hour Reiki Certification Program consists of Reiki Levels I through III (Master Level). Topics covered include the history and uses of Reiki, aspects of human energy systems, how to feel energy, hand placement, meaning and usage of symbols, absentee healing, Master symbols, legal issues, and more.

The sixty-four-hour Touch for Health Certification Program consists of Touch for Health Levels I through IV. Topics covered include balancing pairs of muscles that correspond with Chinese meridians; how to use massage points, holding points, meridians and muscle massage; food testing; language patterns; clearing reactive muscles; techniques for relieving pain; presentation of sound and color to enhance corrections; and more.

Admission Requirements

Certification program applicants must be at least 18 years of age, have a high school diploma, be of good moral character, submit a goal statement, and have a personal interview.

Tuition and Fees

There is a $20 application fee. Tuition for the Clinical Hypnotherapy certification program is $3,315 plus an additional $230 for books and supplies. Tuition for the Reflexology certification program is $2,970 plus an additional $200 for books and supplies.

Tuition and fees for the continuing education certification programs are as follows: Aromatherapy tuition $1,890, lab fees $60; Botanical Health tuition $1,800; Holistic Nutrition tuition $1,155; Iridology tuition $1,800; Neurolinguistic Programming tuition $1,595, tape library $375; Non-Directive Imagery tuition $675; Reiki tuition $730; Touch for Health tuition $900, books and supplies $65.

Financial Assistance

Scholarships, short-term OAH payment plans, and extended bank payment plans are available.

The Qigong and Human Life Research Foundation

Eastern Healing Arts International Training Center
Tian Enterprises, Inc.
2188 Vernon Road
Cleveland, Ohio 44118
PHONE: (800) 859-4343
FAX: (216) 932-2968
E-MAIL: te@modex.com
WEBSITE: www.qi-healing.com

The Qigong and Human Life Research Foundation (QHLRF) is dedicated to the dissemination of information about traditional Chinese qigong. The qigong tradition taught in this system is the Inner Dan Arts and Eastern Healing Technique, introduced to the United States in 1988 by Qigong Master Tianyou Hao. Master Hao has studied and practiced qigong for over fifty years. There are two instructors in the video/correspondence courses and for the three-day intensives; workshops can accommodate as many as fifty students. Students may also select private classes with Master Hao or one of his instructors. (For videos, see page 493.)

Program Description

The Inner Dan Arts' Qigong System focuses on prevention (health and longevity), mind power, and self-healing. The Eastern Healing Arts System focuses on provider-applied, hand Qi healing.

Certification programs to become an Inner Dan Arts Qigong Instructor or to become a Qi Healer are offered year-round as video/correspondence courses. Both programs are offered once a year as classroom intensives with home study, video/correspondence prerequisites.

Community and Continuing Education

Workshops in mind power and self-healing, qigong philosophy and relaxation, Eastern qi healing arts, and the Shao-lin stick healing techniques are offered periodically. Weekly scheduled offerings include Beginning/Intermediate, High I and II, and Super classes, Tai Chi, Qigong Therapy, and Diet Class.

Admission Requirements

Applicants should be in relatively good health.

Tuition and Fees

Tuition for Instructor or Healer video/correspondence courses is $1,250.

Tuition for a three-day Certified Qigong Instructor Intensive Training with video/correspondence prerequisite is $1,250, which includes all video/correspondence materials and three days' accommodations at the Holiday Inn, Cleveland, Ohio.

Tuition for the six-day Certified Qi Healer Intensive Training in Beijing, P.R. China, with video/correspondence prerequisite is $2,950, which includes all video/correspondence materials, tuition, transportation, accommodations, meals, and visiting in China with the cooperation of China Academy of Chinese Traditional Medicine and Beijing Massage Hospital.

SHI Integrative Medical Massage School

P.O. Box 474
130 Cook Road
Lebanon, Ohio 45036
PHONE: (513) 932-8712
FAX: (513) 932-8180
E-MAIL: shischool@aol.com

SHI Integrative Medical Massage School admitted its first students in 1981 and moved to its current location in 1989. There are ten instructors, with a maximum of fifty students per class.

Accreditation and Approvals

The massage program at SHI is approved by the State Medical Board of Ohio for Massage Therapy, and is a member of the AMTA Council of Schools. Graduates are qualified to take the National Certification Examination for Therapeutic Massage and Bodywork (NCETMB).

Program Description

The 600+-hour massage program is available in two formats: the eighteen-month program, which meets for eight hours per week, and the twelve-month program, which meets for fourteen hours per week.

The curriculum is divided into two tracks of study: Anatomy/Physiology and Massage. The Massage curriculum includes Current Psychological Issues, History of Massage, Draping, Terminology, Palpatory Skills, Medical History Taking, Business Practices, and Review for the Ohio State Board exam. Additional hours outside of class are required for both programs. Required weekend courses include Myofascial Therapy, Touch Pro® Chair Massage, Business Practices, Ohio Law for the Professional Massage Therapist, Integrative Medical Massage for the Professional Massage Therapist, and twelve hours of cadaver study. Students must provide therapeutic massage with a preceptor and complete twenty contact hours at an approved outreach site. Students must also complete an Adult CPR/First Aid course prior to graduation.

Admission Requirements

To qualify for admission to the eighteen-month program, applicants should have a high school diploma or equivalent with an overall GPA if 2.5 or better, or have a college GPA of 2.0 or better with a Science GPA of 2.25 or better. Applicants with no science background or a GPA of less than 2.5 may be required to complete a college level course in Human Anatomy/Physiology and/or Medical Terminology prior to being considered for admission.

To qualify for admission to the twelve-month program, applicants should meet all of the requirements for admission to the eighteen-month program plus a minimum of two years of college with a GPA of 2.25 or better, or hold a degree or be employed or have prior employment in an allied health field, Science, Psychology, Education, etc.

All applicants must submit two professional references, a personal history form, and documentation of all legal name changes, and have a personal interview.

Tuition and Fees

Tuition is $6,200. Additional expenses include application fee, $60; estimated books/lab fee, $425; massage table, $400 to $800; five required preceptor massages, $225 to $275; supplies additional.

Financial Assistance

Payment plans are available.

Touch for Health Kinesiology Association

(See Multiple State Locations, pages 415-16)

OKLAHOMA

Oklahoma School of Natural Healing

1660 East 71st Suite 2-O
Tulsa, Oklahoma 74136-5191
PHONE: (918) 496-9401 / (800) 496-9401
FAX: (918) 496-4461
E-MAIL: healing01@sprynet.com

The Oklahoma School of Natural Healing was founded in 1980 by director Robert L. Groves. It is the state's oldest operating licensed school of massage therapy. There are ten instructors; class sizes average twelve to twenty students.

Accreditation and Approvals

The Oklahoma School of Natural Healing has been licensed since 1988. Graduates of the 650- and 1,000-hour programs are qualified to take the National Certification Examination for Therapeutic Massage and Bodywork (NCETMB).

Program Description

The 250-hour Massage Technician Program meets schooling requirements for a City of Tulsa license. Courses include Anatomy and Physiology I and II, Polarity Therapy, Reflexology, Swedish Massage I and II, Business Skills, and 110 hours of Practicum.

The 650-hour Massage Therapist Program includes all of the above courses, as well as Nutrition, Myofascial Release, Hydro/Heliotherapy, Acupressure, Herbology, Deep Tissue Therapies, and 250 hours of Practicum.

The 1,000-hour Master Therapist Course includes all of the Technician and Therapist courses plus Polarity Therapy 1 through 6 (Associate (A.P.P.) level training); the Ortho-Bionomy series of Spine, Extremities, Chapman Reflexes and Advanced; Dalton Myoskeletal Technique; Herbology II; and

Nutrition II, with a total of 260 hours of Practicum. Any of these classes may be substituted for other advanced classes offered such as Homeopathy, On-site Massage, Accelerated Healing Workshop (Taws), Iridology, or any other advanced level course offered at the school to total the necessary hours.

Community and Continuing Education
The school offers a variety of community education courses and advanced training workshops.

Admission Requirements
Applicants must be over 18 years of age, have a high school diploma or GED, be of good moral character, submit a physician's statement of health, and interview with the director.

Tuition and Fees
There is a $25 application fee. The total cost of the 250-hour Massage Technician Program is $1,999, including tuition, books, table, and supplies. The total cost of the 650-hour Massage Therapist Program is $4,235, including tuition, books, table, and supplies. Tuition for the 1,000-hour Master Therapist Course depends on courses selected; the estimated range is $8,000 to $10,000.

Financial Assistance
A prepayment discount is available on professional programs; limited government assistance is available through JPTA or the Department of Vocational Rehabilitation.

Praxis College of Health Arts and Sciences

808 NW 88
Oklahoma City, Oklahoma 73114-2511
PHONE: (405) 949-2244 / (405) 879-0224
FAX: (405) 946-7040

Praxis College was founded in 1988. The school operates a 10,000-square-foot Wellness Center where students provide massage therapy to the public. On-campus student housing is available.

Accreditation and Approvals
Praxis College is licensed by the Oklahoma Board of Private Vocational Schools. Graduates are qualified to take the National

Certification Examination for Therapeutic Massage and Bodywork (NCETMB).

Program Description
The 1,200-hour Certified Massage Therapist Program includes courses in Fundamentals of Professional Practice, Business Ethics, Medical Research, Pathology/Nutrition, Hydrotherapy, Human Performance, Athletic Massage, Psychotherapeutic Massage, Oriental Massage, and Energy Field Massage.

A 500-hour Associate Massage Technician Program prepares students to work in an entry-level position for a certified massage therapist, chiropractor, or physical therapist. Topics covered in this program include basic sports massage, full-body massage, chair massage, reflexology, and beginning skills to safely practice massage. Praxis guarantees that students who complete this program will pass the national certification exam or tuition will be refunded.

Admission Requirements
Admission requirements vary with each program; contact the admissions office for specific information.

Tuition and Fees
Tuition for the 1,200-hour program is $3,000; books and supplies are approximately $300. Tuition for the 500-hour program is $500, including books.

Financial Assistance
Interest-free loans, work-study, and scholarships are available.

OREGON
The American Herbal Institute

3056 Lancaster Drive NE
Salem, Oregon 97305
PHONE: (503) 364-7242
FAX: (503) 585-5995
E-MAIL: raw2103@aol.com
WEBSITE: www.herbsinc.com

The American Herbal Institute (TAHI) was founded in 1992 by Constance and Richard Walker; in 1990 and 1991, TAHI's courses were taught for the National Health Care Institute in Salem. There are seven instructors, with an average of ten (maximum fifteen) students per class. The institute also offers a correspondence course (see page 473).

Program Description

A course in Modern Herbal Studies may be taken for either a Certified Modern Herbalist certificate (139.5 credit hours) or an Advanced Modern Herbalist certificate (154 credit hours).

Required courses for the Certified Modern Herbalist Program include Herbology I through III, Nutrition I, Anatomy/Physiology, Remedies Lab, and two Alternative Modalities seminars.

To earn the Advanced Modern Herbalist Certificate, in addition to the requirements above, students must also complete Herbology IV, Nutrition II, Reflexology, Homeopathy, Field Studies, Independent Master Studies, and three Alternative Modalities seminars.

Classes are held in the evenings at the Herb Lady store.

Admission Requirements

Classes are open to everyone.

Tuition and Fees

Tuition for the Certified Modern Herbalist course is $1,855 and includes books. Tuition for the Advanced Modern Herbalist course is $2,100 and includes books.

Financial Assistance

Payment plans are available.

Animal Natural Health Center

The ANHC Course in Veterinary Homeopathy
1283 Lincoln Street
Eugene, Oregon 97401
PHONE: (541) 342-7665 / (888) 290-8454
FAX: (541) 344-5356
WEBSITE: anhc@pacinfo.com

The Animal Natural Health Center conducts the most extensive accredited training in Veterinary Homeopathy in the United States. Dr. Richard Pitcairn is the primary instructor; there are thirty to sixty students per class.

Accreditation

The ANHC Course in Veterinary Homeopathy is accredited by the Academy of Veterinary Homeopathy.

Program Description

The ANHC Course in Veterinary Homeopathy consists of five four-day sessions about two months apart. The course covers how to take and analyze cases, use repertories and material medica, select remedies and potencies, evaluate responses, and manage both chronic and acute diseases. A comprehensive workbook and extensive case examples are included. Students must complete homework between sessions.

Continuing Education

ANHC offers advanced training in veterinary homeopathy; contact the office for details.

Tuition and Fees

Tuition is approximately $2,500.

Financial Assistance

A payment plan is available.

Ashland Massage Institute

P.O. Box 1233
Ashland, Oregon 97520
PHONE/FAX: (541) 482-5134
E-MAIL: massage@jeffnet.org

The Ashland Massage Institute (AMI) was founded in 1988. AMI cofounder and director Beth Hoffman has studied massage and bodywork since 1979 and has been a practicing massage therapist since 1983. There are fifteen instructors; class sizes range from fifteen to twenty-six students, with a maximum 1:7 teacher:student ratio during technique classes.

Accreditation and Approvals

AMI is licensed by the Oregon Department of Education and the professional massage program is certified by the Oregon

Board of Massage Technicians. Graduates are qualified to take the National Certification Examination for Therapeutic Massage and Bodywork (NCETMB).

Program Description

The 550-hour Massage Prelicensing Program may be completed in one or two years. Classes include Swedish Massage and Fundamentals, Core Communication Skills, Thai Massage and the Healer's Art, Oriental Bodywork, Polarity, Shiatsu, Myofascial Trigger Point Therapy, Counterstrain Technique, Introduction to Deep Tissue, Hydrotherapy, Business and Ethics, Clinical Experience, Observational Forum, Massage for Specific Conditions, and Practical Review, plus the health sciences of Kinesiology, Anatomy and Physiology, and Pathology. Students must receive two professional massages and complete CPR training at a local hospital or Red Cross center.

Community and Continuing Education

One- and two-day classes offered to members of the community include Introduction to Massage, Introduction to Shiatsu, Shiatsu Stretch Massage, and Timeless Face.

One- and two-day classes offered to the massage professional include Introduction to Shiatsu; Introduction to Myofascial Release; Shiatsu Stretch Massage; Mindful Touch; Timeless Face I, II, and III; and Functional Assessment in Massage Therapy. In addition, a three-day Infant Massage Instructor Training Program prepares nurses, physical therapists, massage therapists, and other professionals to conduct the Loving Touch Parent-Infant Massage Program for parents with newborns.

Admission Requirements

Applicants must be at least 18 years of age, submit a completed application form and transcripts, and interview with an admissions representative.

Tuition and Fees

Tuition for the Professional Massage Program is $4,850. Additional expenses include application fee, $50; books, approximately $265; massage table, $400 to $550; two professional massages, $70 to $90; and linens and oil, approximately $20.

Financial Assistance

A payment plan and veterans' benefits are available.

The Australasian College of Herbal Studies

P.O. Box 130
530 First Street, Suite A
Lake Oswego, Oregon 97034
PHONE: (503) 635-6652 / (800) 487-8839
FAX: (503) 636-0706
E-MAIL: achs@herbed.com
WEBSITE: www.herbed.com

Founded in New Zealand in 1978, the Australasian College of Herbal Studies, USA (ACHS) opened in 1991. Formerly exclusively a correspondence school, the college began offering residential modules in Aromatherapy in 1999; see page 462 for correspondence programs. There are two primary instructors for the residential modules with guest lecturers for specific classes; the maximum class size is fifteen.

Accreditation and Approvals

ACHS is licensed with the Oregon Department of Education as a Private Career School and is in compliance with the Oregon Office of Degree Authorization. ACHS courses do not offer transferable or postsecondary credit in the United States at this time. ACHS is approved as a provider of continuing education credits by the AMTA, the Oregon Board of Pharmacy, the Oregon Board of Veterinary Examiners, and the California Board of Registered Nursing.

Program Description

Thus far seven Residential Aromatherapy Modules have been developed. These modules are Aroma 301: Aromatherapy Repertoire and Blending, Aroma 302: Clinical Considerations and Case Studies, Aroma 303: Contraindications and Safety Data, Aroma 304: Natural Health Consulting, Aroma 305: Aromatherapy Chemistry, Aroma 306: Advanced Aromatherapy Repertoire and Blending, and Aroma 307: Aromatherapy Summer School in Provence, France. Aroma 301 through Aroma 306 meet for twenty hours over a weekend; none has a prerequisite. Aroma 307 is held over eight days. Credit is granted toward the Diploma in Aromatherapy.

Admission Requirements

A working knowledge of English is advised.

Tuition and Fees

Tuition for Aroma 301 through Aroma 306 is $15 per credit hour or $300 per module; materials fees are additional. Aroma 307 is $1,800 and includes accommodations, three meals per day, transfers, instruction, tours and trips.

Financial Assistance

Payment plans, an annual scholarship, and Salle Mae Student Loans are available.

Birthingway Midwifery School

4620 North Maryland
Portland, Oregon 97217
PHONE/FAX: (503) 282-5729

The Midwifery Education Program of Birthingway Midwifery Center, Inc., was established in 1993. There are fifteen instructors and guest lecturers; classes are usually limited to nine students.

Accreditation and Approvals

Birthingway Midwifery School is currently in pre-accreditation status with the Midwifery Education Accreditation Council (MEAC) and expects to receive full accreditation in 1999. Upon completion of all midwifery program components, students should have sufficient classroom and clinical knowledge to meet examination and experiential requirements for national (NARM) professional certification and Oregon state licensure as a direct-entry midwife. Other states may have additional clinical requirements; contact the school for more information.

Program Description

Degrees and certifications offered at Birthingway are as follows:

The Certificate in Midwifery requires 158 credit hours in Midwifery Core courses, Midwifery Supplemental courses, and Midwifery Practicum. The Bachelor of Arts in Midwifery requires completion of the Certificate in Midwifery plus twenty-four credit hours from an accredited college or university in English, General Psychology, Humanities, and Liberal Arts courses. The Bachelor of Science in Midwifery requires completion of the Certificate in Midwifery plus twenty-four credit hours from an accredited college or university in English, General Psychology, and Science courses. The Childbirth Educator Certification requires twenty-three credit hours in Midwifery Core courses plus Childbirth Educator Practicum. The Labor Doula Certification requires twenty-seven credit hours in Midwifery Core courses, the Labor Doula course and Practicum, and Emergency Resuscitation. Postpartum Doula Certification requires seventeen credit hours in a Doula course and Practicum, and courses in Breastfeeding, Infancy, and Emergency Resuscitation.

Midwifery Core courses include Antepartum, Intrapartum, Postpartum, Microbiology, Botanicals, Well-Woman Gynecology, Human Genetics, Midwifery Management of Complex Situations, Advanced Skills, Psychosocial Issues and Skills, and Professional Issues. Midwifery Supplemental courses include Breastfeeding, Childbirth Education, Community Resources, Community Service, Doula: Postpartum and Infant Care, Emergency Resuscitation, Infancy, The Labor Doula: Assisting Women with Births, Medical Terminology, Practice Protocols and Risk Assessment, Research Project, Signs and Symptoms, and Synergistic Therapeutics. Practicums are offered in Childbirth Educator, Doula Practicum, Midwifery Practicum, and Labor Doula Practicum.

In addition, for the Midwifery Certificate or Degree, the student must have a passing score on the Comprehensive Exam given after the third year; documentation of midwifery skills; demonstration of Midwifery Integration (the ability to weave together judgment, knowledge, skills, clinical assessment, decision-making, perceptions, and intuition into appropriate action plans); and completion and documentation of clinical requirements which consist of: participant in twenty-five out-of-hospital births, five hospital births, and twenty-five prenatal exams; primary role in twenty-five births, seventy-five prenatal exams, twenty-five newborn exams, and forty postpartum exams; and continuity of care on twenty primary clients.

Admission Requirements

Applicants must have a high school diploma or equivalent and demonstrate proficiency in the English language. Prior to admission, potential students must take a course in Human

Anatomy and Physiology, earning a grade of least B. Students who have not taken this course may meet the requirement by taking Anatomy and Physiology for Midwifery Students offered at Birthingway.

Tuition and Fees

Tuition for the Midwifery Program is $5,000 for the first year, $4,000 for the second year, and $3,000 for the third year. Additional expenses include application fee, $50; annual registration fee, $200; practicum fee, $10 per credit hour. The bachelor's degree evaluation fee is $100.

Financial Assistance

Payment plans and limited work-study positions are available.

Brighid's Academy of Healing Arts

22711 Highway 36
Cheshire, Oregon 97419
PHONE: (541) 998-7986
E-MAIL: gina@herbalism.net
WEBSITE: www.herbalism.net/brighid

Brighid's Academy of Healing Arts was founded in 1997 by Gina McGarry, who has been a professional herbalist for twenty years and a former director of both the California School of Herbal Studies and the Oregon School of Herbal Studies. McGarry is the primary instructor, with local, national and international guests; class sizes average eight to ten students.

Accreditation and Approvals

Students may earn credits toward degree work through an alliance with Evergreen College.

Program Description

The 450-hour, nine-month Professional Herbalist Training Course consists of three trimesters and may be completed on either a weekday or weekend schedule. First Trimester: Foundations covers The Philosophies and Roots of Healing, The Healers Disciplines, Holistic Perspectives of Disease and Wellness, Creating an Organic Medicinal Garden, Wildcrafting and Botany of Medicinals, Medicine Making and Green Pharmacology, and Materia Medica, Materia Magica. The Second Trimester: Intermediate includes Anatomy and Physiology of the Human Body, Empowerment and Self-Esteem, and Therapeutic Applications of Herbal Medicines. The Third Trimester: Advanced covers Becoming a Professional Herbalist, Client Consultation Techniques and Protocol, Bookkeeping, Manufacturing and Authoring, Ceremony and Ritual for Healing, Complementary Medicine, and Maintenance Herbalism.

The seventy-five-hour Celtic Herbcraft Course meets one evening per week for eight months. The program is based on Celtic-European traditions and includes courses in The Philosophies and Roots of Healing, Human Anatomy and Physiology, the systems of the body, Wildcrafting and Botany of Medicinals, The Healer's Disciplines, Creating an Organic Medicinal Garden, Green Pharmacy, Holistic Perspectives of Disease and Wellness, and Materia Medica, Materia Magica, plus scientific data and esoteric and folk knowledge. These coursework hours may be applied toward the Professional Herbalist program requirements.

Community and Continuing Education

A variety of other workshops and symposium are offered.

Admission Requirements

Applicants must complete an application form and have an interview.

Tuition and Fees

Tuition for the Professional Herbalist Program is $3,300. Tuition for Celtic Herbcraft is $700.

Financial Assistance

Payment arrangements are available.

Cascade Institute of Massage and Body Therapies

1250 Charnelton Street
Eugene, Oregon 97401
PHONE: (541) 687-8101
FAX: (541) 687-0285

The Cascade Institute of Massage and Body Therapies (CIMBT) was founded in 1988 by Ruth and Tracy Wise. Ruth

Wise is an R.N. with twenty years of private practice as a massage therapist. There are twenty instructors, with a maximum of twenty students per class.

Accreditation and Approvals

CIMBT is certified by the Oregon Massage Technicians' Licensing Board, licensed by the Oregon Department of Education as a private vocational school, approved by the Washington State Massage Licensing Board, and a member of the American Massage Therapy Association (AMTA) Council of Schools. Graduates are qualified to take the National Certification Examination for Therapeutic Massage and Bodywork (NCETMB).

Program Description

The curriculum for the 565-hour Professional Training Program for Oregon State licensing may be completed in one or two years. Courses include Anatomy and Physiology, Kinesiology, Massage (which covers Swedish, Advanced Swedish, Acupressure Energetics, Deep Tissue Muscle Sculpting, Trigger Point Therapy, Myofascial Release, Proprioseptive Neuromuscular Facilitation (PNF), Posture Basics, Pain Assessment, and Energy Awareness), Massage Clinic, Community Outreach, Pathology, Hydrotherapy, Hydrotherapy-Experiential, CPR, Ethics, Professional Development, Written Exam Review and Practical Exam Review. Classes are held mornings or evenings and some Saturdays.

Continuing Education

Classes are offered to licensed massage professionals in such areas as Muscle Sculpting Bodywork, Shiatsu, Human Cadaver Lab, Myofascial Release, On-Site Massage, and Functional Assessment in Massage Therapy. Additional classes are offered on an ongoing basis.

Admission Requirements

Applicants must be at least 18 years of age; have a high school diploma or equivalent; be capable of financing their education; have received two professional massages; submit an essay, two letters of recommendation, and a letter from a doctor, naturopath, or chiropractor verifying that the applicant is in good health; and interview with an admissions representative.

Tuition and Fees

There is a $150 registration fee. Tuition is $4,970; books and supplies are approximately $250 to $400; three professional massages cost $75 to $135; and a massage table costs (average) $400.

Financial Assistance

A payment plan, veterans' benefits, and state-funded programs are available. A discount is given for early registration.

Center for Herbal Studies

86437 Lorane Highway
Eugene, Oregon 97405
PHONE: (541) 484-6708
E-MAIL: chs@cpplus1.com
WEBSITE: www.cpplus1.com/~chs

The Center for Herbal Studies, founded in 1993 by Cherie Capps, offers on-site classes that are nearly identical to her correspondence program (see page 474). Capps is the only instructor; classes average ten to twelve students.

Program Description

The on-site and correspondence program are each comprised of two courses: the Herbal Studies Diploma and the Clinical Herbology Diploma.

The Herbal Studies Diploma Program consists of two units. Unit I covers Basic Herbal Concepts, Harvesting and Preserving, Historical Perspectives, Legal Issues, Herbal Studies, and Herbal Preparations. Unit II covers Herbal Actions, Botany, Herbal Constituents, Herb Study/Walks, and Course Review.

The Clinical Herbology Diploma consists of two units. Unit I covers Healthy Herbs and Foods, Monitoring the Healing Process, Tissue Cleansing, Nutrition: Vitamins and Minerals, Hydrotherapy, Body Cells and Tissues, and Pharmocokinetics. Unit II consists of eighteen lessons covering the nine major body systems, the immune system, cancer, and treatments using natural therapies.

Tuition and Fees

Tuition for the Herbal Studies Diploma program is $120 for

Unit I and $180 for Unit II. Tuition for the Clinical Herbology Diploma Program is $120 for Unit I and $540 for Unit II.

East-West College of the Healing Arts

4531 SE Belmont Street
Portland, Oregon 97215-1635
PHONE: (503) 231-1500 / (800) 635-9141
FAX: (503) 232-4087
WEBSITE: www.ewcha.com

East-West College of the Healing Arts (EWC) was founded in 1972 as the Midway School of Massage. The college was purchased in 1981 by its current owner, David Slawson. There are eleven instructors; class sizes average sixteen students in massage classes, twenty-four in science classes.

Accreditation and Approvals

EWC is accredited by the Commission on Massage Training Accreditation (COMTA), and approved by the Oregon Massage Licensing Board, the Washington Massage Licensing Board, and the Oregon Department of Education. Graduates are qualified to take the National Certification Examination for Therapeutic Massage and Bodywork (NCETMB).

Program Description

EWC offers both 529-hour and 661-hour Massage Training Programs.

The 529-hour program consists of four academic terms. Courses include Anatomy/Physiology, Kinesiology, Pathology, Massage I: Swedish Massage, Massage II: Massage and Movement, Hydrotherapy, Clinical Practices, and two electives chosen from Craniosacral Massage, Deep Tissue Massage, Massage for Common Injuries, Myofascial Massage, Shiatsu, Sports Massage, and Thai Massage.

The 661-hour program is identical to the 529-hour program with the addition of two elective choices (132 hours), which may be taken in quarters 2–4 or in additional quarters.

Students must also have current First Aid/CPR certification prior to graduation; EWC offers a First Aid/CPR course once per term (at additional cost). In order to apply for a Washington massage license, students must have completed an approved course in AIDS education; EWC offers an authorized audiotape course (at additional cost) to fulfill this requirement.

Admission Requirements

Applicants must be at least 18 years of age, have a high school diploma or GED, have a passing score on the EWC entrance exam, provide proof of receiving one professional Swedish massage, provide a written health clearance, and have a personal interview.

Tuition and Fees

Tuition for the Massage Training programs is $9.90 per clock hour. Tuition plus linen fee for the 529-hour program is $5,437; tuition plus linen fee for the 661-hour program is $6,824. Additional expenses include a $100 application fee; books, $100 to $400; professional treatments, $30 to $60 per session; and massage table.

Financial Assistance

Term and monthly payment plans and full-pay discounts are available.

National College of Naturopathic Medicine

49 SW Porter
Portland, Oregon 97201
PHONE: (503) 499-4343
FAX: (503) 499-0027
E-MAIL: admissions@ncnm.edu
WEBSITE: www.ncnm.edu

Clinic Address:
11231 SE Market Street
Portland, Oregon

The National College of Naturopathic Medicine was founded in 1956 and is the oldest accredited naturopathic school in North America. There are fifty-two full-time and adjunct instructors; class sizes range from up to 120 for lecture to as few as twenty for labs.

Accreditation

National College is accredited by the Council on Naturopathic Medical Education (CNME) and recognized by all state and provincial boards of naturopathic examiners, as well as by the Council of Education of the Canadian Naturopathic Association. The Homeopathic Medicine Certificate Program (part of the N.D. Program) is accredited by the Council on Homeopathic Education (CHE). The Master of Science in Oriental Medicine Program is a candidate for accreditation with the Accreditation Commission for Acupuncture and Oriental Medicine (ACAOM); graduates of this program are eligible to apply for licensure in the state of Oregon and to take both the herb and acupuncture exams administered by the National Certification Commission for Acupuncture and Oriental Medicine (NCCAOM).

Program Description

The four-year, 4,500-hour Doctor of Naturopathy (N.D.) graduate medical program prepares students for state board licensing examinations and the practice of naturopathic medicine. The first two years focus on the standard medical sciences and the history and philosophy of naturopathic medicine. In the third and fourth years, students receive clinical training in diagnosis and naturopathic therapeutics. The N.D. program may also be taken over five years.

The First Year Curriculum includes courses in Anatomy, Gross Anatomy Lab, Physiology, Biochemistry, Medical Histology, Naturopathic Medical Philosophy and Therapeutics, Hydrotherapy, Palpation, Psychology and Counseling, Skills of Communication, Embryology, Neuroanatomy, Microbiology, Research and Statistics, Immunology, Pathology, Psychological Assessment, and Introduction to Clinic.

Second Year Courses include Chinese Medicine, Clinical/Physical Diagnosis, Lab Diagnosis, Pharmacology, Public Health, Clinical Case Presentations, Physiotherapy, Botanical Materia Medica, Homeopathy, Naturopathic Manipulative Therapy, Clinic Education, Nutrition, and others.

Among the Third Year Courses are Diagnostic Imaging, Gynecology, Obstetrics, Clinic Grand Rounds, Clinic Medicinary Practicum, Clinic Lab Practicum, Doctor Patient Relations, Office Orthopedics, Minor Surgery with Lab, Gastroenterology, Environmental Medicine, Cardiology, Pediatrics, First Aid and Emergency Medicine, and others.

Fourth Year Courses include Eye, Ears, Nose and Throat, Clinic X-Ray Practicum, Clinic Field Observation, Dermatology, Endocrinology, Geriatrics, Stress Management, Exercise Therapeutics, Neurology, Urology, Proctology, Business Practice Seminar, Counseling Technique with Lab, Medical Genetics, Jurisprudence and Medical Ethics, Oncology, and more.

Several elective courses are offered each term. The Homeopathic Medicine Certificate Program includes four sequential electives that supplement the required courses in homeopathic medicine. The Naturopathic Obstetrical Certificate Program includes six sequential elective courses. Additional electives are offered in Advanced Minor Surgery, Chronic Viral Disease, Colonics, Northwest Herbs, Natural Pharmacology, Somatic Re-Education, and Clinical Case Presentation.

The three-year, 2,172-hour Master of Science in Oriental Medicine (MSOM) Program is a second-degree program for M.D.s, D.O.s, D.C.s, and anyone who has already taken post-graduate medical sciences and clinical and physical diagnosis. The course of study emphasizes the holistic spirit of the classic teachings of Oriental Medicine. Topics covered include history and philosophy of Oriental medicine; an introduction to the classics and the physicians that introduced the theories or therapeutic methods in question; prescription of herbal formulas; therapeutics exercises (qi gong); and the application of acupuncture, moxibustion, and traditional bodywork techniques.

National College offers a six-year program of study that combines both the N.D. and M.S.O.M. degrees. N.D. students in their second year of study are eligible to apply for the M.S.O.M. program.

Admission Requirements

Applicants to the Doctor of Naturopathy program must have a bachelor's degree from an accredited college with a minimum GPA of 2.5. Students must have completed 20 semester credits of premedical chemistry and biology, one college-level course in physics, six semester credits in the social sciences (including one course in psychology), and six semester credits of humanities, all with a grade of C or better. Preparatory work in anatomy and physiology is also useful. Applicants must submit two letters of recommendation and interview with an admissions representative.

Tuition and Fees
Tuition for the full-time, four-year N.D. track is $14,800 per year. There is a $60 application fee; books and supplies are estimated at $1,310 per year.

Financial Assistance
Federal loans, private scholarships, veterans' benefits, and work-study are available.

Oregon College of Oriental Medicine

10525 SE Cherry Blossom Drive
Portland, Oregon 97216
PHONE: (503) 253-3443
FAX: (503) 253-2701
E-MAIL: lpowell@teleport.com
WEBSITE:www.infinite.org/oregon.acupuncture

The Oregon College of Oriental Medicine (OCOM) was founded in 1983 by licensed acupuncturists Eric Stephens and Satya Ambrose. There are seven full-time and twenty-four part-time instructors, with an average class size of sixty students.

Accreditation and Approvals
The master's degree program in acupuncture and Oriental medicine at OCOM is accredited by the Accreditation Commission for Acupuncture and Oriental Medicine (ACAOM). After passing the National Certification Commission for Acupuncture and Oriental Medicine (NCCAOM) exam, NCCAOM diplomates are eligible to apply to the Oregon State Board of Medical Examiners for Oregon licensing; graduates also successfully apply for licensing in many other states, including California.

Program Description
The four-academic-year Master of Acupuncture and Oriental Medicine Degree Program may be completed in three calendar years.

The first year includes instruction in Traditional Chinese Medical Theory, Point and Channel Location, Medical History: East and West, Living Anatomy, Tui Na, Shiatsu, Western Medical Terminology, Qigong, Anatomy and Physiology, Chinese Herbal Medicine: The Pharmacopoeia, Case Observation and Demonstration, and more.

The second year covers such topics as TCM Pathology and Therapeutics, Point Actions and Indications, Public Health: Community Health and Chemical Dependency, Tai Chi Chuan, Advanced Qigong, Western Medical Pathology, Chinese Herbal Medicine: Formulas, Auricular Acupuncture, Topics in Clinical Research, Dynamics of Illness, and more.

The third year includes Survey of Western Physics, Clinical Internship, Seminar and Section, Herbal Patent Medicine, Jin Shin Do, Structural Diagnosis/Meridian Therapy, Research Practicum, Western Clinical Diagnosis, Diet and Nutrition, Clinical Herbal Internship, Western Pharmacology, Ethics and Practice Management, Introduction to Issues in Public Health, and Community Health Internship.

Admission Requirements
Applicants must have completed at least three years of college (ninety semester credits) at an accredited institution; OCOM recommends that students have completed four years of college. The applicant must have completed college-level courses in general biology, chemistry, and psychology; it is recommended that the applicant also have completed college-level anatomy and physiology. Applicants must submit two personal essays and two letters of recommendation, and have a personal interview.

Tuition and Fees
Tuition is $8,516 per year. Additional expenses include application fee, $50; orientation fee, $50; and books and lab expenses of $75 to $200 per quarter. Total estimated cost for the entire program is $31,500.

Financial Assistance
A payment plan, federal grants and loans, and work-study are available.

Oregon School of Massage

9500 SW Barbur Boulevard #100
Portland, Oregon 97219
PHONE: (503) 244-3420 / (503) 244-1815
FAX: (503) 244-1815
E-MAIL: osm@teleport.com
WEBSITE: OregonSchoolofMassage.com

The Oregon School of Massage was founded in 1984. There are fifteen instructors ; maximum class sizes are sixteen for hands-on classes, twenty-four for lecture classes.

Accreditation and Approvals

The Massage Certificate program has been approved by the Oregon Board of Massage Technicians and by the Washington State Department of Health Massage Program, and prepares the graduate for licensure in Oregon and Washington. Graduates are qualified to take the National Certification Examination for Therapeutic Massage and Bodywork (NCETMB).

Program Description

The 555-hour Massage Certificate program consists of a core curriculum, which includes courses in Anatomy and Physiology, Kinesiology, Pathology, Massage, Hydrotherapy, and Clinic, and 135 hours of electives, which may include Foot Reflexology, Shiatsu, On-Site Massage, Polarity, Deep Tissue, Sports Massage, Body Rock Massage, Side-Lying Massage, Pregnancy Massage, and/or Marketing. Courses in First Aid/ CPR and HIV/AIDS may be required for state licensing; these courses are available at OSM for an additional cost. Students are required to have several professional massages prior to and during training.

Community and Continuing Education

Three-hour Training Previews are held throughout the year and serve as an overview of the profession for prospective applicants.

OSM offers a variety of continuing education courses, including Thai Massage, Massage in a Hospital Setting, ABCs of Chinese Medicine, Spanish Conversation for LMTs, Nutrition, Ecstatic Dance, Chiropractic Assistant Training, Intro to Alexander Technique, Massage for People with Cancer, and more. Courses range from 6.5 to 45 CEUs.

Admission Requirements

Applicants must have a high school diploma or equivalent; one or more years of college is recommended. Applicants must be at least 18 years of age and must have received at least three professional massages during the two years prior to the beginning of training.

Tuition and Fees

Tuition for the 555-hour program ranges from $5,750 to $6,290, depending on payment plan selected. Additional expenses include books, approximately $250; application fee, $100; massage table, $250 to $650 or more; professional massages; oils, sheets, blankets and bolsters.

There is no charge for Training Previews.

Tuition for continuing education courses ranges from $60 to $395.

Financial Assistance

Payment-in-full and early payments discounts, payment plans, and student loans are available.

Oregon School of Midwifery

342 East 12th Avenue
Eugene, Oregon 97401
PHONE: (541) 338-9778 / (888) 815-9692
FAX: (541) 338-9783
E-MAIL: info@oregonmidwifery.org
WEBSITE: www.oregonmidwifery.org

The Oregon School of Midwifery (OSM) was founded in 1993 by Daphne Singingtree, who has been practicing and teaching midwifery since 1974; she is also an author, editor, and founding member of the Oregon Midwifery Council. There are six instructors, with an average of twelve to sixteen students per class. In addition to midwifery training described here, OSM offers comprehensive, certified courses for birth doulas (professional labor support) and postpartum doulas (maternal/child home care providers).

Accreditation and Approvals

OSM is accredited by the Midwifery Education Accreditation Council (MEAC) and meets the standards of education currently set by the Midwives Alliance of North America (MANA) core competencies and the Oregon State Health Division Board of Direct Entry Midwifery. Graduates are eligible to take the Oregon State licensing exam to become a Licensed Direct Entry Midwife and the Certified Professional Midwife (CPM) exam.

Program Description

The three-year, eighty-five-credit Midwifery Program is a combination of classes, self-study and research, community service placement, labor support in the hospital, and supervised internship or apprenticeship in out-of-hospital birth practices. Classes are held two days per week for three eleven-week terms for two years; summer classes are independent study. Outside requirements include a series of childbirth education classes, a La Leche series, and a human anatomy and physiology course; these may be completed before beginning the Midwifery program.

The First Year Curriculum covers such topics as History, Politics, and Ethics of Midwifery; Birth in Various Cultures; Medical Terminology; Reproductive Anatomy and Physiology; Ovulation and Menstruation; Basic Genetics; Embryology and Fetal Development; Principles and Applications of Nutrition; Obstetric Anatomy; Normal Pregnancy Physiology; Use of Herbs and Homeopathics; Prenatal Care, PAP Smears and GYN Exams; Normal Labor; Labor Support; Pain Relief and Comfort Measures; Childbirth Education; Cesarean and VBAC Support; Venipuncture; Fetal Monitoring; Placenta and Third Stage; Communication and Counseling Skills; Sexuality; Newborn; and Lactation.

The Second Year Curriculum includes Microbiology; Research and Statistics; Reproductive and GYN Pathology and Abnormalities; STDs; AIDS; Infertility; Repeated Pregnancy Loss; Complications of Pregnancy; Labor and Delivery Complications; Placental Pathology; Complications in Third Stage; Suturing; Pharmacology; Shock; Principles and Use of IVS; Use of Urinary Catheters; Pathology of the Neonate; Advanced Neonatal Resuscitation; Lactation Disorders; Perinatal and Neonatal Death; Family Planning; Families in Crisis; and Setting Up a Midwifery Practice.

The third year is clinical training or apprenticeship with an independent study component.

A Distance Learning Program is offered to those who already have a preceptor (midwife) who is willing to provide the clinical part of their training. The program integrates apprenticeship with structured academics offered by a combination of print, audio, video, e-mail, and Internet usage. It is not a work-at-your-own-pace home study course; specific timelines for assignments and tests are required. Students are required to come to Eugene once a year for five days of intensive workshops.

Admission Requirements:

Criteria for admission is based primarily on evidence of commitment to direct entry midwifery. In addition, applicants must have a high school diploma or GED; demonstrate proficiency in the English language; have completed a human anatomy and physiology course within the last seven years; show documentation of a current negative TB test; and complete a DONA approved labor support doula course (offered by OSM, may be taken concurrently the first year).

Tuition and Fees

Tuition is $150 per credit or $12,750 for the program. Additional expenses include a $65 application fee; registration fee, $150; books, $200 to $250 per term; and material/lab fees, $40 to $60 per term. Third-year fees vary depending on the clinical site chosen; budget about $2,000 for a high-volume site. In order to keep tuition as low as possible, all students are required to put in two hours per week doing OSM office work; additional fees may be substituted for this requirement.

Financial Assistance

Tuition loans are available from the school in some cases; a limited number of work-study and work-exchange programs and private scholarships may be available. The school has a small scholarship fund for women of color or native Spanish speakers who plan to work in low-income communities.

Sage Femme Midwifery School

(See Multiple State Locations, pages 410-11)

Western States Chiropractic College

2900 NE 132nd Avenue
Portland, Oregon 97230
PHONE: (503) 251-5734 / (800) 641-5641
FAX: (503) 251-5723
E-MAIL: admissions@wschiro.edu
WEBSITE: wschiro.edu

Western States Chiropractic College (WSCC) was founded in 1904 and is located in a residential suburb of Portland. There are forty-two instructors, with an average of fifty students in lectures, eighteen in labs.

Accreditation and Approvals

WSCC is accredited by the Northwest Association of Schools and Colleges and by the Council on Chiropractic Education (CCE).

Program Description

The 4,596-hour Doctor of Chiropractic (D.C.) degree program is typically completed in four years (twelve quarters). The curriculum is a prescribed course of study in which all core classes must be successfully completed in the proper sequence; additional noncredit elective courses may be taken for further study in an interest area.

Courses in the Division of Basic Science include Spinal Anatomy, Gross Anatomy, Cell Biology/Histology, Biochemistry, Embryology, Neuroanatomy, Physiology, Microbiology and Public Health, General Pathology, Neurophysiology, Nutrition, Clinical Microbiology and Public Health, Genetics, Clinic Research Methods, and Toxicology and Pharmacology.

The Division of Clinical Science includes courses in CPR/Emergency Care, Clinical Reasoning and Problem Solving, Physical Diagnosis, Clinical Lab, Dermatology and Infectious Disease, Patient/Practice Management, Clinical Pathology, Chiropractic Physiological Therapeutics, Clinical Nutrition, Jurisprudence and Ethics, Obstetrics, Cardiorespiratory Diagnosis and Treatment, Gastroenterology Diagnosis and Treatment, Genitourinary Survey, Narrative Report Writing, Clinical Pediatrics, Clinical Geriatrics, Clinical Psychology, Minor Surgery/Proctology, and others.

The Department of Radiology includes such courses as Radiographic Anatomy, Bone Pathology, Radiographic Technique, Soft Tissue Manipulation, Soft Tissue Interpretation, and Roentgenometrics.

Courses in the Division of Chiropractic Science include Biomechanics and Palpation, Philosophy and Principles of Chiropractic, Adjustive Technique, Soft Tissue Therapies/Rehabilitation, and Neuromusculoskeletal Diagnosis and Treatment.

The Division of Clinics covers Clinic Observation I through III and Clinic Phase I through IV-C.

The Bachelor of Science in Human Biology degree program is open only to D.C. students; consult the catalog or a WSCC representative for more information.

Continuing Education

The Division of Continuing Education and Postgraduate Studies provides education offerings through seminar, certification, and diplomate programs for D.C. graduates of all accredited chiropractic colleges. Offerings are designed to meet chiropractic relicensure credit as required by the Oregon Board of Chiropractic Examiners and by boards in neighboring states.

Admission Requirements

Applicants must have completed at least two years (sixty semester hours or ninety quarter hours) of course work at a regionally accredited junior college, college, or university with a minimum GPA of 2.25 on a 4.0 scale. Specific course requirements include at least six semester hours each of biology, general chemistry, organic chemistry, and physics; and at least twenty-four semester hours of humanities and social sciences, including at least six semester hours in English composition and three semester hours in psychology.

An on-campus or phone interview may be required. Students must also complete a physical examination and college health evaluation at the Student Health Center before the end of the first year.

Tuition and Fees

Tuition is $4,530 per term; total tuition for the 12-quarter program is $54,360. Other expenses include an application fee of $50, an enrollment fee of $50 per term, and integrated fees of $150 per term; books and equipment are additional.

Financial Assistance

A deferred tuition payment plan, federal loans and work-study, ChiroLoan and Canadian ChiroLoan, scholarships, and veterans' benefits are available.

PENNSYLVANIA

Academy for Myofascial Trigger Point Therapy

1312 East Carson Street
Pittsburgh, Pennsylvania 15203-1510
PHONE: (412) 481-2553
FAX: (412) 481-3279
E-MAIL: amtpt@bellatlantic.net
WEBSITE: www.trfn.clpgh.org/amtpt

Academy for Myofascial Trigger Point Therapy (AMTPT) was founded by Tasso Spanos in 1995. There are two instructors, with an average of ten to fifteen students per class.

Accreditation and Approvals
AMTPT is licensed by the Pennsylvania Department of Education, Division of Private Licensed Schools. Graduates are eligible to take the National Certification Board exam of the National Association of Myofascial Trigger Point Therapists. State licensure is currently being sought for the recognition of Myofascial Trigger Point Therapy as a distinct discipline.

Program Description
The 495-hour Myofascial Trigger Point Therapy Program consists of three trimesters. Courses include History and Principles of Myofascial Therapy, Fundamentals of Physical Evaluation and Palpation, Medical Lectures, Application of Myofascial Therapy, Literature Review, Alexander Technique and Movement Education, Advanced Principles of Myofascial Therapy, Applied Myofascial Therapy, Student Clinic, and Business Skills.

Admission Requirements
Applicants must have a high school diploma or equivalent and submit a physician's statement. An understanding of the human body is essential; nurses, physical therapists, chiropractors, physicians, and massage therapists are eligible. Those without such a background must have completed a course in Anatomy and Physiology; additional recommended courses for such students include Exercise Physiology, Kinesiology, Nutrition, Counseling/Psychology, and Medical Terminology.

Tuition and Fees
Tuition is $7,400. Additional expenses include books, $200; treatment table, $300 to $600; ABMP Practitioner Level membership, $199; additional books, seminars, audio- and videotapes, and wall charts are recommended.

The Alternative Conjunction Clinic and School of Massage Therapy

716 State Street
Lemoyne, Pennsylvania 17043
PHONE: (717) 737-6001
FAX: (717) 737-6607
E-MAIL: melmassag1@aol.com

The Alternative Conjunction Clinic and School of Massage Therapy was founded in 1994 by Melodie A. Adinolfi. There are seven instructors, with an average of eight students per class.

Accreditation and Approvals
The Alternative Conjunction is accredited by the National Accreditation Commission of Cosmetology Arts and Sciences (NACCAS), and approved by the State of Florida and by the National Certification Board for Therapeutic Massage and Bodywork (NCBTMB) as a continuing education provider.

Program Description
The 604-hour Massage Therapy Program may be completed in as little as twenty-four instructional weeks of full-time study; students may complete the program at their own pace. The curriculum includes Massage Theory, Law and Ethics, Business Practices, Chair Massage, Adult CPR and First Aid, Anatomy and Physiology, Advanced Anatomy and Physiology, HIV/AIDS Information, Swedish Massage and Practicum, Esalen Massage and Practicum, Advanced Massage Applications/History Taking/Practicum, Allied Spa Services, Helio/Hydrotherapy, Muscle Testing, and Neuromuscular/Russian/Sports Massage Techniques and Theory.

Admission Requirements
Applicants must be at least 18 years of age, have a high school diploma or equivalent, submit three character references and a physician's statement, and interview at the school with the di-

rector and/or admissions director. Applicants that reside with their parents or legal guardians must be accompanied by them on their visit to the school.

Tuition and Fees

The total cost of the program is $6,295, including tuition, application fee, and table, books, materials, and supplies fee; supplies such as sheets towels, oils, lotions, paper, and pencils are additional.

Financial Assistance

Federal financial aid, payment plans, loans, and veterans' benefits are available.

Career Training Academy

703 Fifth Avenue
New Kensington, Pennsylvania 15068
PHONE: (724) 337-1000
FAX: (724) 335-7140
E-MAIL: jreddy@careerta.com
WEBSITE: www.careerta.com

ADDITIONAL LOCATION:
ExpoMart
105 Mall Boulevard, Suite 300W
Monroeville, Pennsylvania 15146
PHONE: (412) 372-3900
FAX: (412) 373-4262

The Career Training Academy was founded in 1986 and began offering its massage therapy programs in 1993. There are twelve instructors, with an average of twelve students per class (maximum twenty for lab/practicum and twenty-five for lecture).

Accreditation and Approvals

The academy is licensed by the Pennsylvania Department of Education, Division of Private Licensed Schools, and accredited by the Accrediting Commission of Career Schools and Colleges of Technology (ACCSCT). The Therapeutic Massage Technician Program is accredited by the Commission on Massage Training Accreditation (COMTA). The Therapeutic Massage Technician, Comprehensive Massage Therapy, and Advanced Bodyworker Programs are accredited by the Integrative Massage and Somatic Therapies Accreditation Council (IMSTAC). Graduates of massage therapy programs of 500 or more hours are qualified to take the National Certification Examination for Therapeutic Massage and Bodywork (NCETMB).

Program Description

The 300-hour, four-month Swedish Massage Practitioner Program consists of courses in Anatomy and Physiology, Aromatherapy/Homeopathic Remedies, Career Development, Kinesiology, Introduction to Massage, Clinical Evaluation/Client Interaction, Therapeutic Modalities, First Aid/CPR, Practicum, and Swedish Massage I.

The 600-hour, seven-and-a-half-month Therapeutic Massage Technician Program is a more advanced course in Swedish and Therapeutic massage. The curriculum is the same as the 300-hour program, with the addition of Swedish Massage II, Body Reflexology, Sports Massage, Chiropractic Assistance/Nutrition, Basic Shiatsu, Stretching/Acuyoga, Myotherapy, and Chiropractic Assistance/Geriatric Massage.

The 900-hour, eleven-and-a-half-month Comprehensive Massage Therapist Program builds upon the foundation of the Therapeutic Massage Technician Program. Additional courses include Clinic, Business Principles, Intro to Marketing, Pregnancy/Infant Massage, AIDS Awareness, Acupressure, and Public Speaking.

The 1,500-hour, nineteen-month Advanced Bodyworker Program further builds upon the Comprehensive Massage Therapists Program, including additional modalities (Trigger Points: Upper and Lower, Orthopedic Assessment, Myofascial Release, and Craniosacral Therapy) and in-depth general education and business courses including Business English, Diversity in the Workplace, Intro and Advanced Pathology, Principles of Wellness, Psychology, and Nutrition.

The 300-hour, four-month Basic Shiatsu Technician Program is identical to the 300-hour Swedish Massage Practitioner Program with the substitution of Shiatsu I for Swedish Massage I.

The 600-hour, seven-and-a-half-month Advanced Shiatsu Technician Program builds upon the Basic Shiatsu Technician program, with the addition of Shiatsu II, Body Reflexology, Sports Massage, Stretching/Acuyoga, Acupressure, and Myotherapy.

Admission Requirements

Applicants must have a high school diploma or equivalent, submit an evaluation essay and health form, and have an interview.

Tuition and Fees

All programs have the following fees: application fee, $25; insurance fee, $32; and uniforms, $240. A massage table is included with books and supplies in the following figures.

Fees for the 300-hour Swedish Massage Practitioner Program are tuition, $2,100; books and supplies, $941; and lab fee, $75.

Fees for the 600-hour Therapeutic Massage Technician Program are tuition, $4,200; books and supplies, $1,156; and lab fee, $120.

Fees for the 900-hour Comprehensive Massage Therapist Program are tuition, $6,300; books and supplies, $1,491; and lab fee, $180.

Fees for the 1,500-hour Advanced Bodyworker Program are tuition, $10,500; books and supplies, $2,387; and lab fee, $300.

Fees for the 300-hour Basic Shiatsu Technician Program are tuition, $2,100; books and supplies, $913; and lab fee, $75.

Fees for the 600-hour Advanced Shiatsu Technician Program are tuition, $4,200; books and supplies, $1,121; and lab fee, $120.

Financial Assistance

Federal grants and loans, veterans' benefits, and payment plans are available. Aid is also available through the Office of Vocational Rehabilitation, Single Point of Contact, The Negro Educational Emergency Drive, the Department of Public Assistance, and the Private Industry Council.

East-West School of Massage Therapy

504 Park Road North
Wyomissing, Pennsylvania 19610
PHONE: (610) 374-7520
FAX: (610) 375-7554
E-MAIL: ewsmt@talon.net
WEBSITE: www.ewsmt.com

East-West School of Massage Therapy was founded in 1989 by Marilyn McGrath. There are ten instructors, with an average of six students per class.

Accreditation and Approvals

East-West Therapeutic Massage is accredited by the Integrative Massage and Somatic Therapies Accreditation Council (IMSTAC), and is licensed by the Pennsylvania State Department of Education. Graduates are qualified to take the National Certification Examination for Therapeutic Massage and Bodywork (NCETMB). East-West is approved as a continuing education provider by the National Certification Board for Therapeutic Massage and Bodywork (NCBTMB).

Program Description

The 520-hour Massage Therapy/Bodywork Program consists of courses in Swedish/Therapeutic Massage, Anatomy and Physiology, Shiatsu, Reflexology, Sports Massage, Aromatherapy, Polarity Therapy, Chair Massage, Self-Development, Related Studies, Business Practice, and CPR/First Aid.

The 545-hour Shiatsu Bodywork Program consists of three levels. Level One (eighty hours) includes Basic Definitions and Techniques, Classic Meridians, Diagnostic Studies, Anatomy and Physiology, and Related Studies. Topics covered in Level Two (132 hours) include Traditional Oriental Medicine, Seated/Side Position, Diagnostic Techniques, Extended Meridians, Macrobiotics, Advanced Techniques, Anatomy and Physiology II, CPR, and Tai Chi. Level Three (200 hours) includes Pathology, Professional Development, Soft Tissue Release, Compresses, Nutrition, Chi Gong, and Supervised Clinic.

Additional course requirements include 100 hours of Anatomy and Physiology, twenty-five hours of Professional Development, and eight hours of CPR/SFA.

Admission Requirements

Applicants must be at least 18 years of age; have a high school diploma or equivalent; submit two letters of reference, a physician's statement, and a written personal history; and have a personal interview.

Tuition and Fees

There is a $75 application fee. Tuition for the Massage Therapy/Bodywork Program is $4,490; books are $264. Tuition for Shiatsu is $4,700; books are $56.

Financial Assistance

A payment plan is available.

Health Options Institute

1410 Main Street
Northampton, Pennsylvania 18067
PHONE: (610) 261-0880
FAX: (610) 261-2964
E-MAIL: massage8@aol.com
WEBSITE: members.aol.com/massage8

Health Options Institute (HOI) was founded in 1984. There are seventeen instructors, with an average of eight students per class.

Accreditation and Approvals

HOI is licensed by the Pennsylvania Department of Education. Graduates of the 622-hour program are qualified to take the National Certification Examination for Therapeutic Massage and Bodywork (NCETMB).

Program Description

The 500-hour Massage Therapy Program consists of a 104-hour Deep Muscle Massage Program (Block A) followed by two additional blocks of courses, which may be taken in any order or in combination. Students not wishing to commit to the entire program may take Block A alone.

Block A: Deep Muscle Massage Program (104 hours) consists of fifty-six hours of Deep Muscle Massage technique, record keeping, business ethics, basic anatomy, and more, plus forty-eight hours of Group Practical, a guided and supervised group practice session.

In Block B: Clinic (22.5 hours), students work at the clinic on the general public; students need to complete twenty clinic sessions for graduation.

Block C: Complementary Massage Techniques (373.5 hours) covers Shiatsu, Nutrition and Holistic Health, Scentsational Aromatherapy, Reflexology, Multi-Dimensional Human Anatomy, Professional Practice Concepts, Ethics, Therapeutic Touch, Seated Chair Massage, Client Communication Skills, and Polarity.

Continuing Education

A variety of continuing education seminars and classes are offered. Programs offered previously include Wetzig Full Poten-

tial Coordination Training, Neuromuscular Therapy, Mastectomy Massage, Feng Shui Essentials, Functional Cranial Sacral Training, Reiki, Geriatric Massage, Advanced Aromatherapy, Pre- and Post-Natal Massage, and Circles of Life.

Admission Requirements

Applicants must be at least 18 years of age (younger students may be considered on an individual basis) and submit a physician's statement.

Tuition and Fees

Tuition for the Massage Therapy program is $5,995, plus a $100 enrollment fee and $388 for supplies. Tuition for Block A when taken alone is $1,240, plus a $100 enrollment fee and $90 for supplies.

Financial Assistance

Payment plans are available.

The Himalayan International Institute of Yoga Science and Philosophy

RR 1, Box 400
Honesdale, Pennsylvania 18431-9706
PHONE: (800) 822-4547 / (570) 253-5551
FAX: (570) 253-9078
E-MAIL: himalaya@himalayaninstitute.org
WEBSITE: www.himalayaninstitute.org

The Himalayan Institute was founded in 1971 as a nonprofit organization with the goal of helping people to grow physically, mentally, and spiritually. The institute's international headquarters are located on a 400-acre campus in northeastern Pennsylvania.

Other Himalayan Institute centers in the United States are located in New York, Buffalo, Pittsburgh, Glenview, Chicago, Milwaukee, and Dallas/Forth Worth; in Canada, centers are located in Toronto, Canmore, Burnaby, and Regina. Each center has its own schedule of classes and seminars.

Program Description

The Himalayan Institute Teachers' Association (HITA) has been training, certifying, and providing continuing education for hatha yoga teachers for more than twenty years. The program provides a systematic and comprehensive study of raja yoga, the eight-limbed path. This approach to the study and practice of yoga and the development of teaching skills benefits aspiring and experienced teachers, as well as those wishing to advance in their own practice.

The requirements leading to certification include ongoing practice and study in hatha yoga, meditation training in the Himalayan Institute tradition, six home study courses (including Essential Yoga Philosophy, Asana Practice, Science of Breath, Meditation, Anatomy for Yoga, and Diet and Nutrition), two self-study projects, a two-week intensive training (offered annually in the summer), written and practical exams, and eight weeks' teaching experience.

Community and Continuing Education

Weekend and longer seminars are also offered year-round at the international headquarters, and are designed for beginning as well as more advanced students. Among the topics and seminars offered are Dynamics of Meditation, Meditation Retreats, Fundamentals of Hatha Yoga (Levels 1 and 2), Subtle Body Series, Science of Breath, Specialty Yoga, Hatha Yoga Teachers' Retreats, Hatha Yoga Teachers' Training, Homeopathy for Home Use, Ayurveda and Rejuvenation, Biofeedback, Vegetarian Cooking, Herbs, Cleansing and Fasting, Therapeutic and Spiritual Dimensions of Hatha Yoga, Women's Spirituality, and others.

Admission Requirements

Prerequisites for teacher's training include a minimum of one year's experience in intermediate-level hatha yoga, a regular personal hatha yoga practice, and membership in HITA. Certification is valid for three years. Recertification requires specified hours for personal practice, continuing education, and ongoing teaching.

Tuition and Fees

Seminars and the two-week teachers' training intensive range from $100 to $1,000. Call to receive the Himalayan Institute's free *Quarterly Guide to Programs* or for more detailed information. Membership in the Himalayan Institute Teachers Association costs $100 annually, with a $10 application fee.

Lancaster School of Massage

317 North Queen Street
Lancaster, Pennsylvania 17603
PHONE: (717) 293-9698
E-MAIL: lsmassage@redrose.net

Lancaster School of Massage was founded in 1988 by Winona Bontrager, who remains as director and sole proprietor. There are ten instructors, with a maximum class size of eighteen students; the teacher:student ratio for technique classes is 1:5.

Accreditation and Approvals

Lancaster School of Massage is a member of the American Massage Therapy Association (AMTA) Council of Schools, and an affiliate member of Associated Bodywork and Massage Professionals (ABMP). Graduates are qualified to take the National Certification Examination for Therapeutic Massage and Bodywork (NCETMB).

Program Description

The 500-hour Massage Therapy Program consists of courses in Massage Therapy (covering history, theory, contraindications, demonstrations, and modalities that include Swedish Massage, Reflexology, Neuromuscular Therapy, Polarity Therapy, Connective Tissue Massage, Cranio-Sacral, and Sports Massage); Anatomy, Physiology, and Pathology; Awareness and Communication Skills; CPR and First Aid; and Business Practices. Classes are offered mornings and evenings.

Admission Requirements

Applicants must be at least 18 years of age, submit an application with essay, and have a personal interview. Applicants must enroll for the entire 500 hours of training.

Tuition and Fees

Tuition is $5,250. Additional expenses include books, approximately $150, and CPR and First Aid training, approximately $40.

Lehigh Valley Healing Arts Academy

5412 Shimmerville Road
Emmaus, Pennsylvania 18049
PHONE/FAX: (610) 965-6165
E-MAIL: lvhaa@fast.net
WEBSITE: www.illion.com/lvhaa

The Lehigh Valley Healing Arts Academy was founded in 1987 (as the Lehigh Healing Arts Center) by director Bonita Cassel-Beckwith, who has been teaching bodywork since 1984. There are seven instructors plus seventeen guest lecturers; class sizes average twelve to sixteen students (maximum twenty-five students).

Accreditation and Approvals

The academy is licensed by the Board of Private Schools under the Pennsylvania Department of Educatio. Graduates of massage therapy programs of 500 or more hours are qualified to take the National Certification Examination for Therapeutic Massage and Bodywork (NCETMB). The academy is approved by the National Certification Board of Therapeutic Massage and Bodywork (NCBTMB) as a continuing education provider.

Program Description

The 500-hour Bodywork Diploma Program consists of three levels of instruction. Level I includes 150 hours in Anatomy and Physiology, Applied Anatomy, Bodywork Practice and Theory, Remedial Exercises, Business, Pathology and Medical Terminology, Reflexology, Ethics, Boundaries for Bodyworkers, One-To-One Tutorial, and Clinic. Level II (150 hours) includes Anatomy and Physiology II, Deep Tissue Sculpting, Subtle Energy Studies, Body/Mind Integration, Five Elements/Acupressure and Meridian Therapy, One-To-One Tutorial, and Level II Clinic. Level III (200 hours) features courses taught by guest lecturers as well as teachers from the school. Students in the 500-hour program are required to take CPR/AIDS Awareness, Heart-Centered Listening for Bodyworkers, and Body Usage for Bodyworkers; students then elect classes that interest them to complete as many hours as they wish. Elective courses include Carpal Tunnel Massage, Therapeutic Touch (three levels), Reiki (three levels), Reflexology, Body Psychology Through Iridology, Sports Massage, Kinesiology, Spiritual Listening, NLP, Gem-

stone and Color Healing, Yoga, Aromatherapy, Polarity, Craniosacral, Tai Chi, Boundaries for Bodyworkers II, Introduction to Clinical Herbalism, Energy Fundamentals, DansKinetics with Breathwork, Trager® Anatomy, and Trager Intro, Beginning, Intermediate and Practitioner I Trainings. Classes are held days or weekends.

The 200-hour Diploma in Reflexology Program may be taken by itself or as a double diploma program in conjunction with the 500-hour Bodywork Diploma. The Reflexology Program includes in-depth Reflexology courses and clinics; Iridology; Body Psychology; Teeth, Hands and Colon Reflexology; Meditation and Visualization; plus approximately 100 hours of courses taken from the Bodywork program such as Business Practices, Ethics, Boundaries, Medical Terminology, Anatomy and Physiology, and CPR.

Admission Requirements

Applicants must be at least 18 years of age, have a high school diploma or equivalent, and submit a short essay and a letter of recommendation from a health professional.

Tuition and Fees

Tuition for Bodywork Level I is $1,500; for Level II, $1,500; Level III tuition is approximately $2,000 (tuition varies with courses chosen). Additional expenses include books for Level I, $96, and a massage table, approximately $500 to $600.

Tuition for the Reflexology program is $2,000.

Financial Assistance

Payment plans and job partnership trainings are available.

Meridian Shiatsu Institute

998 Old Eagle School Road, Suite 1212
Wayne, Pennsylvania 19087
PHONE: (610) 293-4030
FAX: (610) 971-9860
E-MAIL: caroleepf@aol.com

The Meridian Shiatsu Institute (MSI) was founded in 1983 by Carolee Parker. There are seven instructors, with an average of twelve students per class.

Accreditation and Approvals

MSI is a member of the AOBTA Council of Schools and Programs, licensed as a private school by the Commonwealth of Pennsylvania, and approved as a continuing education provider by the National Certification Board for Therapeutic Massage and Bodywork (NCBTMB).

Program Description

MSI offers 540 hours of Shiatsu training that consists of four levels of Shiatsu, supervised practice, a clinic program, Anatomy and Physiology, and Pathology.

Level I is an introduction to the foundations of Five Element Shiatsu; upon completion of this level, students are able to give a basic full body Shiatsu treatment.

Level II explores in depth the Law of Five Elements, location of key points on the meridians, and energetic assessment techniques of Oriental Bodywork Therapy.

Level III introduces further assessment techniques, intermediate treatment planning skills, professional ethics, and basic business necessities for starting a professional practice.

Level I, II, and III students attend a three-hour supervised practice session once per month; students are required to give a minimum of thirty-six treatments during the first three levels.

Level IV covers the main theories of Classical Chinese medicine in depth, including the Eight Principles, Eight extraordinary meridians, advanced treatment planning, local-distal point theory, and more. Upon completion of Level IV, students are eligible for national certification. All Level IV students take part in a seventy-hour clinical program consisting of fifty one-hour supervised treatments and twenty hours spent in conference, critical review, and discussion of treatment methods.

The 100-hour Anatomy and Physiology for Bodyworkers is designed for Shiatsu and other bodywork therapists and follows the AOBTA Anatomy and Physiology requirement; it may be taken anytime after completion of Level II.

The required ten-week Pathology course covers causes, symptoms, standard medical treatments, and prognoses of common diseases, and may be taken anytime after completion of Level II.

Community and Continuing Education

Courses and workshops are offered on a regular basis to the community and to practitioners. Previously offered topics in-clude Beginners Yoga, Basic Jin Shin Do, Feldenkrais®, Basics of Reflexology, Qi Gong, Reiki, and others.

Admission Requirements

Applicants must have a high school diploma or equivalent, and submit a letter of reference from a health care practitioner.

Tuition and Fees

Tuition for Levels I, II, and III totals $2,535. Tuition for Level IV is $2,070. Tuition for Anatomy and Physiology is $980; for Pathology, $300. Additional expenses include a one-time enrollment fee of $75; books and materials are approximately $190 for all four levels.

Financial Assistance

Tuition may be paid in monthly installments.

Mt. Nittany Institute of Natural Health

301 Shiloh Road
State College, Pennsylvania 16801
PHONE: (814) 238-1121
FAX: (814) 238-8145
E-MAIL: mail2@mtnittanyinstitute.com
WEBSITE: www.mtnittanyinstitute.com

The Mt. Nittany Institute of Natural Health was founded in 1995 by Anne Mascelli, a licensed massage therapist and certified Kripalu yoga teacher. There are twenty instructors. Class sizes are limited as follows: Massage Therapist, twenty-four; Holistic Health Educator, sixteen; Herbal Studies, sixteen; and Reflexology, twelve.

Accreditation and Approvals

The Massage Therapist Training and Holistic Health Educator Training Programs are licensed by the Pennsylvania Department of Education. Mt. Nittany is a member of the American Massage Therapy Association (AMTA) Council of Schools. Graduates of massage therapy programs of 500 or more hours are qualified to take the National Certification Examination for Therapeutic Massage and Bodywork (NCETMB).

Program Description

The 675-hour Massage Therapist Training Program consists of three self-contained modules, which may be completed in seventeen months of part-time study. Module One: Relaxation Work (175 hours) covers Swedish Massage, Foot Reflexology, Anatomy and Physiology (Principles of Support and Movement), Body Mechanics for the Therapist, Communication Skills, Professional Development, Yoga and Relaxation, Movement Re-education, and Practice Sessions. Module Two: Energy Work (200 hours) includes Shiatsu, Polarity Therapy, Anatomy and Physiology (Maintenance Systems of the Body), Tai Chi, Energy Exploration, Professional Development and Practice Sessions. Module Three: Advanced Work (300 hours) covers Connective Tissue Massage, Sports Massage, Neuromuscular Therapy, Hydrotherapy, Applied Technique, Anatomy and Physiology (Control Systems of the Body), Professional Development Project, Marketing and Self Promotion, Business and Tax Issues, Aromatherapy, In-depth Client Charting, and Practice Sessions. Students may attend classes on alternating weekends or one day per week, and may enter the program during Module One or Module Two.

The 250-hour Holistic Health Educator Training Program is an advanced experiential training for health care and helping professionals who desire to teach others to improve their health and well-being through connecting with body, mind, and spirit in everyday life. The program includes training in nutrition, stress management, alternative medicine, and other life-changing skills. Classes are held one weekend per month for one year.

The seventy-eight-hour Herbal Studies Program uses a holistic and hands-on approach to the study of American herbs through in-class instruction and field trips. The program provides an opportunity for health care and helping professionals to augment their professional training, but is open to all. Program themes include Nutritional and Culinary Uses of Herbs, Natural Skin Care and Aromatherapy, Herbal First Aid, and Herbal Gift Making. Students also receive training in herbal preparations and how to apply herbal remedies to specific physical ailments including asthma, allergies, depression, insomnia, and anxiety. Classes meet one Saturday per month for one year.

The 150-hour Reflexology Program consists of three levels of training. Level 1: Basic Skills covers Foot Reflexology: His-tory, Theory and Basic Techniques, Anatomy and Physiology, Pathology, Practitioner Self-Care, Yoga and Relaxation, and Practice Sessions. Level 2: Applied Technique includes Client-Specific Reflexology, Anatomy and Physiology, Pathology, Ethics and Boundaries, Safety and Hygiene, Tai Chi, and Practice Sessions. Level 3: Advanced Work covers Stereognostic Reflexology, Anatomy and Physiology, Pathology, Aromatherapy, Hydrotherapy, Case Studies, In-depth Client Charting, Advanced Practice Sessions, Business Development, Advanced Marketing Strategies, and Community Education Project. Classes are offered one weekend per month for one year.

Admission Requirements

Massage Therapist applicants must be at least 19 years of age, have a high school diploma or equivalent, have received at least one professional massage, submit two letters of recommendation and an essay, and have an admissions interview.

Holistic Health Educator applicants must submit two letters of recommendation and an essay, and have an admissions interview.

Herbal Studies applicants must be at least 18 years of age and have an admissions interview.

Reflexology applicants must be at least 19 years of age, have a high school diploma or equivalent, have received at least one reflexology session, submit two letters of recommendation and an essay, and have an admissions interview.

Tuition and Fees

Tuition for Massage Therapist Training is $5,500 for all three modules; if committed to and paid for one at a time, individual module fees are as follows: Module One, $1,600; Module Two, $1,830; Module Three, $2,745. Additional expenses include application fee and books, $115; supplies, including linens, oils, and a recommended massage table are additional.

Tuition for the Holistic Health Educator Training Program is $2,500, plus a $35 application fee.

Tuition for Herbal Studies is $895.

Tuition for the Reflexology program is $1,850 plus a $35 application fee; books and supplies are additional.

Financial Assistance

Payment plans and early enrollment discounts are available.

Myofascial Release Treatment Centers and Seminars

(See Multiple State Locations, page 402)

Pennsylvania Institute of Massage Therapy

93 S. West End Boulevard, Suite 102–103
Quakertown, Pennsylvania 18951
PHONE: (215) 538-5339
FAX: (215) 538-8896
E-MAIL: drbob@fast.net

The Pennsylvania Institute of Massage Therapy (PIMT) was founded in 1993. The current director, Robert W. Tosh, D.C., has had a private chiropractic practice since 1985; assistant director Terry Ann Tosh is a massage therapist and trained nursing assistant. There are five instructors plus two assistant instructors; the average class size is fifteen students (maximum twenty).

Accreditation and Approvals

PIMT is accredited by the Integrative Massage and Somatic Therapies Accreditation Council (IMSTAC). PIMT is licensed by the Pennsylvania State Board of Private Licensed Schools. Graduates are qualified to take the National Certification Examination for Therapeutic Massage and Bodywork (NCETMB).

Program Description

The 520-hour Massage Therapy Course consists of massage theory and practical application of Swedish and deep muscle therapeutic massage. Allied modalities are covered (including reflexology, sports massage, hydrotherapy, tai chi, shiatsu, and others), as well as massage technique modifications for client conditions. The Anatomy and Physiology segment covers Medical Terminology, Cells and Tissues, Integumentary System, Skeletal System, Muscular System, Nervous System, Endocrine System, Circulatory System, Respiratory System, Digestive System and Nutrition, Urinary System, Reproductive System, Psychology, Business Practices, Deep Muscle Therapy, and a student-run clinic. Classes may be taken on a morning, evening, or weekend schedule.

Continuing Education

Currently under development, pending licensing approval, is a Reflexognosy Program. Reflexognosy is a new technique for realigning the structure of the body through muscle relaxation and joint movement of the foot and lower leg. In addition, Tosh Seminars presents a variety of continuing education seminars taught by other nationally recognized instructors.

Admission Requirements

Applicants must be at least 18 years of age, have a high school diploma or equivalent, and submit a physician's statement of health.

Tuition and Fees

Tuition for the Massage course is $4,450. Additional expenses include $155 for books. Nearby guest house accommodations are available for an additional fee.

Financial Assistance

Payment plans, veterans' benefits, and loan assistance are available.

Pennsylvania School of Muscle Therapy

994 Old Eagle School Road, Suite 1005
Wayne, Pennsylvania 19087-1802
PHONE: (610) 687-0888
FAX: (610) 687-4726
E-MAIL: psmt@psmt.com
WEBSITE: www.psmt.com

The Pennsylvania School of Muscle Therapy (PSMT) was founded in 1982 and moved to its current location in 1994. There are twenty-four instructors, with an average of eighteen students per class.

Accreditation and Approvals

PSMT's Program 104—Professional Swedish Massage is accredited by the Commission on Massage Training Accreditation (COMTA) and by the Integrative Massage and Somatic Therapies Accreditation Council (IMSTAC); graduates are qualified to take the National Certification Examination for

Therapeutic Massage and Bodywork (NCETMB). PSMT is approved by the International Association of Pfrimmer Deep Muscle Therapists (IAPDMT) and by the National Athletic Trainers Association Board of Certification (NATABOC). PSMT is approved by the National Certification Board of Therapeutic Massage and Bodywork (NCBTMB) as a continuing education provider and is licensed by the Pennsylvania State Board of Private Licensed Schools.

Program Description

Courses in the 629-hour, twelve-month Program 104—Professional Swedish Massage include Theory and Practice of Massage, Sports Massage Basics, Business and Professional Ethics, Anatomy and Physiology, Pathology, Hydrotherapy, and CPR/First Aid.

Combinations of basic and advanced training are available in the form of the 737-hour Option 204A—Advanced Medical Massage Program, which combines Professional Swedish Massage and Corrective Medical Massage Techniques, or the 1,043-hour Option 204B—Bodywork Mastery Program, which combimes Professional Swedish Massage, Corrective Medical Massage Techniques, Advanced Anatomy and Physiology, Science of Kinesiology, and Shiatsu.

Continuing Education

Continuing education programs are offered periodically in such areas as aromatherapy, reflexology, massage and bodywork for survivors of abuse, infant massage, basic and advanced sports massage, mother massage, bio-energetic massage, neuromuscular therapy, trigger point therapy, on-site chair massage, and others.

Admission Requirements

Applicants must be at least 18 years of age, have a high school diploma or equivalent, submit three character references, have a physicial certification and personal interview, and pass an entrance exam.

Tuition and Fees

Tuition for Program 104—Professional Swedish Massage is $6,500. Tuition for Program 204A—Advanced Medical Massage Progam is $8,000. Tuition for Program 204B—Bodywork Mastery Program is $11,500. Additional expenses include a $25 application fee and a $125 registration fee; books, supplies, and optional massage table are additional.

Financial Assistance

Payment plans are available through SLM Financial Corporation.

RHODE ISLAND
Apollo Herbs

E-MAIL: apollo@brainiac.com
WEBSITE: www.brainiac.com/apolloherbs

MAILING ADDRESS:
P.O. Box 1885
Kingston, Rhode Island 02881
PHONE: (401) 539-9996
FAX: (401) 539-6115

CLASSROOM ADDRESS:
Olde Allen Farm
840 Old Smithfield Road
North Smithfield, Rhode Island 02896
PHONE: (401) 762-1733

Apollo Herbs, a small business dedicated to the art of natural healing, was founded in 1991 by Michael Ford. Classes are taught by Michael Ford and Jo-Anne Pacheco; classes are limited to twenty students.

Program Description

The nine-month Essence of Herbalism: Herbalist Apprentice Program meets one weekend per month from April to December. Topics covered include Herbal Preparation: Teas, Decoctions, Solar and Lunar Infusions; Determining Good Quality Herbs and Proper Storage; Wild Plant Identification and Herb Walk; Organic Growing, Starting Seeds and Planning Garden; Herbal Therapeutics: The Nervous System; Regenerative Diet and Practices; Herbs and Holism; Terminology of Medicinal Herbs; Herbal Preparation: Tinctures; Plant Anatomy and Physiology; Methods of Wildcrafting; Herbal Pet Care; Compresses and Poultices; Medicinal Plant Chemicals; Working with Flower Essences; Herbs for Children; Syrups and Elixirs; Art Drying, Harvesting and Storing Herbs; Aromatherapy: Medicinal Uses of Essential Oils; Herbs for Winter Health; Capsules, Caplets, Pills and Powders; Herbal Stimulants; Pregnancy and Childbirth; Menopause and Croneship; Natural Skin Care and Cosmetics; and more.

Tuition and Fees

Tuition is $1,200.

SOUTH CAROLINA

Charleston School of Massage

778 Folly Road
Charleston, South Carolina 29412
PHONE: (843) 762-7727
FAX: (843) 762-1392
E-MAIL: charscms@bellsouth.net
WEBSITE: www.charlestonmassage.com

Charleston School of Massage was founded in 1997 by Mark Hendler, D.C., and Denise Hendler. There are three instructors, with a maximum class size of sixteen students.

Accreditation and Approvals

Charleston School of Massage is licensed by the South Carolina Commission on Higher Education, accredited by the American Association of Drugless Practitioners, and a member of the American Massage Therapy Association (AMTA) Council of Schools. Graduates of the 500- and 600-hour programs are qualified to take the National Certification Examination for Therapeutic Massage and Bodywork (NCETMB).

Program Description

The 500-hour Clinical Massage Therapy Program includes Massage History and Therapies; Introduction to Other Bodywork Methods; Anatomy and Physiology; Anatomy Review; Anatomy and Physiology Workshop; Therapeutic Massage Sessions; Introduction to Chair Massage Techniques; Musculoskeletal Examination Procedures; Energy Exchange (Reiki); Nutrition; Rehabilitation and Movement Exercises; HIV/AIDS Education; Marketing, Business and Ethics; First Aid and CPR; Aromatherapy; Facial Massage; Prenatal Massage; Sports Massage; and Supervised Internship.

The 600-hour Clinical Massage Therapy and Spa Therapy Program offers the same coursework as the 500-hour program, with the addition of a 100-hour specialization in Clinical Spa Therapies. This 100-hour program (which is also open to graduates of 500-hour programs from other massage schools) consists of Body Wraps/Masques and Herbal Treatments, Herbal Massage Therapy, Exfoliation and Day Spa Treatments, Facial Steam Vaporizing Procedures, Paraffin/Waxing, Pathology, Spa Therapy Procedures and Skin Products, Spa Therapy and Massage Instrumentation and Procedures, and Supervised Internship.

Programs are offered on both a full-time and part-time basis.

Admission Requirements

Applicants must have at least 18 years of age and have a high school diploma or equivalent.

Tuition and Fees

Tuition for the 500-hour Clinical Massage Therapy Program is $4,975 (includes application and holding fee); books are an additional $225.

Tuition for the 600-hour Clinical Massage and Spa Therapy Program is $6,250 (includes application and holding fee); additional expenses include books, $475, and spa supplies, $275.

Tuition for the 100-hour Clinical Spa Therapy Program taken alone is $1,475 (includes application and holding fee); additional expenses include books, $250, and spa supplies, $275.

Financial Assistance

Payment plans and bank loans are available.

DoveStar Institute

(See Multiple State Locations, pages 391–93)

Pinewood School of Massage

(see Southeastern School of Neuromuscular and Massage Therapy at Spartanburg,
Multiple State Locations, pages 412–13)

Sherman College of Straight Chiropractic

MAILING ADDRESS:
P.O. Box 1452
Spartanburg, South Carolina 29304
PHONE: (864) 578-8770 / (800) 849-8771
FAX: (864) 599-4860
E-MAIL: admissions@sherman.edu
WEBSITE: www.sherman.edu

CAMPUS ADDRESS:
2020 Springfield Road
Boiling Springs, South Carolina 29316

Sherman College of Straight Chiropractic was founded in 1973. "Straight" chiropractic uses vertebral adjusting to correct subluxation, or misalignment of the vertebra; the other school of thought, "mixer" chiropractic, uses manipulation and other methods to accomplish the objective of treating symptoms and disease. The use of the term "straight chiropractic" in the Sherman College name helps to identify it with its total commitment to the teaching, research, and practice relating to vertebral subluxation. There are forty-three instructors, with an average of thirty-five students per class.

Accreditation and Approvals
The Doctor of Chiropractic degree program is accredited by the Council on Chiropractic Education (CCE).

Program Description
The 4,644-hour Doctor of Chiropractic (D.C.) degree program may be completed in thirteen quarters and consists of courses that fall under the general categories of anatomy, physiology and chemistry, radiology, pathology and public health, research, diagnosis, clinic, philosophy, chiropractic technique, and business practices.

Continuing Education
Postdoctoral programs, seminars, and workshops are offered both on campus and through extension. Noncredit courses are offered in the areas of specific adjusting techniques, spinograph analysis and instrumentation, and chiropractic philosophy and communications. Continuing education workshops for license renewal are also offered.

Admission Requirements
Applicants must have completed at least sixty semester hours of undergraduate credit with a minimum 2.50 GPA, including specific courses in English or communication skills, psychology, biology, general and organic chemistry, and physics. In addition, applicants must submit two letters of recommendation.

Tuition and Fees
There is an application fee of $35; tuition is $3,900 per quarter; lab fees are $5 to $25 per course; books and supplies are additional.

Financial Assistance
Scholarships, federal grants, loans, and work-study are available.

Southeastern School of Neuromuscular and Massage Therapy

(See Multiple State Locations, pages 412–13)

TENNESSEE
Cumberland Institute for Wellness Education

500 Wilson Pike Circle, Suite 121
Brentwood, Tennessee 37027
PHONE: (615) 370-9794
FAX: (615) 370-5869
E-MAIL: cumberinst@aol.com

The Cumberland Institute for Wellness Education was established in 1989. There are twenty-three instructors, with an average of twelve to twenty-five students per class.

Accreditation and Approvals

Cumberland Institute is authorized by the Tennessee Education Commission, and the Massage Therapist Program exceeds the 500-hour education requirement for licensing in the State of Tennessee. Graduates are qualified to take the National Certification Examination for Therapeutic Massage and Bodywork (NCETMB).

Program Description

The 500-hour Massage Therapist Program is a self-paced program that may be completed in as little as nine months or as long as thirty-six months. Course offerings include Introduction to Bodywork; Touch Dynamics; Therapist-Client Interdynamics; Bodywork Ethics; Anatomy; Physiology; Kinesiology and Applied Anatomy; Terminology, Pathology, and Documentation; Swedish-Esalen Massage; Lymphatic Drainage Massage; Neuromuscular Therapy; Massage for Injury; Business-Marketing; and Clinical Internship. Classes are held days and evenings

Continuing Education

Up to 283 hours of electives may be taken in addition to the 500-hour program. Courses offered include Advanced Reflexology, Seated Chair Massage, Meridian Theory and Acupressure Massage, Craniosacral Therapy, Cayce-Reilly Massage, and a Spondylopathic Therapy Series.

Admission Requirements

Applicants must be at least 18 years of age, have a high school diploma or equivalent, and interview with the Director.

Tuition and Fees

Tuition for the 500-hour program is $7,290, including books. Other costs include application fee of $35; equipment/supplies, $623; and ABMP insurance, $39. Tuition for elective courses ranges from $190 to $1,250.

Financial Assistance

Payment plans, loans, and a prepayment discount are available.

The Massage Institute of Memphis

3445 Poplar Avenue, Suite #4
Memphis, Tennessee 38111

PHONE: (901) 324-4411
FAX: (901) 324-4470
E-MAIL: massinst@bellsouth.net
WEBSITE: www.themassageinstitute.com

The Massage Institute of Memphis was founded in 1987 by Karen E. Craig. She has produced an instructional cable TV series in Georgia and a commercial instructional massage video. There are sixteen instructors, with a maximum class size of twenty-two students.

Accreditation and Approvals

The Massage Institute of Memphis is authorized by the Tennessee Higher Education Commission. The 600-hour program meets Tennessee licensing requirements and enables students to take the Arkansas State Board of Massage Therapy examination as well as the National Certification Examination for Therapeutic Massage and Bodywork (NCETMB). Continuing education classes provide CEUs for the American Massage Therapy Association (AMTA), Tennessee licensing renewal and the National Certification Board for Therapeutic Massage and Bodywork (NCBTMB).

Program Description

The 600-hour Professional Massage program consists of courses in Anatomy, Physiology, Pathology, Kinesiology, Oriental Anatomy and Physiology, Massage Techniques (including basic massage theory and practice, reflexology, sports massage, chair massage, and clinical practicum), and Health Services Management (including professional development, law, ethics, hydrotherapy, electro/heliotherapy, hygiene/practical demonstration, and AIDS/HIV education). Classes are held days and evenings.

Continuing Education

Guest lectures, seminars, workshops, and specialty classes are offered to massage practitioners and graduates.

Admission Requirements

Applicants must be at least 18 years of age, have a high school diploma or equivalent, be of good moral character and in good health, interview with an admissions representative, and submit two letters of reference.

Tuition and Fees

Tuition is $5,000; individual courses are $10 per hour. Additional expenses include a $30 application fee; books, $250; supplies, approximately $150; massage table, approximately $450; and a hydrotherapy field trip, $100.

Financial Assistance

A payment plan, veterans' benefits, and Tennessee and Arkansas Vocational Rehabilitation are available.

Middle Tennessee Institute of Therapeutic Massage

394 West Main Street, Suite A15
P.O. Box 1200
Hendersonville, Tennessee 37077-1200
PHONE: (615) 826-9500
FAX: (615) 824-1147
E-MAIL: MTITM@Bellsouth.net
WEBSITE: aol@MTITM.com

The Middle Tennessee Institute of Therapeutic Massage (MTITM) was founded by Tami Mercer in 1996. There are twelve instructors, with an average of twenty students per class.

Accreditation and Approvals

MTITM is approved by the Associated Bodyworkers and Massage Professionals (ABMP) and is seeking accreditation from the Commission on Massage Training Accreditation (COMTA). Graduates are qualified to take the National Certification Examination for Therapeutic Massage and Bodywork (NCETMB).

Program Description

The Certified Massage Therapist Program includes over 500 hours of instruction. The curriculum includes Introduction to Massage, Touch Concepts, Client/Therapist Relations, Introduction to Pharmacology, Introduction to Reflexology, Shiatsu, Mind/Body Awareness Education, Anatomy and Physiology, Kinesiology, Nutrition, CPR/First Aid, Swedish Esalen Massage, Sports Massage, Lymphatic Drainage Massage, Business and Marketing, Aromatherapy, and Intern Clinic. Classes are held days, evenings, and weekends.

Continuing and Community Education

Continuing education workshops offered to practicing massage therapists and enrolled students include Intro to Reflexology, Craniosacral Therapy, Neuromuscular Therapy, On-Site Chair Massage, Spa Integration, Connective Tissue, and Carpal Tunnel.

Admission Requirements

Applicants must be at least 18 years of age, have a high school diploma or equivalent, and have an interview.

Tuition and Fees

There is a $25 application fee; tuition is $6,100, including books; and a massage table costs $350 to $500. Fees for workshops range from $75 to $250.

Financial Assistance

School student loans and a payment plan are available.

Tennessee Institute of Healing Arts

5779 Brainerd Road
Chattanooga, Tennessee 37411-4011
PHONE: (423) 892-9882 / (800) 735-1910
FAX: (423) 892-5006
E-MAIL: tiha@aol.com
WEBSITE: www.tiha.com

The Tennessee Institute of Healing Arts (TIHA) was founded in 1989 by massage therapist Alan Jordan as an outgrowth of the Chattanooga Massage Therapy Center. There are sixteen instructors, with an average of twenty students per class.

Accreditation and Approvals

TIHA is accredited by the Commission on Massage Training Accreditation (COMTA) and by the Accrediting Commission of Career Schools and Colleges of Technology (ACCSCT). Graduates are qualified to take the National Certification Examination for Therapeutic Massage and Bodywork (NCETMB).

Program Description

The twelve-month, 1,000-hour Professional Massage and Neuromuscular Therapy Training Program consists of Fundamentals of Massage, Neuromuscular Therapy, Russian Clinical Massage, Massage During Pregnancy, Geriatric Massage, Introduction to Complementary Therapies, Hydrotherapy, Seated Massage, Anatomy and Physiology (lecture and lab), Gross Anatomy Lab (an optional class working with human cadavers at Southern Adventist University), Clinical Pathology, Professional Ethics, Psychology for the Massage Therapist, Relational Bodywork, Self Care Through Movement, Marketing and Business, Nutrition, CPR and First Aid, Statutes/Rules and History of Massage, AIDS/HIV Education, Documented Massage Practice, Student Clinic, Clinical Externship, Documented Professional Massage, and Mid-Term and Final Practical Exams.

Admission Requirements

Applicants must be at least 18 years of age, be in good health, and have a high school diploma or equivalent. In addition, applicants must submit two personal references and have a personal interview.

Tuition and Fees

Tuition is $7,500. Additional expenses include: application fee, $100; books and supplies, approximately $550; optional massage table, $600; liability insurance, $35; lab fee, $35; and three professional massages, approximately $165.

Financial Assistance

Federal grants and loans, veterans' benefits, and payment plans are available.

Tennessee School of Massage

4726 Poplar #4
Memphis, Tennessee 38117
PHONE: (901) 767-8484
FAX: (901) 767-7795
E-MAIL: relax@touchofhealth.com

The Tennessee School of Massage was founded in 1988 by David and Cissie Pryor. There are five instructors, with an average of twelve to fifteen (maximum twenty) students per class. Classes are held at 556 Colonial.

Accreditation and Approvals

Tennessee School of Massage is authorized by the Tennessee Higher Education Commission. Graduates are qualified to take the National Certification Examination for Therapeutic Massage and Bodywork (NCETMB).

Program Description

For the 500-hour Massage Therapy Certification Program, both day and evening classes run over a nine-month period. Courses include Therapeutic Healing Touch, Introduction to Acupressure, On-Site Massage, Anatomy and Physiology, Massage Technique and Practice, Swedish Massage, Kinesiology, Hydrotherapy, Community, Ethics, Sports Massage, Nutrition, and Business Integration. Students must also complete a CPR/First Aid course prior to graduation.

Community and Continuing Education

Community and continuing education classes are ongoing; contact the school for a Community Calendar.

Admission Requirements

Applicants must be at least 18 years of age, have a high school diploma or equivalent, submit two letters of recommendation and a physician's report, receive a professional full-body massage, and have a personal interview.

Tuition and Fees

Tuition is $4,200. Additional expenses include a $50 application fee, $150 for books and class notes, and $400 to $600 for a massage table.

Financial Assistance

Payment plans are available.

TEXAS

Academy of Oriental Medicine - Austin

2700 West Anderson Lane, Suite 117
Austin, Texas 78757
PHONE: (512) 454-1188
FAX: (512) 454-7001
E-MAIL: AcademyOM@aol.com
WEBSITE: www.aoma.edu

The Academy of Oriental Medicine (AOMA) was founded in 1992. President Stuart Watts is the founder of the Southwest Acupuncture College and the International Institute of Chinese Medicine, both in Santa Fe, and has been in clinical practice since 1972. There are eighteen instructors, with an average of twenty-three students per class.

Accreditation and Approvals

The Master of Science in Oriental Medicine is accredited by the Accreditation Commission for Acupuncture and Oriental Medicine (ACAOM), and is approved under the rules of the Texas State Board of Acupuncture Examiners, the New Mexico Board of Acupuncture Examiners, and the Acupuncture Committee of the Department of Consumer Affairs of California. The Oriental Bodywork program is approved by the American Oriental Bodywork Therapy Association (AOBTA).

Program Description

The 2,880-hour Master of Science in Oriental Medicine Program may be completed in three years of full-time study. The program includes 1,044 hours of comprehensive clinical training, seventy-two hours of which is dedicated to herbal prescriptions. The program compares and contrasts Western and Oriental medicine, diagnosis, and procedures, and offers a strong foundation in Traditional Chinese Medicine and a clinically based Western science program. Course work covers Acupuncture and Basic Oriental Medicine, Acupuncture Clinic, Chinese Herbal Training, Western Medical Sciences, Oriental Bodywork, Business and Ethics, and Physical Internal Martial Arts.

The one-year, 596-hour Oriental Bodywork Program provides extensive training in Shiatsu, Tui Na, or Chi Nei Tsang, plus Oriental Medicine Theory, Nutrition, Anatomy and Physiology, Business Management, and the Internal Martial Arts. Students in the Oriental Bodywork Program may apply for transfer credit to the Oriental Medicine Program.

The one-year, 548-hour Medical Qigong Therapy Program covers Medical Qigong, Oriental Medical Theory, Business and Ethics, Western Sciences and Internal Martial Arts.

Classes are taught in English only and are offered days, evenings, and Saturdays.

Continuing Education

A one-year Teacher's Development Program in Oriental Bodywork is open to AOBTA certified practitioners and/or graduates of AOMA's Oriental Bodywork Program or of other AOBTA approved schools. The aim of the program is to enhance teaching skills by drawing on innovations in education beyond Oriental medicine.

Admission Requirements

Applicants to any of AOMA's programs must have completed at least sixty semester credits of general education at the bachelor's level at an accredited college or university, with a minimum GPA of 2.0. Applicants are encouraged to have completed at least six semester credits of Anatomy and Physiology; this requirement must be completed before the second year of Oriental Medicine studies. Further requirements include a high degree of competency in the English language, a personal interview, two letters of reference, a handwritten statement of interest and intent, and a keen desire to become a healer with high ethical standards.

Tuition and Fees

Tuition for all programs is $10.42 per hour for didactic classes and $6.75 per hour for clinic instruction. The approximate total costs for the programs are $27,500 for Oriental Medicine, $5,500 for Oriental Bodywork, $5,250 for Medical Qigong, and $2,950 for Teacher's Development.

Financial Assistance

Scholarships, federal subsidized and unsubsidized loans, and veterans' benefits are available; AOMA is an approved provider of training to clients of the Texas Rehabilitation Commission.

American College of Acupuncture and Oriental Medicine

9100 Park West Drive
Houston, Texas 77063
PHONE: (713) 780-9777 / (800) 729-4456
FAX: (713) 781-5781
E-MAIL: acaom@compuserve.com
WEBSITE: www.acaom.edu

The American College of Acupuncture and Oriental Medicine was founded in 1992 by Shen Ping Liang as the American Academy of Acupuncture and Traditional Chinese Medicine. The college assumed its current name in May 1996. There are sixteen instructors, with an average of twenty students per class.

Accreditation and Approvals
The Master of Science in Oriental Medicine degree program is accredited by the Accreditation Commission for Acupuncture and Oriental Medicine (ACAOM).

Program Description
The four-year Master of Science in Oriental Medicine degree program consists of 1,740 lecture hours and 870 Clinical Training lab hours.

Year One courses include Intro to TCM, History and Philosophy, Physiology of TCM, Etiology and Pathogenesis, Intro to Herbology, Intro to Acupuncture, Anatomy, Diagnosis of TCM, Anatomical Acupuncture, Herbology, Physiology, Research Methodology, Tai Chi and Qi Gong, Medical Terminology, and Histology.

Year Two courses include Differentiation of Syndromes, Herbology, Anatomical Acupuncture, Pathology, CPR and First Aid, Clean Needle Techniques, Health Psychology, Ethics and Patient Communication, Herbal Prescription, Usage of Acupoints, Hygiene and Public Health, Treatment of Common Diseases, Auricular Acupuncture, Acupuncture Techniques, Special Topics, and Clinic Observation.

Year Three courses include Gynecology of TCM, Scalp Acupuncture, Microbiology, Office and Clinic Management, Nutrition and Dietetics, Herbal Clinic Studies, Basic Medical Chinese, Chinese Internal Medicine, Advanced Acupuncture Techniques, Diagnostic Methods of Western Medicine, Pharmacology, Herbal Clinic Studies, Homeopathy, Chronotherapeutics, Medical Referral, Special Topics, Clinic Internship, and Problem-Based Learning.

Year Four consists of TCM Review, Food Therapy, Clinic Internship, Acupressure and Tui-Na, and Problem-Based Learning.

Admission Requirements
Applicants must have completed at least sixty semester hours of general academic college-level courses and submit two letters of recommendation.

Tuition and Fees
There is a $50 application fee; tuition is $160 per credit full-time and $165 per credit part-time. Books and materials cost approximately $300 per semester; graduation fee is $200.

Financial Assistance
Federal grants and loans, a payment plan, and veterans' benefits are available.

Asten Center of Natural Therapeutics

(See Multiple State Locations, page 386)

Austin School of Massage Therapy

2600 West Stassney Lane
Austin, Texas 78745
PHONE: (512) 462-3005 / (800) 276-2768
FAX: (512) 462-3265
WEBSITE: www.asmt.com

The Austin School of Massage Therapy was founded in 1985 and has grown to be the largest in Texas, with classes held in twelve cities: Amarillo, Austin, College Station, Dallas, El Paso, Fort Worth, Lubbock, Midland, San Angelo, San Antonio, and Waco, with more locations coming soon. There are thirty instructors, with an average of twenty-two students per class.

Accreditation and Approvals
The Austin School of Massage Therapy is accredited by the Integrative Massage and Somatic Therapies Accreditation Council (IMSTAC). The 300-hour program meets the requirements of the Texas Department of Health for registration eligibility in the state of Texas. Graduates of massage therapy programs of 500 hours or more are eligible to take the National Certification Examination for Therapeutic Massage and Bodywork (NCETMB).

Program Description

The 300-hour Level One training includes 250 hours of instruction in Massage Technique (topics include Swedish massage, stretching, awareness of energetics, sports massage, trigger points, on-site massage, and others), Anatomy and Physiology, Hydrotherapy, Health and Hygiene, Business Practices and Professional Ethics, Practical Applications, and a fifty-hour internship.

Level Two training adds an additional 900 hours to the program for a total of 1,200 hours. Courses include Sports Massage, Neuromuscular Therapy, Advanced Anatomy, and Internship.

Continuing Education

Continuing education workshops are offered in such areas as myofascial release, trigger point therapy, reflexology, rhythmic massage, energetic techniques, and neuromuscular therapy. Internships and teacher training are also available.

Admission Requirements

Applicants must be at least 18 years old and have a high school diploma or equivalent.

Tuition and Fees

A $200 deposit is due with the application. Tuition for the 300-hour program is $2,950, including handouts, use of a massage table during class, and a polo shirt. Tuition for the 1,200-hour program ranges from $6,000 to $7,000.

Financial Assistance

Payment plans, limited scholarships, veterans' benefits, and limited work-study are available.

Dallas Institute of Acupuncture and Oriental Medicine

2947 Walnut Hill Lane, Suite 101
Dallas, Texas 75229
PHONE: (214) 350-4282
FAX: (214) 350-9056
E-MAIL: DIAOM@Flashnet.com
WEBSITE: www.HolisticNetworker.com/DIAOM

The Dallas Institute of Acupuncture and Oriental Medicine (DIAOM) was founded in 1991 by Stuart Mauro. There are thirteen instructors, with an average of twelve students per class.

Accreditation and Approvals

DIAOM has been granted candidate status with the Accreditation Commission for Acupuncture and Oriental Medicine (ACAOM).

Program Description

The 2,745-hour Oriental Medicine program is a full-time, four-year program taught in a minimum of thirty-six months; a limited number of part-time applicants may be admitted, and must complete the program in a maximum of seventy-two months.

First-year courses include Osteology and Myology, Regional Surface Anatomy, Western Medical Terminology, Oriental Medical Theory, Tui Na, Point Location, Qi Gong, Introduction to TCM Diagnosis, Hygiene and Sanitation, Neurology and Special Senses, Oriental Medical Terminology, Point Energetics, Tongue Diagnosis, Thoracic and Abdominal Systems, Pulse Diagnosis, Clinic Technique, Clinical Observation, and Microbiology.

Second-year courses include Reproduction and Embryology, Zang Fu, Channel Theory, TCM Treatment of Disease, Clinic Technique, Point Energetics, Clinical Observation, Pre-Clinic, Counseling and Communications, Western Diagnosis, Auricular, Materia Medica, Clinic, Pathophysiology and Treatment of Disease, Jin Shin, and Scalp, Face and Foot Acupuncture.

Third-year courses include Pathophysiology and Treatment of Disease, Principles of Nutrition, Materia Medica, Formula, Clinic, TCM Treatment of Disease, Hand Acupuncture, Herbal Internship, Practice Management/Ethics, Botany, Differentiation of Disease, and Clinical Grand Rounds.

Admission Requirements

Applicants must have completed at least sixty semester hours of accredited postsecondary education at the baccalaureate level with a GPA of at least 2.0; be proficient in the English language; submit two letters of recommendation, a statement of intent, and a health certificate signed by a physician; and have a personal interview.

Tuition and Fees
Tuition is $125 per semester hour full-time, $145 per semester hour part-time. Additional expenses include a $50 application fee; approximately $300 per trimester for books and materials; malpractice insurance, at cost; and a graduation fee of $150.

Financial Assistance
Payment plans are available.

Hands-On Therapy School of Massage

PRIMARY SITE:
625 Gatewood Drive
Garland, Texas 75043
PHONE: (972) 240-9288
FAX: (972) 240-9801
E-MAIL: HOTschool@aol.com
WEBSITE: www.handsontherapyschools.com

INTERN CLINIC:
2009 North Galloway
Mesquite, Texas 75149
PHONE: (972) 285-6133

Hands-On Therapy was founded in 1990. Owner/director Carolyn Scott Naile has been practicing bodywork since 1980 and is the past president of the Texas Chapter of the American Massage Therapy Association (AMTA). There are nine instructors, with a maximum of twelve students per class.

Accreditation and Approvals
The Hands-On Therapy massage curriculum is a member of the AMTA Council of Schools and recognized by the Texas Department of Health. Graduates of programs of 500 or more hours are qualified to take the National Certification Examination for Therapeutic Massage and Bodywork (NCETMB). Hands-On Therapy is approved by the National Certificaiton Board for Therapeutic Massage and Bodywork (NCBTMB) as a continuing education provider.

Program Description
The 300-hour Basic Program consists of Swedish Massage, Anatomy and Physiology, Health and Hygiene, Hydrotherapy, Business Practices and Professional Ethics, and a fifty-hour internship.

The 200-hour Advanced Program provides the additional requirements for national certification as well as AMTA membership. Courses include Deep Tissue Massage, Trigger Point, Sports Massage, Chair Massage, Reflexology, and Shiatsu.

Classes are held days, evenings, and weekends, on a slow or fast track.

Continuing Education
A variety of workshops are offered to the massage professional. These include Aromatherapy, Manual Lymph Drainage, Spinal Touch, Trager®, Zen Shiatsu, State Board Test Review, Shiatsu II, Orthobionomy, and any of the advanced program courses.

Admission Requirements
Applicants must be physically, mentally, emotionally, and financially capable of completing the course, be free of criminal convictions, interview with an admissions representative, and tour the school prior to admission.

Tuition and Fees
Basic program is $2,250; books are $184, and supplies are $50. Tuition for the Advanced Program is $1,600. Workshops are individually priced.

Financial Assistance
Early registration discounts, interest-free financing, and long-term financing are available.

The Institute of Natural Healing Sciences

4100 Felps Drive, Suite E
Colleyville, Texas 76034
PHONE: (817) 498-0716 / (800) 448-4954
FAX: (817) 281-1414
E-MAIL: hmmj@nkn.net
WEBSITE: www.mind-body-spirit.com

The Institute of Natural Healing Sciences (INHS) was founded in 1985. The faculty consists of nine members.

Accreditation and Approvals

INHS is a member of the American Massage Therapy Association (AMTA) Council of Schools, and is registered with the Texas Department of Health. Graduates of programs of 500 or more hours are qualified to take the National Certification Examination for Therapeutic Massage and Bodywork (NCETMB).

Program Description

The 300-hour Basic Massage Therapy Course includes classes in Anatomy, Physiology, Health and Hygiene, Business Practices and Ethics, Hydrotherapy, Traditional Swedish Massage Techniques, and a fifty-hour internship. Day and evening classes are offered.

A 290-hour Advanced Course is offered to students who have completed the Basic Course requirements and have graduated from a program approved by AMTA or the Associated Bodywork and Massage Professionals (ABMP). Classes include Reflexology, Sports Massage, Shiatsu and On-Site Chair Massage, Polarity Therapy: Basic and Advanced, Craniosacral Balancing, Myofascial Release, and Clinical Applications of Massage Therapy.

Admission Requirements

Prospective students must be at least 18 years of age; have a high school diploma or equivalent; submit a physician's statement that the applicant is physically capable of participation in the program; have a personal interview; provide two letters of character reference; and be free of any criminal convictions within the past five years.

Tuition and Fees

Tuition for the Basic Course is $2,250. Additional expenses include a $50 application fee; books and supplies, $194; linens and oil, approximately $149; AMTA student membership and liability insurance, $188, or ABMP student membership and liability insurance, $75; massage table additional.

Tuition for the Advanced Course is $2,450; books are $145.

Financial Assistance

A payment plan is available.

The Lauterstein-Conway Massage School

4701-B Burnet Road
Austin, Texas 78756
PHONE: (512) 374-9222
FAX: (512) 374-9812
E-MAIL: info@tlcschool.com
WEBSITE: www.tlcschool.com

The Lauterstein-Conway Massage School (TLC) was founded in 1989, though its core curriculum was developed in 1982 while David Lauterstein taught deep massage and anatomy at the Chicago School of Massage. Lauterstein and John Conway later co-evolved the curriculum at the Texas School of Massage Studies. There are thirty instructors, with an average of twenty-six students per class.

Accreditation and Approvals

TLC's two-semester, 550-hour program is accredited by the Commission on Massage Training Accreditation (COMTA). The school is registered with and regulated by the State of Texas Department of Health. Graduates of programs of 500 or more hours are qualified to take the National Certification Examination for Therapeutic Massage and Bodywork (NCETMB).

Program Description

TLC offers 750 hours of education divided into three semesters. Students may choose between day, evening, or primarily weekend classes.

Semester One consists of the 300 hours required by the Texas Department of Health and is the first semester of the COMTA-accredited program. Courses include Swedish Massage, Human Anatomy, Human Physiology, Hydrotherapy, Human Health and Hygiene, Business Practices and Ethics, and a fifty-hour internship.

Semester Two is the second semester of the COMTA-accredited program. Courses include Advanced Anatomy and Physiology, Sports Massage, Structural Bodywork, Deep Massage, Zen Shiatsu, Integrative Bodywork, Movement Skills, and Professionalism, Ethics, and Business Practice. Semester Two students must have current certification in CPR/First Aid.

Semester Three is a 200-hour program for practicing therapists who want to learn advanced methods of working with clients. Courses include Craniosacral Work, Advanced Structural Bodywork, Clinical Applications in Bodywork, Psychology of Bodywork, Zero Balancing®, and Advanced Integrative Bodywork.

Admission Requirements

Applicants must be at least 18 years of age, have a high school diploma or equivalent, be of sound mind and body, submit a physician's letter, and interview with an admissions representative.

There is no prerequisite training for Semester One. Semester Two requires at least 250 hours of massage therapy training or registration in Texas as a massage therapist. Semester Three requires at least 500 hours of training in massage therapy.

Tuition and Fees

Tuition for Semester One is $2,550 (includes $200 application fee); for Semester Two, $2,550; and for Semester Three, $2,200. Books are approximately $119 for Semester One, $86 for Semester Two, and $98 for Semester Three. Additional expenses include linens and oils, approximately $55 per semester; a massage table, $400 to $600; and CPR/First Aid certification, $35.

Financial Assistance

Payment plans, early registration discounts, and partial scholarships are available.

Maternidad La Luz

1308 Magoffin Street
El Paso, Texas 79901
PHONE: (915) 532-5895
FAX: (915) 532-7127

Maternidad La Luz was founded in 1987 as a community-based birthing center and midwifery school. The staff and students care for approximately forty birthing women per month, 85 percent of whom are Spanish-speaking only. Director Deborah Kaley has been practicing midwifery since 1981. There are eight instructors; approximately twelve students are accepted per quarter.

Accreditation and Approvals

Maternidad La Luz is accredited by the Midwifery Education and Accreditation Council (MEAC) and approved by the State of Texas Department of Health and by the City of El Paso. Completion of the first four quarters will meet NARM requirements for a Certified Professional Midwife.

Program Description

The Direct Entry Midwifery Program consists of four quarters; students requiring a three-year program will need to successfully complete all nine quarters. Students learn practical midwifery skills beginning the first day of classes, and can expect hands-on birth experience within the first month. Students attend approximately twenty-five to thirty-five births per quarter (100 to 140 per year); the clinical experience during the year program far exceeds the NARM requirements to become a Certified Professional Midwife.

First Quarter academic classes include Communication Skills, Regulation and Ethics, Infection Control and Applied Microbiology, HIV/AIDS/HBV, Maternal Assessment, Venipuncture/Lab, Pap/GC/Chlamydia, Spanish for Midwives, Basic Labor Support, Basic Emergency Skills, Basic Newborn Skills, Basic Postpartum Skills, Initial Interviews, Nutrition, Family Planning, Breastfeeding, Medical Terminology for Midwives, Pelvimetry, Understanding Labwork, Gestational Diabetes, Common Prenatal Complications, and others.

The Second Quarter curriculum includes Neonatal Resuscitation, Physiology of Labor, Fetal Heart Tones, Normal Birth and Labor, Normal Postpartum, Hemorrhage and Shock, Newborn Adaptation, Risk Assessment, Prematurity/Postmaturity, Premature Rupture of Membranes, Unusual Presentations, Placenta Problems, Death/Grief, Water Birth, Uterine Complications, Postpartum Complications, and Homebirth and Establishing a Private Practice.

Third Quarter topics include Current Midwifery Issues, Childbirth Education and Counseling, Childbirth Education Classes, Choosing On-Call Clients, Peer Review, and Birth Talks/Midwifery Issues.

Fourth Quarter topics include Principles of Preventative and Community Health in Well Woman Care, Physical Assessment, Pharmacology, Embryology, Genetics, IV Practicum, Ultrasound, Multiple Births, Alternative Therapies, Advanced Suturing, Breeches, and more.

Topics covered in quarters Five through Nine include Social and Cultural Aspects of Midwifery Care, Research, Methods and Analysis, Epidemiology, Clinical Synthesis, and Past, Present and Future of Midwifery plus seminars in Prenatal Care, Labor, Birth, Newborn Care, and Postpartum Care.

Admission Requirements

Applicants must be at least 18 years of age and have a high school diploma or equivalent. A thorough understanding of English is required. Before beginning classes students must have proof of a current CPR card, proof of a negative TB tine test, a car and a valid driver's license. A basic understanding of Spanish is an asset. It is strongly recommended that applicants obtain a Neonatal Resuscitation Certificate before coming to the center; the certification is offered at Maternidad La Luz only during the Second and Ninth Quarters.

Tuition and Fees

Tuition is $2,250 for the First and Second Quarters (combined fee); $2,250 for the Third and Fourth Quarters (combined fee); and $1,450 for each of the Fifth through Ninth Quarters.

Financial Assistance

Past students have been able to arrange college credit for their training at Maternidad La Luz and have thus been able to get financial aid through their sponsoring university. Maternidad La Luz offers one full tuition scholarship to assist women of color; some work-study scholarships are available for the Fifth through Ninth Quarters.

Parker College of Chiropractic

2500 Walnut Hill Lane
Dallas, Texas 75229-5668
PHONE: (972) 438-6932 / (800) GET-MY-DC (admissions)
FAX: (214) 902-2413
E-MAIL: admissions@parkercc.edu
WEBSITE: www.parkercc.edu

Parker College of Chiropractic was founded in 1978. The college is named for Dr. James William Parker, who established eighteen chiropractic clinics in Texas and founded the Parker Chiropractic Resource Foundation, which has held nearly 350 four-day postgraduate seminars (the Parker School for Professional Success) attended by over 200,000 chiropractors. There are 122 instructors, with a student:teacher ratio of 13:1.

Accreditation and Approvals

Parker College of Chiropractic is accredited by the Southern Association of Schools and Colleges and by the Council on Chiropractic Education (CCE).

Program Description

The 4,852½-hour Doctor of Chiropractic (D.C.) degree program may be completed in nine trimesters of full-time study.

Trimesters I through III include Seminars for Success, Systemic Anatomy, Embryology, Histology, Cell Biology, Introduction to Chiropractic, Chiropractic Philosophy, Ethics, Gross Anatomy, Physiology, Biochemistry, Palpation, Spinal Biomechanics, Normal Radiographic Anatomy, Fundamentals of Diagnostic Imaging, Research and Statistics, Neuroscience, Microbiology, Diversified Technique, and Extra-Spinal Biomechanics.

Trimesters IV through VI include Assembly, Physiology, Pathology, Public Health, Neuroscience, Thompson Technique, Clinical Orthopedics, Physical Diagnosis, Radiographic Exam Technique, Pharmacology/Toxicology, Diagnosis, Lab Diagnosis, Clinical Neurology, Bone Pathology, Gonstead Technique, Upper Cervical Technique, Student Clinic, Building a Student Clinic Practice, Emergency Care, Physiological Therapeutics, Chiropractic Theories, EENT, and Bone Pathology.

Courses in trimesters VII through IX include Chiropractic Theories, Clinical Nutrition, Physiological Therapeutics, Clinical Psychology, Sacro-Occipital Technique, Soft Tissue Pathology, OB/GYN, Dermatology, Internship Lecture and Practicum, Risk Management/Malpractice, Chiropractic Philosophy, Geriatrics/Pediatrics, Flexion/Distraction, Activator, Applied Kinesiology, Rehabilitation Procedures, Chiropractic Economics, Jurisprudence, and Communications.

A Bachelor of Science degree in anatomy may be earned simultaneously with the D.C. degree; consult the catalog or a college representative for additional information.

The Chiropractic Assistant Program is an ongoing two-year course of study leading to licensure in Florida; contact the college for additional information. Other C.A. courses are presented in relevant areas of interest.

Continuing Education

Postgraduate education programs are offered in Chiropractic Orthopedics, Clinical Neurology, Chiropractic Roentgenology, The Evaluation of Sports Injuries and Their Management, Chiropractic Principles and Technique, Clinical Diagnosis, Practice Management, Special License Renewal Symposia, Physiological Therapeutics in Chiropractic, Meridian Therapy/Acupuncture, Clinical Nutrition, and Chiropractic Assistant.

Postgraduate courses leading to diplomate status include Diplomate American Board of Chiropractic Orthopedists (DABCO); Diplomate American Chiropractic Academy of Neurology (DACAN); and Diplomate American Chiropractic Board of Nutrition (DACBN). Each requires 300 to 360 hours or approximately three years to complete. The college also offers a 100-hour Certification in Sports Injuries.

Admission Requirements

Applicants must have completed at least sixty semester hours (two academic years) of college-level credit at an accredited institution with an overall GPA of at least 2.50 on a 4.0 scale and a grade of C or better in each science course. Specific course requirements include at least six semester hours each in biological science, general or inorganic chemistry, organic chemistry, physics, and English or communicative skills; at least three semester hours of psychology; at least fifteen semester hours of humanities or social sciences; and from four to twelve semester hours of electives. It is highly recommended that a student take anatomy and physiology prior to attendance. Texas licensure laws require additional hours of prerequisite science courses beyond those listed above; see the catalog for details.

Applicants must also be physically capable of performing manipulative procedures and submit three letters of recommendation (one preferably from a Doctor of Chiropractic).

Tuition and Fees

Tuition and fees are $5,087 per trimester. Additional expenses include application fee, $35; books and supplies, approximately $618 per trimester; and graduation fee, $130.

Financial Assistance

Federal grants, loans, and work-study; state grants; scholarships; ChiroLoan; Bureau of Indian Affairs; and veterans' benefits are available.

Texas Chiropractic College

5912 Spencer Highway
Pasadena, Texas 77505-1699
PHONE: (713) 487-1170 / (800) GO-TO-TEX
FAX: (713) 487-2009
E-MAIL: amonsegue@txchiro.edu
WEBSITE: www.txchiro.edu

Texas Chiropractic College was founded in San Antonio in 1908 by Dr. J. N. Stone, a pioneer in the field of chiropractic. There are thirty-eight full-time and seven part-time faculty members, with an average of fifty students per class.

Accreditation and Approvals

Texas Chiropractic College is accredited by the Council on Chiropractic Education (CCE) and by the Commission on Colleges of the Southern Association of Colleges and Schools. The college is also recognized by the Federation of Chiropractic Licensing Boards.

Program Description

The ten-trimester, 4,605-hour Doctor of Chiropractic (D.C.) degree program may be completed in five years (attending fall and spring trimesters) or as little as three and one-third years by also attending summer trimesters.

First-year (trimesters 1 through 3) classes include Histology, Gross Human Anatomy, Chiropractic Principles, Human Biochemistry, Palpation, Research Methodology, Spinal Anatomy, Physiology, Clinic Clerkship, Human Embryology, General Microbiology, Spinal Biomechanics, Human Neuroanatomy, Adjusting Procedures, Pathogenic Microbiology, Abnormal Psychology, and Pathology.

Second-year (trimesters 4 through 6) courses include Pathology, Physiology, Clinic Clerkship, Chiropractic Principles, Adjusting Procedures, Public Health and Hygiene, Appendicular Biomechanics, Toxicology/Pharmacology, X-Ray Physics, Physical Exam and Diagnosis, Introduction to Radiology, Nutrition, Obstetrics and Gynecology, Pediatric and Geriatric Diagnosis, X-Ray Positioning, Clinical Neurology, Clinical Case Applications, Orthopedics, Skeletal Imaging, and Internal Diagnosis.

Third-year (trimesters 7 through 9) classes include Spinal Imaging, Clinical Lab Diagnosis, Orthopedics, Student Clinic,

Dermatology, Internal Diagnosis, Adjusting Procedures, Physical Medicine and Rehab, Case Management, Emergency Procedures, Ethics and Jurisprudence, Insurance and Office Procedures, and Clinic.

The tenth trimester consists of Clinic and Preceptorship.

Students may also complete a Bachelor of Science degree in Human Biology. See the catalog for specific information.

Continuing Education

A range of continuing education opportunities is offered to the Doctor of Chiropractic, from extensive diplomate-level classes of 300 or more hours to twelve-hour weekend seminars. Programs are offered that, upon completion, make the doctor eligible for examination leading to diplomate status in Diagnosis, Internal Disorders and Preventive Medicine (DABCI), neurology (DACAN) or orthopedics (DABCO). In addition, the college offers certification programs in Certified Chiropractic Sports Physician (CCSP), clinical nutrition, and Manipulation Under Anesthesia (MUA). Numerous weekend programs are also offered both on and off campus in such areas as physical medicine, modern concepts of pain management, behavioral medicine, personal injury, Myofascial Trigger Point Therapy, AIDS, surface EMG, and other areas.

Admission Requirements

Applicants must have completed at least two years (sixty semester hours or ninety quarter hours) of prechiropractic college work at a regionally accredited college or university, with a minimum GPA of 2.5 on a 4.0 scale for all college work; all prerequisite science courses must carry a grade of C or better. Applicants must have completed, or must complete by the term of enrollment, the following courses: six semester hours of biological science with lab; six semester hours of inorganic chemistry; six semester hours of organic chemistry; six semester hours of physics; six semester hours of English or communication skills; three semester hours of psychology; and fifteen semester hours of social sciences/humanities electives. Course work in computer skills and statistics is strongly recommended.

Applicants must also submit an essay and two personal references, one of which must be from a Doctor of Chiropractic; interview with an admissions representative; and have the physical strength and bodily coordination to perform chiropractic manipulative techniques, the manual dexterity to perform safely and effectively in the laboratories and in diagnosis, and sufficient auditory sense and speaking ability to conduct health history interviews and clinical examinations. Physically disabled students who cannot meet the physical qualifications will be subject to a review/evaluation for admission eligibility.

Tuition and Fees

Tuition is $4,600 per trimester.

Financial Assistance

Federal grants, loans, and work-study; scholarships; state grants; ChiroLoan; other loan sources; veterans' benefits; and aid from state rehabilitation agencies are available.

Texas College of Traditional Chinese Medicine

4005 Manchaca Road, Suite 200
Austin, Texas 78704
PHONE: (512) 444-8082 / (800) 252-5088
FAX: (512) 444-6345
E-MAIL: texastcm@taxastcm.edu
WEBSITE: www.texastcm.edu

The Texas College of Traditional Chinese Medicine held its first class in January 1990, and is the oldest school of acupuncture and Oriental medicine in Texas. A sister-school relationship is maintained with the Heilongjiang University of Traditional Chinese Medicine in Harbin, People's Republic of China. There are twelve instructors; class sizes range from eight to twenty-five students.

Accreditation and Approvals

The Oriental Medicine Program is accredited by the Accreditation Commission for Acupuncture and Oriental Medicine (ACAOM) and approved by the Texas State Board of Acupuncture Examiners.

Program Description

The 2,645-hour Master of Science in Oriental Medicine Program runs eight semesters.

The first-year curriculum includes such classes as Fundamental Theories of TCM; Chinese Terminology and Phonetics; Point Location; Diagnosis and Differentiation; Five Element Theory and Application; Qigong; Anatomy, Physiology, and Histology; CPR; Biomedical Concepts and Terminology; Special Acupuncture Techniques; TCM Herbology; Meridian Theory; and Clinical Observation and Evaluation.

Year Two consists of Meridian Acupoint Energetics and Application; TCM Prescriptionology; Internal Medicine (Acupuncture); Biomedical Diagnosis: Lab Test; Clinical Internship; Scalp and Ear Acupuncture; Food, Diet, and Vitamins; Biomedical Pathology and Bacteriology; and more.

In Year Three, the curriculum includes Classics: Shang Han Lun; Patent Herbs and Herbal Prescription Preparation; Tui Na; Directed Research: Acupuncture; Practical Herbal Formulations; Biomedical Pharmacology; Internal Medicine: Herbology; TCM Gynecology; Practice Management and Ethics; Counseling and Communications; Licensure Requirements and Examination Preparation; Hygiene, Public Health, and Referral Modalities; Clinical Internship; and more.

Classes are held Monday through Friday nights and during the day on Saturday. Most students hold full-time jobs.

Admission Requirements

Applicants must have completed at least sixty semester hours of accredited college-level course work. Applicants must also interview with an admissions representative and submit a letter explaining why they wish to attend.

Tuition and Fees

Didactic tuition is $135 per semester credit; clinic tuition is $210 per semester credit. Additional expenses include a $75 application fee; registration fee, $50 per semester; herb use fee, $100; clinic use fee (third to sixth semesters), $75 per semester; liability insurance (third through sixth semesters), approximately $200 per semester; books and supplies, approximately, $150 per semester; and time payment fee, $25 to $50. Total costs are approximately $3,560 per semester in the first year and $3,770 per semester thereafter.

Financial Assistance

Federal loans and payment plans are available. Federal grants are available for undergraduate students who have not earned a bachelor's or professional degree.

The Winters School

4625 Southwest Freeway, Suite 142
Houston, Texas 77027
PHONE: (713) 626-2200
FAX: (713) 626-2230
E-MAIL: TWSdirectr@aol.com

The Winters School was founded in 1984 by owner and president Nancy Winters. Ms. Winters has served on the Advisory Council on Massage Therapy for the Texas Department of Health. The faculty consists of sixteen members. Maximum student:instructor ratios are 50:1 for lectures and 30:1 for hands-on training.

Accreditation and Approvals

The Winters School is a Texas State–registered massage school, and is approved by the National Certification Board for Therapeutic Massage and Bodywork (NCBTMB) as a continuing education provider. Students who complete both the Basic and Associate programs are eligible to take the National Certification Examination for Therapeutic Massage and Bodywork (NCETMB).

Program Description

The 300-hour Basic Massage Therapy Program (BMTP) includes Human Anatomy, Human Physiology, Hydrotherapy, Human Health and Hygiene, Business Practices and Professional Ethics, Swedish Massage Therapy, and Internship. Classes meet several times per week for four to eight months.

An additional 250 hours of training are offered through the Associate Massage Therapy Program (AMTP). Courses include Program Orientation, Polarity Therapy, Business Development, Somatics: Deep Tissue, Intermediate Anatomy and Physiology, Shiatsu, and Session Design.

Part-time students may enroll in individual topics.

Admission Requirements

Applicants must submit a completed application form and verification that the applicant has received at least one professional bodywork session from a registered massage therapist.

Tuition and Fees

Basic Massage Therapy Program tuition is $2,600 including a $200 application fee; total estimated cost for the entire program including tuition, books, supplies, and two bodywork sessions is $3,582. Tuition for the Associate Program is $2,500; total estimated cost for the program including tuition, books, and supplies is $2,670. Part-time tuition is $10 per hour for Basic Level courses, $12 per hour for Associate Level courses.

Financial Assistance

Payment plans and veterans' benefits are available.

UTAH

Myotherapy College of Utah

1174 East 2700 South #19
Salt Lake City, Utah 84106
PHONE: (801) 484-7624
Fax (801) 484-1928
E-MAIL: myo@xmission.com

Myotherapy College of Utah was founded by Jim and Shirley Foster in 1987. Vaughn L. Belnap is the current president/director. There are 16 instructors, with an average of fifteen students per class.

Accreditation and Approvals

Myotherapy College of Utah is accredited by the Accrediting Commission of Career Schools and Colleges of Technology (ACCSCT), and approved by the Utah Nurses Association and by the National Certification Board for Therapeutic Massage and Bodywork (NCBTMB) as a continuing education provider. Graduates are qualified to take the National Certification Examination for Therapeutic Massage and Bodywork (NCETMB).

Program Description

The 780-hour Basic Core Course in massage therapy consists of Swedish Massage, including theory, lab, clinical practice, and specialized massage; Anatomy, including anatomy and physiology, functional anatomy, and common pathology; General Education, consisting of study skills, practice building and Utah

law, and psychology for the massage therapist; Bodywork, including therapeutic principles, survey of bodywork modalities, acutherapy, polarity, introduction to shiatsu, and Touch for Health I; and electives that include Shiatsu II, Touch for Health II, Basic Sports Massage, Business Practices, and others.

Continuing Education

Continuing education classes are offered in Spinal Touch, Aromatherapy, Sports Massage, Herbology, Personology, Tui Na, Cranial, and more.

Admission Requirements

Applicants must have a high school diploma or equivalent and interview with the admissions director. Advanced course applicants must have a license to perform massage or similar qualifications in a health care field; applicants who have not graduated from the Basic Course must pass an extensive anatomy exam and practical hands-on evaluation before taking any advanced classes.

Tuition and Fees

There is a $25 application fee and a $100 registration fee. Tuition is $165 per quarter credit, or $6,435 total for the 39-credit Basic Core Course. Books are approximately $675; an optional massage table and supplies are additional.

Financial Assistance

A payment plan and financial aid are available to those who qualify.

The School of Natural Healing

P.O. Box 412
Springville, Utah 84663
PHONE: (801) 489-4254 / (800) 372-8255
FAX: (801) 489-8341
E-MAIL: snh@avpro.com
WEBSITE: www.schoolofnaturalhealing.com

While the School of Natural Healing emphasizes home study, four- and six-day certification seminars in Utah are offered to complement the correspondence programs in herbology and iridology. See pages 476-77 for a complete description of both home study programs and seminars.

Utah College of Massage Therapy

(See Multiple State Locations, page 417)

Utah College of Midwifery

230 West 170 North
Orem, Utah 84057
PHONE: (801) 764-9068 / (888) 489-1238
E-MAIL: midwife@uswest.net

Utah College of Midwifery (UCM) was founded in 1980. There are twenty instructors, with an average of six students per class. In addition to the programs described here, UCM offers the following additional certifications: Certified Childbirth Educator (CCE); Certified Doula (CD); and Certified Birth Attendant (CBA) Level I, II, and III; contact the college for details about these programs.

Accreditation and Approvals

Utah College of Midwifery is accredited by the Midwifery Education Accreditation Council (MEAC). UCM's curriculum is in compliance with the Midwives' Alliance of North America (MANA) core competencies and the North American Registry of Midwives (NARM) practical skills. Graduates are eligible to apply for NARM Certification and to take the NARM exams.

Program Description

UCM programs described here are the undergraduate degrees Associate of Science in Midwifery (A.S.M.) and Bachelor of Science in Midwifery (B.S.M.), the certification Certified Traditional Midwife (C.T.M.), the graduate degree Master of Science in Midwifery (M.S.M.), and the graduate-level certification Certified Master Midwife (C.M.M.).

There are three levels of undergraduate core requirements; each level takes one year to complete. Level I core courses are Introduction to Anatomy; Anatomy and Physiology of Obstetrics; Herb Identification, Horticulture, and Preparations; Holistic Health; Pediatrics; Labor and Birth; Postpartum Care;

Postpartum Care Lab; Neonatal Resuscitation; and Reflexology. Level II core courses are Genetics; Medical Terminology; Body Systems Analysis; Diagnostic Tests; Prenatal Care; Prenatal Care Lab; Complications; Suturing; Labor and Birth Lab; History of Midwifery; and Massage. Level III core courses are Chemistry and Nutrition; Applied Microbiology Lab; Embryology and Neonatology; Clinical Epidemiology; Symptomology; Homeopathy for Midwives; Natural Family Planing; Obstetrical Pharmacology; Suturing; Well Woman Care; Communication Skills for Health Professionals; Client Handbook; and Midwifery Services. Core courses are also available through correspondence; contact UCM for details.

Associate of Science in Midwifery (A.S.M.) requirements include completion of Level I and II core courses; completion of a total of sixty-six semester credits (twenty or more credits must be UCM courses); a minimum GPA of 2.0 in all core courses, with an overall minimum GPA of 2.5; completion of parts I–V of the Practical Skills Guide for Midwifery; completion of clinical experience, including seventy-five prenatal exams, fifty births, twenty newborn exams, and forty postpartum exams; current CPR certification; plus additional requirements.

Bachelor of Science in Midwifery (B.S.M.) requirements include completion of all of the A.S.M. requirements above plus completion of Level III core courses; completion of an additional sixty semester credits beyond the associate's degree (twenty or more credits must be UCM courses); plus additional requirements.

Certified Traditional Midwife (C.T.M.) requirements include completion of the Associate of Science in Midwifery (A.S.M.) degree, completion of Level III core courses, and additional requirements.

The Master of Science in Midwifery (M.S.M.) is an individually constructed program. Students must take at least thirty-two credits from the graduate curriculum, which is divided into the following modules: Professional Development Module; Midwifery Module; Holistic Health Module; Clinical Module; Thesis and/or Project Module; and Closing Module. Students must also verify or complete the clinical requirements for NARM certification, take a comprehensive exam, and meet additional requirements.

Certified Master Midwife (C.M.M.) requirements include

completion of the Master of Science in Midwifery (M.S.M.) degree, statistical analysis of personal midwifery practices, primary care giver for fifty women, and additional requirements.

Community and Continuing Education

UCM offers classes to the public which include Childbirth Classes, Natural Family Planning, Reflexology, CPR Certification, Certified Childbirth Educator, and Certified Doula.

Admission Requirements

Undergraduate degree applicants must have a high school diploma or equivalent, be proficient in English, submit two letters of recommendation, and interview with the registrar. Prior to the start of or within the first year of midwifery training, applicants should be a Certified Childbirth Educator or Certified Doula (available through UCM).

Graduate degree applicants must have a minimum GPA of 3.0 for their last sixty hours of undergraduate work or take the GRE General Test if grades are lower; have a bachelor's degree in Midwifery or a bachelor's degree with a major in pre-med, nursing, biological sciences, or health sciences, or a bachelor's degree with NARM certification or 100 documented birth experiences, or have M.D., Ph.D. in Naturopathy, or Doctor of Chiropractic degree; submit a letter of intent and two letters of recommendation; and interview with the graduate director.

Tuition and Fees

Undergraduate tuition is $85 per credit. Additional expenses include application fee, $25; clinical credits, $220; student fees, $150; certificates, $75 to $150; catalogs, $30; syllabi, $400; lab fees, $140; CPR certificate, $45; membership in midwifery organization, $60; books, $1,800; midwifery supplies, $1,000; off-site clinical training, $2,500. Total expenses for the three-year CTM program, $11,020.

Graduate tuition is $95 per credit. Additional expenses include application fee, $75; books, $500 to $1,500; comprehensive exam, $75; diploma fee, $25; MANA membership, $60; NARM certification, $700; and video expenses, $400 to $1,000.

Continuing education classes vary in price; Certified Childbirth Educator and Certified Doula courses are each $275.

Financial Assistance

Students may apply for personal loans at local banks.

VERMONT

Sage Mountain Herbal Retreat Center

P.O. Box 420
East Barre, Vermont 05649

The Sage Mountain Retreat Center was cofounded in 1989 by Rosemary Gladstar, author and founder of both the California School of Herbal Studies and United Plant Savers (see pages 451–52).

Program Description

A variety of programs in herbal education are offered in Vermont, around the world, and by correspondence (see page 476).

The Spirit and Essence of Herbs: An Herbal Apprentice program is offered both as a seven-month program and a two-week intensive apprenticeship limited to thirty students. Topics include identification of wild edible and medicinal plants; wild food cooking; herbal preparations, such as infusions, decoctions, solar and lunar infusions, salves, oils, and tinctures; materia medica: herbal therapeutics; field trips; plant walks; and more. This program is also offered one weekend per month over seven months.

Beyond Herbology 101, a five-day program in advanced herbal studies, features well-known teachers and focuses each year on a different aspect of herbalism.

Admission Requirements

There are no minimum age or educational requirements.

Tuition and Fees

Tuition for the Spirit and Essence of Herbs Herbal Apprentice program is $1,200 for the two-week intensive program, and $1,050 for the seven-month program. Tuition for both programs includes the Science and Art of Herbalism correspondence course, all materials and handouts, vegetarian meals, camping, and/or dormitory-style lodging. The cost of Beyond Herbology 101 is $450, including vegetarian meals, camping, and/or dormitory-style lodging.

Financial Assistance

A few work-study scholarships are available for each program.

Vermont College of Norwich University

Adult Degree Program
Montpelier, Vermont 05602
PHONE: (802) 828-8500 / (800) 336-6794
FAX: (802) 828-8508
E-MAIL: vcadmiss@norwich.edu
WEBSITE: www.norwich.edu/vermont college

Vermont College is part of Norwich University, founded in 1819. While the main campus is in Montpelier, the college also has an adult learning center in Brattleboro.

Accreditation and Approvals

Norwich University is accredited by the New England Association of Schools and Colleges, which permits Vermont College to provide fully accredited programs of study.

Program Description

The Adult Degree Program allows students to earn a Bachelor of Arts degree primarily by studying at home. Each semester, students choose a topic or subject area to study in depth for six months, and work with a faculty mentor to develop a detailed study plan involving reading and writing as well as other forms of creative expression, field work, or educational experiences. Students should expect to commit twenty hours per week to the program and to attend a nine-day residency in Montpelier at the beginning and end of every semester or one weekend each month.

Self-directed study is available in the area of holistic studies. Students have designed study projects that include An Exploration of Holistic Health Practices, Transpersonal Psychology, Substance Abuse Counseling and Movement Therapy, Herbology, Shamanic Healing, and Body/Mind Healing with a Focus on Visualization Techniques.

Requirements of the degree include study in the humanities, fine arts, social sciences, math, and science. Transferred credits may be used toward these requirements. Fifty percent of ADP graduates go on to graduate school; some use the ADP bachelor's degree as preparation for continued education in acupuncture, homeopathy, movement therapy, and other holistic therapies.

Admission Requirements

Applicants must submit official high school or college transcripts, a personal essay, and three letters of recommendation, and interview with an admissions representative.

Tuition and Fees

There is a $35 application fee; tuition is $4,310 per semester, including residency room and board.

Financial Assistance

Federal grants and loans, state grants, loans, scholarships, and specialized grants are available.

Vermont School of Herbal Studies

P.O. Box 232
Marshfield, Vermont 05658
PHONE: (802) 456-1402

The Vermont School of Herbal Studies was founded in 1991 by Janice M. Dinsdale. There are ten instructors, with an average of 14 students per class.

Program Description

The seven-month Foundations of Herbalism program meets one weekend per month and emphasizes a hands-on, folkloric approach. Topics covered include Herbal Applications, Culinary Uses of Herbs, Wild Foods Foraging, Flower Essences, Herbal Case Histories, Ethical Wildcrafting, Medicinal Terminology, Herbal Preparations, Aromatherapy, Planning and Planting an Herb Garden, Field Trips, Business Practices, Herbal First Aid, Spring Tonics, Natural Cosmetics, Chinese Herbs, Creating an Herbal Pharmacy, Herbs to Dry, Plants as Teachers, Ancient Wisdom, and The Art of Simplicity.

Tuition and Fees

Tuition is $975 and includes handouts, herb teas, products made in class, a complete first-aid kit, and guest speakers.

The Vermont School of Professional Massage

14 Merchant Street
Barre, Vermont 05641
PHONE: (802) 479-2340 / (800) 287-8816
FAX: (802) 479-2340

The Vermont School of Professional Massage was founded in 1989 by Faeterri Silver, who has been licensed for the practice of massage since 1981. In this small family-oriented school, Faeterri is the administrator and primary instructor, with occasional guest lecturers. Classes are limited to twelve students.

Accreditation

The Vermont School of Professional Massage is recognized by the State of Vermont, and graduates are qualified to take the National Certification Examination for Therapeutic Massage and Bodywork (NCETMB).

Program Description

The 600-hour full-time Professional Massage Therapy Program runs Monday through Wednesday for nine months. The curriculum includes Human Anatomy and Physiology, Massage Theory (including general relaxation massage, neuromuscular therapy, myofascial release, and an exposure to craniosacral therapy, lymphatic drainage techniques, shiatsu, chair, sports, Trager, and more), Massage Practicum Clinic, Eastern Bodywork, Medical Terminology, Office Procedures and Business Practices, Adjuncts (Practitioner Health, Ethics, CPR/First Aid, and Community Service), Assessment and Pathology.

Admission Requirements

Potential applicants are evaluated on desire and ability; a personal interview is encouraged.

Tuition and Fees

Tuition is $4,100 and includes books and practicum materials.

Financial Assistance

Monthly payment plans and Vermont Student Assistance Corporation (VSAC) grants are available.

Wellness College of Vermont

11 Bausch Lane
Chittenden, Vermont 05737
PHONE: (802) 483-2415
E-MAIL: Diana@NewWorldPractices.com
WEBSITE: NewWorldPractices.com

The Wellness College of Vermont was founded in 1998 by Diana Moore, who is currently the only instructor. Classes range from a minimum of four to a maximum of twelve students. Classes are held in Bradford, Vermont.

Accreditation and Approvals

The college is registered in Vermont. Graduates are qualified to take the National Certification Examination for Therapeutic Massage and Bodywork (NCETMB).

Program Description

The 871-hour, five-semester Massage and Bodywork Certification Program consists of courses in Anatomy and Physiology, Pathophysiology, Adjunct Counseling, Wellness Lifestyles, CPR and First Aid, Swedish Massage, Hydrotherapy, Reflexology, Acupressure, Polarity, Deep Tissue, Energy Massage, Integrated Massage and Bodywork Internship, Professional Practitioner Internship, Health Services Management and Business Practices, and Statues, Rules, Professional Standards and Ethics.

The 637-hour, four-semester Botanical Systems Certification Program consists of courses in Anatomy and Physiology, Pathophysiology, Adjunct Counseling, Wellness Lifestyles, CPR and First Aid, Introduction to Biochemistry and Plant Anatomy and Physiology, Herbology and Lab, Aromatherapy, Essences and Homeopathy, Internship, Health Services Management and Business Practices, and Statues, Rules, Professional Standards and Ethics.

The 845-hour, five-semester Energy Systems Program consists of courses in Anatomy and Physiology, Pathophysiology, Adjunct Counseling, Wellness Lifestyles, CPR and First Aid, Energy Systems, Acupressure, Polarity, Energy Massage, Integrated Energy Internship, Professional Practitioner Internship, Health Services Management and Business Practices, and Statues, Rules, Professional Standards and Ethics.

Admission Requirements

Applicants must have a high school diploma or equivalent.

Tuition and Fees

Tuition for the Massage and Bodywork program is $5,000. Tuition for the Botanical Systems program is $3,656. Tuition for the Energy Systems program is $4,850.

Financial Assistance

Payment plans are available.

VIRGINIA

Advanced Fuller School of Massage

3500 Virginia Beach Boulevard
Virginia Beach, Virginia 23452
PHONE: (757) 340-7132
FAX: (757) 486-7769
E-MAIL: Nbender102@aol.com

Advanced Fuller School of Massage was founded in 1983. There are thirty-five instructors, with an average of twenty students per class and a 1:10 teacher:student ratio.

Accreditation and Approvals

Advanced Fuller School of Massage is approved by the Virginia Association of Schools and is a member of the American Massage Therapy Association (AMTA) Council of Schools; graduates of massage therapy programs of 500 or more hours are qualified to take the National Certification Examination for Therapeutic Massage and Bodywork (NCETMB). The school is approved as a continuing education provider by the National Certification Board for Therapeutic Massage and Bodywork (NCBTMB).

Program Description

A 500-hour Massage Therapy Program consists of a 250-hour Basic Massage Program, which includes courses in Anatomy and Physiology, Therapeutic Massage, Reflexology, Hydrotherapy, Aromatherapy, Clinical Massage, Deep Tissue Techniques, Myotherapy, Neuromuscular Therapy, Sports and Injury Therapies, Chair Massage, Business Management, Professional

Ethics, and CPR/First Aid, plus an additional 250 hours taken before, during or after the Basic Program and selected from such offerings as Advanced Anatomy and Physiology, Mind/Body Integrative Therapy, Injury Assessment and Therapy, Shiatsu Massage, Medicinal Herbs and Nutrition Healing, Prenatal and Infant Massage, Neuromuscular, Craniosacral, Applied Kinesiology, and others.

The 250-hour Aromatherapist Practitioner Program consists of three levels. Level I: The Foundation covers the use of more than twenty essential oils and the importance of combining, preparation, and presentation, and how oils interact on physical and emotional levels and with skin types, lymphatic system and limbic brain. Level II: The Aromatherapist Practitioner Program covers history, chemistry, and philosophy of healing with essential oils, plus education in the botanical, musculoskeletal, cardiovascular, digestive and urinary diseases. Level III: The Professional Aromatherapist Program covers aromafacials, scalp treatments, and massage with special blends.

The 225-hour Reflexologist Training Program consists of two levels. Level I: The Foundation covers foot and hand reflexology movements and reflex meanings, auriculotherapy with ions, and ear candling. Level II: Reflexologist Program covers history, benefits and contraindications, kinesiology, targeting physical ailments, essential oil effects and color therapy, pathologies, anatomy, business management, documented client sessions and more.

Community and Continuing Education

Personal Use Workshops are scheduled once each month in Swedish Massage, Reflexology, and Acupressure. Continuing education workshops are offered to practicing massage therapists and bodyworkers and include those topics listed under the 500-hour program (above) and others.

Admission Requirements

Applicants must be at least 18 years of age; have a high school diploma; and interview with an admissions representative. Massage Therapy applicants must have received at least two professional massages within the previous six months.

Tuition and Fees

Tuition for the 500-hour Massage Therapy Program is $3,150, plus $310 for books (the 250-hour Basic Massage Program may be taken alone for $1,650 plus $70 for books). Additional expenses include a massage table (approximately $450) and supplies.

Tuition for the Aromatherapy Practitioner Program is $260 for Level I (plus $20 for books); $490 for Level II (plus $13 for books); and $850 for Level III.

Tuition for the Reflexologist Training Program is $210 for Level I (plus $17 for books), $990 for Level II (plus $63 for books).

Financial Assistance
Payment plans and veterans' benefits are available.

Applied Kinesthetic Studies

462 Herndon Parkway, Suite 208
Herndon, Virginia 20170
PHONE: (703) 464-0333
FAX: (703) 464-5999
E-MAIL: AKSmassageschool@erols.com
WEBSITE: www.AKSmassageschool.com

Applied Kinesthetic Studies (AKS) was founded in 1992 by V. Wendell Driggers; the current owner/director is H. Katharine Hunter. There are three theoretical instructors and over ten practical instructors, with an average class size of eighteen to twenty students.

Accreditation and Approvals
AKS has a Certificate to Operate from the Virginia Board of Education. Graduates are qualified to take the National Certification Examination for Therapeutic Massage and Bodywork (NCETMB).

Program Description
The ten-month, 602-hour Massage and Bodywork Program consists of Human Anatomy and Physiology, Structural Kinesiology, Recognition of Various Conditions, Massage/Bodywork (including Observation Techniques, Hands-on Practical Work, Seated Massage, Range of Motion, Client Positioning and Draping, and Stretching Techniques), Adjunct Techniques (including Stress Management, Non-Western Techniques, and exposure to Reflexology, Rolfing, Shiatsu, Energy Work, and Chiropractic), and Professional Training (including Business Practices and Ethics). Classes meet twice a week (mornings or evenings) with one all-day Saturday per month.

Admission Requirements
Admission is by application and mutual interview.

Tuition and Fees
Tuition is $3,850. Additional expenses include books, CPR and First Aid training, required professional massages, and a massage table.

Financial Assistance
Payment plans and veterans' benefits are available.

Aromatherapy Center

4016 Lake Glen Road
Fairfax, Virginia 22033
PHONE: (703) 222-0960
FAX: (703) 222-1308
E-MAIL: aroma@erols.com
WEBSITE: www.aromatherapy-center.com

The Aromatherapy Center was founded in 1989 by Mireille Nedelec and Clydette Clayton, leading practitioners of aromatherapy in the United States and France. There are two instructors, with a maximum class size of fifteen students.

Program Description
The 150-hour Aromatherapy Certification Program: The French School consists of sixty-six classroom hours (over eight one-day classes and one three-hour class) and eighty-four hours of homework, class project, and practicum. Topics covered include history of aromatherapy, pathologies, principles of holistic treatment, aromatic botany and biochemistry, raw products used in aromatherapy, method of application and use of essential oils, monographs of the main essential oils and their practical uses, aromatherapy and the Chakra System, techniques of blending, the ethical practice of aromatherapy, and more.

The 150-hour AromaYoga™ Auric Aromatherapy Certification Program teaches AromaYoga, an energetic healing system of yoga using aromas. The goal of the program is to heal oneself and to reach "The Perfection" in the physical body and soul and to heal others through the use of special perfumes transmitted by Masters, simple postures, and special breathing techniques. The Certification Program includes study and work on the purification of each energy center using specific perfumes, study of the interaction of the perfumes on different chakras and minor energy centers, perfection of auric breathing methods using aromas, diagnosis using perfumes, diverse applications of AromaYoga treatments, and more. In order to practice AromaYoga Auric Aromatherapy, students must complete the Certification Program classwork of eight full days and three two-hour workshops; pass a final exam; complete a practicum and thesis/project; and complete all homework assignments over nine months.

Admission Requirements

Applicants must have a high school diploma or equivalent and submit an application with essay.

Tuition and Fees

Tuition for the Aromatherapy Certification Program is $1,000; tuition for the AromaYoga Program is $1,000. There is a $25 application fee.

Cayce/Reilly School of Massotherapy

215 67th Street at Atlantic Avenue
Virginia Beach, Virginia 23451-0595
PHONE: (757) 437-7202
FAX: (757) 428-0398
E-MAIL: cayceschool@are-cayce.com
WEBSITE: www.are-cayce.com/masso

The Cayce/Reilly School of Massotherapy was founded by Dr. James Windsor and Dr. Harold Reilly in 1987 as the Harold J. Reilly School of Massotherapy. The school is a department of the Association for Research and Enlightenment (ARE), a nonprofit organization founded in 1931 and dedicated to helping people better their lives through the Edgar Cayce readings. There are twenty-four instructors, with an average of twenty students per class.

Accreditation and Approvals

The Cayce/Reilly School of Massotherapy is accredited by the Commission on Massage Training Accreditation (COMTA) and licensed by the Commonwealth of Virginia Department of Education. Graduates are qualified to take the National Certification Examination for Therapeutic Massage and Bodywork (NCETMB).

Program Description

The unique curriculum, with a basis in Swedish massage, focuses on personal transformation and emphasizes a balanced lifestyle as recommended in the Edgar Cayce readings. The program is designed to train individuals not only as massage therapists, but as healers desiring to integrate mind, body, and spirit.

The 600-hour massage program may be completed in six months of full-time study (twenty-five to thirty hours per week), or may be taken on a part-time basis. Classes offered in the Evening Studies Program consist of all classes in the 600-hour program plus more than 600 additional hours in electives.

Classes offered include Beginning Massotherapy: Fundamentals of Cayce/Reilly Massage, Intermediate Massage, Sports Massage, Therapeutic Massage, Swedish, Integrative Massage, Clinical Experience/ Practicum, Applied Kinesiology, Chair Massage, Geriatric Massage, Pregnancy Massage, Reflexology, Jin Shin Do, Therapeutic Touch, Anatomy and Physiology I and II, Body/Mind/Spirit, Hydrotherapy, Professional Business Development and Ethics, Cayce Home Remedies, and Dreams and Meditation.

Community and Continuing Education

A variety of specialized workshops are offered throughout the year including Beginner's Massage Workshops, Advanced Cayce/Reilly, Manual Lymph Drainage, First Aid/CPR, and others.

Admission Requirements

Applicants must have a high school diploma or equivalent; be able to speak and understand English; submit a physician's statement of health and two letters of reference from professional persons; and interview with an admissions representative.

Tuition and Fees

Tuition and fees for the 600-hour Massage Program are $4,500. Tuition for the Evening Studies Program is $8 per hour. Additional expenses include a $50 application fee; books and supplies, $300 to $375; two professional massages, $60 to $90; CPR/First Aid training, $36; and a recommended massage table, $300 to $600.

Financial Assistance

Payment plans, scholarships, and partial scholarships are available.

Dreamtime Center for Herbal Studies

P.O. Box 215
Flint Hill, Virginia 22627
PHONE: (540) 636-3078
E-MAIL: drmtime@shentel.net
WEBSITE: www.dreamtimeherbschool.com

Dreamtime Center for Herbal Studies was founded in 1996 by Kathleen Maier and Teresa Boardwine. There are six instructors; class sizes average twenty to twenty-five students (eight students for clinic).

Program Description

Dreamtime I: Foundations is a nine-month intensive program of herbal medicine. Classes meet one weekend per month from March through November. The first weekend module covers Holistic Herbalism, Herbal Actions, Intro to Phytochemistry, Herbal Preparations, Organic/Biodynamic Gardening Techniques, and Ethical Wildcrafting Issues. Each successive month will cover an organ system through the study of Anatomy and Physiology, Materia Medica, Clinical Applications, Labs for Specific Botanical Preparations, and Nutrition. Included are field trips to a working herb farm and other ecosystems. The class is limited to twenty students.

Dreamtime II: Clinical Internship is open to those who have completed Dreamtime I or can demonstrate equal competency. Classes meet every Wednesday, March to November. Classes include Assessment Skills, Medical Histories, Advanced Medical Terminology, Phytopharmacology, Advanced Formula Making, Stocking the Apothecary, Client Relations and Confidentiality,

Working in a Holistic Practice, Referring Complementary Therapists, guest teachers, and weekly case studies. The class is limited to eight students.

Dreamtime is in the process of developing a three-year program to train new herbalists and to prepare students to qualify for professional status with the American Herbalists Guild. The first two years are described above; the third year is forming through the teachings of guest herbalists as described below.

Continuing Education

Dreamtime offers advanced workshops by guest teachers in The Master Series: Above and Beyond. Topics have included Doctrine of Signatures, Diagnostics, and Plant Wisdom; Clinical Skills Intensive; and Sacred Plant Medicine.

Admission Requirements

Applicants must submit answers to application questions in essay or story form.

Tuition and Fees

Tuition for Dreamtime I: Foundations is $3,000, including natural gourmet meals, rustic lodging or camping, texts, medicine making materials, and lab fees. Tuition for Dreamtime II: Clinical Internship is $2,000; equipment and text not included.

Tuition for workshops in The Master Series ranges from $225 to $495.

Financial Assistance

Payment plans and limited work-study are available.

Eastern Institute of Hypnotherapy

P.O. Box 249
Goshen, Virginia 24439-0249
PHONE: (540) 997-0325 / (800) 296-MIND
FAX: (540) 997-0324
E-MAIL: HypTrainer@aol.com
WEBSITE: members.aol.com/EIHNATH

The Eastern Institute of Hypnotherapy (EIH) was founded in 1989 and is the sister organization to the National Association of Transpersonal Hypnotherapists (see page 454). Allen S. Chips, D.C.H., the primary instructor for the hypnotherapy training program, pioneered the Chips and Associates Hypnotherapy Centers and has conducted over 7,000 hours in clinical private practice.

There are two instructors plus guest lecturers, with an average of twenty-five and a maximum of forty students per class.

Accreditation and Approvals

The Certification Program is approved by the National Association of Transpersonal Hypnotherapists (NATH) and licensed by several state boards of education for proprietary schools.

Program Description

The 100-hour Hypnotherapy Certification Program consists of forty hours of in-class instruction and sixty home-based hours. Topics covered include History, Misconceptions, Susceptibility, Rapport, Suggestibility Tests, Induction Methods, Mind/Brain Testing, Post-Hypnotic Suggestion, Ericksonian Methods, NLP Therapy, Weight Loss, Introduction to Regression, Case Histories, Research Studies, Hypnosis Phenomena, Self-Hypnosis, Deepening Trance, Dangers, Signs of Hypnosis, Suggestive Therapy, Smoking Cessation, "Past Life" Therapy, and others. Students are required to submit a short research assignment, an induction assignment and a final exam.

The 150-hour Master Hypnotherapist Certification is designed for the professional hypnotherapist who is familiar with and wants to specialize in hypnotic regression therapy. Topics covered include Regression Scripts, Methodology and Review; Strategic Therapy and Pattern Detection; Multi-Session Format; Unconscious Triggers; Goal Management and Clinical Formatting; Advanced Abstract "Past Life" Models; Emotional Clearing Techniques, Time Line Induction, and Regression Methods; Advanced Study in Transformational Models; Blending the Wounded Child; Retrieving Fragmented Selves (Soul Retrieval); Generational Time Lines and Forgiveness; Archetypes, Alternate Realities, and Higher Guidance Therapies; and more.

A Hypnotherapy Trainer's Training is offered to Certified Hypnotherapists. The program covers Effective and Dynamic Public Speaking Skills, Various Training/Workshop Designs, How to Effectively Utilize Group Dynamics, How and When to Select Demonstrations, Certifying Professionals in Hypnotherapy, and more.

EIH's Transpersonal Reiki Institute Trainings include Reiki I Certification, Reiki II Certification, and Reiki Master Certification.

The First Degree of training expands one's experience of life through the Reiki initiation process, which reawakens one's own natural healing channel; this energy "attunement" occurs in four ceremonial acts shared by the Reiki Master with each student. The student is instructed in the history of Reiki, the basic hand positions, how to treat oneself, and how to use Reiki in service to others.

The Second Degree level of training involves one attunement by the Reiki Master and instruction in the conscious use of ancient symbols to increase the power of treatments, reach the subconscious mind, and send the energy to someone from a distance.

Reiki Master training is for those who wish to certify others in the Usui system of Reiki. The course is taught once per year on an individual basis; contact the institute for additional information.

Admission Requirements

Registration, a deposit, and a goal statement are required.

Tuition and Fees

Fees listed are for students who preregister; a $50 fee is added for those who don't preregister.

Tuition for the 100-hour Hypnotherapy Certification Program is $895, including all materials. Tuition for the 150-hour Master Hypnotherapist Certification is $995. Tuition for the Hypnotherapy Trainer's Training is $1,495. Tuition for NLP Certification is $995. Tuition for Reiki I is $195; for Reiki II, $250; and for Reiki Master Certification, $995.

Financial Assistance

Group discounts are available.

Equissage

P.O. Box 447
Round Hill, Virginia 22141
PHONE: (540) 338-1917 / (800) 843-0224
FAX: (540) 338-5569
E-MAIL: equissage@webtv.net
WEBSITE: www.equissage.com

The Equissage company was founded in 1989 by Mary A. Schreiber for the purpose of offering massage therapy services to the equine athlete. The company initially marketed its services to East Coast racetracks. After gaining national media exposure, the company produced two full-length instructional videos (see page 494), and in 1991, introduced the nation's first training program in equine sports massage therapy. There are three instructors, an average of ten students per class, and more than 2,000 graduates worldwide.

Accreditation and Approvals

The program is accredited by the International Association of Equine Sports Massage Therapists.

Program Description

The sixty-hour Certificate Program in Equine Sports Massage Therapy consists of classroom study and individualized practical applications, and is limited to seven students. Topics include history of the use of massage on animals, introduction to sports massage for humans, demonstration of Equissage® on equine subjects, equine muscle anatomy and physiology, stress point therapy, hands-on application, and business and marketing plans.

Admission Requirements

A love of animals is the most important qualification for success. A background in massage therapy is preferable but not mandatory.

Tuition and Fees

Tuition is $875.

National Center for Homeopathy

801 North Fairfax Street, Suite 306
Alexandria, Virginia 22314
PHONE: (703) 548-7790
FAX: (703) 548-7792
E-MAIL: info@homeopathic.org
WEBSITE: www.homeopathic.org

The National Center for Homeopathy (NCH), a nonprofit organization, is the largest homeopathic organization in the United States. The center offers seminars and training programs for both the consumer and the licensed health care professional, and also promotes health through homeopathy via a number of other professional services (see page 453).

The center's summer instruction program is an outgrowth of the Postgraduate School for Physicians in Homeopathy, established in 1922. Since that time, courses have been held almost every year. Courses are held at Johns Hopkins University in Baltimore, Maryland, but NCH is not affiliated with Johns Hopkins.

Accreditation and Approvals

The National Center for Homeopathy's beginning-level postgraduate courses are accredited by the Council on Homeopathic Education (CHE).

Program Description

Courses for consumers include Homeopathy 101—Foundations in Homeopathy, a two-day seminar providing a solid foundation in homeopathy; Homeopathy 102—Basic Acute Homeopathy, a five-day course providing practical instruction in the use of homeopathy for cuts, burns, sprains, dental problems, and more; Homeopathy 103—Intermediate Acute Homeopathy, a five-day course exploring more advanced acute remedies; and Study Group Workshop, a two-day seminar offering practical instruction in starting a study group, attracting members, sponsoring speakers, teaching the use of materia medica, and more.

Courses for health care providers include Homeopathic Prescribing I for Professionals, a five-day course concentrating on the treatment of the most common acute problems seen in a general practice, including first aid, otitis media, gastroenteritis, backaches, and more; and Homeopathic Prescribing II for Professionals, a five-day course covering treatment of pneumonia, hepatitis, kidney diseases, and other acute and chronic conditions.

Seminars open to both consumers and health care professionals include Introduction to Homeopathic Animal Care (two days), Intermediate Homeopathic Animal Care (four days), and Advanced Homeopathic Prescribing for Animals (two days), and Philosophy of Homeopathic Medicine, a two-day seminar that offers a comprehensive examination of the roots and philosophy of homeopathy. Admission to successive course levels requires appropriate prerequisites.

A certificate of attendance will be furnished upon completion of each course; no degrees or diplomas are given.

Admission Requirements

It is an NCH educational ethic that it will freely share homeopathic knowledge with all persons and will not deny it to anyone because of his or her professional background.

In order to be eligible for professional courses, health care professionals need a current health care license from a state licensing board; allied health care professionals need a letter from their physician-employer; full-time students enrolled in a course of study that leads to eligibility to be licensed as a health care provider must present proof of enrollment; foreign health care providers must submit copies of valid licenses to practice medicine in their country.

Tuition and Fees

The NCH membership fee is $40. Courses range from $180 to $230 for two-day seminars and $435 to $545 for the five-day courses. Tuition for professionals is $545 per course, or $1,040 for both Prescribing courses. The Study Group Workshop is $30. Required books must be purchased separately. Room and board is available in college-style dormitories (single occupancy) for $124 to $310 per course.

Financial Assistance

Tuition discounts are available to spouses/domestic partners of registrants (50 percent), full-time students enrolled in a course leading to eligibility to be licensed as a health care provider (50 percent), other full-time students (10 percent), and senior citizens age 62 and up (10 percent). Discounts do not apply to room and board. A limited number of tuition grants and loans are available.

The Polarity Center and Shamanic Studies

309 Williamsburg Road
Sterling, Virginia 20164
PHONE: (703) 471-4014

The Polarity Center was founded in 1980 by Rose Diana Khalsa, a polarity therapist, shamanic healer, and former vice president of the Board of Directors for the American Polarity Therapy Association.

Accreditation and Approvals

Training at the Polarity Center and Shamanic Studies is approved by the American Polarity Therapy Association (APTA).

Program Description

The A.P.P. (Associate Polarity Practitioner) Program is a 155-hour, first-level program that leads to A.P.P. certification in accordance with APTA standards. The principles of polarity therapy are introduced through classes in Nutrition and Cleansing Techniques, Polarity Theory, Bodywork, Polarity Yoga, Communication Skills, and Energetic Anatomy.

The R.P.P. (Registered Polarity Practitioner) Program is a 495-hour, twenty-four-month program focusing on developing skills necessary for becoming a professional practitioner. Students gain an understanding of the Five Elements and learn to integrate body, mind, and spirit in healing work. Training includes supervision and feedback on craniosacral, nutritional counseling, polarity yoga, and counseling skills, and extensive work with the nervous systems, structural balancing, and sound. Upon completion of the program, students may apply to APTA for R.P.P. status. R.P.P. certification requires fifty hours of anatomy and physiology, which is provided in the training.

Community and Continuing Education

Ongoing classes are offered in shamanic healing. These include Shamanic Art: Mask and Shield Building; Basic and Advanced Shamanic Journeying; Nature Rituals; Rites of Passage; Medicine Wheel teachings; Sacred Songs and Shamanic Dancing; and Soul Retrieval Training.

Admission Requirements

The most important requirement is the applicant's sincerity and commitment to polarity therapy. Students applying for the A.P.P. Program must complete an application and interview with the director. Students applying for the R.P.P. Program must have completed an A.P.P. Program or equivalent, complete an application, and interview with the director.

Tuition and Fees

Tuition for the A.P.P. Program is $1,650, including APTA membership; books are additional. Tuition for the R.P.P. program is $4,500, including retreat; books are approximately $80.

Financial Assistance

Payment plans are available; a ten percent discount is given for full payment upon registration for the A.P.P. program only.

Richmond Academy of Massage

2004 Bremo Road, Suite 102
Richmond, Virginia 23226
PHONE: (804) 282-5003
FAX: (804) 288-7356

The Richmond Academy of Massage was founded in 1989. There are four instructors, with an average of twenty students per class.

Accreditation and Approvals

The Richmond Academy of Massage has been issued a certificate to operate by the Virginia State Board of Education. Graduates are qualified to take the National Certification Examination for Therapeutic Massage and Bodywork (NCETMB).

Program Description

The 500-hour Professional Training for Certification in Massage Therapy Program covers such topics as anatomy, physiology, Swedish and therapeutic massage, sports massage, geriatric massage, shiatsu, trigger point therapy, on-site corporate massage, and First Aid/CPR. The program, coupled with an estimated 600 hours of out-of-class work, leads to certification as a massage therapist. Classes meet two evenings per week and on twelve Saturdays for a full year.

Admission Requirements

There is no minimum age or educational requirement.

Tuition and Fees

Tuition is $3,900 plus a $50 application fee. Additional expenses include a massage table ($60 to $600), books and supplies.

Financial Assistance

A payment plan and veterans' benefits are available.

Satchidananda Ashram—Yogaville

Buckingham, Virginia 23921
PHONE: (804) 969-3121 / (800) 858-9642
FAX: (804) 969-1303
E-MAIL: iyi@yogaville.org
WEBSITE: www.yogaville.org

Sri Swami Satchidananda (Sri Gurudev) founded Integral Yoga International in 1966. Integral yoga teaches that peace is within each one of us, and that to realize that peace and to live a useful life, we need a healthy and easeful body and a clear mind. There are forty-three instructors/administrators, with an average of twenty-five to thirty-five students per class.

Program Description

Satchidananda Ashram—Yogaville offers yoga teacher training in several formats.

The month-long Basic Hatha Yoga Teacher Training is a comprehensive certification program in which the student will learn to instruct a beginner level class. The program explores all aspects of yoga, including asanas, pranayama, anatomy and physiology, and the study of yoga philosophy.

Additional teacher training programs include Intermediate Hatha Yoga Teacher Training, Advanced Teacher Training, Prenatal Teacher Training, Postpartum Teacher Training, Stress Management Teacher Training, Peer Counseling Teacher Training, Yoga of the Heart: Cardiac Teacher Training, Meditation Teacher Training, and Raja Yoga Teacher Training.

Community and Continuing Education

A number of courses, workshops, and retreats are offered which address such topics as Natural Healing and Wellness, Alternative Approaches to Health, Meditation for Regular Practitioners, Yoga and Psychotherapy, Wilderness Yoga Adventure, Introduction to Integral Yoga, Children are Natural Yogis, Feng

Shui plus Yoga, A Spiritual Approach to Grief, Disease and Death, Native American Traditions and Ceremonies, and many more.

Tuition and Fees

Tuition figures for all programs include tuition, dormitory, and vegetarian meals; in some courses, books are also included.

Tuition for the Basic Hatha Yoga Teacher Training is $1,950.

Tuition for Intermediate Hatha Yoga Teacher Training is $1,200; for Advanced Teacher Training, $990. Intermediate and Advanced may be taken sequentially for a total of $1,995.

Tuition for Prenatal Teacher Training is $795; for Postpartum Teacher Training, $350. Prenatal and Postpartum may be taken sequentially for $1,050.

Tuition for Stress Management Teacher Training is $1,200.

Tuition for Peer Counseling Teacher Training is $600.

Tuition for Yoga of the Heart: Cardiac Teacher Training is $1,250.

Tuition for Meditation Teacher Training is $1,200.

Financial Assistance

Discounts are available for seniors and full-time students.

Virginia School of Massage

2008 Morton Drive
Charlottesville, Virginia 22903
PHONE: (804) 293-4031 / (888) 599-2001
FAX: (804) 293-4190
E-MAIL: registrar@vasom.com
WEBSITE: www.vasom.com

SATELLITE LOCATION:
2820 Valley Avenue
Winchester, Virginia
106-B Southpark Drive
Blacksburg, Virginia

The Virginia School of Massage (VSM) was founded in 1989 by Jerry Toporovsky, a massage therapist who also founded the Baltimore School of Massage. The school graduates an average of eighty students per year. There are sixteen instructors with an average of twelve students per class.

Accreditation and Approvals

The Virginia School of Massage is accredited by the Accrediting Commission of Career Schools and Colleges of Technology (ACCSCT), a member of the American Massage Therapy Association (AMTA) Council of Schools, and approved by the National Certification Board for Therapeutic Massage and Bodywork (NCBTMB) as a continuing education provider. Graduates of massage therapy programs of 500 or more hours are qualified to take the National Certification Examination for Therapeutic Massage and Bodywork (NCETMB).

Program Description

The twenty-week, part-time Basic Massage Course offers an introduction to massage therapy and serves as a foundation for the trainings offered in the Intermediate and Advanced Courses. Students may take the avocational Basic Course only, or continue their studies after completing the Basic Course by enrolling in either the 510-hour or 610-hour program beginning at the Intermediate Level.

The 510-hour, part-time Massage Therapy Training Program consists of the Basic, Intermediate and Advanced Courses, the Intermediate and Advanced Weekends, five one-day trainings, and all required lab and student clinic hours. Students must take CPR and First Aid training, available through community Red Cross courses, prior to graduation.

The 610-hour Professional Medical Massage Therapy Program may be taken on either a part-time or full-time basis. It includes the Basic, Intermediate, Advanced, and Medical Massage Courses, the Intermediate and Advanced Weekends, five one-day trainings, and all required lab and student clinic hours at the School. Students must take CPR and First Aid training, available through community Red Cross courses, prior to graduation.

Admission Requirements

Applicants must be at least 18 years of age and have a high school diploma or equivalent.

Tuition and Fees

Tuition for the Basic Course is $775; additional expenses include a $50 application fee and $80 for books and lab fees.

Tuition for the 510-hour Massage Therapy Training Program is $4,600. Additional expenses include a $100 application fee and a $300 textbooks and supply fee.

Tuition for the 610-hour Professional Medical Massage Program is $5,700; additional expenses include a $100 application fee and a $400 supply fee.

Other expenses for the 510- and 610-hour programs include approximately $85 for linens and oils, approximately $25 for CPR/First Aid certification, $8 for a VSM T-shirt.

Financial Assistance

Federal grants and loans, payment plans, and veterans' benefits are available.

WASHINGTON

Alexandar School of Natural Therapeutics

4032 Pacific Avenue
Tacoma, Washington 98408
PHONE: (253) 473-1142
FAX: (253) 473-3807

The Alexandar School of Natural Therapeutics was founded in 1980 by Aliesha Alexandar, who served for eight years as president of the Washington State Massage Therapy Association Board. There are twelve instructors; massage classes may accommodate twenty-five to thirty students, although the average class size is fourteen to eighteen.

Accreditation and Approvals

The 650-hour Massage Therapy Program exceeds the State of Washington professional licensing requirement. Graduates are qualified to take the National Certification Examination for Therapeutic Massage and Bodywork (NCETMB).

Program Description

The eleven-month, 650-hour Massage Therapy program includes Swedish Massage I and II; Anatomy and Physiology; Basic Muscle Anatomy and Kinesiology; Advanced Muscle Anatomy, Kinesiology, and Remedial Exercise; Clinical Treatment; Living Kinesiology; Body Psyche/Advanced Deep Bodywork; Student Clinic/Treatments; Onsite Massage; Fundamentals of Oriental Medicine; Sports Massage; Aromatherapy and Herbal

Facial and Body Spa Treatments; Hydrotherapy; and Practice Management/ Business Practice.

Admission Requirements

Applicants must be at least 18 years old, have a high school diploma or equivalent, and be in good health.

Tuition and Fees

Tuition is $6,900, including a $100 application fee. Additional expenses include books, approximately $325; First Aid/CPR, $25; AIDS training, $35; classroom massage supplies, $150; and a massage table, $300 to $700.

Financial Assistance

Payment plans, veterans' benefits, Dept. of Vocational Rehabilitation, Employment Security, and Labor and Industries retraining programs are available.

Ashmead College School of Massage

WEBSITE: www.ashmeadcollege.com

CORPORATE OFFICES:
444 NE Ravenna Boulevard, Suite 401
Seattle, Washington 98115
PHONE: (206) 524-3605
FAX: (206) 729-4306

EVERETT:
2721 Wetmore Avenue
Everett, Washington 98201
PHONE: (415) 339-2678
FAX: (415) 258-2620

SEATTLE:
2111 N Northgate Way, Suite 218
Seattle, Washington 98133
PHONE: (206) 527-0807
FAX: (206) 527-1957

TACOMA:
5005 Pacific Highway East, Suite 20
Fife, Washington 98424
PHONE: (253) 926-1435
FAX: (253) 926-0651

VANCOUVER:
120 NE 136th Avenue, Suite 220
Vancouver, Washington 98684
PHONE: (360) 885-3152
FAX: (360) 885-3151

Ashmead College (formerly Seattle Massage School) was founded in 1974 and is owned by High Tide, Inc., wholly owned by Paul Rerucha and Nancy Ashmead Rerucha. There are approximately seventy instructors in four locations, with a maximum class size of twenty-four students for practicum and thirty-five for lecture; the usual class size is twenty-two students.

Accreditation and Approvals
Ashmead College is accredited by the Accrediting Council for Continuing Education and Training (ACCET) and the Commission on Massage Training Accreditation (COMTA). Graduates of the Professional Licensing Program are eligible to take the Washington and Oregon State Massage Licensing Examinations, and/or the National Certification Examination for Therapeutic Massage and Bodywork (NCETMB).

Program Description
The 1,038-hour, five-term Professional Licensing and Specialist Program may be completed in fifteen months and consists of four terms of Professional Licensing course work followed by a Term Five Specialist Program in either Sports Massage Specialist, Aromatherapy and Spa Specialist, Hospital and Long Term Care Specialist. The 795-hour, four-term Professional Licensing Program may also be taken over twelve months without the Term Five specialization.

Professional Licensing courses offered in terms one through four include Anatomy and Physiology, Kinesiology, Massage Theory and Practice, Professional Development, Seated Massage, Student Development, AIDS Education, First Aid/CPR, Hydrotherapy, Pregnancy Massage, Business Skills, Sports Massage, Student Clinic, Chronic Pain, Hospital Internship, and Student Project.

The Term Five Sports Massage Specialist Program covers Anatomy and Physiology, Kinesiology, Massage Theory and Practice, Business, Advanced Orthopedic Injury and Assessment, First Aid/CPR, and Sports Massage.

The Term Five Aromatherapy and Spa Specialist Program includes Aromatherapy Theory and Practice; Botany, Essential Oils and Blending; Basic Chemistry and Aromachemistry; and Spa Therapies.

The Term Five Hospital and Long Term Care Specialist program covers Massage Practice, Hospital/Nursing Home Internship, Anatomy and Physiology, Massage Therapy and Psychosocial Issues, Geriatric Massage Practice, Business Marketing to Facilities, Massage in the Labor Room, and Advanced First Aid/CPR.

Classes are held mornings, afternoons, and evenings.

Admission Requirements
Applicants must be at least 18 years of age upon graduation from Ashmead College, and must have a high school diploma or equivalent; previous experience in massage is helpful but not required. Applicants may be denied admission on the basis of health problems, poor hygiene, lack of financial capability, insufficient motivation, or exhibiting no ability to benefit from the college's programs.

Tuition and Fees
Total tuition and fees for the Four Term Professional Licensing Program is $9,874 plus $1,240 for books and supplies; for the Five Term Professional Licensing, $12,574 plus $1,460 for books and supplies; and for Term Five only, $2,800 plus $920 for books and supplies.

Financial Assistance
Federal grants and loans, Washington State Need Grants, and payment plans are available; veterans' benefits are available in Everett, Seattle, and Tacoma, and will be available in 2001 in Vancouver.

Bastyr University
14500 Juanita Drive Northeast
Kenmore, Washington 98028-4966
PHONE: (425) 823-1300
FAX: (425) 823-6222
WEBSITE: www.bastyr.edu
E-MAIL: admiss@bastyr.edu

Bastyr University was founded in 1978 as the John Bastyr College of Naturopathic Medicine. In 1994, the university received an $840,000 grant from the National Institutes of Health Office of Alternative Medicine to establish a Center for Alternative Medicine Research in HIV/AIDS. In 1996, the university moved from its Seattle location to nearly fifty acres of woods and fields on the northeast shore of Lake Washington. The 186,000-square-foot complex includes a whole foods, vegetarian cafeteria and expanded classroom, research, and laboratory facilities. The university operates the Natural Health Clinic of Bastyr University in Seattle's Wallingford neighborhood.

Accreditation and Approvals

Bastyr University is accredited by the Commission on Colleges of the Northwest Association of Schools and Colleges. The Naturopathic Medicine Program is accredited by the Council on Naturopathic Medical Education (CNME). The master's degree programs in Acupuncture and Oriental Medicine are accredited by the Accreditation Commission for Acupuncture and Oriental Medicine (ACAOM). The Didactic Program in Dietetics is approved by the American Dietetic Association Council on Education. Bastyr is approved as a provider of continuing education by the Washington State Nurse's Association and by the American Council on Pharmaceutical Education.

Program Description

The four-year, 322-credit Doctor of Naturopathic Medicine Program prepares students to take the Naturopathic Physicians Licensing Exam (NPLEX). Results of this exam are used in all states that license naturopathic physicians. Departments within the Naturopathic Medicine Program include the departments of Ayurvedic Medicine; Botanical Medicine; Homeopathic Medicine; Physical Medicine; Spirituality, Health and Medicine; and Naturopathic Midwifery. The program consists of two years of preclinical curriculum, two years of clinical naturopathic medicine curriculum, fifteen credits of electives, and 1,332 hours (forty-seven credits) of clinical experience. Topics covered in the preclinical curriculum include Human Anatomy, Physiology, Biochemistry, Histology, Living Anatomy, Embryology, Human Pathology, Immunology, Infectious Diseases, Genetic Counseling, Research Methods and Design, Physical and Clinical Lab Diagnosis, Pharmacology, Fundamentals of Traditional Chinese Medicine, Naturopathic Philosophy, Hydrother-

apy, Massage, Botanical Medicine, Fundamentals of Ayurvedic Medicine, Basic Foods/Diet Assessment, Homeopathy, and more. The clinical naturopathic medicine curriculum covers such areas as Addictions and Disorders, Botanical Medicine, Gynecology, Psychological Assessment, Pediatrics, Cardiology, Minor Surgery, Geriatrics, Sports Medicine, Endocrinology, Diagnostic Imaging, Oncology, and more. Clinical experience includes Preceptorships, Clinic Assistant Shifts, Patient Care Clinic Shifts, and Physical Medicine Shifts.

A one-year, thirty-credit graduate Professional Certificate Program in Spirituality, Health and Medicine is offered to professionals in health care, counseling, the ministry and related fields who wish to study the connection between spirit and healing. Course work includes study of diverse religions and spiritual traditions and their impact on health.

The Master of Science Degree in Acupuncture and Oriental Medicine (MSAOM) is a four-year program offering training in acupuncture, Oriental medicine, Chinese herbal medicine, and the health sciences. The curriculum includes Organic Chemistry; Biochemistry; Anatomy and Physiology; Western Clinical Science and Disease Processes; Acupuncture Techniques, Diagnosis, Pathology, and Therapeutics; and Chinese Herbal Materia Medica and Therapeutics. Clinical training is integrated with course work beginning with the second year.

The Master of Science Degree in Acupuncture (MSA) is a three-year program in acupuncture, Oriental medicine, and the health sciences. The curriculum is the same as that of the MSAOM, with the omission of requirements in Chinese herbal medicine and language.

A one-year Certificate in Chinese Herbal Medicine is offered to acupuncturists, N.D.s, currently enrolled N.D. students, MSA students, or individuals with equivalent background. The course work includes clinical training.

The Master of Science Degree in Nutrition balances a "whole foods" approach with an understanding of human behavior, human biochemistry, and nutrient metabolism, and emphasizes patient education and motivation. Course work includes Nutritional Assessment, Diet Therapy, Disease Processes, Principles of Whole Foods, Research Methodology, and Community Practicum. Graduates work as nutrition counselors, clinical nutritionists, researchers, and as consultants to the food and fitness industries.

The Didactic Program in Dietetics and Dietetic Internship

Program are designed to fulfill the American Dietetics Association's academic requirements for Registered Dietitians and to provide performance requirements for entry-level dietitians through supervised practice.

Bastyr offers an undergraduate Bachelor of Science Degree in Psychology, in Herbal Sciences, and in Natural Health Sciences with majors in Nutrition, Oriental Medicine, and Exercise Science and Wellness to upper-division undergraduates.

Community and Continuing Education

Bastyr offers a variety of courses that are open to the public, including Introduction to Natural Medicine, Whole Foods Production, Traditional Chinese Medicine Fundamentals, Psychology of Human Relations, and numerous basic science courses.

Health care professionals can participate in Bastyr's continuing professional education programs through home study. Contact the Continuing Education Department at (425) 602-3152 for more information.

Bastyr has discontinued its distance learning correspondence program but is interested in offering web-based courses and programs. Online programs are in the research and planning stages. Check the university web site for updated information.

Admission Requirements

All applicants must submit official transcripts and letters of recommendation; graduate school applicants must also interview with an admissions representative.

Applicants to the Doctor of Naturopathic Medicine Program must have completed a bachelor's degree or at least 135 quarter credits (eighty semester credits) and significant life experience. The mean GPA for entering students is 3.2. Prerequisite courses include college-level algebra or precalculus; statistics; general chemistry with labs; organic chemistry with labs; general biology or a combination of courses to include cell and molecular biology, genetics, botany, and taxonomy with labs; physics; psychology; English; and humanities. Required science courses must have been taken within seven years of matriculation. Scores on standardized tests (GRE or MCAT) are not required. Students entering the program who have graduated from an accredited professional school or program (including M.D., D.O., D.C., and others) and who are legally qualified to practice may apply for advanced standing.

Applicants to the Professional Certificate Program in Spirituality, Health, and Medicine must be practicing professionals or have a bachelor's degree and considerable work experience in their fields.

Applicants to the Master of Science programs in Acupuncture or Acupuncture and Oriental Medicine must have completed a bachelor's degree. Prerequisite courses include college-level algebra or precalculus, general chemistry, general biology with lab, and general psychology.

The Certificate in Chinese Herbal Medicine Program is open to currently enrolled students of acupuncture and Oriental or naturopathic medicine, acupuncturists, N.D.s, and other health care professionals. Current students or graduates of Bastyr University need only submit the application form and a brief statement regarding their interest in Chinese herbal medicine. All others must submit a current résumé, two letters of recommendation, and transcripts.

Applicants to the Master of Science in Nutrition Program must have completed a Bachelor's degree. Prerequisite courses include college-level algebra or precalculus, general chemistry, general biology with lab, general psychology, anatomy and physiology, organic chemistry with lab, nutrition, foods, microbiology, and biochemistry.

Students transferring into the Bachelor of Science programs must have completed ninety quarter credits (sixty semester credits) with an overall GPA of 2.25. Prerequisites include at least fifty-four general education quarter-credits, including English and public speaking, college-level algebra or precalculus, general biology with lab, and general psychology.

Tuition and Fees

The catalog costs $5; there is a $60 application fee for undergraduate degree and certificate programs, a $75 application fee for graduate programs, and a $25 fee for nonmatriculated and/or nondegree programs.

Tuition for clinic credits is $220 per credit hour and for other credits, $192 per credit hour. Total first-year costs, including tuition, fees, books, and supplies, are as follows: four-year N.D., $16,742; five-year N.D., $13,158; MSAOM or MSA, $14,420; MSN, $9,953; BSNHS-OM, $14,000; and BSNHS-Nutrition, Psychology, Herbal Sciences or Exercise Science and Wellness, $10,200.

Tuition for the Professional Certificate Program in Spirituality, Health, and Medicine is $5,760; books and fees are additional.

Financial Assistance

Federal loans, federal and Washington State work-study programs, federal grants, limited scholarships, Canadian federal student loans programs, most Canadian provincial loans, and private loans are available.

Brenneke School of Massage

160 Roy Street
P.O. Box 9886
Seattle, Washington 98109
PHONE: (206) 282-1233
FAX: (206) 282-9183
E-MAIL: brenneke@halcyon.com
WEBSITE: www.brennekeschool.com

The Brenneke School of Massage was founded in 1974 by Director Heida F. Brenneke, an author and former Director of Education for the American Massage Therapy Association—Washington. There are fourteen core faculty members, with a maximum of thirty-six students per class and a teacher:student ratio of 1:5 during hands-on classes.

Accreditation and Approvals

The Brenneke School of Massage programs are accredited by the Accrediting Council for Continuing Education and Training (ACCET) and by the Commission on Massage Training Accreditation (COMTA); the programs are approved by the Washington State Massage Board, and graduates are qualified to take the National Certification Examination for Therapeutic Massage and Bodywork (NCETMB). Brenneke is approved by the National Certification Board for Therapeutic Massage and Bodywork (NCBTMB) as a continuing education provider.

Program Description

The 650-hour, twelve-month Professional Licensing Program (PLP) includes Swedish Massage, Anatomy and Physiology, Professional Development, Business, Advanced Massage Techniques, Kinesiology, Pathology, Event Sports Massage, Intro-

duction to Myofascial Technique, Trigger Point Therapy, AIDS Education, Clinical Hydrotherapy, Teaching Clinic, and Treatment Case Studies. Electives include Therapeutic Touch; Polarity; Manual Lymph Drainage; Reiki; Lomi Lomi; Shiatsu; Foot Reflexology; Introduction to Herbology; Cadaver Anatomy; Introduction to Body, Mind, and Spirit; and more.

The 1,000-hour, twelve-month Expanded Professional Licensing Program (EPLP) includes all of the instruction offered in the PLP program with the addition of Introduction to Oriental Massage, Lymphatic Massage, Pregnancy Massage, Ways of Learning, and Field Experience in a variety of professional health care settings.

Continuing Education

Nationally known massage therapists present specialty workshops at Brenneke throughout the year. Brenneke also offers continuing education workshops on a monthly basis for the licensed massage practitioner; topics may include Shiatsu, Foot Reflexology, Herbology, Lomi Lomi, Infant Massage, Running Injuries, Advanced Sports Massage, Reiki, Introduction to Craniosacral Therapy, Bob King Seminars, and many others.

Massage Therapy for the Novice is a two-day introductory course in Swedish massage that is open to the public, and is also a prerequisite for both Professional Licensing Programs.

Admission Requirements

Applicants must be at least 18 years of age by the beginning of class, be physically and emotionally capable of performing and receiving massage, have a high school diploma or equivalent, interview with the director of admissions, and successfully complete the Massage Therapy for the Novice class.

Tuition and Fees

There is a $100 application fee, and the Massage Therapy for the Novice Course costs $100. Both fees are applicable toward tuition if the student enrolls in either licensing program.

Tuition for the PLP is $7,645. Tuition for the EPLP is $10,950. Additional expenses include a massage table, approximately $500 to $700, and one professional massage per term, $30 to $50. Several elective classes require a copayment.

Financial Assistance

Payment plans, federal grants and loans, and veterans' benefits are available.

Brian Utting School of Massage

900 Thomas Street, Suite 200
Seattle, Washington 98109
PHONE: (206) 292-8055/ (800) 842-8731
FAX: (206) 292-0113
E-MAIL: admissions@busm.com
WEBSITE: www.busm.com

The Brian Utting School of Massage was founded in 1982 by Brian Utting. The school's mission is to produce outstanding massage practitioners with a deeper sense of their humanity, accomplished through accommodation of individual learning styles, personal attention, and guidance. There are thirteen instructors with a maximum of forty-four students per class.

Accreditation and Approvals

The Professional Massage Licensing Program is accredited by the Commission on Massage Training Accreditation (COMTA), and certified by the Washington State Department of Health and Division of Professional Licensing, the Washington State Board of Massage, and the Oregon Board of Massage Technicians. Graduates are qualified to take the National Certification Examination for Therapeutic Massage and Bodywork (NCETMB). The school is approved by the National Certification Board for Therapeutic Massage and Bodywork (NCBTMB) as a continuing education provider.

Program Description

The 1,000-hour Licensing Program includes theoretical grounding in Anatomy and Physiology, Kinesiology, Pathology, and Pathophysiology; Theoretical Applications, including body mechanics and movement analysis, cadaver anatomy at Bastyr University, First Aid, CPR, AIDS/HIV training, hydrotherapy theory and applications, indications and contraindications, palpation skills, and muscle palpation; Professional Preparation, including business and marketing skills, communication skills, internship program, professional ethics, and student clinic; and Bodywork Techniques that include Swedish massage, deep tissue massage, circulatory massage, art and technique of deep touching, deep muscle therapy, clinical massage, injury evaluation and treatment, connective tissue massage, neuromuscular technique, foot reflexology, pregnancy massage, and sports massage. Classes may be taken on a day or evening schedule.

Optional student support classes include Introduction to Anatomy for Massage Students, Conditioning for Massage Students, and Learning Skills Tutorial.

Community and Continuing Education

The One-Day Introductory Workshop is a hands-on introduction to Swedish massage; the course is a prerequisite for application.

Continuing education courses are typically offered in areas such as manual lymph drainage, craniosacral, on-site (chair) massage, injury assessment and treatment, Ben Benjamin: Survivors of Abuse, shiatsu, and Trager®.

Admission Requirements

Applicants must have a high school diploma or equivalent, have no criminal convictions, submit a certificate of health, and be able to give and receive massage. Applicants must also participate in the One-Day Introductory Workshop and interview with one or more admissions committee members. A prior class in anatomy is recommended.

Tuition and Fees

Tuition is $9,300, including a $100 registration fee and a $200 enrollment fee; books, massage table, and supplies cost approximately $1,300. Tuition for the One-Day Introductory Workshop is $40.

Financial Assistance

Payment plans, personal loan assistance, veterans' benefits, and aid from the Washington State Worker Retraining Program are available.

Cedar Mountain Center for Massage

5601 NE St. Johns Road
Vancouver, Washington 98661
PHONE: (360) 696-2210
FAX: (360) 696-0130

Cedar Mountain Center for Massage was founded in 1984 as Southwest Washington Massage Therapy School. There are seven instructors; class sizes are limited to twelve.

Accreditation and Approvals
The Cedar Mountain Center for Massage training program is approved by the Washington State Board of Massage and the Oregon State Board of Massage. Graduates are qualified to take the National Certification Examination for Therapeutic Massage and Bodywork (NCETMB).

Program Description
The 710-hour Massage Licensing Program consists of three fifteen-week trimesters. Trimester I courses include Anatomy and Physiology, Business Skills, Massage, Hydrotherapy, Pathology, Structural Kinesiology, Educational Kinesiology (Brain Gym), an Independent Study Project and Office Practicum. Trimester II consists of Anatomy and Physiology, Deep Tissue and Palpation Skills, Shiatsu Theory, Introduction to Electives, Kinesiology, Pathology, Hydrotherapy, Student Clinic, and Independent Study Project. Trimester III includes Postural Analysis, Business Skills: Marketing, Student Clinic, Independent Study Project, Office Practicum, and a minimum of 115 hours of electives chosen from Shiatsu Form and Clinic, Touch for Health, AMMA Seated Massage, Basic Aromatherapy, Polarity Therapy, Reflexology, Syntropy, Pregnancy/Side-Lying, and Hospital Massage. Students may enroll for morning or evening classes.

Admission Requirements
Applicants must be at least 18 years of age, have a high school diploma or equivalent, be physically capable of performing and receiving massage techniques, and have a personal interview.

Tuition and Fees
Total cost of the program, including tuition, student service fee, and registration fee, is $6,550. Additional expenses include books, $350; massage table, $700 (new); linens, oils, and other supplies, $150; and exam and licensing fees at completion of program, $210.

Financial Assistance
Payment plans, loans, and prepayment discount are available.

Institute for Therapeutic Learning

9322 21st Avenue NW
Seattle, Washington 98117
PHONE: (206) 783-1838
E-MAIL: jelias@sprynet.com
WEBSITE: home.sprynet.com/~jelias

The Institute for Therapeutic Learning was founded in 1988 by Jack Elias, a licensed clinical hypnotherapist, certified NLP practitioner, and author of *Finding True Magic*. Elias is the only instructor, with an average of fourteen students per class.

Accreditation and Approvals
Completion of the 150-hour program will enable students to qualify for certification and membership as clinical hypnotherapists in state and national hypnosis associations. At this time, 150 hours is the generally recognized minimum level of training.

Program Description
The 150-hour Transpersonal Clinical Hypnotherapy/NLP Program consists of six twenty-five-hour phases: Full Spectrum Hypnosis Training; Transpersonal Regression Therapy; Transpersonal Therapy; Transpersonal Hypnotherapy Applications; Comprehensive Work with Inner Archetypes, NLP, Ericksonian Hypnosis, Couples, and Groups; and Releasing Unwanted Influences: Future Progression. Upon completion of each of the second-through-sixth phases, students must conduct a one-hour hypnotherapy session. Training is offered in both a weekend format and a 150-hour summer intensive.

The 150-hour program may also be taken through correspondence, either for certification or for personal growth without certification.

After the live training, students may take an additional 150 hours of independent study (with tapes), and receive certification in recognition of 300 hours of training. Certification at 450 hours of training and beyond is also available.

Admission Requirements
A high school diploma or equivalent are prerequisites for enrolling.

Continuing Education
Continuing education, mentorship classes, and supervision are available.

Tuition and Fees
Tuition for the Transpersonal Clinical Hypnotherapy Program ranges from $1,500 prepaid to $1,800; books are approximately $120. Tuition for the same program by correspondence ranges from $1,665 to $1,835, depending on payment schedule; books cost $104. Tuition for the noncertification correspondence program is $760 to $935 (this is for training manuals and tapes only; omits tutorials and submission of homework).

Financial Assistance
The institute is on the approved training list of the Division of Vocational Rehabilitation.

The Institute of Dynamic Aromatherapy

2000 2nd Avenue, Suite 206
Seattle, Washington 98121
PHONE: (206) 374-8773 / (800) 260-7401
FAX: (360) 651-8859
E-MAIL: jades@accessone.com
WEBSITE: www.TheIDA.com

The Institute of Dynamic Aromatherapy (IDA; formerly the New England Center for Aromatherapy) was founded in 1990 by Jade Shutes. There are four instructors; maximum class size is twenty-four students.

Accreditation and Approvals
IDA is licensed by the Washington State Board for Vocational Education, and recommended by the American Alliance of Aromatherapy. The IDA is approved by the National Certifica-

tion Board for Therapeutic Massage and Bodywork (NCBTMB) as a continuing education provider.

Program Description
The IDA Nine-Month Apprenticeship Program: A Practitioner's Diploma Training consists of 108 hours of live instruction plus 200 hours of home study via the IDA Correspondence Program. The Apprenticeship core curriculum includes nine modules covering such topics as From Plant to Essential Oil, Materia Medica, Phytols and Floral Waters, Base Material and Oils, Dynamic Blending Technique, Consultation Procedures, The Chemistry of Essential Oils, Specific Treatment Blending, Reflexology Weekend, Business Practices and Ethics, Herbal Infusions, Flower Essences, Presentation of Research Papers, and much more. Other requirements include ten case studies, research paper and presentation, final exam, fourteen hours of electives, and completion of the Correspondence Program.

The IDA Correspondence Program may be taken independently or as part of the Apprenticeship program. The twelve-chapter program includes Anatomy and Physiology, Common Disorders of Each System, Best Applications for Each System, Materia Medica Specific to Individual Systems, Introduction to Dynamic Aromatherapy, Olfaction and the Psychotherapeutic Properties of Essential Oils, Therapeutic Uses of Olfaction, Disorders of Olfaction, The Energy of Essential Oils, and much more.

Admission Requirements
Applicants must be at least 18 years of age; it is recommended that applicants have a high school diploma or equivalent.

Tuition and Fees
Tuition for the Apprenticeship Program (including Correspondence Program) is $2,025. Tuition for only the Correspondence Program is $625.

Financial Assistance
Payment plans are available.

Institute of Integrative Aromatherapy

(See Multiple State Locations, pages 395-96)

Northwest Institute of Acupuncture and Oriental Medicine

701 North 34th Street, Suite 300
Seattle, Washington 98103
PHONE: (206) 633-2419
FAX: (206) 633-5578
E-MAIL: mmcghee@niaom.edu
WEBSITE: www.niaom.edu

The Northwest Institute of Acupuncture and Oriental Medicine (NIAOM) was founded in 1981 as a nonprofit educational organization. The institute moved to its present Fremont neighborhood location in January 1999. There are forty instructors, with a maximum of thirty-five students per class.

Accreditation and Approvals

The Master of Acupuncture and the Master of Traditional Chinese Medicine Programs are accredited by the Accreditation Commission for Acupuncture and Oriental Medicine (ACAOM). The institute is also approved by the Washington State Department of Licensing. The acupuncture and herbal programs are approved by the Acupuncture Examining Committee in California. Although chemistry and physics are not requirements to enter the Northwest Institute, graduates of the program need these two courses to sit for the California Acupuncture Exam.

Program Description

The three-year, 132-credit Master of Acupuncture (M.Ac.) Program focuses on the study of traditional Chinese medical theory, diagnosis, meridians and points, therapeutics and techniques, as well as Western anatomy, physiology, pathology, and Western clinical sciences. There are also elective course sequences in Chinese dietary therapy, auricular medicine, medical Qi Gong, Chinese medical language, and Tui Na. The 850 hours of clinic work includes observation and supervised clinical practice throughout the three-year program.

The four-year, 165-credit Master of Traditional Chinese Medicine (MTCM) Program combines the study of acupuncture and Chinese herbology and includes 900 clinical internship hours. Many of the Oriental Medicine Theory and Western Science courses in the MTCM Program are identical to the courses in the three-year M.Ac. Program (above). MTCM students also take specialized courses which combine acupuncture and herbal medicine in the areas of herbal studies foundations, therapeutics, and clinical problem-solving.

Continuing Education

Postgraduate certificate programs are offered in TCM Pediatric Acupuncture, Japanese Acupuncture, Toyo Hari, and Community and Public Health. These programs are open to licensed acupuncturists. Each certificate program has its own entrance requirements and length of study.

NIAOM plans to introduce additional advanced study certificate programs in the areas of Women's Health, Oriental Bodywork, Geriatric Health, and Medical Qi Gong.

Approximately twenty continuing education workshops are offered each year in such topics as Qi Gong, Chinese Herbal Patent Medicine, Energy Field Medicine, Japanese Acupuncture, Detox Acupuncture, Pulse Diagnosis, Treatment of Pain, and others.

Admission Requirements

Applicants for the Master of Acupuncture Program must have completed three years (ninety semester or 135 quarter credits) of accredited college or university study (bachelor's degree recommended), including one course in both general biology and general psychology. Applicants must also submit an essay and two letters of recommendation, and complete a personal interview.

Applicants for continuing education in acupressure, traditional Chinese medicine, Western academic courses, and clinical training will undergo specific evaluation of their educational background in order to ascertain whether it is sufficient for the requested area of continuing education.

Tuition and Fees

Total cost of tuition for the three-year M.Ac. degree is $26,600. Total cost of tuition for the four-year MTCM degree is $31,950. Books and supplies for the degree programs are approximately $1,000 to $1,250.

Financial Assistance

Federal financial aid, loans, veterans' benefits, and Canada student loans are available.

Seattle Institute of Oriental Medicine

916 NE 65th Street, Suite B
Seattle, Washington 98115
PHONE: (206) 517-4541
FAX: (206) 526-1932
E-MAIL: info@siom.com
WEBSITE: www.siom.com

The Seattle Institute of Oriental Medicine (SIOM) was founded in 1994 by Directors Dan Bensky and Paul Karsten. There are twenty-five instructors, with an average of twelve students per class.

Accreditation and Approvals
The Master's in Acupuncture and Oriental Medicine degree program is accredited by the Accrediting Commission for Acupuncture and Oriental Medicine (ACAOM).

Program Description
The three-year, 2,730-hour Master's in Acupuncture and Oriental Medicine degree program consists of 1,065 Oriental Medicine hours, 345 Western Clinical Sciences hours, and 1,320 Clinic hours. All students are expected to attend full-time. Classes are taught in English.

Clinical Training begins in the First Year with 405 hours of Clinic Skills Lab, Clinic Preceptorship, and Case Discussion. Courses include Fundamentals Intensive, Zang-fu Pathology, Six Stages/Four Levels, Eight Extra Channels: Manaka Approach, Five Phase Acupuncture: Meridian Therapy, Body Fluid Metabolism, Channel Pathways, Point Location and Anatomy, Point Groups, Introduction to Needling, OSHA/CNT/Safety, Materia Medica/Herbal Formulas, Food Therapy, Pharmacognosy, Chinese Medical Language, Acupressure, Qi Gong, Tai Chi, Emergency Protocols, Surface Anatomy, Pathology and Assessment, Microbiology, and Medical Terminology.

The Second Year includes 405 hours of Clinical Training in the form of Clinic Internship and Case Discussion. Courses include Diagnosis and Treatment, Microsystems, Chinese Acupuncture Techniques, Japanese Acupuncture Techniques, Electroacupuncture, Chinese Medical Language, Medical Communication and Referral: Internal Medicine, Biochemistry and Nutrition, Pharmacology, and Biophysics.

The Third Year includes 510 hours of Clinical Training in the form of Clinic Internship, Case Discussion, Acupuncture Detox Clinic, and Specialty Clinic. Courses include Neuromusculoskeletal Conditions, Gynecology, Special Topics, Professional Issues, Practice Management, Research in Oriental Medicine, Survey of American Medicine, Counseling and Referral, Chinese Medical Language, Chinese Medical Philosophy, Medical Communication and Referral: NMS, Medical Communication and Referral: Gynecology, Physical Assessment, and Public Health and Chemical Dependency.

Students take a series of written and practical comprehensive exams at the end of each year. At the end of the third year, students must complete a clinical skills checklist.

Admission Requirements
Applicants must have completed three years (ninety semester credits) of successful college study. At least ten semester credits must have been in the basic sciences, with at least one course each in General Biology, Chemistry, and Psychology, and at least eight semester credits must have been in Anatomy and Physiology with lab. In addition, applicants must have current Red Cross CRP and First Aid certification. One semester of Chinese language is highly recommended. Applicants must submit an essay and have a personal interview.

Tuition and Fees
Total tuition for students entering in 1999 is $30,150; for students entering in 2000, total tuition is $31,410; for those entering in 2001, total tuition is $32,760. Additional expenses include a $50 application fee; an estimated $800 for books and supplies; and malpractice insurance fees of $100 per trimester in the second and third years.

Financial Assistance
SIOM is applying for approval for financial aid, which would allow students to apply for federal guaranteed student loans.

Seattle Midwifery School

2524 16th Avenue South, Room 300
Seattle, Washington 98144-5104
PHONE: (206) 322-8834 / (800) 747-9433
FAX: (206) 328-2840

E-MAIL: info@seattlemidwifery.org
WEBSITE: www.seattlemidwifery.org

The Seattle Midwifery School (SMS) was founded in 1978. SMS has graduated over 120 midwives, nearly 2,000 doulas, and more than 100 doula trainers. There are seventeen faculty members; classes are limited to twenty students. The Midwifery Education Program is offered in Seattle and New England.

Accreditation and Approvals

SMS is accredited by the Midwifery Education Accreditation Council (MEAC), by the Accrediting Council for Continuing Education and Training (ACCET), and by the Washington State Department of Health meeting the criteria for midwifery educator. Graduates are eligible for licensure in Washington and several other states as well as certification by the North American Registry of Midwives (NARM).

Program Description

In addition to the training program for direct-entry midwives described here, SMS offers training for labor and postpartum doulas and childbirth educators (see Community and Continuing Education below).

The 125.5-credit Midwifery Education Program may be completed in nine quarters of study; the program is offered in a monthly seminar format. Courses include Assessment of Women, Basic Health/Nursing Skills, Basic Practicum, Counseling Skills for Midwives, Education Skills for Midwives, Embryology and Fetal Development, Gynecology/Women's Health, Perinatal Epidemiology, Professional Issues, Basic and Perinatal Nutrition, Basic Clinical Seminar, Genetics, Midwifery Care, Basic Practicum, Pharmacological and Alternative Treatments, Advanced Clinical Seminar, and Advanced Practicum. First-year students are exposed to a broad spectrum of practice styles and sites, which may include gynecology/family planning clinics, hospital labor and delivery units, prenatal/postpartum clinics, newborn nurseries and others, where they may work with licensed midwives, certified nurse-midwives, nurse practitioners, naturopaths, or physicians. Student clinical activities occur primarily in community-based preceptorships where clients are followed through the entire childbearing year. Students generally work with at least two preceptors in North America during this year; in addition, most students go overseas for one to three months of intensive training in various high-volume hospitals staffed by midwives. It is usually necessary for students to relocate for at least a portion of their clinical training.

Community and Continuing Education

A two-part, four-day Labor Support Course (LSC) meets the training standards to become a certified doula and is offered to the community as well as being a prerequisite for the Midwifery Education Program. Part I, required for students with little or no experience in childbirth education or labor and birth care, covers reproductive anatomy, fetal development, components of perinatal care, clinical terminology, pain management and techniques. Part II focuses on the emotional and psychological aspects of giving birth and its significance in women's lives; topics covered include scope of practice, culturally sensitive support, coping with complications of pregnancy and labor, newborn care, and breastfeeding.

Postpartum Doula Training is a four-day program that includes discussion of the doula's role and the scope of postpartum care, home visit protocol, cultural aspects, communication and listening skills, and how to help a new family with infant feeding and breastfeeding support, newborn and mother care, and more.

A three-day Childbirth Educator Training Program provides basic training to begin a career as a childbirth educator and meets training requirements for certification with Birth Education Northwest (BEN).

A three-day Doula Trainer Course: Training the Trainer is offered to those who have attended a minimum of ten births as a doula and have either two years or ten class series experience as an educator. The course consists of Part II of the Labor Support Course (described above) and one day of teacher training. The focus is on content and teaching effectiveness, analysis of different teaching styles, development of objectives, and exploration of ways to convey values relating to ethical issues, scope of practice, and professional standards.

Admission Requirements

Applicants for the Midwifery Education Program must have a high school diploma or equivalent; demonstrate proficiency in the English language; complete forty-five quarter credits or twenty-seven semester credits of college work with a cumulative GPA of 2.8 or better; complete a Labor Support Course approved by Doulas of North America or equivalent or have relevant birth experience with documentation; complete specific requirements in Math, English, Human Anatomy, Microbiology, Social Science, and Biology or pass equivalent Challenge Exams; attend a personal interview and Admissions Day; and submit three letters of reference. Relevant life experience, such as midwifery or other health-related work, childbirth education, labor support experience, and other involvement in women's health or social services may be considered in lieu of college work. It is also strongly recommended that all applicants attend a series of Childbirth Educator classes; complete advanced first aid and CPR certification; complete courses in Communication Skills or Women's Studies; attend midwifery courses and workshops; join midwifery organizations; pursue basic health care experience or education; and participate in the care of pregnant, birthing or postpartum women.

Tuition and Fees
Total tuition for the Midwifery Educator Program is approximately $24,000. Additional expenses include application fee, $50; registration fee, $100; copyright and photocopy expenses, $9 per credit; books and materials, approximately $1,000 for the program; supplies and equipment, approximately $400; and lab supplies fee, $40. Students may be required to purchase liability insurance.

Tuition for the Labor Support Course is $375 for both parts, $225 for Part I or Part II individually; books are additional.

Tuition for Postpartum Doula Training is $375; books are additional.

Tuition for Doula Trainer Course: Training the Trainer is $350.

Tuition for Childbirth Educator Training is $575; books are additional.

Financial Assistance
Midwifery students are eligible for Title IV federal financial aid. Private scholarships and grants are available. Students who make a commitment to serve in one of the state's "Midwife Shortage Areas" may qualify for the Washington State Health Professional Scholarship and Loan Repayment Program.

Soma Institute
730 Klink Road
Buckley, Washington 98321
PHONE: (360) 829-1025
FAX: (360) 829-2805
E-MAIL: soma@nwrain.com
WEBSITE: www.soma-institute.com

The Soma techniques were developed and the institute founded in 1978. Karen Bolesky and Marcia Nolte have codirected the Soma Institute since 1986. Soma Neuromuscular Integration, or Soma bodywork, is a ten-lesson process of body therapy that structurally rebalances the body and reconditions the nervous system. There are three full-time instructors plus adjunct instructors; classes have from five to a maximum of fourteen students.

Accreditation and Approvals
In order to practice Soma Neuromuscular Integration in the State of Washington, one must hold a Washington massage license or other license that allows external touch. Graduates of massage therapy programs of 500 hours or more are qualified to take the National Certification Examination for Therapeutic Massage and Bodywork (NCETMB).

Program Description
The Soma Institute offers a twofold training program. Students who hold a state license or are from states that do not require a license may take the Soma Neuromuscular Integration training (Soma training) alone. Those who do not hold a license in either massage or physical therapy take both the Foundation Training and the Soma Training, which will prepare the student to take the Washington State Board of Massage licensing exam.

The Foundation Training consists of 200 hours of classroom instruction that, when combined with Soma Training, meets the 500-hour requirement for Washington State licensing. Courses include Anatomy and Physiology, Contraindications, Pathophysiology, Kinesiology, Basic Technique of Massage, and Psychology for the Bodyworker.

The 368-hour Soma training consists of Principles of Soma Neuromuscular Integration (including myofascial anatomy and physiology, skeletal anatomy, and structural integration),

Soma Neuromuscular Integration Training (which includes two demonstrations of each of the ten session series and hands-on practice), Social and Psychological Integration, Clinical Application of Soma Principles, Structural and Anatomical Assessment, Student Development, Client Development and Practice, and Somassage Technique.

Admission Requirements

Applicants must have a high school diploma or equivalent, be examples of health, and interview with an admissions representative. Admission to Soma training is based, in part, on assessment of the student's commitment to succeed as a Soma practitioner as demonstrated by a college degree, state licensing, self-employment, or other criteria. Applicants must have received the ten sessions of Soma bodywork or, in some cases, another form of structural integration.

Tuition and Fees

Tuition for the Soma Training is $7,500; for the Foundation Training, $2,500. The Institute supplies a manual, BodyCushion®, and other supplies; books, massage table, linens, and First Aid/CPR/AIDS training are additional.

Financial Assistance

A payment plan is available, and a discount is given for full payment before classes begin.

Spectrum Center School of Massage

MAILING ADDRESS:
1001 North Russell Road
Snohomish, Washington 98290
PHONE: (206) 334-5409 / (800) 801-9451
E-MAIL: spctrmcntr@aol.com

SCHOOL ADDRESS:
12506 18th Street NE, Suite 1
Lake Stevens, Washington 98258-9728

The Spectrum Center School of Massage was founded in 1981 and is owned by Director Barbara Collins. There are twelve instructors, with an average of eighteen students per class.

Accreditation and Approvals

The Spectrum Center is approved by the Washington State Board of Massage. Graduates are qualified to take the National Certification Examination for Therapeutic Massage and Bodywork (NCETMB).

Program Description

The ten-month, 660-hour Professional Massage training course is composed of two five-month semesters. The curriculum includes Anatomy, Physiology, and Pathology, Business Practices, Clinical Treatments, Deep Tissue/Advanced Techniques, Human Behavior, Hydrotherapy, Indications and Contraindications, Kinesiology, Lymphatic Drainage, Massage Theory and Practice, Medical Terminology, On-Site, Polarity, Shiatsu, Sports Massage, Study Skills, AIDS Training, Pregnancy Massage, Foot Reflexology, and Student Clinic. Classes are held days and evenings.

Admission Requirements

Applicants must be at least 18 years of age, have a high school diploma or equivalent, and interview with an admissions representative.

Tuition and Fees

Tuition is $6,000. There is a $150 registration fee, supplies and insurance are $250, books cost approximately $300, and a massage table costs $450 to $700.

Financial Assistance

Payment plans, veterans' benefits, and Division of Vocational Rehabilitation assistance are available.

Tri-City School of Massage

26 East 3rd Avenue
Kennewick, Washington 99336
PHONE: (509) 586-6434
E-MAIL: PJKruschke@aol.com

The Tri-City School of Massage was founded in 1968 by Ruth Williams, who has been an American Massage Therapy Association (AMTA) member since 1947 and served as AMTA's national president, historian, and national education director.

There are two instructors, with an average of twenty students per class.

Accreditation and Approvals

The Tri-City School of Massage curriculum is approved by the Washington State Board of Massage. Graduates are qualified to take the National Certification Examination for Therapeutic Massage and Bodywork (NCETMB).

Program Description

The 850-hour Massage Therapy Program consists of 500 classroom hours and 350 independent study hours. Courses include Anatomy and Physiology, Health and Hygiene, Pathology, Hydrotherapy, AIDS Awareness, Massage Theory (Swedish), Applied Anatomy and Kinesiology, Business and Professional Ethics, Medical Gymnastics, Body Mechanics, Massage-Related Techniques (such as connective tissue, positional release, reflexology, sports massage, acupressure, magnetic therapy, massage in pregnancy, baby massage, and on-site massage), Thesis, and Clinical Application (150 massages). Classes are held in the evenings, with daytime study halls.

Admission Requirements

Students must have a high school diploma or equivalent, should be financially and mentally stable, and in good physical health. There is no age requirement.

Tuition and Fees

There is a $100 registration fee; tuition is $4,500. Additional expenses include: massage table, $450 to $600; linens and bolsters, $160 to $210; uniform, $35; massage oil, $30; optional field trip, $25 to $35; optional AMTA student membership and Washington chapter fee, $178; and optional flash cards, $20.

The Wellness Institute

(See Multiple State Locations, pages 418–20)

Yoga Centers

2255 140th Avenue NE, Suite F
Bellevue, Washington 98007
PHONE: (425) 746-7476

FAX: (425) 746-3961
E-MAIL: yoga@oz.net
WEBSITE: www.yogacenters.com

Yoga Centers was founded in 1992 by Aadil Palkhivala, who has studied with B. K. S. Iyengar for over thirty years. The name Yoga Centers means yoga "centers" you in your body/life/mind. Yoga Centers offers the advanced kedric wall-rope system, pelvic swings, abundant props, two studios, and a retail store. There are fifteen instructors with a maximum of fifteen to thirty students per class.

Program Description

The seven-day Beginning Teacher Training is for beginning teachers or serious students interested in the basics of props, adjustments, therapeutic application of poses, and daily asana practice. It includes over forty hours of teacher training, plus over ten hours of regular classes.

The Intermediate/Advanced Teacher Training is held over nine days (sixty hours plus over ten hours of regular classes) and offers a deeper understanding of the use of props, adjustment, and therapeutic applications of poses, as well as pranayama, yoga philosophy, and meditation.

Admission Requirements

At least one year of practice is suggested prior to enrollment in Beginning Teacher Training. Permission is required for the November Intermediate/Advanced class only.

Tuition and Fees

The Beginning Teacher Training Course costs $495 to $595, depending on the registration date. The Intermediate/Advanced Teacher Training Course costs $645 to $745, depending on the registration date.

Financial Assistance

Payment plans and early registration discounts are available.

WEST VIRGINIA
Mountain State School of Massage

MAILING ADDRESS:
P.O. Box 4487
Charleston, West Virginia 25364
PHONE: (304) 926-8822
FAX: (304) 926-8837
E-MAIL: info@mtnstmassage.com
WEBSITE: www.mtnstmassage.com

FACILITY:
3407 Riverlane Drive
Malden, West Virginia 25306

Mountain State School of Massage was founded in 1995 as an affiliate of the Florida School of Massage. Directors Robert Rogers and Mary E. Mangus-Rogers, D.C., graduated from the Florida School of Massage in 1986. There are eight instructors, with an average of twenty students per class.

Accreditation and Approvals
Mountain State School of Massage has been awarded a certificate to operate by the State College Systems of West Virginia, and is approved by the National Certification Board for Therapeutic Massage and Bodywork (NCBTMB) as a continuing education provider. Graduates of either the Resident or Home Study Program are eligible to sit for the National Certification Examination for Therapeutic Massage and Bodywork (NCETMB) and to apply for massage therapy licensure in West Virginia.

Program Description
The 750-hour, six-month Resident Therapeutic Massage Program includes instruction, supervised practice, and directed independent study. The curriculum consists of Massage Therapy (covering Swedish Massage, Connective Tissue Therapy, Neuromuscular Therapy, Shiatsu, Polarity Therapy, Reflexology, Seated Chair Massage, and Sports Massage); Hydrotherapy; Anatomy and Physiology, Kinesiology and Pathology; Awareness and Communication Skills; Professional Standards, Ethics and Business Practices; CPR, First Aid, and Preventing Communicable Diseases; and Massage Practicum. Classes are held weekdays.

A Home Study Program consists of self-paced learning as well as required hands-on training at the school and covers the same material as the Resident Program, with the exception of Shiatsu and CPR classes. The eighteen-month program begins with a weekend of communications and awareness training. An additional sixteen weekends of hands-on training is interspersed throughout the program, with all theoretical content studied at home at the pace of one lesson per week.

Community and Continuing Education
Continuing education workshops are offered throughout the year. These have included Present-Centered Awareness Therapy, Connective Tissue, and Light Touch Therapy.

The 250-hour Structural Integration Certification Program consists of 180 hours of classroom instruction and seventy hours of supervised clinical practice and directed independent study. Topics covered include theory and practice of the ten-session structural integration bodywork, anatomy and kinesiology of sleeve and core muscles, models of structural and functional relationships and body observational skills, advanced connective tissue and myofascial release techniques, and body-centered awareness and communication skills. Classes meet in a series of four-day sessions conducted over six months. Clinic internship is scheduled after class of weekends.

Admission Requirements
Therapeutic Massage applicants must be at least 19 years of age (this requirement may be waived through personal interview), have a high school diploma or equivalent, and submit a biographical essay. An interview may be required.

Structural Integration applicants must be at least twenty years of age; have graduated from a massage or bodywork program with a curriculum of at least 500 hours, or have equivalent health care training in other disciplines and have taken a basic connective tissue therapy class; and have a willingness to explore their own personal growth and value systems in both group and individual settings.

Tuition and Fees
Tuition for the Therapeutic Massage Program is $5,700; tuition for the Home Study Program is $5,300. Additional expenses for either program include a $50 application fee; books, approximately $300; one massage from an instructor, $35 to $50; an op-

tional massage table, $400 to $600; and liability insurance, $150 to $200. Supplies are additional.

Tuition for the Structural Integration Program is $2,500.

Financial Assistance
A payment plan is available.

WISCONSIN

Blue Sky Educational Foundation

Professional School of Massage and Therapeutic Bodywork
220 Oak Street
Grafton, Wisconsin 53024
PHONE: (414) 376-1011
FAX: (414) 692-6387

The Blue Sky Professional School of Massage was founded in 1985 by Blair and Karen Lewis. There are twenty-two instructors, with an average of sixteen to thirty-six students per class.

Accreditation and Approvals
The Professional School of Massage is recognized by the International Myomassethics Federation (IMF) and is a member of the American Massage Therapy Association (AMTA) Council of Schools. Graduates are qualified to take the National Certification Examination for Therapeutic Massage and Bodywork (NCETMB). The City of Milwaukee has approved the curriculum.

Program Description
The 625-hour, ten-month Professional Massage Program consists of courses in Learning Strategies, Experiential Anatomy and Physiology: The Return of Joy, Muscles and Bones, World of Natural Medicine, Juicing for Health, Introduction to Massage: Full Body Relaxation Techniques, Reflexology/Foot Massage, Facial Massage, Polarity, Hatha for Health Professionals, Healthy Cooking, Healthy Life, Clinical Anatomy and Physiology, Neuromuscular Therapy, Ayurvedic Facial Massage, Lymphatic Massage, Sports Massage, Tai Chi Chuan, Allied Health Sciences Review, Clinical Pathology in the Massage Practice, Medical Terminology and Writing Progress Notes, Therapeutic Techniques and Specialty Areas, Introduction to the Business

World, Professional Field Placement, Community Service, and Student Clinic Experience. Students must also choose four electives from Jin Shin Do, Reiki, Sports Massage, Seated Therapeutic Massage, Neuromuscular Therapy, Whole Body Herbal Massage, Touch for Health, and others. Other graduation requirements include CPR/First Aid certification, human anatomy coloring book, a written report, thirty massages on teaching staff, an oral classroom presentation, homework, and exams. Classes are held days and evenings; weekend seminars are required for all students. The program may also be taken on a part-time basis.

Community and Continuing Education
Many courses are open to the general public. The Please Touch Program meets once a week for ten weeks, and offers an introduction to massage for the public or for potential students.

Nationally recognized continuing education seminars are offered on such topics as myofascial release, sports massage, NMT, Ayurvedic massage, advanced massage, polarity, and on-site chair massage.

Admission Requirements
Applicants must be at least 18 years of age; have a high school diploma or equivalent; be emotionally, mentally, and physically able to give and receive massage; have received two professional massages, submit two letters of recommendation (preferably one from a health professional), and have a personal interview.

Tuition and Fees
There is an application/interview fee of $35; tuition is $5,675. Supplies cost $500, including books, charts, lab fees, and materials; an optional massage table costs $400 to $850; and IMF and/or AMTA membership, national exams, and license cost $100 to $300. The Please Touch Program costs $275, or $400 for household couples.

Financial Assistance
A payment plan is available.

Lakeside School of Massage Therapy

1726 North 1st Street, Suite 100
Milwaukee, Wisconsin 53212
PHONE: (414) 372-4345
FAX: (414) 372-5350
E-MAIL: lakeschool@aol.com

Lakeside School of Massage Therapy (formerly the Lakeside School of Natural Therapeutics) is a nonprofit organization established in 1985. There are ten instructors. The school maintains a minimum teacher:student ratio of 1:14 in all bodywork classes and 1:6 during the supervised clinical experience.

Accreditation and Approvals

The Massage Therapy training program at Lakeside School is accredited by the Commission on Massage Training Accreditation (COMTA) and approved by the Wisconsin State Educational Approval Board. Graduates are qualified to take the National Certification Examination for Therapeutic Massage and Bodywork (NCETMB).

Program Description

The 600-hour Massage Therapy Training Program consists of Anatomy, Physiology, and Pathology; Kinesiology; Theory and Practice of Massage (with an emphasis on Swedish Massage, but also including an introduction to Reflexology, Sports Massage, Trigger Point Therapy, Shiatsu, Connective Tissue Manipulation, Range of Motion, Stretching, and Joint Mobilization); CPR; First Aid; Hydrotherapy; HIV Awareness; Business and Professional Practice Issues; and Body Mechanics/Clinician Self-Care. Classes are offered days, evenings, and weekends.

Admission Requirements

Applicants must be at least 18 years of age, have a high school diploma or equivalent, be physically capable of providing massage, be capable of effective interpersonal communication, and interview with an admissions representative.

Tuition and Fees

Tuition is $5,200. Additional expenses include an application fee of $30 and $275 for books; uniforms and supplies are additional.

Financial Assistance

Payment plans are available.

Midwest College of Oriental Medicine

WEBSITE:: www.acupuncture.edu

MAIN CAMPUS:
6226 Bankers Road, Suite 5 and 6
Racine, Wisconsin 53403
PHONE: (414) 554-2010 / (800) 593-2320
FAX: (414) 554-7475

ADDITIONAL CLASSROOMS:
4334 North Hazel # 206
Chicago, Illinois 60613
PHONE: (773) 975-1295

Midwest College was founded in 1979. The governing body of Midwest College is Acupuncture Center Inc.; the corporate officers and owners are William Dunbar and Robert Chelnick. Both the Oriental Medicine and Acupuncture Programs are offered in Racine; only first-year classes in acupuncture, evening classes in biomedicine, and internship are offered in Chicago. There are eighteen faculty members; class sizes average twelve students in practicum classes, forty in lecture classes.

Accreditation and Approvals

Midwest College is accredited by the Accreditation Commission for Acupuncture and Oriental Medicine (ACAOM) and approved by the State of Wisconsin Educational Approval Board. Graduates of the Master of Science in Oriental Medicine Program are eligible to sit for both the Acupuncture and Herb examinations given by the National Commission for the Certification of Acupuncture and Oriental Medicine (NCCAOM). Graduates of the Acupuncture Program are eligible to sit for the Acupuncture examination given by the NCCAOM.

Program Description

Midwest College offers a Master of Science in Oriental Medicine (MSOM) and a master's-level certification in Acupuncture. Both programs focus on the Chinese eight principle system of physiology, pathology, diagnosis, and treatment strategy used in the practice of Oriental medicine. Students in the OM program also study the classical herbal theories and traditions as well as new developments using herbs in Chinese medicine. Students in the OM program begin studying herbs in the fifth quarter. The minimum completion time for the 2,556-hour Oriental Medicine Program is thirty-six months (four academic years); the minimum completion time for the 2,028-hour Acupuncture Program is twenty-seven months (three academic years). Many students continue to work full-time while attending school evenings and weekends.

Courses offered include Fundamentals of Oriental Medicine, Chinese Medical Pathology, Point Location, Accessory Techniques, Physical Assessment, Anatomy, Oriental Massage Therapy, Oriental Philosophy, Needle Technique, Chinese Differential Diagnosis, Eight Principle Treatment Strategy, Neurology, Physiology, Pathology, Physical Examination, Treatment Strategy, Orthopedics/Traumatology, Survey of Nutrition, Survey of Pharmacology, Chinese Medicine Clinic Review, Acupuncture Practice Management, Introduction to Herbs/Chinese Materia Medica, Formulation, Internal Medicine, and Oriental Medicine Practice Management. Other requirements include directed learning papers in Chinese Medical History, Holistic Medical Systems, and Pathology Research; a major paper; and Acupuncture and/or Herbal Internship. Foreign internships are offered at Guangzhou Medical University in the Guangdong province of China.

Admission Requirements

Applicants must have an associate's degree or two years of postsecondary education from an accredited school (sixty semester credit hours), submit two letters of recommendation, and complete an admissions interview.

Tuition and Fees

The total minimum cost of the Oriental Medicine Program is $30,285; with foreign internship, $35,385. The total minimum cost of the Acupuncture Program is $24, 687; with foreign internship, $29,787. The application fee is $30 (included in totals). Books are an additional $1,500 for the OM program, $1,200 for the Acupuncture Program; supplies are an additional $500 for either program.

Financial Assistance

Students are eligible to apply for federal grants and loans.

Wisconsin Institute of Chinese Herbology

6921 Mariner Drive
Racine, Wisconsin 53406
PHONE: (414) 886-5858

The Wisconsin Institute of Chinese Herbology was founded in 1990 by Arthur D. Shattuck, a national board-certified acupuncturist, Chinese herbalist, and noted author and lecturer in the areas of Chinese medicine and Chinese herbology. The institute shares a building with the Wisconsin Institute of Natural Wellness (see page 352).

Accreditation and Approvals

All courses offered by the institute are approved by the National Commission for the Certification of Acupuncturists (NCCA) to provide continuing education units for acupuncturists and Chinese herbologists.

Program Description

An eight-month Chinese Herbology Course meets one evening per week and offers a comprehensive program in the science and art of Chinese herbology. The course combines lectures, practicums, related reading assignments, fieldwork, three original papers, and successful completion of thirty case studies for over 450 hours of participation. Topics covered include anatomy, physiology, Chinese diagnostic techniques, Chinese herbal botany, and chemistry. Each student will develop a collection of raw herbs, many harvested from the Institute's own herbal gardens.

Community and Continuing Education

Several one-day and weekend seminars are offered in topics related to Chinese herbology.

Tuition and Fees

Contact the institute for current tuition.

Financial Assistance

A discount is given for payment in full by the first class; a payment plan is available.

Wisconsin Institute of Natural Wellness

6921 Mariner Drive
Racine, Wisconsin 53406
PHONE: (414) 886-5858

The Wisconsin Institute of Natural Wellness was founded in 1995 by Anne M. Frontier, a certified massage therapist, and Arthur D. Shattuck, a national board certified acupuncturist, Chinese herbalist, and noted author and lecturer in the areas of Chinese medicine and Chinese herbology. The institute shares a building with the Wisconsin Institute of Chinese Herbology (see page 351).

Accreditation and Approvals

The institute is approved by the Educational Approval Board of the State of Wisconsin. Graduates are qualified to take the National Certification Examination for Therapeutic Massage and Bodywork (NCETMB) as well as the National Commission for the Certification of Acupuncturists Diplomate of Chinese Bodywork board certification exam.

Program Description

The 650-hour Professional Massage Therapy Certification Program combines the treatment principles of Chinese medicine with Western massage modalities. The curriculum includes Hands-On Therapy: Massage Theory and Techniques; Massage Anatomy: Bones and Muscles; Meditation and Personal Growth: A Self-Exploration; Anatomy and Physiology: East Meets West; Clinical Experience; Tai Chi; Independent Study; CPR Training; and weekend intensives in the areas of Shiatsu, Reiki, Jin Shin Do, Tui Na, Business and Marketing, Feng Shui, SoMove (a movement therapy that incorporates the work of Thomas Hanna, Alexander, and Feldenkrais®), and medical Intake, Assessment, and Record Keeping. Students may choose evening classes or same-day afternoon and evening classes.

Continuing Education

Many weekend intensives are offered in additional Chinese

medical modalities such as feng shui, Chinese herbology, and tuina.

Admission Requirements

Applicants must have a high school diploma or equivalent; be physically able to perform the required work; be free of communicable disease as documented by a physician; have had two documented full body massages; submit two character references, an essay, and two photos; visit the institute; and interview with an admissions representative.

Tuition and Fees

Tuition for the Professional Massage Therapy Program is $5,500, including a $300 deposit; books and materials cost approximately $200, and a massage table costs $300 to $600.

Financial Assistance

A payment plan is available.

WMB Hypnosis Training Center

831 West Main Street, Upper Left Suite
Lake Geneva, Wisconsin 53147
PHONE: (414) 249-8802
FAX: (414) 249-0587
E-MAIL: wmb@PowerandQui.com
WEBSITE: www.PowerandQui.com

WMB Hypnosis Training Center was founded in 1999 by Walter Matthew Brown. There are three instructors, with a maximum of thirty students per class.

Accreditation and Approvals

WMB Hypnosis Training Center is endorsed by the International Medical and Dental Hypnotherapy Association (IMDHA).

Program Description

The forty-hour Basic Hypnosis Program covers such topics as History of Hypnosis, Suggestibility Testing, Induction Methods, Guided Mental Imagery, Group Hypnosis, Principles of Suggestion, Pre-Induction Talk, Relaxation/Stress Management, Self-Hypnosis, Setting Up a Practice, Directed Independent Study, and more.

The forty-hour Advanced Hypnosis Program covers Advanced Methods, Waking Hypnosis, Rapid Inductions, Hickman Method, Age Regression, Amnesia and Surgery, Hypnotherapy, Dreams and Meaning, Post Hypnotic Suggestion, Visual Hallucination, Glove Anesthesia and Dentistry, Introduction to NLP, The Elman Method, and more.

The forty-hour Hypnoanalysis Program covers Fundamentals of Hypnoanalysis, Subconscious Order of Importance, Basic Communication Type, Word Association in Hypnosis, Hypnoanalysis Goals in Therapy, Spiritual Cleansing/Healing, Subconscious Motivation of Health and Disease, Sexual Disorders, Theology in Hypnosis, Regression Therapy, and more.

Admission Requirements

Applicants must be at least 18 years of age and have a high school diploma. The training is open both to students new to the field and to those who wish to refine their skills.

Tuition and Fees

Tuition for each forty-hour course is $595.

Financial Assistance

Discounts are offered for spouse or assistant and for payment in full fourteen days prior to class.

Canada

Tuition at Canadian schools is in Canadian dollars unless otherwise noted. Prices shown do not reflect the required GST (Goods and Services Tax).

ALBERTA
Alberta Institute of Massage

7644 Gaetz Avenue
Red Deer, Alberta T4P 2A8
Canada
PHONE: (403) 346-1018
FAX: (403) 346-0606
WEBSITE: members.xoom.com/AIofM

The Alberta Institute of Massage was founded in 1990 by Bob Layden. There are four instructors, with an average class size of twenty-two (maximum thirty).

Program Description

The 1,000-hour Massage Therapy Program consists of coursework in Anatomy and Physiology (emphasizing the skeletal, muscular, nervous and circulatory systems), Massage Practical (including basic relaxation massage, trigger point therapy, assessment, injury care, treatment, PNF stretching and related studies), CPR, First Aid, Advanced Assessment, Student Clinic, and more. Classes are held during the day; clinical practicum hours and supplementary classes are held evenings and weekends.

Admissions Requirements

Applicants should have a grade 12 diploma, have completed Biology 30 or equivalent, and have a personal interview; exceptions to the educational requirements may be made, depending on the applicant's other qualifications.

Tuition and Fees

Tuition is $7,100. Additional expenses include a $100 registration fee and approximately $300 for books; linens and liability insurance are additional.

Financial Assistance

Student financing is available.

Edmonton School of Swedish Relaxation Massage

290 Kaska Road
Sherwood Park, Alberta T8A 4G7
Canada
PHONE: (780) 464-8548
FAX: (780) 417-1248

Edmonton School of Swedish Relaxation Massage has four faculty members.

Accreditations and Approvals

Edmonton School of Swedish Relaxation Massage is licensed under the Private Vocational Schools Act of Alberta.

Program Description

The 1,000-hour Massage Therapy Program consists of Terminology, Osteology, Myology, Splanchnology (the study of organs), Angiology, Cytology/Histology, Syndesmology/Arthrology (the study of joints and ligaments), Neurology, Physiology, Pathology, Massage Theory, Assessment, Principles of Treatments, Clinical Practice, Outreach, Remedial Exercise, and Hydrotherapy Theory and Practice. The program may be completed in six months of full-time study.

Admission Requirements

Applicants must be at least 18 years of age and have a high school diploma. Applicants over 23 years of age may qualify as mature students (personal interview in lieu of diploma).

Tuition and Fees

Tuition is $5,800 and includes books, linens, and use of school equipment. There is a $75 registration fee due with application.

Financial Assistance

Tuition may be paid in two installments.

Foothills College of Massage Therapy

Suite 400, 7330—Fisher Street SE
Calgary, Alberta T2H 2H8
Canada
PHONE: (403) 255-4445
FAX: (403) 255-4074
E-MAIL: info@fcomt.com
WEBSITE: www.fcomt.com

The Foothills College of Massage Therapy was founded in 1994 by Beth Checkley. There are ten instructors, with a maximum of thirty students per class.

Accreditation and Approvals

Foothills College is a Private Vocational School; both massage programs are licensed programs.

Program Description

The 1,000-hour Massage Therapy Program includes Massage Theory and Technique, Advanced Massage Techniques, Assessment of Musculoskeletal Disorders, Massage Treatments, Self-Care, Human Relations and Communications, Hydrotherapy, Therapeutic Exercise, Splanchnology (medical terminology and overview of all bodily systems), Myology, Osteology, Syndesmology (classification of joints), Neurology, Systems Anatomy and Physiology, Pathology, and Business.

Students of the 2,200-hour Massage Therapy Program must first complete the 1,000-hour program at Foothills or possess equivalent training. Courses offered beyond the 1,000-hour program include Advanced Myology, Advanced Osteology, Advanced Syndesmology, Biomechanics, Regional Anatomy, Pathology, Systems Anatomy and Physiology, Nutrition and Public Health, Human Relations and Communication, Business, Assessment and Treatment, Therapeutic Exercise, Ergonomics, Hydrotherapy, Clinical Practicum, Myofascial Release, Proprioceptive Neuromuscular Facilitation (PNF), On-Site Massage Marketing and Practice, and Aromatherapy.

Admission Requirements

Applicants must be at least 18 years of age, be a high school graduate with grade 12 biology, and have a personal interview. Applicants over 23 years of age qualify as mature students and may be admitted without a diploma upon review of past experience and study.

Tuition and Fees

There is a $50 application fee.

Tuition for the 1,000-hour program is $6,500 and includes required texts, linen package, use of school equipment, clinic space and outreach supervision.

Tuition for the 2,200-hour program is $7,260 and includes required texts, use of school equipment and clinic space.

Financial Assistance

Both programs qualify for Government Student Assistance Programs; tuition may be paid in two installments.

Grant MacEwan Community College

P.O. Box 1796
Edmonton, Alberta T5J 2P2
Canada
PHONE: (403) 497-5188
FAX: (403) 497-5170
E-MAIL: bowmanc@infinity.gmcc.ab.ca
WEBSITE: www.gmcc.ab.ca

The Holistic Health Practitioner Program at Grant MacEwan Community College was founded in 1992. The Holistic Health Practitioner Program faculty consists of thirteen instructors; the Massage Therapy Program has twenty instructors. Class sizes average forty students.

Program Description

The 645-hour Holistic Health Practitioner Program may be completed in two years (six trimesters) of full-time study; some options for part-time study are available. Year One courses include The Multidimensional Being Part I, Therapeutic Relationships, Introduction to Complementary/Alternative Modalities Part I, Awakening the Inner Healer: Self Healing Practices, Philosophical and Theoretical Foundations of Holistic Healing, Counseling and Teaching, Complementary/Alternative Clinical Practice, and Health and Healing: Unitary Person Assessment. Year Two courses include Establishing a Collaborative Practice, Introduction to Complementary/Alternative Modalities Part II, The Multidimensional Being Part II, Complementary/Alternative Clinical Practice, and Clinical Internship.

The Massage Therapy Program is based on a 2,200-hour curriculum and may be completed in two years (six trimesters) of full-time study; the program may also be taken on a part-time basis. Year One courses include Massage Therapy as a Profession, Terminology for Massage Therapists, Communication Skills for Massage Therapists, Functional Survey for Massage Therapists, Body Structure, Body Functioning, Techniques, Developing Therapeutic Relationships, The Human Lifespan, Body Movements, Human Disease Processes, Assessment for Massage Therapists, Introduction to Business Management, and Clinical Practice. Year Two courses include Techniques, Massage Therapy for Special Populations, Individual Field Project, Sports Massage, Nutrition/Pharmacological Concepts, Treatments and Planning, and Clinical Practice.

Admission Requirements

Holistic Health Practitioner applicants must have a high school diploma or equivalent and must have taken basic human anatomy and physiology or human physiology (ninety hours). Students are required to have taken ENGL 111 prior to completion of the program; CPR at the Basic Rescuer Level is required before the commencement of the spring session in the first year and is to be updated annually.

Massage Therapy applicants must have a high school diploma or equivalent and must have taken Biology 30 or Chemistry 30 or Science 30; mature students who have not taken one of these courses must take a fifteen-hour self-study course in Physiology Basics after admission into the program. Mature students may be considered on an individual basis. CPR at the Basic Rescuer Level and a First Aid certificate are required prior to taking Clinical Practice I and must be maintained.

Tuition and Fees

Tuition is $8,900. Additional expenses include books, supplies, SA fees, and health plan fees.

Financial Assistance

Federal and provincial government student grants and loans are available.

Mount Royal College

Centre for Complementary Health Education
Continuing Education and Extension
2204 2 Street SW
Calgary, Alberta T2S 1S5
Canada
PHONE: (403) 503-4886/ (403) 503-4888
FAX: (403) 503-4899
E-MAIL: aghani@mtroyal.ab.ca
WEBSITE: www.mtroyal.ab.ca/programs/conted/certindex.html

Mount Royal offered its first massage course in 1982. In 1997, the program was extended to 1,000 hours. There are twenty instructors, with a maximum of twenty-six students per class.

Accreditation and Approvals

Each province has its own licensing requirements; students are encouraged to investigate the requirements of the province in which they intend to practice prior to enrolling.

Program Description

The 1,000-hour Massage Therapy Program includes courses in Massage-Related Terminology and Concepts, Introduction to Therapeutic Massage, Anatomy and Physiology, Advanced Studies of Joints and Soft Tissues, Pathology, Advanced Massage Techniques, Clinical Practicum, Kinesiology and Remedial Exercise, Orthopedic Assessment, Professional Role of the Massage Therapist, Marketing and Career Development, and Integrated Studies. Full- and part-time programs are offered.

A four-course Acupressure Therapy Certificate Program meets two evenings and one Saturday per week from September to May. Topics covered include anatomy and physiology, pathology, and Oriental principles of assessment and treatment based on acupressure techniques. Students apply their knowledge in a clinical setting.

A four-course Reflexology Therapy Certificate Program meets two evenings and one Saturday per week from September to May. Topics covered include anatomy and physiology, pathology, and Oriental principles of assessment and treatment based on reflexology techniques. Students apply their knowledge in a clinical setting.

A four-course Aromatherapy Certificate Program meets two evenings and one Saturday per week from September to May. Topics covered include anatomy and physiology, pathology, materia medica, aromassage techniques, the energetics of oils, assessment and treatments. Students apply their knowledge in a clinical setting.

Continuing Education

A three-course Sports Massage Certificate Program is offered to massage therapists. Topics covered include pre- and post-event principles, orthopedic assessment and treatment of sports injuries, training principles, and more.

Professional Development courses are offered on a regular basis to massage therapists and health care practitioners. Topics have included Introduction to Herbology for the Health Professional, Assessment and Treatment of Headaches, Iridology, Assessment and Treatment Using Muscle Energy Techniques, and others.

Admission Requirements

Applicants must have an Alberta high school diploma or equivalent or be a mature student age 23 or older. A grade 12 biology credit would be beneficial, but is not required.

Tuition and Fees

Tuition is charged on a per-course basis and ranges from $135 to $650 per course; the total cost of thirteen courses and two clinical practicums is $6,250. Books and supplies are approximately $650.

Tuition for the Acupressure Therapy Certificate is $1,875. Tuition for the Reflexology Therapy Certificate is $1,875. Tuition for the Aromatherapy Certificate is $1,675 plus approximately $200 for supplies.

Tuition for the Sports Massage Certificate is $735. Most Professional Development courses are $50.

Financial Assistance

Financial assistance is available; contact the Financial Aid office for specific information.

The Northwestern School of Massage

(see The Orthopaedic Massage Therapy Institute, below).

The Orthopaedic Massage Therapy Institute

2424 4th Street SW, Suite 920
Calgary, Alberta T2S 2T4
Canada
PHONE: (403) 228-6307
FAX: (403) 228-4651

The Orthopaedic Institute was founded in 1979. The Northwestern School of Massage is an affiliate of the Orthopaedic Institute. Stillpoint Clinics is the parent company of the Orthopaedic Institute.

Accreditation and Approvals

The 250-hour course is a licensed course under Private Vocational Schools. M1000, M1500, and M2200 courses are recognized by all the major associations for eligibility for membership.

Program Description

The Northwestern School of Massage is an affiliate of the Orthopaedic Institute and offers a 250-hour program (M250) in Swedish Relaxation Massage. The curriculum covers the professional practitioner-client relationship, partial and full body massages, health club and spa work, postural awareness, muscle strength, range of motion, basic anatomy, basic nutrition, and physiology of the muscular and skeletal system. Enrollment in this course or the equivalent is a prerequisite for the Orthopaedic Institute's 1,000-, 1,500-, and 2,200-hour programs.

Advanced Therapeutic Massage Programs M1000, M1500, and M2200 consist of 1,000, 1,500, and 2,200 hours of training, respectively. M1000 is an evening and weekend certificate program and meets the minimum requirement for a therapist in Alberta. M1500 is a daytime diploma program which may be completed in twelve months. M2200 is a more advanced daytime diploma program which may be completed in eighteen months. Courses differ in the amount and depth of material covered. Course content offered includes Massage for Small Animals, Jin Shin Do, Shiatsu/Acupressure/Trigger Point, Equine Massage, Massage for Immobilized Patients, Myofascial Release, Traditional Chinese Medicine, Insurance Billings, Manual Lymphatic Drainage, Sports Massage, Orthopaedic (Soft Tissue) Assessment and Treatment, Anatomy and Physiology, Histology and Basic Pathology, Energy Metabolism, Hydrotherapy, Kinesthetic Movement, Measuring Muscle Strength, Palpation, Massage Therapy Treatment with Thermal Techniques, Basic Practice Management, Practice in Public Clinic, and more.

Admission Requirements

Applicants must have a high school diploma or equivalent or be a mature student (twenty years old) or take an entrance exam; have a personal interview; and submit two character references.

Tuition and Fees

Tuition for M250 is $1,499; for M1000, $5,850; for M1500, $8,500; for M2200, $12,500. Books and supplies are additional.

Financial Assistance

Scholarships and payment plans are available.

Somatic Arts Institute

6304 109A Street
Edmonton, Alberta T6H 3C7
Canada
PHONE: (403) 438-3757
E-MAIL: Somatic.Arts.Institute@telusplanet.net
WEBSITE: telusplanet.net/public/mvdg/somatic_arts_institute.html

The Somatic Studies Program began offering graduate training in fall 1998; the Somatic Therapist Program is scheduled to begin September 2000.

Accreditation and Approvals

Graduates are qualified to take the National Certification Examination for Therapeutic Massage and Bodywork (NCETMB) and/or applicable state licensing exams. Somatic Therapist graduates will have the academic credentials to practice under massage licensing laws in Alberta.

Program Description

The Somatic Therapist Program is a part-time, two-year training in integrated massage and bodywork. Classes meet Sunday, Monday, and one weekday evening, forty weeks per year. Training includes study of the theory and practice of modern massage therapies, somatic education, Eastern therapeutic modalities, and healing through movement. Courses include Manual Manipulation and the Therapeutic Relationship, Somatic Therapies, Western Therapeutic Treatment, Pathology and Dysfunction, Physical Assessment, Movement Education, Pharmacology, Nutrition and Metabolism, Hydrotherapy and Spa Treatments, Anatomy and Physiology, Business and Practice Management, Therapeutic Relations/Interactive Skills Group, Synthesis/Integration, Clinical/Outreach, and Self Integration.

The Somatic Studies Program is a part-time, two-year

graduate program for health care practitioners. Classes meet Sunday and Monday once a month, ten months each year. Courses include Somatic Therapies (Western), Somatic Psychologies, Experiential Anatomy and Physiology, Expressive Arts, Eastern Practices, Psychodynamics and the Relational Field, Contemporary Health Problems, Somatic Practice I: The Body in Relationship, Somatic Practice II: The Body as a System, Somatic Practice III: Working with the Imaginal/Dreaming Body, and Integrative Project.

Continuing Education

The institute offers a variety of courses, workshops, and seminars throughout the year; ask to be placed on the mailing list or check the website for current offerings.

Admission Requirements

Somatic Therapist applicants are required to have at least a high school diploma or a college-level course in biology. Some prior personal work with a counseling therapist and with bodywork is highly recommended. During the program students who do not have a prior personal bodywork practice will select and practice a personal bodywork practice such as tai chi or yoga to further the integration of learning into embodied understanding.

In addition to the above requirements, Somatic Studies applicants should also be a graduate of either a helping/ healing profession or a somatic practice.

Tuition and Fees

Tuition for the Somatic Therapist Program is $9,950. Tuition for the Somatic Studies Program is $3,200.

Financial Assistance

For the Somatic Therapist Program, monthly payment plans and early payment discounts are available. For the Somatic Studies Program, tuition may be paid in two annual payments ($1,600 each).

University of Alberta, Faculty of Extension

93 University Extension Centre NW
Edmonton, Alberta T6G 2T4
Canada

PHONE: (780) 492-3037 / (800) 808-4784
FAX: (780) 492-1857
E-MAIL: health.wellness@ualberta.ca
WEBSITE: www.extension.ualberta.ca/acupuncture

The Certificate Program in Medical Acupuncture was first offered at the University of Alberta in 1990.

Accreditation and Approvals

Successful completion of the Certificate Program in Medical Acupuncture is recognized as a qualification to practice acupuncture by the College of Physicians and Surgeons of Alberta, College of Physicians and Surgeons of British Columbia, College of Physicians and Surgeons of Saskatchewan, Yukon Medical Council, Alberta Dental Association, and the Colleges of Physical Therapists of Alberta, British Columbia, Manitoba and Saskatchewan.

Continuing Education

The Certificate Program in Medical Acupuncture consists of 200 credit hours of intensive graduate-level instruction in the theory and clinical practices of acupuncture and Oriental medicine. The program is designed to be taken on a part-time basis and can be completed in one year. The four modules each consist of two three-day weekends.

The program consists of Module I: Basic Elementary Acupuncture; Module II: Fundamental Acupuncture; Module III: Microsystems of Acupuncture; and Module IV: Clinical Acupuncture. A practical and oral exam follows each of the first three modules, and a two-day final comprehensive written, oral and clinical exam is offered once each year.

Admission Requirements

The program is open to fully licensed physicians, dentists, and physiotherapists.

Tuition and Fees

Tuition is $995, including lab fee, for each of the four levels; the final exam is an additional $395.

BRITISH COLUMBIA

Academy of Classical Oriental Sciences

420 Railway Street
Nelson, British Columbia V1L 1H3
Canada
PHONE: (250) 352-5887/ (888) 333-8868
FAX: (250) 352-3458
E-MAIL: acos@acos.org
WEBSITE: www.acos.org

The Academy of Classical Oriental Sciences (ACOS) was founded in 1994 by Warren Fischer and Michael Smith. There are seven faculty members; the average class size is typically twenty-five students in the first year.

Accreditation and Approvals

ACOS will meet or exceed all academic and clinical requirements laid out by the regulating body of the Health Professions Council of British Columbia's newly formed College of Acupuncture.

Program Description

The four-year program in Traditional Chinese Medicine consists of 216 credits. Year One courses include Fundamentals of TCM, Yang Sheng Fa (Nourishing Life Principles), History of Chinese Medicine, Dao Yin, Qi Gong, Anatomy, Tai Chi Chuan, Chinese Language, TCM Diagnostics, Meridians, Differential Diagnosis, Tui Na, Physiology, and Qi Gong Systems and Styles. Year Two courses include Acupoints, Qing Zhi Bing (Mental and Emotional Disharmony Patterns), Zhong Yao Xue (Chinese Herbs), Classmate Case Study, Western Medical Pathology, Qi Gong as Practical Therapy, Chinese Language, Techniques of Acupuncture and Moxibustion, Yao Fang Xue (Herbal Formulae), Comparable Syndromes, Clinical Observation, Acupressure, Tui Na and Kinesiology, and Introduction to Western Clinical Medicine. Year Three courses include Therapeutics, Advanced Diagnostic Methods and Counseling Skills, Nei Ke (Chinese Internal Medicine), Theory Comparison, Clinical Observation and Discussion, Qi Gong for Medical Practitioners, Selected Classics, Wai Ke (Chinese External Medicine), Gynecology and Pediatrics, Supervised Clinical Practice, Advanced Tui Na, and Accreditation Preparation. Year Four courses include Therapeutics, Clinical Reference Techniques, Understanding Yao Fang (Herbal Prescriptions), Business Management and Ethics, Supervised Clinical Practice, Instructors Course in Tuina, Qi Gong and Dao Yin, Research Techniques, Thesis Project and Clinical Internship.

Admission Requirements

Applicants must have completed two years of postsecondary education in the Arts or Sciences; Mature students who are 19 years of age and/or have been out of school for fifty-two weeks and have not completed two years of postsecondary education are offered the full-time program and are under academic probation for the first year (a cumulative GPA of less than 2.0 will result in withdrawal). Applicants must also be proficient in oral and written English. Preference is given to full-time applicants.

Tuition and Fees

Tuition for first-year full-time students is $121 per credit; for part-time students, $150 per credit; for audit students, $135 per credit. Additional expenses include books, approximately $1,100 per year; administration fee, $33 per term; student fee, $13 per term; library endowment fee, $13 per term; and campus amenity fee, $13 per term.

Financial Assistance

Financial assistance may be available to qualifying students.

Canadian Acupressure Institute

301-733 Johnson Street
Victoria, British Columbia V8W 3C7
Canada
PHONE: (250) 388-7475
FAX: (250) 383-3647
E-MAIL: caii@tnet.net
WEBSITE: come.to/cai

The Canadian Acupressure Institute Inc. (CAII) was founded in 1994 by Kathy de Bucy and Arnold Porter. There are thirteen instructors plus seven teaching assistants; classes average twenty to twenty-two students.

Accreditation and Approvals

CAII is accredited by the Private Post-Secondary Education Commission of British Columbia. Program I graduates are eligible to apply for certification by the Jin Shin Do Foundation, the American Oriental Bodywork Therapy Association (AOBTA), and the British Columbia Acupressure Therapists' Association. Program II graduates are eligible to apply for certification by the AOBTA, the British Columbia Acupressure Therapists' Association, and the Shiatsu Therapy Association of British Columbia upon completion of a two-part examination.

Program Description

The 725-hour Program I: Jin Shin Do Acupressure curriculum consists of Basic Jin Shin Do Acupressure, Intermediate Jin Shin Do, Advanced Jin Shin Do, Counseling Skills, Module II (covering advanced study of the strange flows and five elements, specific application to common conditions, and an introduction to traditional Chinese medicine), Module III (covering counterindications for acupressure, ethical and legal considerations, and supervised clinical practice), Anatomy and Physiology, Extended Jin Shin Do Therapeutics, Communication Skills, Bodymind Energetics, and Pal Dan Gum (Taoist yoga movements).

The 1,000-hour Program II: Shiatsu curriculum consists of Shiatsu Theory and Practice: Module I and II, General Oriental Bodywork Therapeutics, Clinical Practice, Anatomy, Physiology and Pathology, Personal and Professional Development, Communication Skills, and Jin Shin Do.

A 250-hour Jin Shin Do Certification Program is offered in weekend modules over a two-year period.

Admission Requirements

Applicants must be at least 18 years of age with grade 12, or a mature student (nineteen years of age or older and out of school at least one year) with life experience demonstrating responsibility; be fluent in spoken and written English; be physically and mentally healthy; have received at least two Jin Shin Do or Shiatsu sessions prior to acceptance; submit a certificate of health and two letters of reference; answer a series of essay questions; and have a personal interview. Applicants must also have completed a fifteen-hour course in bodywork such as Reiki, Reflexology, Massage, etc.

Tuition and Fees

Tuition for Program I is $6,400. Tuition for Program II is $8,500. Additional expenses for both programs include approximately $450 for books and $600 for acupressure sessions from practitioners and teachers as part of examination requirements.

Tuition for the 250-hour Jin Shin Do Certification Program is $2,800.

Financial Assistance

Payment plans and early payment discounts are available. Government financial assistance may be available for eligible students.

Canadian College of Acupuncture and Oriental Medicine

855 Cormorant Street
Victoria, British Columbia V8W 1R2
PHONE: (250) 384-2942 / (888) 436-5111
FAX: (250) 360-2871
E-MAIL: ccaom@islandnet.com
WEBSITE: www.islandnet.com/~ccaom/

The Canadian College of Acupuncture and Oriental Medicine (CCAOM) was founded in 1985 as the School of Traditional Chinese Medicine. In 1991, the East West Medical Society, a nonprofit organization, was formed to take over administration of the college. There are twelve instructors, with an average of twenty-five students per class.

Accreditation and Approvals

The college is registered with the Private Post-Secondary Education Commission of British Columbia. Graduates are eligible to take the acupuncture examination of the National Commission for the Certification of Acupuncturists (USA).

Program Description

The 2,592.5-hour Acupuncture and Oriental Medicine program may be completed in four years of full-time study; part-time study is possible if space permits. First Year courses include TCM: Foundations, TCM: History, Doctrines and Theories, Acupuncture: Meridians and Points, Herbology: Materia Medica, Biomedical Physical Assessment, Clinical Observation, Medical Mandarin Terminology, Tai Qi, and Jin Shin Do. Second Year courses include TCM: Internal Medicine, TCM: Clinical Diagnosis, Acupuncture: Therapeutics and Techniques, Acupuncture: Point Energetics, Herbology: Formulas and Strategies, Biomedical Pathology, Clinical Observation, Professional Clinical Observation, and Tui Na. Third Year courses include TCM: Inner Classic of the Yellow Emperor, TCM: Gynecology and Pediatrics, Acupuncture: Treatmentology, Herbology: Formula Combinations and Modifications, Herbology: Treatise on Febrile Diseases Caused by Cold, Biomedical Clinical Diagnosis, Biomedical Physical Assessment, Clinical Practicum, and Counseling Skills. Fourth Year courses include TCM: Comprehensive Review, TCM: Clinical Lectures, TCM: Dermatology, External and Five Sense Diseases, Acupuncture: Microsystems, Acupuncture: Case Studies, Acupuncture: Sports/Physical Trauma, Herbology: Chinese Dietary Systems, Herbology: Synopsis of Prescriptions of the Golden Chamber, Herbology: Study of Warm Illnesses, Clinical Practicum, Practice Management, and Ethics and Legal Issues.

Admission Requirements

Applicants must have completed two years of postsecondary education in humanities or sciences or the equivalent in education, work experience, and professional training, plus a credit course in basic anatomy and physiology, the equivalent of a two-semester college or university anatomy and physiology course. In addition, applicants must be proficient in oral and written English, have financial resources to complete the program, submit two letters of reference and a certificate of health, and a personal essay. Preference is given to full-time applicants. Preference may be given to students who have taken courses in Sciences, Healing Practices, Psychology, Eastern Philosophy, and/or Mandarin.

Tuition and Fees

Tuition is $6,000 per academic year. Other expenses include an application fee of $100; books and supplies are additional.

Financial Assistance

Full-time students may apply for a Canada Student Loan and/or a provincial student loan.

Canadian College of Massage and Hydrotherapy/West Coast College of Massage Therapy

(See Multiple State Locations, pages 420–21)

Dr. Vodder School—North America

(See Multiple State Locations, pages 422–23)

Dominion Herbal College

7527 Kingsway
Burnaby, British Columbia V3N 3C1
Canada
PHONE: (604) 521-5822
FAX: (604) 526-1561
E-mail: herbal@uniserve.com
WEBSITE: www.dominionherbal.com

Dominion Herbal College (DHC) was founded by Dr. Herbert Nowell, a naturopathic physician, in 1926. There are thirty instructors, with an average of twenty-five students per class. DHC offers classroom programs in Vancouver and Toronto, as well as several self-paced home study programs (see pages 474–75).

Accreditation and Approvals

DHC is a registered Post-Secondary School in the Province of British Columbia. Graduates of the Clinical Herbal Therapist program are eligible for membership in the Canadian Herbalists' Association of British Columbia and the American Herbalist Guild as Registered Clinical Herbal Therapists.

Program Description

The three-year Clinical Herbal Therapist diploma program is a full-time program consisting of over 2,000 classroom hours and 500 practical clinical hours. The curriculum includes Anatomy and Physiology, Chemistry for Herbalists, Biochemistry, Botany, History and Philosophy, Nutrition, Introduction to Pharmacokinetics, Introduction to Pharmacognosy, Pharmacy: Herbal, Pathology, Medical Terminology, Clinical Assessment, Laboratory Analysis, Materia Medica, Therapeutics,

Pharmacology, Business Practice, and Principles of Practice and Ethics. Students must also complete a St. Johns CPR Course.

Continuing Education

A Clinical Aromatherapy Program is offered to graduates of the Clinical Herbal Therapist or the Clinical Phytotherapy Program or other health care professionals with clinical experience. The course meets for eighty classroom and sixteen clinic hours and consists of Principles of Natural Therapeutics, Physio-Medicalism, Materia Medica, Practical Procedures, Full Body Manual Lymphatic Draining, Chartered Herbalist Course: Materia Medica, and Clinic Practicum.

Admission Requirements

Clinical Herbal Therapist Program applicants must have a high school diploma, including courses in Introductory Chemistry and either Biology or Anatomy/Physiology. Applicants without background in these subjects may take a prerequisite home study course from DHC.

Tuition and Fees

Tuition for the Clinical Herbal Therapist Program is $9,300 for Year One; $9,300 plus $2,000 for clinical hours in Year Two; and $9,300 plus $300 for a practical exam in Year Three.

Tuition for the Clinical Aromatherapy program is $2,500.

Financial Assistance

Payment plans are available.

International College of Traditional Chinese Medicine of Vancouver

1508 West Broadway, #201
Vancouver, British Columbia V6J 1W8
Canada
PHONE: (604) 731-2926
FAX: (604) 731-2964
E-MAIL: info@tcmcollege.com
WEBSITE: www.tcmcollege.com

The International College of Traditional Chinese Medicine of Vancouver was founded in 1986.

Accreditation and Approvals

The International College of Traditional Chinese Medicine of Vancouver is registered with the Private Post-Secondary Education Commission of British Columbia. It is designated in British Columbia as an "Eligible Institution" under the Canada Student Loans Act, and recognized by the Ministry of Education in the Province of Quebec and in the Province of Ontario for student loans under the Student Financial Aid Programs. Graduates are prepared to meet all of the qualifying examinations and regulations concerning acupuncture and traditional Chinese medicine.

Program Description

Diploma programs are offered in Traditional Chinese Medicine, Chinese Acupuncture, and Chinese Herbology.

The Four-Year Diploma Program in Traditional Chinese Medicine consists of 2,942 hours of instruction. First Year courses include Foundation of TCM, Diagnosis of TCM, Chinese Herbology, Chinese Acupuncture, Foundation of Chinese Language, Directed Reading, Western Anatomy, Chinese Tui Na/Qi Gong, Surface Anatomy and Acupuncture Points, History of TCM, and Dispensing Procedures Practicum. Second Year courses include Internal Medicine, Chinese Herbology, Chinese Acupuncture, Chinese Herbal Formulas, Dermatology and External Diseases in TCM, Directed Reading, Western Physiology, Clinical Procedures Practicum, Techniques and Modern Systems of Acupuncture, Clinical Observations, and Orthopedics and Traumatic Injuries in TCM. Third Year courses include Gynecology in TCM, Chinese Acupuncture, Directed Reading, Internal Medicine, Chinese Herbal Formulas, Diseases of Five Senses in TCM, Clinical Practices, Studies of Clinical Cases, and Western Diagnosis. Fourth Year courses include TCM Classics, Acupuncture Classics, Advanced Acupuncture, Advanced Herbology, Clinic Practices in China, Foundations of Western Pharmacology, Western Nutrition and Chinese Food Cure, Studies of Clinical Cases, Methodology of Clinical Research, Clinical Practices, and Graduation Thesis.

The Three-Year Diploma Program in Chinese Acupuncture consists of 2,072 hours of instruction. First Year courses include Foundation of TCM, Diagnosis of TCM, Foundation of Chinese Language, Chinese Acupuncture, Directed Reading, Western Anatomy, Chinese Tui Na/Qi Gong, Surface Anatomy and Acupuncture Points, History of TCM, and Chinese Herbology.

Second Year courses include Internal Medicine, Western Diagnosis, Chinese Acupuncture, Acupuncture Classics, Dermatology and External Diseases in TCM, Directed Reading, Western Physiology, Clinical Procedures, Techniques and Modern Systems of Acupuncture, Clinical Observations, and Orthopedics and Traumatic Injuries in TCM. Third Year courses include Gynecology in TCM, Chinese Acupuncture, Directed Reading, Internal Medicine, TCM Classics, Diseases of Five Senses in TCM, Clinical Practices, Studies of Clinical Cases, and Advanced Acupuncture.

The Three-Year Diploma Program in Chinese Herbology consists of 2,072 hours of instruction. First Year courses include Foundations of TCM, Diagnosis of TCM, Foundation of Chinese Language, Chinese Acupuncture, Directed Reading, Western Anatomy, Chinese Tui Na/Qi Gong, Dispensing Procedures Practicum, History of TCM, and Chinese Herbology. Second Year courses include Internal Medicine, Chinese Herbology, TCM Classics, Chinese Herbal Formulas, Dermatology and External Diseases in TCM, Directed Reading, Western Physiology, Clinical Procedures, Clinical Observations, Orthopedics and Traumatic Injuries in TCM, and Methodology of Clinical Research. Third Year courses include Gynecology in TCM, Studies of Clinical Cases, Directed Reading, Internal Medicine, Chinese Herbal Formulas, Diseases of Five Senses in TCM, Clinical Practices, Western Diagnosis, and Advanced Herbology.

Continuing Education

The Medical Acupuncture for Physicians, Dentists, and Physiotherapists Program totals 300 hours of instruction at three levels. The program covers philosophy and theory of acupuncture, diagnosis, point locations, techniques of acupuncture, acupuncture treatment of various diseases, acupuncture classics, modern research of acupuncture, clinical training, and more.

Admission Requirements

Applicants must have a minimum of two years of college education or the equivalent and a sincere desire to pursue knowledge in traditional Chinese medicine.

Those applying for the Medical Acupuncture for Physicians, Dentists, and Physiotherapists program must submit documentation to substantiate his or her professional status.

Tuition and Fees

Tuition for the three diploma programs is payable as follows: $970 on the first of August accompanied by five postdated checks for $970 each (October 1 though February 1). Part-time students pay on an hourly basis with $275 for a one-hour course, $550 for a two-hour course, $825 for a three-hour course for one entire academic year. Full-time students should allow $700 per year for books.

Total tuition for the Medical Acupuncture for Physicians, Dentists, and Physiotherapists Program is $4,800 ($1,300 for Level One, $1,600 for Level Two, and $1,900 for Level Three).

Financial Assistance

Tuition may be paid in full for a 10 percent discount. Loans and additional financial assistance may be available.

Okanagan Valley College of Massage Therapy Ltd.

200, 3400 - 30th Avenue
Vernon, British Columbia V1T 2E2
PHONE: (250) 558-3718
FAX: (250) 558-3748
E-MAIL: ovcmt@telus.net
WEBSITE: www.ovcmt.com

The Okanagan Valley College of Massage Therapy Ltd. was founded in 1994 by Douglas R. Fairweather and Ken Andrusiak. The faculty consists of twenty-four instructors and teaching assistants. Maximum class size is forty-four.

Accreditation and Approvals

OVCMT is accredited by both the Private Post-Secondary Education Commission and by the College of Massage Therapists of British Columbia.

Program Description

The 3,000-hour Massage Therapy curriculum may be completed in three years.

Year One Practical Courses include Professionalism: Jurisprudence, Massage Theory and Practice (consisting of Swedish, Neuromuscular Therapy, and Stress Management Techniques), Sports Massage, Hydrotherapy, Communications,

Introduction to Musculoskeletal Assessment and Self Awareness, and Clinical Practicum. Year One Academic courses include Human Anatomy, Human Physiology, Public Health and Self Care.

Year Two Practical Courses include Actino Therapy (the use of rays of light for therapeutic benefit), Clinical Theory and Practice, Clinical Practicum, Specific Outreach, and Advanced Massage Techniques and Integration (consisting of Lymph Drainage, Connective Tissue Techniques, and Neuromuscular Therapy). Year Two Academic courses include Human Anatomy, Human Physiology, Advanced Neurology, Pathology, and Kinesiology and Therapeutic Exercise.

Year Three Practical Courses include Clinical Outreach, Advanced Technique Development, and Clinical Theory and Practice. Year Three Academic Courses include An Introduction to Medicine, An Introduction to Research Methods and Statistics, Pathology, Small Business Management, Nutrition, Professionalism: Jurisprudence, and Integrated Science.

Students are required to obtain and/or hold a valid CPR/First Aid certificate by the end of Term 1, Year 2.

Admission Requirements

Applicants must have graduated grade 12 (or have a GED) with chemistry 12 and English 12 or a passing mark on an English competency exam for college entrance, plus a minimum of three credits in a university or college level biology for science majors. Applicants are required to have a minimum level of experience in introductory massage; this can be accomplished by attending a weekend workshop. Applicants must also submit three references, a résumé, a physician's statement, and a brief essay.

Tuition and Fees

Tuition is $7,500 per year. Additional expenses include a $75 application fee; a $500 deposit, which will be applied toward textbooks and miscellaneous supplies (approximate textbook costs are $500 to $525 in Year One, $700 to $725 in Year Two, and $200 to $275 in Year Three); a massage table, approximately $600 to $800; and additional supplies.

Financial Assistance

Tuition is payable in monthly installments.

Vancouver Homeopathic Academy

P.O. Box 34095
Station D
Vancouver, British Columbia V6J 4M1
Canada
PHONE: (604) 708-9387
FAX: (604) 708-1547
WEBSITE: www.homeopathyvancouver.com

The Vancouver Homeopathic Academy was founded in 1994 by Murray Feldman, C.C.H., RSHom. There are four instructors, with an average of twenty-five students per class.

Accreditation and Approvals

The Vancouver Homeopathic Academy is registered with the Private Post Secondary Education Commission of British Columbia.

Program Description

Two options are available for training in classical homeopathy: a one-year Foundation Course and a four-year Homeopathy Program; the Foundation Course is the first year of the four-year program, but may be taken independently.

Year One—Foundation Course will not train students to be homeopathic practitioners, but will provide a sound systematic understanding of homeopathic philosophy and principles. Students will learn how to apply homeopathy effectively as a means of self-help in simple first aid and everyday acute situations. This course also provides a basis for further study. A Certificate of Attendance will be given at the end of the first year.

Year Two provides a deepening of first-year concepts. Live cases will be taken and discussed with students. Topics include remedy reaction, second prescription, different forms of case analysis, potency and repetition, case management, miasms and nosodes, obstacles to cure, case taking, hierarchy of symptoms, and pathology.

Year Three covers different aspects of case taking and analysis, different views of miasms, long-term and difficult case management, repertory work and interpretation of symptoms, family groupings of remedies, therapeutics, and practical issues in practice. Those who meet the requirements will receive a Diploma of Classical Homeopathy (D.C.H.) at the end of the fourth year.

Year Four is a support year featuring students' live and paper cases and providing opportunities to discuss issues that arise in practice, including case management.

Classes meet in Vancouver on 11 weekends per year for the first three years, and on six weekends in Year Four.

Admission Requirements

Applicants for the first year must be at least 21 years of age, have a high school diploma, be fluent in written and spoken English, and have a strong desire to study homeopathy. Students entering the second year must have taken or must take concurrently a college-level course in anatomy and physiology. Students entering the third year must have taken a First Aid and CPR course.

Tuition and Fees

Tuition for Year One, Two and Three is $2,800 per year (including GST); books are additional. Tuition for Year Four is $1,200.

Financial Assistance

Payment plans are available.

Yasodhara Ashram

Box 9
Kootenay Bay, British Columbia V0B 1X0
Canada
PHONE: (250) 227-9224 / (800) 661-8711
FAX: (250) 227-9494
E-MAIL: yashram@netidea.com
WEBSITE: www.yasodhara.org

The Yasodhara Ashram was founded in 1963 by Swami Sivananda Radha, an authority on Kundalini yoga and Eastern yoga psychology. Swami Radha has written many books on yoga and spiritual life and has established a number of Radha Centres that offer workshops and ongoing classes. There are six to ten instructors, with six to twenty students per class.

Accreditation and Approvals

Yasodhara Ashram is registered with the Private Postsecondary Education Commission of British Columbia.

Program Description

The ashram offers a wide range of options for training, upgrading, or certification in Kundalini yoga, dreams, Hidden Language of Hatha Yoga, and hatha. The Yoga Development course is a prerequisite for all teacher training. Classes include the week-long Hatha Training for Teachers and the two-week Hidden Language of Hatha Yoga Teacher Certification.

The Yoga Development Course (YDC) is an intensive three-month program in all aspects of yoga and self-development. The courses in this program are dedicated to the investigation of mind and consciousness through Kundalini yoga, prayer dance, hatha yoga, mantra yoga, satsang, dream work, and growth workshops.

A variety of other courses are offered throughout the year, including a week-long immersion in the Kundalini system, the 10 Days of Yoga, Karma yoga work opportunities, mantra, music and consciousness, and a program for youth and teens. Retreats are offered year-round.

Continuing Education

Annual refresher courses are offered to those who have completed certification programs.

Tuition and Fees

Tuition for the Yoga Development course is $6,000; for the Hatha Training for Teachers, $690; and for the two-week Hidden Language of Hatha Yoga, $940. These costs include three meals per day and shared accommodations; private rooms are available at additional cost. A children's program of activities, including swimming, crafts, hiking, music, and yoga costs $20 per day. The Youth Program is free, by application.

Financial Assistance

Limited scholarships are sometimes available.

ONTARIO

Aromaflex Centre of Healing Arts

511-2055 Carling Avenue
Ottawa, Ontario K2A 1G6
Canada
PHONE: (613) 725-9226
FAX: (613) 725-3402
E-MAIL: aromaflx@home.com
WEBSITE: www.comsearch-can.com/aromaflx.htm

The Aromaflex Centre of Healing Arts was founded in 1990 by Patricia Hall, the primary instructor. There is a maximum of six students per class. A correspondence program is also offered; see page 466.

Accreditation and Approvals

Graduates of the Standard and Advanced Level Aromatherapy programs are eligible to apply for Certified Aromatherapy Health Therapist or Registered Aromatherapy Health Practitioner designations from the Canadian Examining Board of Health Care Practitioners.

Program Description

The 215-hour, five-month Standard Level Aromatherapy Program is a certification course in Aromatherapy Lymphatic Drainage Massage with in-depth usage of essential oils. Courses include Introduction to Essential Oils; Essential Oil Chemistry; Essential Oil Workshops: Top, Middle and Base Notes; Carrier Oil Workshop; Designing and Prioritizing Treatments; Hands-On Aromatherapy Massage; Reflexology Assessment; Anatomy and Physiology; The Business of Aromatherapy; Aromatherapy Applications; Business Internship; 30 Case Studies; Thesis Project; and Exams.

The 174-hour, five-month Advanced Aromatherapy Program is an in-depth study and practice of aromatherapy massage, using various forms of bodywork including Swedish Massage, Advanced Lymphatic Drainage, and Problematic Aroma Solutions. The program includes a Thesis Project, Class Lectures, Spa Weekend, Case Studies, Business Orientation, Theory Exam, and Practical Exam.

The 170-hour, four-month Wholistic Reflexology Program covers Reflexology Through the Ages, Basic Anatomy and Physiology as it Pertains to the Feet and Hands, Pain Management Techniques, Diseases of the Feet and Nails, Emotions and the Feet, Assessment Procedure Techniques, Foot Care: Exercises and Infusions, How to Locate and Balance the Chakras, Wholistic Foot Reflexology, Introduction to Hand Reflexology, Body Energy Release, and more. The program consists of twelve in-class practical lessons, Anatomy and Physiology, Case Studies, The Business of Reflexology, Thesis Project, and Exams (Theory and Practical).

Community and Continuing Education

One-day and weekend workshops are offered in such topics as Introduction to Essential Oils, Back Massage for Family and Friends, Introduction to Reflexology, Le Petit Spa, and others.

Admission Requirements

Applicants must be at least 18 years of age (or have written permission from their parent or guardian) and have a high school diploma or equivalent.

Tuition and Fees

Tuition for Standard Level Aromatherapy is $1,850. Tuition for Advanced Aromatherapy is $1,850. Additional expenses for these programs include a portable massage table and accessories, $725; essential and carrier oils and supplies, $85 to $400; and charts, $28.

Tuition for Wholistic Reflexology is $450.

Canadian College of Massage and Hydrotherapy/West Coast College of Massage Therapy

(See Multiple State Locations, pages 420–21)

The Canadian College of Naturopathic Medicine

1255 Sheppard Avenue East
North York, Ontario M2K 1E2
Canada
PHONE: (416) 498-1255

FAX: (416) 498-1576

E-MAIL: info@ccnm.edu

WEBSITE: www.ccnm.edu

The Canadian College of Naturopathic Medicine (CCNM), founded in 1978 as the Ontario College of Naturopathic Medicine, is the only recognized college of naturopathic medicine in Canada. There are approximately forty-five instructors, with a maximum of 120 students per class.

Accreditation and Approvals

CCNM is a candidate for accreditation with the Council on Naturopathic Medical Education (CNME). The college is recognized by the four Canadian provinces that license naturopathic physicians (British Columbia, Manitoba, Ontario, and Saskatchewan). Students who plan to practice in the United States should contact their states' naturopathic licensing boards for more information.

Program Description

CCNM offers a four-year, full-time professional program in naturopathic medicine leading to the Doctor of Naturopathic Medicine (N.D.) diploma. The major areas of study are basic medical sciences and clinical and naturopathic disciplines.

First-year courses include Anatomy; Histology; Physiology; Biochemistry; Naturopathic Medical History, Philosophy, and Principles; Soft Tissue Manipulation; Public Health; Homeopathy; Immunology; Introduction to Pathology; Nutritional Biochemistry; Counseling; Hydrotherapy; and Introduction to Oriental Medicine.

Second-year courses include Pathology, Differential Diagnosis, Laboratory Diagnosis, Homeopathic Medicine, Acupuncture and Oriental Medicine, Clinical Nutrition, Botanical Medicine, Radiology, Microbiology, Pharmacology, Naturopathic Manipulation, and Clinic.

Third-year courses include Orthopedics, Acupuncture and Oriental Medicine, Homeopathic Medicine, Botanical Medicine and Pharmacognosy, Counseling Skills, Clinical Nutrition, Naturopathic Manipulation, Women's Health Issues, Diagnostic Imaging, Counseling, Obstetrics, Pediatrics, and Clinic.

Fourth-year courses include Case Studies in Naturopathic Medicine, Skills of Communication, Study of Treatments, Practice Management, Jurisprudence/Ethics, Minor Surgery, and Clinic.

Admission Requirements

Prerequisites for admission to the program include three years of full-time university studies at an accredited institution (a Bachelor of Science degree is recommended); required courses include general biology, general chemistry, organic chemistry, biochemistry, and general psychology, all completed with a grade of C or better. Additional requirements include official transcripts, two letters of reference, a personal statement, and an interview with the admissions team.

Potential applicants may attend orientation evenings and/or the Student for a Day program.

Tuition and Fees

Tuition for the regular full-time program is $13,500 per year.

Financial Assistance

Students may be eligible for the Canada Student Loan Program (CSL) or the Ontario Student Loan Program (OSL), or may be eligible for U.S. financial aid. A limited number of bursaries are available at the College.

Canadian Holistic Therapist Training School/ Mississauga School of Aromatherapy

(See Multiple State Locations, pages 421–22)

Canadian Memorial Chiropractic College

1931 Bayview Avenue

Toronto, Ontario M4G 3E6

Canada

PHONE: (416) 482-2340

FAX: (416) 482-9745

WEBSITE: www.cmcc.ca

The Canadian Memorial Chiropractic College (CMCC) was founded in 1945 and is Canada's largest chiropractic college. Approximately 80 percent of the chiropractors in Canada are graduates of CMCC. There are fifty-nine full-time and forty-seven part-time faculty members, with an undergraduate enrollment of approximately 620 full-time students distributed almost equally among the four years of study.

Accreditation

CMCC is accredited by the Council on Chiropractic Education of Canada (CCEC). Through a reciprocal agreement among CCEC, CCE (U.S.A.), the Australian Council of Chiropractic Education, and the European Council on Chiropractic Education, this status is recognized in the United States, Australasia, and Europe, and allows CMCC graduates to apply for licensure in most countries around the world.

Program Description

The 4,500-hour Undergraduate Professional Program consists of three nine-month periods and one twelve-month period over four years. The curriculum is distributed among four divisions: Biological Sciences (Anatomy, Physiology, Biochemistry, Pathology, and Microbiology); Chiropractic/Clinical Sciences (Applied Chiropractic Studies, Chiropractic Principles and Practice, Clinical Diagnosis, and Radiology); Clinical Education, on campus at the Herbert K. Lee Walk-In Clinic and in six other community clinics; and Research (Applied Research, Biometrics, and Investigative Projects).

Community and Continuing Education

A postgraduate residency program is offered in three areas of special study: clinical sciences, radiology, and sports sciences. Upon completion, students are eligible to take examinations leading to certification as a Fellow of the College of Chiropractic Sciences (Canada), Fellow of the College of Chiropractic Radiology (Canada), or Fellow of the College of Sports Sciences (Canada).

Both on- and off-campus programs are offered for continuing education credit for licensure. These weekend programs include current basic and clinical research, technique updates, philosophy, principles, and practice management issues. In addition, Continuing Education programs are offered to field practitioners, chiropractic support staff, and the general public.

Admission Requirements

Applicants to the Undergraduate Professional Program must have completed at least three years of study (ninety credit hours) in any discipline at a Canadian university or its equivalent. It is strongly recommended that applicants have completed courses in organic chemistry, biology, psychology, humanities, and/or social sciences. Applicants will also be interviewed by an admissions team and must submit two essays, three references, and an autobiographical sketch.

Tuition and Fees

Tuition is $11,816 per year; tuition for international students is $14,636 per year. Additional expenses include Student Activity fee, $125 per year; Student Canadian Chiropractic Association fee, $20 per year; books, approximately $1,050 per year; spinal column model, approximately $210; and diagnostic equipment, approximately $450.

Financial Assistance

Canada Student Loan Program, provincial student loans, and private scholarships are available.

Canadian School of Natural Nutrition

10720 Yonge Street, Suite 220
Richmond Hill, Ontario L4C 3C9
Canada
PHONE: (905) 737-0284 / (800) 569-9938
FAX: (905) 737-7830
E-MAIL: info@csnn.ca
WEBSITE: www.csnn.ca

CORRESPONDENCE COURSE DIVISION:
PHONE: (905) 852-9660 / (800) 328-0743 / (888) 837-0337 (en français)
FAX: (905) 852-4616

The Canadian School of Natural Nutrition (CSNN) was founded by Danielle Miscampbell, RNC, in 1995. Classes are held at Richmond Hill, Toronto, Scarborough, Mississauga, Halifax and Vancouver. There are thirty instructors; classes are limited to fifteen students. A correspondence program is also offered; see page 491.

Accreditation and Approvals

The Diploma in Natural Nutrition is approved by the Nutritional Consultants Organization of Canada (NCOC). Graduates with a cumulative average of 80 percent or higher are asked to submit an application to NCOC; no further exams are necessary. Upon acceptance of the application by the NCOC, graduates are given the RNC designation.

Program Description

The Diploma Course in Natural Nutrition consists of 234 hours of classroom instruction, 250 hours of clinical studies (including fifteen client assessments), and 100 hours of in-class practicum. The program may be completed in one year of day classes or two years of evening classes. Courses include Fundamentals of Nutrition, Anatomy and Physiology, Nutritional Symptomatology, Preventive Nutrition, Body-Mind-Spirit, The Connection, Chemistry and Biochemistry, Cellular Biology, Pathology and Nutrition, Lifecycle Nutrition, Ecology and Nutrition, Allergies, Alternative/Comparative Diets, Nutritional Literature Research, and Fundamentals of Business. Graduates are granted the designation Registered Holistic Nutritionist (RHN) and qualify for the designation Registered Nutritional Consultant (RNC).

Continuing Education

A 116-hour program in Bio-Energy Feedback Screening is offered to graduates of the Nutrition Program and other interested professionals. The program leads to the designation Certified Bio-Energy Technician and consists of courses in Health Kinesiology, Electrodermal Screening, and a practicum component.

Admission Requirements

A high school diploma or mature student status for those 19 years of age or over is required.

Tuition and Fees

Tuition for the Natural Nutrition program is $4,355. Tuition for the Bio-Energy Feedback Screening program is $2,000. Books are additional.

Financial Assistance

Flexible payment plans within the study periods are available.

Centennial College

P.O. Box 631
Station A
Scarborough, Ontario M1K 5E9
Canada
PHONE: (416) 289-5000
FAX: (416) 694-1503
E-MAIL: success@Lmail.cencol.on.ca
WEBSITE: www.cenco1.on.ca

Centennial College was founded in 1966 and offers certificate, diploma, post-diploma certificate, and apprenticeship programs in a variety of fields. There are ten full-time and numerous part-time instructors in the Massage Therapy, Complementary Care, and Wellness and Lifestyle Management Programs; the average practice class size is twenty students. There are four campuses in Scarborough.

Accreditation and Approvals

Graduates of the Massage Therapy Program are eligible to write the registration exams administered by the College of Massage Therapists of Ontario. Graduates of the Shiatsu Therapy Program may become members of the Shiatsu Therapy Association of Ontario. The Complementary Care Program is an approved and funded program of the Ontario Ministry of Education.

Program Description

Programs offered relating to the field of alternative health care include Massage Therapy, Shiatsu Therapy, and Complementary Care.

The Massage Therapy diploma program may be completed in six semesters (three years). First-year courses include Massage Theory and Practice, Body-Mind-Spirit Connection, The Therapeutic Relationship, Stress Management and Self-Care, Practicing College English Skills/Reading and Writing Prose, Introduction to Complementary Therapies, Introduction to Hydrotherapy, Clinical Anatomy, Physiology, Business Skills for the Health Care Entrepreneur, and Reading and Writing Prose/Approaches to Literature. Second-year courses include Massage Theory and Practice, Clinic, Clinical Anatomy, Remedial Exercise and Kinesiology, Nutrition, Outreach, Pathophysiology, Neuroanatomy and Physiology, and two General Education electives. Third-year courses include Outreach, Massage Theory and Practice, Pathophysiology, The Therapeutic Relationship, Trends and Issues in Massage Therapy, Clinic, Creating an Independent Practice, and two General Education electives.

The Shiatsu Therapy diploma program may be completed in six semesters (three years). First-year courses include Shiatsu Theory and Practice, Introduction to Complementary Care, Holistic View of Health, Clinical Anatomy, Stress Management and Self-Care, Practicing English Skills/Reading and Writing Prose, Traditional Chinese Medical Theory, Physiology, and Reading and Writing Prose/Approaches to Literature. Second-year courses include Shiatsu Theory and Practice, Neuro-Anatomy and Physiology, Chinese Medical Theory, Client/Therapist Relationship, Clinic, Pathophysiology, Outreach, Business Skills for the Health Care Entrepreneur, Kinesiology, and an General Education elective. Third-year courses include Shiatsu Theory and Practice, Pathophysiology, Client/ Therapist Relationship, Trends and Issues in Shiatsu Therapy, Clinic, Nutrition, Pathophysiology, Creating an Independent Practice, Outreach, Auxiliary Modalities, and a General Education elective.

The one-year Complementary Care post-diploma certificate program is designed for those who wish to establish a private practice or want to augment their current health care practice to offer greater client choice. Courses include Body-Mind-Spirit Connection, Introduction to Complementary Therapies, Business Skills for the Health Care Entrepreneur, Ethical and Professional Relationships, Stress Management and Self-Care, Therapy Theory and Practice, Complementary Therapies, Creating and Independent Practice, Stress Management and Client Care, Natural Nutrition, and Complementary Care Field Placement. After completing the Field Placement, students may be certified in Aromatherapy or Reflexology, study Therapeutic Touch, or receive additional training in other therapies.

Only Canadian students may be classified as part-time students; international students must enroll as full-time students.

Admission Requirements

Massage Therapy and Shiatsu Therapy applicants must have an Ontario Secondary School Diploma or equivalent or be age 19 or older; have satisfactory grades (70 percent general level, 60 percent advanced level) in two senior-level sciences (biology, chemistry, or physics) and grade 12 English; have satisfactory results in a communications, mathematics, and science skills assessment; submit a statement of health from a medical doctor; have CPR/First Aid certification; and attend an information session.

Complementary Care applicants must have a university degree, college diploma, or relevant work experience; submit a statement of health from a medical doctor; have CPR/First Aid certification prior to entering Semester 2; submit references, a résumé, and a completed questionnaire; and attend an application review and information session.

Tuition and Fees

Tuition is $1,620 per year for Canadian students, $9,575 per year for international students. Additional expenses for all students include a student activity fee, $184; program incidentals fee, $70 (varies by program); student services fee, $50; and technology/copyright fee, $85.

Financial Assistance

Scholarships, grants, loans, work-study, and payment plans are available.

D'Arcy Lane Institute School of Massage Therapy

627 Maitland Street
London, Ontario N5Y 2V7
Canada
PHONE: (519) 673-4420
FAX: (519) 673-0645
E-MAIL: darcyinc@serix.com
WEBSITE: www.serix.com/~darcyinc/

The D'Arcy Lane Institute was founded in 1986. The D'AL School of Equine Massage Therapy was introduced in January 1997. There are twenty-two instructors, with a maximum of forty-five students per class.

Accreditation and Approvals

D'Arcy Lane is registered and approved as a Private Vocational School with the Ministry of Education and Training in Ontario.

The Massage Therapy Program is approved by the College of Massage Therapists of Ontario. The Equine Massage Therapy Program is approved by the International Federation of Registered Equine Massage Therapists.

Program Description

The 2,200-hour Massage Therapy Program may be completed in eighteen or twenty-two months and consists of courses in Human Relations, Professionalism and Ethics, Anatomy, Physiology, Pathology, Massage Theory and Techniques, Massage Treatments and Assessments, Hydrotherapy, Nutrition and Public Health, Kinesiology and Remedial Exercises, Business Management, Clinical Problem Solving, Student Clinic, and Outreach.

The 2,200-hour program in Equine Massage Therapy is a full-time, comprehensive program consisting of courses in Terminology, Human Relations, Professionalism and Ethics, Anatomy, Physiology, Pathology, Massage Theory and Techniques, Massage Treatments, Hydrotherapy, Kinesiology (Conformation and Movement), Business Management, Equine Behavior, Equine Management, and Externship.

Classes for both programs meet three days per week.

A one-day Introduction to Massage Therapy Class, offered to prospective students and a prerequisite for the 2,200-hour program, includes Basic Anatomy, Swedish Massage Techniques, Effects and Uses of Massage, Relaxation Techniques, Sport Techniques, and a massage given by a therapy student.

A one-day Introduction to Equine Massage Therapy Class, offered to prospective students and a prerequisite for the 2,200-hour program, covers Equine Massage Therapy, Basic Anatomy, and Effects and Uses of Massage.

Admission Requirements

Applicants are expected to have a high school diploma or to write an entrance exam; to be a Canadian citizen, landed immigrant, or have a student visa; to speak, write, and understand English; to have completed the eight-hour Introduction to Massage Therapy/Equine Massage Therapy Course; to have a doctor's medical certificate and three character references from professional sources; to have current CPR and First Aid certificates; and to submit a personal letter and photos.

Tuition and Fees

Tuition for either program is $14,000. In addition, the mandatory material package (which includes books, linens, liability insurance, uniforms, and more) for the Human Program is $2,477; for the Equine Program, $2,413.

The Introduction to Massage Therapy Course is $60. The Introduction to Equine Massage Therapy Course is $70.

Financial Assistance

Student loans are available to qualified students.

Homeopathic College of Canada

280 Eglinton Avenue East
Toronto, Ontario M4P 1L4
Canada
PHONE: (416) 481-8816
FAX: (416) 481-4444
E-MAIL: info@homeopath.org
WEBSITE: www.homeopathy.edu

The Homeopathic College of Canada (HCC) was founded in 1995; in 1996, HCC and Humber College (one of Canada's largest community colleges, founded in 1966) formed a partnership to develop a full-time homeopathy program. In 1999, HCC entered into a leasing agreement with the University of Toronto to hold classes at the downtown campus. There are twenty-five instructors, with a maximum of fifty students per class.

Accreditation and Approvals

HCC is accredited by the Manitoba Homeopathic Association, the Ontario Homeopathic Association, and the Pacific Homeopathic Association of British Columbia. Canadian college and university credits are given for some courses.

Graduates of the 3,045-hour Homeopathic Program receive a Diploma in Homeopathic Medicine and Science (DHMS) and are eligible to take either the OHA or PHABC Board Qualifying Examination in order to register as a Homeopathic Doctor. Graduates should ascertain whether the title Homeopathic Doctor (H.D.) is permitted by the government in the jurisdiction of their practice.

Program Description

The 3,045-hour Homeopathic Medicine and Science Program is a four-year, full-time program that includes an intensive clinical internship, a research project on environmental health, and a thesis on homeopathy. The curriculum includes Anatomy and Physiology, Biochemistry, Botany, Clinical Externship, Community Health, Complementary Modalities, Differential Diagnosis, Emergency Medicine, Environmental Medicine, Ethics and Law, Homeopathy, Homeopathic Therapeutics, Lab Analysis, Nutrition, Pathology, Pharmacology, Physical Examination, Practice Management, Psychology, Stress Management, and Toxicology.

The Homeopathic Medicine and Science Program for Physicians and Health Care Practitioners is open to doctors and consists of 662 hours of homeopathic instruction, plus 506 hours of clinical internship. The classroom course may be completed in two academic years or twenty months. Courses include Botany, Clinical Externship, Complementary Modalities, Environmental Medicine, Ethics and Law, Homeopathy, Homeopathic Therapeutics, Lab Analysis, Nutrition, Pharmacology, Practice Management, Psychology, and Stress Management.

Classes are held evenings and weekends. The teaching clinic runs throughout the year on weekdays at both the Etobicoke and Toronto locations. Under special circumstances, students may apply for a partial load.

The First Aid/Acute Correspondence certificate is a home study course open to pharmacists, pharmacist's assistants, and others. The program consists of twenty-four lessons to be completed within twelve months, and is not intended to produce homeopathic practitioners. The course includes Introduction and History, Principles, Symptomatology, Repertories, Case Taking, Classical and Contemporary Materia Medica, Homeopathic First Aid for Children, Allergic Reactions, Sprains and Fractures, Preparing for Surgery and Dental Operations, Spinal Injuries, Homeopathy for Pets, and more. It is the student's responsibility to find HCC-approved proctors to supervise examinations.

Admission Requirements

All applicants must submit a résumé, a handwritten letter, and two letters of reference.

Applicants to the Homeopathic Medicine and Science Program must have, at minimum, an Ontario secondary school diploma including Ontario academic credits in English, math, biology, and chemistry, BC Dogwood Diploma or equivalent, plus two years of study at the college/university level; a bachelor's degree is recommended. Those who do not meet these requirements may apply as a special applicant; contact the registrar for further information.

Applicants to the Homeopathic Doctorate program for physicians and health care practitioners must hold an N.D., M.D., D.C., D.O., D.D.S., D.V.M., or Ph.D. degree.

Tuition and Fees

Tuition for the Homeopathic Medicine and Science program is $3,000 per semester. Tuition for the Homeopathic Medicine and Science Program for Health Care Practitioners is $10,000. Tuition for the First Aid/Acute Correspondence certificate program is $950. Other costs include application fee, $50; Ontario Homeopathic Association membership, $50 per year; graduation fee, $35; Homeopathic Board Examination, $1,100; and malpractice insurance, $100. Books and diagnostic equipment are additional.

Financial Assistance

Payment plans and a prepayment discount are available.

ICT Kikkawa College

1678 Bloor Street West
Toronto, Ontario M6P 1A9
PHONE: (416) 762-4857
FAX: (416) 762-5733
E-MAIL: kcadmissions@ictschools.com
WEBSITE: www.ictschools.com

ICT Northumberland College

1660 Hollis Street
Halifax, Nova Scotia
PHONE: (902) 425-2869
FAX: (902) 762-5733
E-MAIL: ncadmissions@ictschools.com
WEBSITE: www.ictschools.com

Founded in 1981, International Complementary Therapy (ICT) owns and operates two schools in two Canadian provinces.

There is a maximum of twenty-five students in practical classes; students work in pairs with one to twelve students per instructor.

Accreditation and Approvals

The massage therapy programs at both ICT schools are accredited by the Commission on Massage Training Accreditation (COMTA).

Program Description

The 2,200-hour program in Massage Therapy may be taken over eighty-two or seventy-three weeks. First-year courses include Anatomy, Clinical Assessment and Treatment Skills, Massage and Hydrotherapy Techniques, Pathophysiology, and Teaching Clinic. Second-year courses include Advanced Techniques, Clinical Assessment and Treatment Skills, Clinical Skills Laboratory, Field Placement Practicum, Pathophysiology, and Practice Management.

Prior to entrance into the program, the schools offer a preparatory forty-hour course to help ensure student success. The Preadmission Course: Study for Success focuses on science and study skills.

Community and Continuing Education

An Introduction to Massage Therapy as a Career Workshop is offered to the public on a regular basis.

Admission Requirements

Applicants must have a secondary school diploma (grade 12) or equivalent. Applicants who do not meet this requirement but who are age 19 or older may apply as a mature student and will be required to successfully complete a Mature Student Admission Test. Most applicants are required to take the school's Preadmission Course, although candidates with university degrees are generally exempted from this requirement.

Tuition and Fees

Tuition for the full program is $14,200 ($7,100 per academic year); tuition for the Preadmission Course is $260. (Students who have successfully completed the Preadmission Course and Year One of the Massage Therapy program will have a $200 credit applied against their tuition balance upon registering for Year Two.) Additional expenses include a $60 application fee; books, materials, uniforms, linen, and supplies are approximately $1,800 over the two years of study.

Financial Assistance

A Scholarship Program, Bursary Program, payment plan, and provincial assistance under the Ontario Student Assistance Program and the Nova Scotia Student Assistance Program are available.

The Institute of Aromatherapy

2206 Queen Street East
Toronto, Ontario M4E 1E7
Canada
PHONE: (416) 698-5850 / (888) 578-7815
FAX: (416) 698-8684
E-MAIL: aromashp@rogers.wave.ca
WEBSITE: www.aromashoppe.com

The Institute of Aromatherapy, founded in 1986 by Jan Benham, is the oldest school of aromatherapy in Canada. There are six instructors; classes are limited to eight students.

Accreditation and Approvals

Diplomas issued by the Institute of Aromatherapy for the Career Courses and the Certification Courses are recognized by the Federal Ministry of Human Resources, Government of Canada, by the Canadian Examining Board of Health Care Practitioners, and by many associations of professional aromatherapists.

Program Description

The Institute of Aromatherapy offers several Certification Courses which may be taken individually or combined with other courses into comprehensive Career Courses resulting in designations.

The Registered Aromatherapy Health Practitioner (RAHP) Designation Program is a part-time program consisting of two three-month semesters. This course of study includes the Standard Aromatherapy, Advanced Aromatherapy, and Anatomy and Physiology certification courses, plus Essential Oil Seminar, Reflexology Seminar, Creamy Craft of Cosmetic Making,

Business Orientation (Practical), St. John's Ambulance, and Spa Weekend. Two thesis projects and sixty case studies are also required.

The Holistic Health Practitioner designation program is a part-time program consisting of one nine-month school year with three trimesters. This course of study includes the Standard Aromatherapy, Reflexology, Advanced Aromatherapy, and Anatomy and Physiology certification courses, plus Essential Oil Seminar, Creamy Craft of Cosmetic Making, Soap Making, Reflexology Seminar, St. John's Ambulance, Business Orientation (Practical), and Spa Weekend. Three thesis projects and ninety case studies are also required.

The Certified Natural Health Practitioner (CNHP) designation program is a full-time program consisting of one nine-month school year with three trimesters. This course of study includes the Standard Aromatherapy, Reflexology, Advanced Aromatherapy, Aroma Cosmetology, Advanced Bodywork, Anatomy and Physiology, Nutrition, and Thai Massage certification courses, plus Tai Chi, Meditation, Guest Speaker Seminar, Creamy Craft of Cosmetic Making, Soap Making, Essential Oil Seminar, Reflexology Seminar, Aromatherapy Hand and Foot Treatments, Business Orientation (Practical), St. John's Ambulance, School Clinic, Supervised Community Care, and Spa Weekend; students also choose three courses from Hypnosis for Healing, Nutritional Herbs, Dance of the Goddess and the Warrior, Reiki I, Therapeutic Touch, and Herbs with Jan. Five thesis projects and 135 case studies are also required.

The Certified Reflexology Health Practitioner (CRHP) designation program is a part-time program consisting of one three-month semester. This course of study includes the Reflexology and the Anatomy and Physiology certification courses, plus Essential Oil Seminar, Reflexology Seminar, St. John's Ambulance (recommended), and Business Orientation (Theory and Practical). One thesis project and thirty case studies are also required.

Community and Continuing Education

Certification courses in Standard Aromatherapy (175 hours), Advanced Aromatherapy (176 hours), Aroma Cosmetology (159 hours), Reflexology and Foot Care (144 hours), Anatomy and Physiology (forty-three hours), Basic Nutrition (twenty hours), and Thai Massage (thirty-two hours) may be taken individually, outside of the longer designation programs above.

Special interest courses, many five to ten hours in length, may also be taken individually and are open to the public. These include Therapeutic Touch, Reiki I, St. John's Ambulance, Essential Oil Seminar, Reflexology Seminar, The Creamy Craft of Cosmetic Making, Aromatherapy Spa Weekend, Nutritional Herbs, Hypnosis for Healing, Basic Herbology, The Art of Soap Making, Tai Chi, Meditation, and Dance of the Goddess and the Warrior.

Admission Requirements

Applicants must have a high school diploma.

Tuition and Fees

Tuition for the Registered Aromatherapy Health Practitioner (RAHP) designation program is $3,495. Tuition and course materials for the Holistic Health Practitioner designation program total approximately $4,500. Tuition for the Certified Natural Health Practitioner (CNHP) designation program is $6,950. Additional estimated costs for each of these three programs are $785 for a portable massage table and accessories, $50 to $200 for essential and carrier oils, and $14 to $22 for books.

Tuition and course materials for the Certified Reflexology Health Practitioner (CRHP) designation program is $1,050.

Tuition for the individual certification courses is as follows: Standard Aromatherapy, $1,600; Advanced Aromatherapy, $1,600; Aroma Cosmetology, $1,850; Reflexology and Foot Care, $1,050; Anatomy and Physiology, $600; Basic Nutrition, $495; and Thai Massage, $750.

Tuition for special interest courses ranges from $95 to $295.

Financial Assistance

Payment plans are available.

The Michener Institute for Applied Health Sciences

222 St. Patrick Street
Toronto, Ontario M5T 1V4
Canada
PHONE: (416) 596-3177 / (800) 387-9066
FAX: (416) 596-3168
E-MAIL: info@michener.on.ca
WEBSITE: www.michener.on.ca

The Michener Institute was founded in 1958 for the training of medical laboratory technologists based at Toronto General Hospital, and moved into its current location in 1972. Over 80,000 students have graduated from forty-three full- and part-time programs. In addition to the programs described below, diploma and post-diploma programs are offered in such areas as Nuclear Medicine Technology, Radiography, Respiratory Therapy, Genetics Technology, Ultrasound, and many others. The Acupuncture Program was established in 1997. Distance learning courses are offered in various fields of complementary health; see page 462. There are eight instructors, with an average of twenty students per class.

Accreditation and Approvals
The Michener Institute is accredited by the Canadian Medical Association.

Program Description
A four-year, 140-week diploma program is offered in Acupuncture. Year One courses include The Foundations of Traditional Chinese Medicine (TCM), Special Topics on TCM, The Human Body, Applied Microbiology, Computer Literacy, Qi Gong and Tai Ji Quan Exercise, Acupuncture and Moxibustion, Anatomy and Neuroanatomy for Acupuncturists, The Diagnostics of TCM, Health Preservation and Rehabilitation in TCM, and Clinical Practicum. Year Two courses include Acupuncture and Moxibustion, Physiology and Research Methods for Acupuncturists, Special Topics on TCM, Chinese Herbal Medicine, Clinical Acupuncture, Pathophysiology, and Clinical Practicum. Topics covered in Year Three include Clinical Acupuncture, Special Topics on TCM, Tui Na (Traditional Chinese Therapeutic Massage), Pharmacology, Clinical Features of Disease (Western Medicine), Counseling for Acupuncturists, and Clinical Practicum. Year Four consists of Clinical Acupuncture, Professional Issues, and Clinical Practicum. The program provides opportunities to study elsewhere for a portion of the final year (Beijing, Tianjin, Melbourne, San Francisco).

Community and Continuing Education
Courses offered as part of the pending Herbal Medicine certificate programs may be taken as continuing education; however, students must meet eligibility requirements for the programs.

Admission Requirements
Acupuncture applicants must have completed at least two years postsecondary education with a minimum of 60 percent in each course. Academically qualified applicants will be asked to visit a clinical site, may be interviewed and/or write an admission/aptitude test, and may be given a test of English proficiency.

Tuition and Fees
Tuition for the Acupuncture Program is $8,500 per year; books are approximately $400. Equipment deposits, lab coats, uniforms, and professional society fees are additional.

Financial Assistance
Scholarships, bursaries, Canada Student Loans, and Ontario Student Loans are available.

Reaching Your Potential

11181 Yonge Street, Room 141
Richmond Hill, Ontario L4S 1L2
Canada
PHONE: (905) 474-1848
FAX: (905) 944-8869
E-MAIL: wharris@reachingyourpotential.com

Reaching Your Potential was founded in 1996; founder Sherry Smith has been involved with holistic healing since 1979. Ms. Smith is the past president of the Ontario Polarity Therapy Association. There are five instructors, with five to twenty students per class.

Accreditation and Approvals
Trainings are approved by the American Polarity Therapy Association (APTA).

Program Description
Introduction to Polarity Therapy is a one-weekend workshop designed for those who are interested in polarity therapy either as a potential career or on a recreational level. It is a prerequisite for those who plan to continue with the Level 1 training. Topics include Basic Polarity Theory; the General Session; Balancing the Five Elements and Seven Chakras; Basic Polarity Ex-

ercise; Food, Energy, and Polarity; and Attitude, Energy, and Polarity.

The Level 1 Polarity Therapy certification training consists of 125 classroom hours; graduates are qualified to apply for Associate Polarity Practitioner (A.P.P.) registration with APTA. Topics include General, Functional, and Structural Contacts (fifty hours); Theory (thirty hours); Assessments (five hours); Polarity Exercise (five hours); Diet (five hours); Attitude (five hours); Managing Your Practice (five hours); and Clinical Feedback (twenty hours). For registration as an A.P.P., five personal polarity sessions are required.

The Level 2 Polarity Therapy certification training consists of 360 classroom hours; graduates are qualified to apply for Registered Polarity Practitioner (R.P.P.) registration with APTA. Topics include General, Functional, and Structural Contacts (100 hours); Theory (seventy hours); Assessments (twenty hours); Polarity Exercise (twenty hours); Diet (twenty hours); Attitude (forty-five hours); Managing Your Practice (thirty-five hours); and Clinical Feedback (fifty hours). For registration as an R.P.P., ten personal polarity sessions are required.

Admission Requirements

There are no formal admission requirements, only a willingness to learn. Introduction to Polarity Therapy is the prerequisite for Level 1. Level 1 is the prerequisite for Level 2.

Tuition and Fees

Tuition for the Introduction to Polarity Therapy course is $200.

Tuition for the Level 1 training is $1,800; this includes the Introduction to Polarity Therapy workshop. Books cost $150, and personal polarity sessions are additional. Tuition for the Level 2 Training is $4,400; books and personal polarity sessions are additional.

Financial Assistance

Extended payment plans are available.

Sault College of Applied Arts and Technology

P.O. Box 60
443 Northern Avenue
Sault Ste. Marie, Ontario P6A 5L3

PHONE: (705) 759-6700 / (705) 759-6774 / (800) 461-2260
FAX: (705) 759-3273 / (705) 759-1319
WEBSITE: www.saultc.on.ca

Sault College of Applied Arts and Technology, established in 1965, offers more than fifty one-, two-, and three-year diploma and certificate programs in such areas Applied Sciences, Aviation, Business, Engineering, Health Sciences, and other areas. The college enrolls about 2,700 full-time students. The Massage Therapy Program at Sault College was started in 1996, and enrolls fifty to sixty students per year.

Program Description

The three-year, six-semester Massage Therapy Program includes courses in Anatomy and Physiology, Communications Skills, Personal Wellness, Professional Human Relations, Computers in Health Care, Massage Theory, Massage Lab, Professional Growth, Nutrition, Introduction to Psychology, Massage Practice, Pathophysiology, and Entrepreneurship.

Admission Requirements

Applicants must have an Ontario Secondary School Diploma or equivalent including grade 12 technical math, English, senior-level biology, and one other senior science with 70 percent at the general level or 60 percent at the advanced level for the four course requirements. Applicants who are 19 years of age or over and who lack the academic entrance requirements may be considered for entrance as mature students; each application will be considered on an individual basis.

Students must have current CPR (Level C) and First Aid Certificates.

Tuition and Fees

Tuition and fees for full-time students are $1,785 per year. Books, professional supplies, and additional fees for the first and second semester are $1,200–$1,800 (estimated); for the third and fourth semester, $1,200–$1,800 (estimated); and for the fifth and sixth semester, to be established. There are extra fees for registration exams in Toronto and for registration with the College of Massage Therapists of Ontario.

Financial Assistance

The Ontario Student Assistance Program, scholarships, bursaries and awards, the Emergency Loan Fund, other student loans, and work-study programs are available to those who qualify.

Shiatsu Academy of Tokyo

320 Danforth Avenue, Suite 206
Toronto, Ontario M4K 1N8
Canada
PHONE: (416) 466-8780
FAX: (416) 466-8719
E-MAIL: sait131@attglobal.net
WEBSITE: www.toronto.com/shiatsuacademy

The Shiatsu Academy of Tokyo was founded in 1990 by Kensen Saito. There are thirteen instructors, with a maximum of twenty students per class.

Accreditation and Approvals
The Shiatsu Academy of Tokyo operates under the governing auspices of the Private Vocational Schools Division of the Ontario Ministry of Colleges and Universities.

Program Description
The two-year, 2,200-hour Professional Shiatsu Practitioner Course leads to a Shiatsu Practitioner Diploma. Courses include Shiatsu Theory, Shiatsu Technique, Shiatsu Practice, Anatomy, Physiology, Pathology, Professional Ethics, Communications, Nutrition, Public Health, and Business Practice. Students are required to practice shiatsu at the school clinic after the second semester.

Admission Requirements
Applicants must have completed high school or may qualify as mature students.

Tuition and Fees
Tuition is $9,000; books, uniforms, and clinic supplies are approximately $920.

Financial Assistance
Financial aid is available from the Ontario Student Assistance Program.

Shiatsu School of Canada

547 College Street
Toronto, Ontario M6G 1A9
Canada
PHONE: (416) 323-1818 / (800) 263-1703
FAX: (416) 323-1681
E-MAIL: info@shiatsucanada.com
WEBSITE: www.shiatsucanada.com

The Shiatsu School of Canada (SSC) was founded in 1986 by Kaz and Yasuko Kamiya and teaches shiatsu to the 2,200-hour standard, comparable to shiatsu programs in Japan. The School teaches both the Namikoshi Thumb and Meridian styles of shiatsu. There are twenty-two instructors, with an average of twenty-eight students per class. (For information on Shiatsu School of Canada instructional videos, see page 488.)

Accreditation and Approvals
The Shiatsu School of Canada is registered and approved as a private vocational school under the Private Vocational Schools Act.

Program Description
The 2,200-hour Career Training in Shiatsu Therapy Diploma Program may be completed in two years of full-time study or three years of part-time study. The curriculum includes Shiatsu Practice, Shiatsu Treatment, Shiatsu Theory, Eastern Medical Theory, Student Clinic, Human Anatomy, Human Physiology, Human Pathology and Symptomatology, Auxiliary Modalities, Communication Skills, Public Health, Self-Care, Ethics and Jurisprudence, Nutrition, and Business.

Community and Continuing Education
Free information sessions and shiatsu demonstrations are held at least once per month.

Health professionals such as Registered Massage Therapists, chiropractors, and graduates of a 2,200-hour diploma in shiatsu therapy may apply for admission to the 450-hour, sixteen-month Postgraduate Career Training in Acupuncture Therapy Program, held one evening per week and one weekend per month. Both Chinese and Japanese acupuncture techniques are taught, in classes that include Introduction to

Eastern Medical Theory, Shiatsu, Point Location and Indication, Meridian Theory, Advanced Diagnosis, Differential Diagnosis, Needling and Other Techniques, Clinical Practicum, and Japanese Acupuncture and Moxibustion Theory and Practice.

Admission Requirements

Applicants to the 2,200-hour Shiatsu Therapy Diploma Program should be at least 18 years of age; have a high school diploma or equivalent; have had some exposure to bodywork; have audited two SSC classes (one practical and one science); submit two letters of reference, a physician's statement, and an essay; and have an interview. Mature students at least 19 years of age and out of school for at least one year may be admitted after passing a grade 12 equivalency test or GED.

The 450-hour Postgraduate Acupuncture Therapy Program is designed exclusively for health professionals who have a Western science background such as Registered Massage Therapists, physiotherapists, nurses, chiropractors, etc., and those who have a 2,200-hour diploma in shiatsu therapy. Contact the school regarding specific prerequisite requirements.

Tuition and Fees

Tuition for the 2,200-hour Shiatsu Therapy Program is $11,500. Additional expenses include books, approximately $500 to $700; shiatsu kit, approximately $225; plus uniforms and school supplies.

Tuition for the Postgraduate Acupuncture Therapy Program is $4,000. Additional expenses include books, approximately $200 to $300; final exam, $50; plus materials and clinic uniform.

Financial Assistance

Students enrolled in the Shiatsu Therapy Diploma Program may be eligible for the Canada Student Loans Program or the Ontario Student Loans Plan.

Spirit of the Earth Centre for Herbal Education and Earth Awareness

5871 Bells Road
London, Ontario N6P 1P3
Canada

PHONE: (519) 652-0230
FAX: (519) 652-9190
E-MAIL: shantree@hotmail.com
    alliance@spirit-earth.com
WEBSITE: www.spirit-earth.com

Spirit of the Earth Centre for Herbal Education and Earth Awareness, formerly known as Balance Life Gardens, was founded by Walter Kacera in 1983. There are fifteen faculty members, with an average class size of fifteen students (maximum twenty). For home study courses, see page 477.

Program Description

The one-year program, Therapeutic Herbalism: Clinical Protocols in Herbal Administration/Application combines apprenticeship with classroom instruction. Included as the core of the program is the correspondence course, *Therapeutic Herbalism*, written by David Hoffman. The curriculum covers Herbalism, Gaia in Action; Classification of Medicinal Plants; Actions Strengths and Chemistry; Medicinal Formulations; Traditional Pharmacology; Materia Medica; Botany; Pharmacy and Dispensing; Emergency Applications; Immunity, Holism and Phytotherapy; Research Updates; and Phytotherapy for Children and the Elderly. Course Projects include Clinical Case Studies, Botanical Profile, Formulation Protocols, and Writing a Research Thesis.

The one-year course, Practical Herbalism: Hands-On Application and Experience Using Herbs for Health, includes Wild Plant Identification, Garden Design, Herb and Nature Walks, Wild Food Cooking, Preventative Medicine, Safe and Unsafe Herbs, Determining Herbal Quality, Herbal Medicine-Making, Earth Awareness and Ceremony, Herbal Pet Care, Natural Skin and Body Care, Aromatherapy and Flower Essences, and Kitchen Pharmacy. Course projects include Designing a Medicinal Garden, Creating an Herbarium, Herb Presentation, and Making a First Aid Kit.

Practical Iridology is offered as two two-day intensives. The curriculum covers Eye Anatomy and Physiology, Physical Integrity and Constitution, Bridging the Gap Between American and European Iridology, Biological and Psychological Iris Models, Case Studies, In-Depth Study of the Collarette, Syndromes: Cardio-Abdominal and Cardio-Renal, Deviation in Contraction Furrows, and Sclera and Conjunctiva Signs. Also offered are a Pre-Certification Course for NIRA (National Iridology Research Association) and a Certification Course for NIRA, upon completion of which the student will receive a Certification certificate from NIRA.

The one-year course Constitutional Medicine: A Comparative Study of Eastern and Western Protocols of Constitutions covers The Human Constitution, Your Unique Prakruti, Understanding Tridoshas, Diagnosis: Pulse, Tongue, Facial, Lip, Nail and Eye, Urine Constitutional Analysis, Dietary Assessment, Herbal Energetics, The Healing Tastes, Nutritional Medicine, Treatment Protocols, Remedial Measures, Modern Energetic Formulas, and Lifestyle and Routine. Course projects include Case Studies with Protocols, Comparative Family Analysis, Constitutional Research Thesis, and Family Tree Presentation.

Each course meets for eight full weekends; on the ninth weekend, there is an exam and students present their thesis projects.

Community and Continuing Education

A number of workshops, celebrations, and herb/earth walks are scheduled throughout the year on such topics as Full Moon Meditation and Drumming, Herbal Spa Day, A Woman's Cycle: Herbal Healing for Women, Herbal Aphrodisiacs, Ayurveda: The Science of Self Healing—Practical Applications, and others.

Tuition and Fees

Tuition for Therapeutic Herbalism is $1,995. Tuition for Practical Herbalism is $1,995. Tuition for Clinical Iridology is $1,995; the Pre-Certification Course is $495; the Certification Course is $695. Tuition for Constitutional Medicine is $1,995.

Financial Assistance

Payment plans are available. NIRA members receive a $20 discount on the Pre-Certification and Certification courses.

Sutherland-Chan School and Teaching Clinic

330 Dupont Street, 4th Floor
Toronto, Ontario M5R 1V9
Canada
PHONE: (416) 924-1107

FAX: (416) 924-9413
E-MAIL: admissions@sutherland-chan.com
WEBSITE: www.sutherland-chan.com

Grace Chan and Christine Sutherland founded the Sutherland-Chan School and Teaching Clinic in 1978. Graduates have consistently earned the highest marks on the Board exams of all the massage therapy schools in Ontario. There are fifty instructors. The teacher:student ratio for academic classes is 1:75 or less; for practical classes, 1:18 or less; for student clinic, 1:12; and for outreach, 1:10 or less.

Accreditation and Approvals

The diploma program offered by Sutherland-Chan is approved by the Ontario Ministry of Training, Colleges and Universities, and by the College of Massage Therapists. Graduates are eligible to take licensing exams throughout Canada and the United States. Sutherland-Chan is also a member of the Ontario Association of Career Colleges, the National Association of Career Colleges, and the American Massage Therapy Association (AMTA) Council of Schools.

Program Description

The two-year (or 18-month), 2,200-hour full-time Massage Therapy Program is designed to provide a balance between academic knowledge and clinical competence. Year One focuses on fundamentals; courses include Anatomy, Techniques, Hydrotherapy, Body Awareness, Clinical Theory, Therapeutic Relationship, and Rhythmic Techniques. Year Two focuses on integration and the refinement of clinical skills; courses include Neurology, Remedial Exercise, Clinical Assessment, Business and Massage Therapy Regulation and Ethics, Nutrition, Peripheral Joint Mobilization, Regional and Pregnancy Massage, Point Therapy, elective courses, and the Outreach Program, in which students work with members of the community who face physical, emotional, mental, and/or socioeconomic challenges to health and wellness. Physiology, Pathology, and Massage Treatments, and Clinical Practicum are part of the curriculum for both Year One and Year Two.

The sixteen-hour Introduction to Massage course is a general interest course for the public and a prerequisite for applicants to the 2,200-hour program.

A forty-eight-hour Preadmission Science Course is designed for the diploma applicant with identified weakness in basic science background. The course focuses on principles of biochemistry, cell structure and function, and an overview of body systems. This course is also available by correspondence.

Admission Requirements

Applicants must have a high school diploma or equivalent, and must have completed a recent science course and the Introduction to Massage course or equivalent sixteen-hour basic massage course. Applicants must also submit a résumé and two letters of reference.

Tuition and Fees

Tuition for the two-year Massage Therapy Program totals $14,700 (including $100 registration fee). Additional expenses include a $65 application fee; books, supplies, and uniform, approximately $2,100; Introduction to Massage Course, $200; Preadmission Science Course or Correspondence Course, $400.

Financial Assistance

Students may be eligible for assistance under the Canadian Student Loans and/or Ontario Student Assistance Programs.

Toronto School of Homeopathic Medicine Ltd.

17 Yorkville Avenue, Suite 200
Toronto, Ontario M4W 1L1
Canada
PHONE: (416) 966-2350 / (800) 572-6001
FAX: (416) 966-1724
E-MAIL: info@homeopathycanada.com
WEBSITE: www.homeopathycanada.com

The Toronto School of Homeopathic Medicine (TSHM) was founded in 1994 by Raymond Edge. There are six core homeopathy instructors, with a maximum of fifty students per class. Classes are held at Victoria College in the University of Toronto and the Canadian College of Naturopathic Medicine, and are also offered in home study format.

Accreditation and Approvals

TSHM is accredited by the Council on Homeopathic Education (CHE). TSHM is certified as an educational institution by the Ministry of Employment and Immigration, and has adopted the core curriculum guidelines of the International Council for Classical Homeopathy (ICCH).

Program Description

The three-year professional Homeopathic Practitioner Diploma Program consists of approximately 3,000 hours of lecture, clinical training, and study time. The curriculum consists of Fundamental Principles and Philosophy, History of Homeopathy, Case Taking, Case Analysis, Materia Medica, Homeopathic Repertory, Case Management, Clinical Externship, Counseling Skills, Pathophysiology, Ethics and Practice Management, and Physical Examination. Classes are held two weekends per month. Supervised clinical training begins in the second year and is held on Fridays at the Yorkville Avenue administrative offices.

Community and Continuing Education

The Homeopathic First Aid Program is geared toward the layperson and meets one evening per week for ten weeks. Topics covered include the history of homeopathy, comparison of homeopathy with other health care disciplines, discussion of the vital force, principles, homeopathic pharmacy, acute case-taking, how and when to take the remedies, cautions and antidotes, and treating physical trauma, acute conditions, children, and more.

The Year Four Post-Graduate Program is offered to students who have competed foundational training in homeopathy and consists of five weekends of study. The course is intended to immerse the student in the practical application of classical Hahnemannian principles. The focus of the course is on Case Taking (developing interviewing skills), Case Analysis (case assessment and symptom hierarchy), and Case Management (problem cases and troubleshooting).

The Professional Home-Study Certification Program is based on the accredited lecture program and consists of three levels (Foundation, Intermediate, and Advanced) corresponding to approximately 700 hours of study for each level plus extensive clinical training. A professional diploma in classical homeopathy is awarded upon completion of all three levels plus approved anatomy, physiology, and pathology courses and clinical training. Personal tutors facilitate the learning process. Lessons are augmented with audiotapes.

Admission Requirements
Applicants to the three-year professional diploma program must have a high school diploma or equivalent plus a minimum of two years of study at the college/university level; it is recommended that students be at least 21 years of age. Applicants must also submit a life history sketch, essay, and two letters of reference, and have a personal interview. Prospective students may attend the Student-For-A-Day Program prior to enrollment.

Year Four Post-Graduate Program applicants should have completed at least a three-year diploma program in homeopathy with medical sciences and clinical exposure.

Tuition and Fees
Total course fees for all three levels (classroom or home study) are $5,850; if paid in advance, $4,850. Books are additional. For the home study program, clinical training is additional and varies with options selected.

Tuition for the Homeopathic First Aid Program is $150; students may choose to pay $15 per class on a drop-in basis. Tuition for the Year Four Post-Graduate Program is $950.

Financial Assistance
Prepayment discounts, payment plans, and limited scholarships are available.

Toronto School of Traditional Chinese Medicine

2010 Eglinton Avenue West, Suite 302
Toronto, Ontario M6E 2K3
Canada
PHONE: (416) 782-9682
FAX: (416) 782-9681
E-MAIL: info@tstcm.com
WEBSITE: www.tstcm.com

The Toronto School of Traditional Chinese Medicine (TSTCM) was founded in 1995 by Dr. Mary X. Wu, who is a member of the Government Advisory Panel on Natural Health Products and the Expert Committee on Complementary Medicine of Health Canada. There are ten instructors, with ten to twenty students per class.

Accreditation and Approvals
Acupuncture and Traditional Chinese Medicine is not currently regulated in Ontario, and standards of education and practice have yet to be established. However, the program at TSTCM exceeds the number of hours required for taking the licensing exam in Alberta, British Columbia, and Quebec.

The Doctor of Traditional Chinese Medicine Diploma Program meets the requirements of the National Certification Commission for Acupuncture and Oriental Medicine (NCCAOM), which accepts transcripts from TSTCM as documentation of education obtained by students applying for national certification in the United States. However, students enrolling on or after July 1, 1999, should note that as of date, candidates who apply for certification through NCCAOM's Formal Education route of eligibility must have graduated from a school that is accredited, in candidacy for accreditation, or approved through an equivalent evaluation at the graduation date.

Program Description
The four-year, 2,800-hour Doctor of Traditional Chinese Medicine (DTCM) Diploma Program may be completed in three years (nine terms) in an accelerated schedule and is the equivalent of the master's degree programs offered in the United States. Courses include TCM Theory I–IV, Acupuncture I–VI, Chinese Herbal Medicine I–V, TCM Clinics I–IV, Anatomy, Physiology, Pathology, Pharmacology, Western Diagnosis, Western Clinic, Tui Na I–III, Taiji-Qigong, Chinese TCM Language, Special Needling Techniques, Treatment of Addictions, Ethics and Business Management, Research and Thesis, Seminar, TCM Dietetics, Special Topics, Review and Graduation Exam, Clinical Observation, Clinical Assistance, and Clinical Internship.

An 860-hour Diploma in Chinese Herbal Medicine prepares graduates for membership in Chinese medical associations, entitles them to malpractice insurance, and may be credited toward the DTCM Diploma. Courses include TCM Theory I–IV, Chinese Herbal Medicine I–V, TCM Clinics I–IV, and Clinical Training.

Upon request, students may also obtain Certificates in Acupuncture (280 hours) or Chinese Herbal Medicine (360 hours). The Acupuncture Certificate covers TCM Theory I and II, Acupuncture I and II, and Clinical Training. The Chinese Herbal Medicine Certificate includes TCM Theory I and II, Chinese Herbal Medicine I–III, and Clinical Training.

Students may choose between full-time day classes or part-time evening/weekend classes.

Admission Requirements

Applicants must have completed two or more years of postsecondary education at a recognized university or institute, or equivalent professional experience; be proficient in the English language; and show evidence of maturity, a keen interest in TCM, and financial stability. In addition to transcripts, applicants must also submit two letters of recommendation and a statement of purpose.

Tuition and Fees

Full-time tuition is $2,500 per term; half-time students (eight to fifteen hours per week) pay $11 per hour and part-time students (four to seven hours per week) pay $12.50 per hour. Other expenses include application fee, $30; books, $400 per year; student membership fee, $25 per year; and clinic supplies, $100 per year.

QUEBEC

Feldenkrais Institute of Somatic Education

P.O. Box 363, Station Delorimier
Montreal, Quebec H2H 2N7
Canada
PHONE/FAX: (514) 529-5966

The Feldenkrais® Institute of Somatic Education offers a four-year training program accredited by the Feldenkrais Guild®. No new trainings are planned at this time; contact the institute for information on future programs.

Le Centre Psycho-Corporel

675, Marguerite Bourgeoys
Quebec (Quebec) G1S 3V8
Canada
PHONE: (418) 687-1165 / (800) 473-5215
FAX: (418) 687-1166
E-MAIL: opsante@mlink.net
WEBSITE: www.mlink.net/~opsante

Le Centre Psycho-Corporel was founded in 1980. All instruction, as well as the catalog, is in French. There are fifteen instructors, with an average of twelve to sixteen students per class.

Accreditation and Approvals

Le Centre Psycho-Corporel is accredited by the Federation Quebecoise des Massotherapeutes (FQM) and the Association des Ecoles de Massotherapie du Quebec (AEMQ).

Program Description

Le Centre Psycho-Corporel offers two levels of instruction: a 432-hour (minimum) Massage Program and a 1,000-hour (minimum) Massotherapy Program. Required courses for both programs include Introduction to Massage (Californian, shiatsu, and Swedish); Anatomy, Physiology, and Pathology; Professional Aspects; Interview Techniques; and Helping Relationship. Electives include Manual Lymph Drainage, Trager®, Sports Massage, Reflexology, Shiatsu, Qigong, Relaxation, Hygiene, and more.

Admission Requirements

Applicants must be at least 18 years of age, have a high school diploma or equivalent, submit a résumé and recent photograph, and have taken a twelve-hour introductory course in massage.

Tuition and Fees

Tuition for the 432-hour program is $4,295; tuition for the 1,000-hour program depends on the courses chosen. There is a $75 application fee.

Financial Assistance

Financial assistance is available through the Bank of Montreal.

Sivananda Ashram Yoga Camp

(See Multiple State Locations, pages 423-24)

SASKATCHEWAN

McKay School of Massage and Hydrotherapy

226, 20th Street East
Saskatoon, Saskatchewan S7K 0A6
Canada
PHONE: (306) 652-7878
FAX: (306) 653-1808
E-MAIL: ccampus@sk.sympatico.ca

The McKay School of Massage and Hydrotherapy was founded in 1994 as part of McKay Technical Inc., which was founded in 1982. There are eighteen instructors in the massage program, with an average of twenty students per class.

Accreditation and Approvals

McKay is registered with Saskatchewan Post-Secondary Education and Training. Graduates are qualified to take the entry exam for professional regulation in Saskatchewan and other provinces.

Program Description

The two-year, 2,400-hour Massage and Hydrotherapy Program includes courses in Gross Anatomy, Systems Anatomy/Physiology, Pathology, Massage Theory and Techniques, Clinical Assessment, Massage Treatments, Hydrotherapy, Clinical Internship/Field Placement, Advanced Techniques Workshops (including sports massage, manual lymph drainage, craniosacral therapy, myofascial release, infant massage, visceral manipulation, and connective tissue work), Applied Kinesiology, Body Awareness, Remedial Exercise, First Aid/ CPR, Business, Study Management Skills, and Personal/Professional Development.

Admission Requirements

Applicants must have a high school diploma or equivalent, demonstrate proficiency in biology and either chemistry or physics, and complete an eight-hour appraisal session which includes a hands-on massage techniques workshop and interview. Mature students over 19 years of age and lacking certain educational requirements may be admitted under certain circumstances.

Tuition and Fees

The cost of tuition, books, and fees is approximately $7,500 per year. The appraisal session costs $75.

Financial Assistance

Canada and Saskatchewan student loans and in-house financing may be available.

MULTIPLE STATE LOCATIONS

The programs listed in this section either have branches in more than one state or province, or are seminars or workshops that travel to different states or provinces in any given year. These programs are broken down into United States and Canadian listings, and are listed alphabetically.

United States

American Academy of Environmental Medicine

American Financial Center
7701 East Kellogg, Suite 625
Wichita, Kansas 67207-1705
PHONE: (316) 684-5500
FAX: (316) 684-5709
E-MAIL: aaem@swbell.net
WEBSITE: www.healthy.net/pan/pa/NaturalTherapies/aaem/

The American Academy of Environmental Medicine was founded to study and treat people with illnesses or health problems caused by adverse, allergic, or toxic reactions to a variety of environmental substances. Over 400 physicians in the United States and around the world are members; for membership information, see pages 449-50.

Accreditation and Approvals

AAEM is accredited by the Accreditation Council for Continuing Medical Education to sponsor continuing medical education for physicians.

Program Description

AAEM offers seminars and courses intended for M.D.s and D.O.s.

The Annual Meeting of the Academy is an open forum introducing the latest ideas in the diagnosis and treatment of environmental illness. These advanced seminars have been held throughout the United States and Canada. Educational formats include plenary sessions, panels, Q & A sessions, case presentations, workshops, concurrent sessions, a syllabus, and audiotapes.

The academy also presents instructional courses each year. Basic courses provide the physician with the fundamental tools of diagnosis and treatment, and emphasize inhalant allergy and intracutaneous serial end point titration. Advanced courses concentrate on diagnosis of food and chemical sensitivities, yeast-related problems, autoimmune disorders, endocrine imbalances, and nutritional deficiencies.

Admission Requirements

Seminars and courses are intended for M.D.s, D.O.s, and all other health professionals interested in enhancing the outcomes of many complex issues using the cause-oriented, patient-centered concepts and practices of Environmental Medicine.

Tuition and Fees

Instructional courses are approximately $495 per course for members, $595 for nonmembers.

American Academy of Medical Acupuncture

5820 Wilshire Boulevard, Suite 500
Los Angeles, California 90036
PHONE: (323) 937-5514

FAX: (323) 937-0959
E-MAIL: jdowden@prodigy.net
WEBSITE: www.medicalacupuncture.org

The American Academy of Medical Acupuncture (AAMA) was founded in 1987 by a group of physicians who were graduates of the Medical Acupuncture for Physicians training programs sponsored by UCLA School of Medicine. AAMA serves as both a professional (see pages 445-46) and certifying (see page 435) organization. The symposium and review classes are held at locations throughout the country.

Accreditation and Approvals

AAMA has created a proficiency examination for physicians who have incorporated acupuncture into their medical practice; the Board of Directors awards a Certificate of Proficiency in Medical Acupuncture to those who successfully pass this exam. The exam is the first step toward establishing a formal recognized board certification program.

Both the symposium and the examination review course have been approved for continuing medical education (CME) credits.

Program Description

An annual four-day Medical Acupuncture Symposium addresses the use of acupuncture in the practice of contemporary medicine for physicians (M.D.s or D.O.s) with little or no acupuncture knowledge, as well as for those with years of experience. Workshops typically cover such topics as an introduction to acupuncture, energetics and manual medicine, applications of medical acupuncture in the management of disease, research, and more.

A two-day Examination Review Course has been developed by John Reed, M.D., who has taught the clinical portion of the introductory program at the symposium for several years. This course requires some advance home study work and two full days on-site prior to the exam.

Admission Requirements

The symposium is open to physicians (M.D.s and D.O.s) interested in or already practicing acupuncture. The review course is for physicians already proficient in medical acupuncture.

Tuition and Fees

Registration for the Medical Acupuncture Symposium costs approximately $475 to $675, depending on AAMA membership status and date of registration; discounts are given for early registration. Registration for the Examination Review Course is $425; the examination costs $500.

American Viniyoga Institute

P.O. Box 88
Makawao, Hawaii 96768
PHONE: (808) 572-1414
E-MAIL: info@viniyoga.com
WEBSITE: www.viniyoga.com

American Viniyoga Institute was founded in 1983 by Gary Kraftsow, who was the first American certified to train teachers in the Viniyoga lineage. Viniyoga is defined as the appropriate application of asana, pranayama, sound, visualization, meditation, and relaxation respecting individual needs. Gary and Minka Kraftsow are the primary instructors; classes average fifty students per training. Workshops are held on Maui and in various locations throughout the mainland United States and Europe.

Program Description

The Viniyoga Teacher Training program consists of eight nine-day sessions. The first seven sessions are nonresidential training sessions; the eighth is a residential retreat. Topics covered include Principles of Breath and Movement, Forward Bends, The Science of Sequence, Principles of Adaptation, Backward Bends, Observation: Reading the Body, Human Energy System, Twists and Lateral Bends, Introduction to Pranayama, Bandhas and Mudras, Extension, Sound and Chanting, Meditation, Inversion, Developing the Personal Ritual, Introduction to Teaching Methodology, Balance, and Introduction to Yoga Therapy. The curriculum is covered through group practice, lecture, discussion and group processes. Students are also required to take a minimum of eight 1½ hour private sessions.

The Viniyoga Therapist Training Program for Viniyoga Therapist Certification consists of four nine-day sessions. The first three sessions are nonresidential training sessions; the fourth is a residential retreat. The subject matter is organized in the categories of Common Aches and Pains, Chronic Disease, and Emotional Health. Students are also required to take a minimum of four 1½ hour private sessions.

New programs will be starting in 2000; contact the institute for details.

Admission Requirements

Contact the institute for admission requirements and opportunities to begin Viniyoga studies prior to starting the formal training program.

Tuition and Fees

Contact the institute for information regarding tuition.

American Yoga Association

P.O. Box 19986
Sarasota, Florida 34276
PHONE: (941) 927-4977
FAX: (941) 921-9844
E-MAIL: yogamerica@aol.com
WEBSITE: users.aol.com/amyogaassn

The Easy Does It Yoga program was created by the American Yoga Association's founder, Alice Christensen, for use with people with physical limitations due to age, convalescence, injury, or substance abuse recovery. There are ten instructors, with an average of twelve students per class.

Program Description

The American Yoga Association's Easy Does It Program consists of specially adapted classical yoga exercises, breathing techniques, and guided relaxation. The Easy Does It Trainer Program is geared toward geriatric health practitioners, nurses, physical therapists, nursing home staff, and others who care for the elderly or those with physical limitations. The association offers on-site programs at various colleges or continuing education programs throughout the country. The curriculum may be adapted to cover several weeks or days.

Instruction includes goals and objectives of the Easy Does It Program; the physical, mental, and emotional benefits; how to teach a variety of seated and standing exercises; how to practice and teach two breathing techniques; how to teach relaxation; how to apply the techniques to those recovering from substance abuse or injury; and how to motivate clients to continue with the program.

Tuition and Fees
Fees vary with the length and sponsor of the course.

Asten Center of Natural Therapeutics

TEXAS LOCATIONS
797 North Grove Road, Suite 101
Richardson, Texas 75081-2761
PHONE: (972) 669-3245
FAX: (972) 669-1191
E-MAIL: Astenctr@flash.net
700 South Cooper, Suite 1
Arlington, Texas 76001
PHONE: (817) 233-0782

MONTANA LOCATION
121 West Legion
P.O. Box 1009
Whitehall, Montana 59759-1503
PHONE: (406) 287-5670
FAX: (406) 287-7900

The Asten Center of Natural Therapeutics was founded by Paige Asten in Texas in 1983. The Whitehall, Montana, school was opened in 1990; the Arlington, Texas, school was opened in 1999. There are fifteen instructors, with a maximum of twenty students per class.

Accreditation and Approvals
The Asten Center is recognized by the Texas Department of Health, licensed by the Montana Department of Commerce, and approved by the State of Iowa. Graduates of massage therapy programs of 500 or more hours are qualified to take the National Certification Examination for Therapeutic Massage and Bodywork (NCETMB).

Program Description
Offered in Texas, the 550-hour Massage Therapy Program is divided into Basic and Specialized Sections. The Basic Section consists of 300 hours of instruction and is the minimum required by the Texas Department of Health for registration. The Basic Section includes instruction in Anatomy and Physiology, Health and Hygiene, Hydrotherapy, Swedish Massage, Business Practices and Ethics, and Internship. The Specialized Section adds instruction in Reflexology; Trigger Point Therapy; Sports Massage; Practice Specialty Classes that include Chair Massage, Manual Lymphatic Drainage, Polarity, Nurturing Massage, First Aid/CPR, and Pregnancy, Infant and Elderly Massage; and Clinical Application Classes that include treatment for sprained ankle, carpal tunnel syndrome, whiplash, headaches and migraines, TMJ dysfunction, sciatic pain, tennis elbow, spinal deviations, and other dysfunctions.

Offered in Montana, the 605½-hour Massage Therapy Program is also divided into two sections. The Basic Section consists of 286 hours and includes instruction in Anatomy and Physiology, Swedish Massage, Hydrotherapy/Cryotherapy, Health and Hygiene, Business Practices and Ethics, and Externship. The Specialized Section consists of 319½ hours and includes Anatomy and Physiology, Reflexology, Trigger Point Therapy, Sports Massage, Special Problems, and Clinical Applications.

Admission Requirements
Applicants must complete an admissions application, be free of contagious disease, and interview with an admissions representative.

Tuition and Fees
In Texas, tuition and books for the Basic Section is $2,630; tuition and books for the Specialized Section is $2,421. Additional expenses include linens, $45; towels, $40; lotion, $20; clothing, $40; and an optional portable massage table, $289.

In Montana, the total course fee is $5,080, which includes tuition, massage table and travel bag, face cradle, books, AMTA student membership, massage lotion, and CPR training; linens are additional.

Financial Assistance
Payment plans, student loans, and aid from the Texas Rehabilitation Commission, the Texas Commission for the Blind, and JTPA are available. Students in Texas who register for both sections consecutively receive a reduction in tuition.

Biofeedback Instrument Corporation

255 West 98th Street
New York, New York 10025
PHONE: (212) 222-5665
FAX: (212) 222-5667
E-MAIL: ac@inx.net

The Biofeedback Instrument Corporation, founded in 1981, registers students for a number of biofeedback courses offered in several states and countries. There are one to six instructors, depending on the course, and a maximum of fifty students per class.

Accreditation and Approvals
The eight-day BCIA Certification Training Series meets the educational requirement for BCIA certification.

Program Description
The two- to six-day EEG Biofeedback Training Course for Professionals, founded in 1969 by Siegfried and Susan Othmer, is designed for practitioners and researchers who work in fields such as ADD/ADHD, Specific Learning Disabilities, Sleep Disorders, Depression and Anxiety, Addictive Behavior, and others. The program covers EEG Fundamentals, History of EEG Biofeedback, Analysis of the EEG, Discussion of EEG Biofeedback for Specific Conditions, New Frontiers of EEG Biofeedback, Training Outcomes, Practical Considerations, and Practicum.

An eighty-hour, eight-day BCIA Certification Training Series Program, founded by Adam Crane, consists of three modules. Module A (thirty hours) covers Introduction to Biofeedback, Preparing for Clinical Intervention, Neuromuscular Intervention: General, Central Nervous System Interventions: General, Autonomic Nervous Systems: General, Instrumentation, and Professional Conduct. Module B (thirty hours) covers Neuromuscular Intervention: Specific, Autonomic Nervous System: Specific, Biofeedback and Distress, Instrumentation, Adjunctive Techniques and Cognitive Interventions, Professional Conduct, and Supervised Personal Training on EMG and Temperature. Module C (twenty hours) includes Preparing for Clinical Intervention, Autonomic Nervous System Interventions: Specific, Biofeedback and Distress, Adjunctive Techniques and Cognitive Interventions, Professional Conduct, and Case Conference.

Dr. Brotman offers a one-day Introductory Course to Clinical Biofeedback that includes Menninger Foundation videotapes; hands-on use of temperature, EMG, EEG, and GSR biofeedback instrumentation; demonstration of computerized biofeedback systems; supplementary relaxation techniques; and more.

Dr. Brotman also offers a one-day course, Biofeedback Supplementary Techniques including Traditional and Ericksonian Hypnosis, Cognitive Restructuring, and Their Applications.

Students may also register through Dr. Brotman for the BCIA-accredited Professional Biofeedback Certificate Program described under Stens Corporation, page 414.

Admission Requirements
The courses are designed for professionals such as psychologists, psychiatrists, social workers, counselors, psychotherapists, and others.

Tuition and Fees
Tuition for the EEG Biofeedback Courses is $995 for five-day comprehensive and specialty courses, $595 for three-day specialty courses.

Tuition for the eight-day BCIA Certification Training Series is $1,585.

Tuition for the one-day Introductory Course is $250 plus $80 for course materials. Tuition for the one-day Supplementary Techniques Course is $350.

Financial Assistance
A tuition discount of approximately 10 percent is available to students.

BioSomatics

P.O. Box 206
Grand Junction, Colorado 81502
PHONE: (970) 245-8903
FAX: (970) 241-5653
E-MAIL: biosomatics@gj.net
WEBSITE: www.biosomatic.com

Educational director Carol Welch has been devoted to developmental movement since 1979 and is one of only thirty-eight individuals trained by Thomas Hanna. BioSomatics blends Welch's own distinctive approach to Somatic Movement reeducation, which combines principles from Hanna Somatics with the worlds of dance and yoga. Welch is the primary instructor; class sizes range from 16 to 30 students. Seminars are held across the United States and Canada in such cities as Seattle, Denver, Albuquerque, Tucson, Des Moines, Maui, Vancouver, and Regina (Saskatchewan). For information on instructional videos, see pages 485–86.

Program Description

There are six seminars offered in BioSomatics Movement Education in the tradition of Thomas Hanna.

The Posture and Movement Seminar runs two and a half days and is a primer in somatic education. Topics include use of the pandicular response (the primary hands-on method of clinical education) for the reeducation of habitual flexion and extension patterns, how habitual postural patterns are the underpinning of many physical problems, movement to avoid or reverse stuck posturing, and relanguaging problems in sensory terms. This seminar must be taken before any of the subsequent seminars.

The three-day Landau Seminar covers clinical somatic education to address habituation of the Landau reflex, movements for senile posture, how to build somatic education into your practice, and more.

The three-day Trauma Reflex Seminar covers clinical somatic education to address habituation of the startle and trauma reflexes, explorations in verbal and mental imagery, movements in the reeducation of the relationship of the ankle, knee, and hip to the torso, and more.

The three-day Startle Reflex Seminar teaches releasing deeper effects of the startle reflex, movements for joints, developmental stages of movement, roller work to self-adjust tension, and more.

The three-day Renegotiating and Transforming Trauma Seminar teaches neurological coordination/tension patterns, control over evolutive scoliosis through sustained position traction, renegotiating birth trauma, and more.

The two-day Pure Movement Seminar covers the use of movement to create healthy spines, moving the body to adjust the emotions, increasing sensitivity for feeling the movements of the spine, tissues, and bones, and more.

A certificate of completion will be awarded after attending all seminars twice and passing an evaluation of hands-on skills. Two years of practice and application, six case history studies, and ten private somatic sessions are required before taking the certification evaluation. The certificate of completion entitles the practitioner to be known as a Resource for Bio-Somatic Education.

Admission Requirements

The certification/evaluation Program is intended for practitioners in orthodox or complementary medicine, therapy, or education. A knowledge of anatomy and physiology is recommended, as is experience in some form of body-oriented therapy and/or psychotherapy or movement education. Applicants must answer a brief questionnaire and submit a résumé and a letter of recommendation.

Tuition and Fees

Tuition for the Posture and Movement Seminar is $275; for the Landau Seminar, $350; for the Trauma Reflex Seminar, $350; for the Startle Reflex Seminar, $350; for the Renegotiating and Transforming Trauma Seminar, $350; and for the Pure Movement Seminar, $250.

Financial Assistance

A discount is given for early registration.

Blue Cliff School of Therapeutic Massage

WEBSITE: www.bluecliffschool.com

NEW ORLEANS CAMPUS:
1919 Veterans Boulevard
Kenner, Louisiana 70062
PHONE: (504) 471-0294
FAX: (504) 466-8514

LAFAYETTE CAMPUS:
103 Calco Boulevard
Lafayette, Louisiana 70503
PHONE: (318) 269-0620
FAX: (318) 269-0688

SHREVEPORT CAMPUS:
3823 Gilbert Drive
Shreveport, Louisiana 71104
PHONE: (318) 861-5959
FAX: (318) 861-5957

GULFPORT CAMPUS:
942 East Beach Boulevard
Gulfport, Mississippi 39507

Blue Cliff School of Therapeutic Massage was founded in 1987 by Vernon Smith. The Blue Cliff Sports Massage Team participates in local athletic events, including the Mardi Gras Marathon. There are fifteen to thirty instructors per campus, with an average of fifteen to twenty-five students per class.

Accreditation

All Louisiana campuses are licensed by the Proprietary School Commission of the Louisiana Department of Education. Additionally, the New Orleans campus is accredited by the Accrediting Commission of Career Schools and Colleges of Technology (ACCSCT); its 600-hour program is accredited by the Commission on Massage Training Accreditation (COMTA); and its 300-hour Shiatsu Practitioner Program is approved by the American Oriental Bodywork Therapy Association (AOBTA) as qualifying graduates for practitioner-level membership in the AOBTA. The Gulfport campus is licensed by the State of Mississippi under its Commission on Proprietary School and College Registration. The programs at the Lafayette, Shreveport, and Gulfport schools are modeled after the programs at Blue Cliff in New Orleans.

Program Description

The New Orleans campus offers both a 600-hour Massage Therapist Program and a 750-hour Clinical Massage Therapist program; the other three campuses offer a 600-hour program.

The New Orleans 600-hour Massage Therapist curriculum includes Swedish Massage, Anatomy and Physiology, HIV, Tai Chi, Therapeutic Communication, Supervised Clinical Practice, Marketing and Professionalism, Laws and Legislation, Ethics, Reflexology, Sports Kinesiology, Pathophysiology, Deep Tissue Massage, Chair Massage, Craniosacral Therapy, Hydrotherapy, Healing Touch, Neuromuscular Therapy, CPR/ First Aid, Sports Massage, Basic Shiatsu, Point Energetics, Sports Shiatsu, and Community Outreach.

The New Orleans 750-hour Clinical Massage Therapist Program has a strong orthopedic, functional assessment orientation with an emphasis on application of techniques in Supervised Clinical Practice and participation in athletic events. The curriculum includes most of the courses in the 600-hour program plus Charting, Caring for the Self, Medical Terminology, Applications of Neuromuscular Therapy, Functional Assessment, additional training in Sports Kinesiology and Sports Massage, and Supervised Clinical Practice in NMT.

The Lafayette, Shreveport, and Gulfport campuses each offer a 600-hour Massage Therapist Program whose curriculum varies slightly from campus to campus. The Shreveport and Lafayette programs are prelicensing programs with a Western perspective; the Gulfport curriculum also includes a significant emphasis on Spa Therapy, reflecting the demands of the local resort market.

Each campus offers day, night, and weekend schedules.

Community and Continuing Education

One-day introductory Eastern- and Western-style technique classes are offered to the public. A variety of continuing education workshops are offered to the massage community; many of these satisfy state and national CEU requirements.

The New Orleans campus also offers a 300-hour Oriental Bodywork Practitioner Program for those who have completed the 600-hour Massage Therapist Program or its equivalent. The curriculum includes Body Systems Balancing, Intermediate Shiatsu, Supervised Clinical Practice, Assessment, Qigong, Zang Fu, Extraordinary Vessels, Point Energetics, Pulses and Tongues, Five Transformations, and Comprehensive Review and Finals, plus ten hours of Community Outreach.

Admission Requirements

Applicants must be at least 18 years of age, have a high school diploma or the equivalent, be in good health and physically capable of performing massage, complete an application with essay questions, and have a personal interview. Students are strongly encouraged to have had at least one professional massage prior to the start of classes.

Tuition and Fees

Tuition and fees for the New Orleans campus are as follows: Tuition for the 750-hour program is $6,000; tuition for the 600-hour program is $4,900; tuition for the 300-hour Oriental Bodywork program is $2,500.

Tuition for the 600-hour program offered at the Lafayette and Shreveport campuses is $4,900.

Tuition for the 600-hour program offered at the Gulfport campus is $4,400.

Additional expenses for any of the 600-hour or 750-hour programs include application fee, $25; registration fee, $75; student liability insurance fee, $15; and textbook and instructional materials fee, $435. Linens and oils are additional.

Financial Assistance

Payment plans, veterans' benefits, and aid from Louisiana Rehabilitation Services are available.

Creativity Learning Institute

30819 Casilina Drive
Rancho Palos Verdes, California 90275
PHONE: (310) 541-4844 / (800) 366-7908
E-MAIL: sstockwell@earthlink.net

Creativity Learning Institute was founded in 1978 by Shelly Stockwell, Ph.D. Stockwell teaches all classes; visiting adjunct instructors include Ormond McGill and Charlene Acherman. Classes range from fifteen to 100 students. Courses are offered in Rancho Palos Verdes, California; Sedona, Arizona; Bali, Indonesia, and other locations around the world.

Accreditation and Approvals

Creativity Learning Institute is endorsed by the International Medical and Dental Hypnotherapy Association (IMDHA), the American Board of Hypnotherapy (ABH), and the International Hypnosis Federation (IHF).

Program Description

The 200-hour Hypnotherapy Program consists of four 50-hour segments. Classes include Hypnotist Certification, Master Hypnotist Certification, Hypnotherapist Certification, Transpersonal Hypnotherapist Certification, Past Life Certification, Weight Loss Instructor Certification Training, American Smoke Out Certification Training, Pain and Stress Management Certification Training, Motivational and Sales Hypnotherapy, Master of Stage Hypnosis Certification, and Medical and Dental Hypnotherapy Certification. Intensives are held from Wednesday to Sunday and weekend courses Friday through Sunday.

Community and Continuing Education

The institute offers motivational speakers, full-day workshops, weekend retreats, corporate training, and consulting. Specialty classes are offered in Urban Shamanism, Vision Quests, Abundance and Psychic Development, and other topics.

Correspondence courses are available upon request; these require a written thesis and exam.

Admission Requirements

The minimum age for attendance is ten years; minors require parental permission.

Tuition and Fees

Tuition is $600 for each fifty-hour course segment. Tuition varies for traveling training courses.

Financial Assistance

Payment plans are available; early registration discounts are usually offered on touring certification courses.

The Day-Break Geriatric Massage Project

P.O. Box 1815
Sebastopol, California 95473-1815
PHONE: (707) 829-2798
FAX: (707) 829-2799
E-MAIL: daybreak@monitor.net
WEBSITE: www.daybreak-massage.com

Day-Break was founded in April 1982 as Day-Break Stress and Pain Control by Dietrich Miesler, a former nursing home administrator. The institute develops treatment programs, instructional materials and training classes directed at such age-related health conditions as poor circulation, muscle and joint pain and stiffness, and stroke recovery, and ongoing research studies on the effect of massage on Parkinson's and peripheral vascular disease. There are six instructors, with 12 to 20 students per class.

Day-Break also offers books, videos, and other products; see page 486.

Accreditation and Approvals
Day-Break is approved as a continuing education and instructor training provider by the National Certification Board for Therapeutic Massage and Bodywork (NCBTMB), the Florida State Massage Therapy Association, and the College of Massage Therapists of British Columbia.

Program Description
The Day-Break Certification Program in Geriatric Massage is a modular program consisting of a basic workshop, a correspondence course, and an advanced geriatric massage workshop.

The two-and-one-half-day, seventeen-hour Level One Day-Break Geriatric Massage Workshop is the basis of the training program in geriatric massage. Topics covered in the Workshop include physiological, psychological, and sociological aspects of aging; client assessment, cautions and contraindications; modification of standard massage techniques; and practical hands-on work with older people. Workshops are held at massage schools throughout the country.

The Distance Learning Course CC'96 serves as a follow-up for therapists who have attended the Level One Workshop. Topics covered in this video-based course include information on age-induced health conditions and how they can be addressed with hands-on techniques.

The Level Two Advanced Geriatric Massage Workshop involves supervised hands-on work with nursing home patients.

Admission Requirements
Applicants must be an insured member of ABMT, AMTA, IMA, NANMT, or NCBTMB and should be a mature massage therapist with a minimum of 150 hours of formal massage training, including Swedish massage. In addition, applicants should have worked with seniors in either a family or health care setting, should have some teaching experience or talent for teaching, must have easy access to a computer and fax machine, and must have an e-mail address.

Tuition and Fees
Costs are as follows: enrollment fee, $200; membership fee, $35; Level One Workshop, $290; distance learning course, $285; Level Two Workshop, $290.

DoveStar Institute

NEW HAMPSHIRE LOCATION:
50 Whitehall Road
Hooksett, New Hampshire 03106-2104
PHONE: (603) 669-9497 / (603) 669-5104
FAX: (603) 625-1919
E-MAIL: 1stdovestar@mediaone.net
WEBSITE: www.dovestar.edu

MASSACHUSETTS LOCATION:
120 Court Street
Plymouth, Massachusetts 02360
PHONE: (508) 830-0068
FAX: (508) 830-0288

SOUTH CAROLINA LOCATIONS:
20 Palmetto Parkway
Hilton Head Island, South Carolina 29928
PHONE: (843) 342-3362
FAX: (843) 342-3639
119 Main Street
Lake City, South Carolina 29560
PHONE: (843) 394-7922
7900 Porcher Drive
Myrtle Beach, South Carolina 29572
PHONE: (843) 449-9194

In 1973, Kamala Renner started the Yoga Retreat Center and Massage School in Hooksett, New Hampshire. In 1978, the center became known as the EarthStar Holistic Center and DoveStar Institute, and was licensed as a holistic therapy school in 1981. Training is held in Hooksett, New Hampshire; Plymouth, Massachusetts; and in Lake City, Hilton Head, and Myrtle

Beach, South Carolina. There are twenty instructors, with ten to twenty students per class.

Accreditation and Approvals

DoveStar Institute is licensed by the New Hampshire Postsecondary Education Agency, the Commonwealth of Massachusetts Department of Education, and the South Carolina Commission on Higher Education. Graduates of massage therapy programs of 500 or more hours are qualified to take the National Certification Examination for Therapeutic Massage and Bodywork (NCETMB). The curriculum is designed to meet New Hampshire state licensing requirements, and is approved by the American Council of Hypnotist Examiners (ACHE).

Program Description

The 300-hour Reiki-Alchemia Core Energy Work Program integrates the healing techniques of alchemia, which utilizes transformational and transmutational life force energy qualities, with the Usui method of reiki, which activates universal life force energy with the Usui master keys. Required courses include Intuitive Development, Alchemia Bodywork, Reiki First Degree, Hypnotherapy, Alchemia Breathwork, RENEW, Four Forces, Alchemy and Physiology, plus a four-day intensive and four electives.

Kriya massage incorporates the universal four forces (centripetal, centrifugal, gravity, and electromagnetic) into classical massage techniques. The Kriya Massage Program for New Hampshire licensure is a 750-hour program. Required courses include Kriya Massage, Alchemia Bodywork, Client Pathology, Sports Hydrotherapy, Spa Hydrotherapy, Detox Hydrotherapy, Health Services Management, Business and Marketing, State Rules and Regulations, Adult CPR, and Anatomy and Physiology, plus the choice of two courses each in the areas of Oriental, energy work, somato-emotional release, and anatomy and movement, plus seven electives. Six supervised kriya bodywork practicums and clinical are also required.

The Kriya Massage Program for national certification is a 500-hour program that includes Kriya Massage, Alchemia Bodywork, Health Services Management, and Anatomy and Physiology, plus the choice of one course each in the areas of Oriental, energy work, and somato-emotional release, plus seven electives. Six supervised kriya bodywork practicums and clinical are also required.

The goal of Alchemical Synergy is to connect with the "inner master" or "inner adult" and reclaim responsibility for oneself. The 500-hour Alchemical Synergy Program includes required courses in Hypnotherapy (1 through 6), Four Forces, Inner Alignment, Inner Commitment, Inner Harmony, Inner Power, and Four Forces Counseling, plus nine electives, six supervised hypnotherapy practicums, assisting with Hypnotherapy Courses 1 through 6, and receiving forty-four hours of hypnotherapy sessions.

The HypnoSynergy Certification is a 400-hour program consisting of required classes in Induction Methods, Emotional Clearing, Inner Resources, Past Lives, Conference Room 1 & 2, Business and Marketing, Four Forces and HypnoSynergy and Bodywork, seven electives, three supervised practicums, assisting at six HypnoSynergy Seminars and receiving twenty hours of HypnoSynergy sessions.

The 1,500-hour Holistic Practitioner Program involves extensive training in holistic health care. Requirements include at least 500 hours of training in each of the Bodywork, Synergy, and Reiki-Alchemia Programs, and clinical practice in each of these areas.

The Reiki Master Teacher Program consists of Reiki First, Second, and Third Degree Therapist required courses, as well as forty hours of supervising healing circles, assisting in Reiki First, Second, and Third Degree classes, Four Forces, attending Master Teacher classes, and receiving Reiki Master Teacher Attunement. Completion requires a minimum of one year of study with a Reiki Master Teacher.

Alchemia yoga is a form of physical movement that incorporates the holistic approach to physical fitness. The 523-hour Alchemia Yoga Teacher Program consists of required courses in Alchemia Yoga, Strain/Counterstrain, Acupressure, Alchemia Bodywork, Reiki First Degree, Alchemy and Physiology, Hypnotherapy, Alchemia Breathwork, RENEW, Four Forces, Kinesiology Theory, and Anatomy and Physiology, as well as assisting at alchemia yoga classes and practice teaching.

A DoveStar Teacher Training Program is offered that emphasizes holistic health. Students must monitor a variety of classes, attend teacher training classes, complete certification in a field of choice, assist at two-day seminars, supervise practicums, and attend a week-long teacher training intensive.

Admission Requirements

Applicants must interview with an admissions representative.

Tuition and Fees

Tuition for the Reiki-Alchemia Program is $3,640, plus a $200 enrollment fee.

Tuition for the Kriya Massage Program for New Hampshire licensure is approximately $7,000. Additional expenses include a $200 enrollment fee; books, approximately $300; supplies, $100; and a massage table.

Tuition for the Kriya Massage Program for national certification is approximately $4,200. Additional expenses include a $200 enrollment fee; books, approximately $250; supplies, $100; and a massage table.

Tuition for the Alchemical Synergy Program is $4,775; there is a $175 enrollment fee, and books are $100.

Tuition for the Holistic Practitioner Program varies with courses; there is a $600 enrollment fee.

Tuition for the HypnoSynergy Program is $3,425, and for the Alchemical Synergy Program, $4,775.

Tuition for the Reiki Master Teacher Program is $1,940, plus a $125 enrollment fee.

Tuition for the Alchemia Yoga Teacher Program is $4,095, plus a $175 enrollment fee.

The cost of the DoveStar Teacher Certification Program varies depending on the classes selected and the area of certification; contact DoveStar for more information.

East West Academy of Healing Arts/ Qigong Institute

P.O. Box 31211
San Francisco, California 94131
PHONE: (415) 285-9400
E-MAIL: eastwestqi@aol.com
WEBSITE: www.eastwestqi.com

The East West Academy of Healing Arts was founded in 1973 by Dr. Effie Poy Yew Chow, an acupuncturist and psychiatric nurse. Dr. Chow is the primary instructor, and uses the Chow Integrated Healing System in which modern Western practices are blended with ancient Eastern healing arts. Seminars are held in San Francisco, Spokane, Ottawa, Toronto, Vancouver, and other locations in the United States, Canada, and around the world. The academy, in association with the World Qigong Federation, also sponsors an annual World Congress on Qigong. The American Qigong Association is a subsidiary of the East West Academy of Healing Arts (see page 460).

Program Description

Three-day weekend seminars in Qigong Miracle Healing include an Introductory Seminar and Basic Skills Seminar; 100-hour Intensive Training Seminars are held one weekend per month for four months. Topics covered include the theory of Qi, energy therapy, overview of the Chow Integrated Healing System, Qipressure points, basic exercises, and hands-on techniques.

Tuition and Fees

Tuition varies with location; contact the academy for details.

Feldenkrais® Resources

830 Bancroft Way, Suite 112
Berkeley, California 94710
PHONE: (510) 540-7600 / (800) 765-1907
FAX: (510) 540-7683
E-MAIL: feldenres@aol.com
WEBSITE: www.feldenkrais-resources.com

MAILING ADDRESS:
PO Box 2067
Berkeley, California 94702

Feldenkrais Resources was founded in 1983. It is the leading school for the postgraduate training of Feldenkrais practitioners, and also the publisher of Dr. Feldenkrais' audio- and videotape programs, and books and audiotapes of leading Feldenkrais practitioners (see pages 486-87). There are generally four to six instructors per segment of classroom instruction, with an average of forty students; students are also required to arrange individual lessons as part of the program. The programs are held in Montclair, New Jersey; Baltimore, Maryland; and Berkeley, California.

Accreditation and Approvals

The Feldenkrais Professional Training Program is fully accredited by the Feldenkrais Guild and recognized by all international Feldenkrais teacher organizations throughout Europe, Australia, Israel, and South America.

Program Description

The Feldenkrais Professional Training Program meets forty days per year over three and a half years in a weekend-based format. The program offers extensive practical experience and in-depth training in both Awareness Through Movement® and Functional Integration®, as well as a thorough exploration of the theory underlying the Feldenkrais method through lectures, discussions, study groups, and readings.

Upon completion of the second year of training, qualified students will be authorized to teach Awareness Through Movement to the public. At the end of the fourth year, students become practitioners of both Awareness Through Movement and Functional Integration, and will be eligible for full membership in the Feldenkrais Guild®.

Community Education

One-day Feldenkrais Method workshops for prospective training program participants and the general public are held in New York, New Jersey, Delaware, the Washington, D.C./Baltimore area, and Berkeley, California.

Admission Requirements

There are no prerequisites.

Tuition and Fees

Tuition is $3,600 per year, plus a $50 application fee. The one-day workshops cost $65 with preregistration and $75 at the door as space permits.

Financial Assistance

Payment plans are available, as well as a limited number of work-scholarships and tuition reduction plans for students traveling from Canada.

The Foundation for Aromatherapy Education and Research

1900 West Stone Avenue
Fairfield, Iowa 52556
PHONE: (515) 472-2422, ext. 220
FAX: (515) 472-8672
E-MAIL: info@amrita.net
WEBSITE: www.amrita.net

The Foundation for Aromatherapy Education and Research (a division of the wholesale business Amrita Aromatherapy) was founded by Dr. Christoph Streicher in 1997. There are three instructors; classes range from a minimum of twelve students to a maximum of thirty. Courses are offered throughout the country; contact the foundation to sponsor a course.

Program Description

The Basic Foundations of Aromatherapy course is based on the Holistic Paradigm and consists of four sequential certification classes.

Class I is a two-day seminar. The students review twenty basic essential oils, basic physiology, interaction of oils on physical and emotional levels, use of oils in skin care, how to create a blend, methods of application, and very basic and simple massage techniques. For those pursuing certification, labs and homework must be completed prior to acceptance into Class II.

Class II is a two-day seminar. This class is for those desiring to treat individuals in consultation. It includes study of aromatherapy practice, essential oil chemistry, essential oil safety and hazards, essential oil profiles, and therapeutic blends; students review twenty-six essential oils. Labs and homework must be completed prior to Class III.

Class III is a two-day seminar. The level of study is for those seeking to use aromatherapy as an adjunct to their profession. It includes history of aromatherapy, systems and disease management with essential oils, advanced blending principles and practice, internal use of essential oils (safety and hazards), and advanced essential oil chemistry; students review nine essential oils. Students wishing to complete certification are assigned a research paper.

Class IV is a one-day seminar that includes student presentation of research papers and advanced special topics; students may choose instead an optional phone interview/presentation. A certificate is awarded upon completion of Class IV.

Admission Requirements

Class I is open to students wishing to care for themselves and their families, retail business owners and their employees, those desiring general basic knowledge of aromatherapy, as well as those pursuing certification and integration of aromatherapy into their aesthetic or health care practice. Each class builds upon the foundation of knowledge given in the previous class, and must be taken sequentially.

Tuition and Fees

Tuition is $275 for Class I; $275 for Class II; $275 for Class III; and $150 for Class IV.

Financial Assistance

Scholarships may be awarded; prepayment discounts are available.

Hellerwork International

406 Berry Street
Mount Shasta, California 96067
PHONE: (530) 926-2500 / (800) 392-3900
FAX: (530) 926-6839
E-MAIL: Hellerwork@aol.com
WEBSITE: www.hellerwork.com

Hellerwork, created by Joseph Heller in 1979, is a discipline that includes bodywork, movement, and dialogue as a step in developing consciousness. Like Rolfing, the massage component of Hellerwork focuses on the connective tissue, or fascia, and attempts to correct body misalignment by releasing tension in the fascia. Today there are over 300 certified Hellerwork practitioners in twenty-nine states and seven foreign countries. Training is offered by practitioners located throughout the United States (including Hawaii), as well as Europe, Japan, and New Zealand.

Program Description

The Hellerwork Practitioner Training is a 1,250-hour certification program. The curriculum is the same for every training

although the format may vary. The curriculum includes Human Evolution and Gravity, Introduction to Body Systems, Applied Human Anatomy and Physiology, Myofascial Anatomy, Principles and Techniques of Structural Bodywork, Gross Anatomy Lab, Structural and Functional Assessment, Deep Tissue Bodywork Practicum, Body Awareness and Movement Lab, Psycho-Somatic Movement Analysis, Hellerwork Movement and Practicum, Communicating Movement Lessons, Ergonomics, Introduction to Psychological Inquiry, Fundamentals of Dialogue, Intra/Interpersonal Communications, Client Development, Business Standards/Ethics, and Marketing Your Practice.

Special training is offered for the health care professional.

Admission Requirements

Applicants must be at least 21 years of age, have a high school diploma or equivalent, have received the Hellerwork series, interview with the director of the chosen training, and complete any educational prerequisites required for the chosen training.

Tuition and Fees

Tuition is approximately $12,995, but varies with location.

Financial Assistance

A payment plan is available.

Institute of Integrative Aromatherapy

WEBSITE: www.integratedaroma.com

WEST COAST HEADQUARTERS:
P.O. Box 18
Issaquah, Washington 98027
PHONE: (877) FMEDICA
FAX: (425) 557-0805
E-MAIL: floramed@aol.com
WEBSITE: www.aroma-m.com

MIDWEST HEADQUARTERS:
1750 30th Street, # 333
Boulder, Colorado 80301
PHONE: (888) 282-2002
E-MAIL: laraink9@idt.net

The Institute of Integrative Aromatherapy was founded in May 1998 by Valerie Cooksley, R.N., and Laraine Kyle, R.N., M.S., C.M.T. Courses are held regularly in Bellevue, Washington, and Boulder, Colorado, and may be scheduled at other locations throughout the United States. There are two instructors, with an average of six to twelve students per class.

Accreditation and Approvals

The course offered by the Institute of Integrative Aromatherapy has been approved for 156 contact hours of continuing education by the American Holistic Nursing Association, which is an approver of continuing education in Nursing by the American Nursing Center's Commission on Accreditation.

Program Description

The Integrative Aromatherapy Program is taught in five two-day trainings. The course includes an in-depth study of a minimum of fifty essential oils. Topics covered include Holism in Health Care; History; Extraction Methods; Safety and Precautions; Beginning Botany and Chemistry; Blending Theories and Practicum; Methods of Application; Carriers for First Aid and Skin Care; Essential Oil Applications for Women's Care, Pain Relief, Lymphatic System, Endocrine and Nervous Systems, and more; Comfort Touch Techniques; Case Study Presentations; Monographs on Unusual Essential Oils; Aromatherapy Protocol Design; Research Reviewed; Professional Issues; and more. Completion of the course requires attendance at all trainings, satisfactory completion of twenty case studies, the construction of two Aromatherapy Protocols for a specific focus, a ten-page theme paper, and two detailed essential oil monographs on an unusual essential oil.

Admission Requirements

The program is open both to health professionals wanting to integrate the use of aromatic extracts in their healing work, as well as individuals who desire to practice integrative aromatherapy safely for their family.

Tuition and Fees

Tuition and materials is $250 for each two-day training.

Integrative Yoga Therapy

1207 Lincoln Avenue
Galena, Illinois 60136
PHONE: (815) 777-6629
E-MAIL: iyt@yogatherapy.com
WEBSITE: www.yogatherapy.com

Founded in 1992, Integrative Yoga Therapy (IYT) blends timeless yoga techniques with the concepts of mind-body health. The two-week residential program is offered in a variety of locations, including California, Massachusetts, England, Brazil, New Zealand, and Argentina. Classes have an average of thirty students (maximum forty).

Program Description

The Integrative Yoga Therapy Training Program consists of a two-week residential program followed by a four-month internship and home study course. In the residential program, students work in small groups with a personal mentor who will continue to guide them during the internship phase. The internship includes teaching the eight-week IYT yoga program, completing eight individual sessions, studying the IYT manual, and completing the accompanying workbook.

The main areas of study are the Art and Science of Yoga, Understanding the Mind-Body Connection, and Awakening the Spirit of Yoga. Students become certified teachers of the IYT Yoga and Stress Management Program, learn a methodology for one-on-one yoga therapy sessions, gain an understanding of the traditional psychology of yoga, explore the field of mind-body health, study key yoga postures in depth and understand how the asanas work with the mind and emotions, learn guided imagery techniques and a variety of deep relaxation techniques, learn the relationship between yoga and Ayurveda, and more.

Admission Requirements

Applicants must submit an application and have prior yoga experience.

Tuition and Fees

Tuition and fees vary with location and accommodations, ranging from $2,200 to $2,800. This includes tuition, accommodations, vegetarian meals, training manual, workbook, and personal supervision for the four-month internship/home study.

International Alliance of Healthcare Educators®

11211 Prosperity Farms Road, Suite D-325
Palm Beach Gardens, Florida 33410-3487
PHONE: (561) 622-4334 / (800) 311-9204
FAX: (561) 622-4771
E-MAIL: iahe@iahe.com
WEBSITE: www.iahe.com

The International Alliance of Healthcare Educators (IAHE) is a coalition of health care educators dedicated to the advancement of progressive therapeutic modalities. The alliance shares the staff expertise and established resources of the Upledger Institute, an educational, clinical, and research center founded in 1985 by John E. Upledger, D.O., O.M.M., who developed CranioSacral Therapy more than twenty-five years ago. Workshops are held throughout the United States, Canada, Europe, the Far East, and the Caribbean. There are 161 instructors, with an average of twenty-five to thirty students in hands-on workshops. IAHE also sells educational tapes and related products (see page 487).

Accreditation and Approvals

Practitioners use workshops to fulfill continuing education requirements for a variety of different professions. Participants are advised to consult their professional state board prior to registration.

Program Description

IAHE offers continuing education workshops to health care providers such as physical, occupational, and massage therapists, osteopathic physicians, chiropractors, M.D.s, nurses, and others.

Three-, four-, and five-day workshops are offered through IAHE in such areas as Upledger CranioSacral Therapy®, SomatoEmotional Release®, Visceral Manipulation, Zero Balancing, Process Acupressure, Mechanical Link, Trauma Release Therapy, Energy Integration, Fascial Mobilization, Lymph Drainage Therapy, and Therapeutic Imagery and Dialogue.

CranioSacral Therapy certification is offered at two levels.

Certification in CranioSacral Therapy Techniques is offered after completion of the four-day CranioSacral Therapy I and II courses and successful testing. In these courses, students explore the anatomy and physiology of the craniosacral system, develop light-touch palpation skills and fascial release techniques, learn to evaluate and treat cranial-base dysfunction, and more.

CranioSacral Therapy Diplomate Certification is offered after completion of CranioSacral Therapy I and II, Somato-Emotional Release I and II (each four days in length), the five-day Advanced I CranioSacral Therapy Course, and successful testing. In the SomatoEmotional Release classes, students learn to integrate hands-on techniques with verbal dialoguing, help the patient identify and expel negative emotional experiences, participate in class exercises designed to strengthen the relationship between the conscious and nonconscious mind, and more. The Advanced I CranioSacral Therapy Course is an in-depth experience for the serious practitioner, in which students observe and participate in therapy sessions.

Admission Requirements

In most cases, workshop admission requires participants to hold a current health care license or certificate, or to be enrolled in an educational program granting licensure or certification.

Tuition and Fees

Tuition varies by course and ranges from $350 to $1,500.

Financial Assistance

A discount is given to documented full-time health care students.

International Ayurvedic Institute

111 Elm Street, Suites 103-105
Worcester, Massachusetts 01609
PHONE: (508) 755-3744
FAX: (508) 770-0618
E-MAIL: ayurveda@hotmail.com

The International Ayurvedic Institute (formerly the New England Institute of Ayurvedic Medicine) was founded in 1994 by

Dr. Abbas Qutab and is affiliated with Westbrook University (distance education). There are six faculty members with a maximum of fifty students per class. Classes are offered in Worcester and Boston, Massachusetts; Phoenix, Arizona; Detroit, Michigan; and Washington, D.C.

Accreditation and Approvals
The institute is in the process of applying for accreditation; contact the institute for details.

Program Description
The 500-hour Diploma Course in Ayurvedic Health Sciences includes 117 hours of classroom instruction and clinical training in seminar format and 383 hours of the Independent Guided Study Program. Courses include Ayurvedic Anatomy and Physiology, Etiology and Pathology of Disease, Ayurvedic Nutrition/Dietary Therapy, PanchaKarma/Ayurvedic Massage, Ayurvedic Herbology and Clinical Case Management, and Advanced Pulse Diagnosis and Clinical Evaluation.

Admission Requirements
Applications are accepted from both graduate and nongraduate applicants. Applications must be made in the form of a letter or request to the administration office. Nondegree candidates will need to submit three letters of recommendation.

Tuition and Fees
Tuition is $4,200 plus an additional $90 to $150 for books.

Financial Assistance
Early payment discount of 5 percent and payment plans for those with demonstrated financial hardship are available.

International Institute of Reflexology

5650 First Avenue North
P.O. Box 12642
St. Petersburg, Florida 33733
PHONE: (727) 343-4811
FAX: (727) 381-2807
E-MAIL: ftreflex@concentric.net
WEBSITE: www.reflexology-usa.net

Foot reflexology was originally developed by the late Eunice Ingham, whose nephew is president of the International Institute of Reflexology (IIR). The institute serves as both a professional organization and an educational institution, as it offers a worldwide referral service, educational seminars, certification programs, and advanced training.

Accreditation and Approvals
The program at IIR is approved for continuing education credits by the Florida Board of Massage, Florida and California Nurses boards, and the National Certification Board for Therapeutic Massage and Bodywork (NCBTMB).

Program Description
Two-day seminars are offered throughout the United States and Canada to both professionals and laypersons. Seminars include lecture and practical, film graphics, and charts.

A certification exam may be taken by those who have attended at least two full two-day seminars and have completed one year of practice after the first seminar. The exam includes both written and practical components.

Tuition and Fees
Two-day seminars cost $295, or $110 for former students. The certification exam costs $180.

International Veterinary Acupuncture Society

P.O. Box 1478
Longmont, Colorado 80502-1478
PHONE: (303) 682-1167
FAX: (303) 682-1168
E-MAIL: ivasoffice@aol.com

The International Veterinary Acupuncture Society was founded in 1974 as a nonprofit educational organization. Class locations may vary. The 1999–2000 course will be held in San Diego, California.

Accreditation and Approvals
The veterinary acupuncture course qualifies for sixty hours of continuing education credits for 1999 and sixty hours for 2000.

Program Description

A 120+-hour course, divided into four sessions, in basic veterinary acupuncture is offered to licensed graduate veterinarians. The course covers small and large animal acupuncture equally, as well as TCM and scientific aspects of acupuncture. Session One provides a basic understanding of TCM principles, their relationship to Western medicine, and the fundamentals of needling technique. Session Two provides a working knowledge of TCM diagnostic approaches and small animal and equine acupuncture. Session Three integrates the diagnostic and treatment regimens, and Session Four enables attendees to incorporate the basic knowledge of acupuncture into clinical practice.

Topics covered include the Meridian Pathways, Fundamental Substances, Zang-Fu Organs, Causes of Disease, Special Action Points, Acupuncture Points and Meridians, the Circadian Clock, the Five Phases (Elements), the Eight Principles, Zang-Fu Pathology, Bi Syndrome, TCM, Points and Clinical Applications, Empirical Point Use and TCM Applications, Small Animal and Large Animal Western Acupuncture, Neurophysiology, Applied Neurology, Incorporating Acupuncture into Your Practice, Legal Aspects, Dealing with Failures, Electro-Acupuncture, History of Acupuncture, and practical laboratories.

Upon completion of the course, graduates are eligible to take the IVAS certification exam. Requirements for certification include being a licensed veterinarian in good standing; attendance at all four seminars; payment of the examination fee and passing scores on written and practical exams; submission and approval of the required case report; and forty hours spent with a certified member with approved case load or at IVAS-approved regional clinical workshops.

Admission Requirements

The course is open only to licensed graduate veterinarians.

Tuition and Fees

Tuition is $3,500 for all four sessions, including course notes, examination fees, and a one-year membership in IVAS.

International Yoga Studies

13833 South 31st Place
Phoenix, Arizona 85048

PHONE: (602) 759-1972
FAX: (602) 704-9656
E-MAIL: IYSUSA@aol.com

International Yoga Studies (IYS) was founded as a not-for-profit organization in 1994 by Sandra Summerfield Kozak and is based on the European Union of Yoga's four-year teacher training requirements. Workshops are held throughout the United States and Canada by many different instructors. Class sizes average twelve to forty students.

Program Description

The 500-hour IYS Teacher Certification Program is an "out-of-walls" adult education program that typically takes four years to complete. Requirements include nine hours of Foundation (Overview of Ancient Texts, Historical Overview, Outline of Yoga Theory, Basic Practices, and Self-Awareness and Personal Growth); 131 hours of Practical Knowledge (Asana, Pranayama, Meditation, Anatomy and Physiology, Developing Personal Practice, Applied Principles of Movement, and Mudras and Kriyas); 100 hours of General Theoretical Knowledge (Eastern History and Culture, Intro to Ayurveda, Samkhya Philosophy, Hatha Yoga Pradipika, The Main Paths, Bhagavad Gita, Holistic Health, Psychological Thought, Nutrition, and more); 100 hours Professional (Asana, Warm-up, Toning, Relaxation, Communication and Language Clarity, Yoga Therapy, Program and Class Design, Sanskrit, Ethics, The Art of Teaching, and Internship and Private Instruction); and 160 hours of Electives/Major Field of Study (Ayurveda, Yoga Philosophy, Energy Systems, Yoga Therapy, Vedic Studies, Sanskrit, Research, Meditation, Pranayama, Special Populations, Physiology, Yoga Psychology, Restorative Yoga, or Ancient Texts). The weekend workshops and four-day intensives make use of training weekends and workshops in the student's own locale; allow students to select a major field of study; receive credit at IYS for study or training programs around the world; and receive IYS credit for prior training and education. IYS has direct student contact through annual IYS four-day intensives and a mentoring process.

Admission Requirements

After two years of prior yoga training and completion of an IYS intensive, students may apply for the Teacher Certification Program. Applicants must submit a biography and letter of recommendation from their current yoga teacher.

Tuition and Fees
Tuition for the required four-day intensive is $396 to $468 per year; administrative tuition fee is $504 per year. Other fees include a $63 application fee; $504 induction process fee; and final exam and diploma fee, $252. Workshop fees, travel, accommodations, and supplies are additional.

Jin Shin Jyutsu®

8719 East San Alberto
Scottsdale, Arizona 85258
PHONE: (480) 998-9331
FAX: (480) 998-9335
WEBSITE: www.jinshinjyutsu.com

Jin Shin Jyutsu® physio-philosophy is an ancient art of harmonizing the body's life energy. The art was revived in the early 1900s by Master Jiro Murai in Japan and given to Mary Burmeister, who brought it to the United States in the 1950s. Jin Shin Jyutsu does not involve massage or manipulation; it is a gentle art in which the fingertips are placed (over clothing) on safety energy locks to harmonize and restore the energy flow. It can be applied as self-help or by a trained practitioner. Seminars are held throughout the world.

Accreditation and Approvals
The full basic seminar and the Now Know Myself seminar are approved for continuing education credits by the California Board of Registered Nursing and the National Certification Board for Therapeutic Massage and Bodywork (NCBTMB). The Instructor Training in Self-Help seminar is approved for continuing education units by the California Board of Registered Nursing.

Program Description
Each five-day basic seminar consists of two parts: Part I introduces the dynamic qualities of the twenty-six safety energy locks, the trinity flows, the concepts of depths within the body, and the physio-philosophy of Jin Shin Jyutsu, through lecture and hands-on application. Part II introduces the twelve organ flows, listening to pulses, the special body flows, and how these contribute to harmonizing body, mind, and spirit. Once a student has completed three full basic seminars, a certificate is issued signifying attainment of minimum practitioner-level training.

The five-day Now Know Myself Seminar further examines the wealth of information in Parts I and II. Participants experience "hands-on" daily as both practitioners and receivers.

The three-day Jin Shin Jyutsu Instructor Training in Self-Help (IT IS) is designed for those who wish to share self-help in a class setting or with friends. IT IS teaches how to present Jin Shin Jyutsu self-help confidently and in a clear and simple way.

Admission Requirements
For the Basic Seminars, Part I is a prerequisite for Part II. Applicants to the Now Know Myself Seminar must have completed the Basic Seminar three times. Applicants to the IT IS Seminar must have completed the Basic Seminar three times and have a basic knowledge of Mary Burmeister's self-help books.

Tuition and Fees
Tuition for Part I is $350 for new students and $180 for review students. Tuition for Part II is $250 for new students and $120 for review students. The Now Know Myself seminar is $600. The Instructor Training in Self-Help Seminar is $275 for new students and $150 for review students.

Kali Ray TriYoga®

P.O. Box 946
Malibu, California 90265
PHONE: (310) 589-0600
FAX: (310) 589-0783
E-MAIL: info@kaliraytriyoga.com
WEBSITE: www.kaliraytriyoga.com

The original Kali Ray TriYoga® Center was established in 1986. In 1997, a TriYoga teacher training center was opened in Santa Cruz, where there are fifteen instructors. Kali Ray founded the complete system of teachings known as TriYoga, a proven method of personal transformation. Classes are offered on a private, semiprivate, and group basis in Santa Cruz, and in Great Barrington, Massachusetts; retreats and programs are also offered in various locations both nationally and internationally.

Program Description

The Kali Ray TriYoga Teacher Training Program consists of teacher training weekend intensives, an internship program, and classes at the center or with a certified teacher. The training emphasizes understanding the postures; the connecting movements; and the sequencing of Kali Ray TriYoga Flows®. The TriYoga Flows are systematic sequences of postures synchronized with breath and mudra. One posture flows into another in a precise manner, with an emphasis on spinal wavelike movements. The sequences are systematized over seven levels, basic to advanced.

Practice teaching skills workshops and private instruction are integral to the training, and support those in the internship program who are working toward certification. Topics covered include practical anatomy, practice in speaking and teaching skills, sensitivity in alignment assistance, alignment practice, creating the class environment, and learning organizational aspects of creating classes. Other classes include Natural Alignment, Pranayama, Meditation, Mudra, Trinity Practice, Yoga Nidra, Vegetarian Nutrition, Sanskrit, Chanting, Kirtana, and Vedic Philosophy.

The Internship Program is designed to give guidance in preparation for teacher certification. Interns learn the TriYoga Flows, gain a thorough understanding of the method, and develop teaching skills through practice. The program may be personalized to fit individual needs.

A certification final is arranged after completion of certification requirements and with a teacher recommendation. The time required for certification varies with previous experience, ability, and time devoted to the program.

Admission Requirements

All students are welcome, from those who have no prior yoga experience to those who have been certified teachers for many years.

Tuition and Fees

Tuition for Teacher Training Weekend Intensives is in the range of $135 to $165; individual sessions range from $30 to $75. The Internship Program fee, recommended for those working toward certification, is $108 per level of certification.

The Michael Scholes School for Aromatic Studies

4218 Glencoe Avenue #4
Marina Del Ray, California 90292
PHONE: (310) 827-7737 / (800) 677-2368
FAX: (310) 827-6068
E-MAIL: mhscholes@aol.com

The Michael Scholes School for Aromatic Studies was founded in 1989 as a resource for essential oil education for both personal and professional use. Courses are held throughout the United States and Canada. There are three instructors, with twenty to thirty students per class. Home study courses are described on page 468. Books, videos, blending kits, and other products are also available; see page 466.

Program Description

A one-year Aromatherapy diploma course (held in Los Angeles, New York, and Calgary, Alberta) consists of ten weekends or sixty evening classes. The course focuses on the practical applications of over one hundred essential oils, forty perfume absolutes, and over twenty-five carriers, presented through live lectures and demonstrations, video review, essential oil comparison, slide presentations, and practical blending. Topics include History, Distillation, Safety and Toxicology, Chemistry, Botany, Blending, the Aromatic Consultation, Designing Treatments, Basic Anatomy and Physiology, Massage Demonstration, Reflexology, Case Study Review, Hands-On Treatment, Anatomy of Skin and Hair, Child Care and First Aid, Ritual Use, Subtle Energy, the Chakra System, Fragrance and the Mind, Business of Aromatherapy, and more. Classes may also be taken individually.

A five-day certification program (offered in Miami, Vancouver, New York, Los Angeles, and Atlanta) offers instruction in the Botanical Families Approach, the Chemistry of Essential Oil Constituents, Hippocratic Temperaments, Blending, Aromatherapy and Massage, Subtle Aromatherapy, Aromatherapy and Skin and Hair Care, Aromatherapy for Pregnancy and Child-Care Workshop, AromaFitness Workshop, Psycho-Aromatherapy, the Business of Aromatherapy, and Hands-On Application.

Other specialty courses, educational tours, and residential programs are offered.

Admission Requirements

Those wishing to enroll in the five-day certification program must have taken one of the home study courses or attended a live class and completed all course requirements.

Tuition and Fees

Tuition for the one-year diploma course is $2,300 to $2,700. Tuition for the five-day certification program is $575.

Financial Assistance

A payment plan and work-study are available.

Myofascial Release Treatment Centers and Seminars

222 West Lancaster Avenue
Paoli, Pennsylvania 19301
PHONE: (800) FASCIAL
FAX: (610) 644-1662
E-MAIL: fascia@erols.com
WEBSITE: www.vll.com/mfr/

Myofascial Release Treatment Centers and Seminars was founded in 1966. Physical therapist John F. Barnes originated the myofascial release approach and teaches all of the Myofascial Release I and II, Cervical-Thoracic, and Myofascial Unwinding Seminars. There is one instructor for every fifteen to twenty students. Seminars are held throughout the country.

Accreditation and Approvals

Myofascial Release Seminars are approved for continuing education credits by many organizations, including the California Board of Registered Nursing, the National Certification Board for Therapeutic Massage and Bodywork (NCBTMB), several state boards of massage therapy, physical therapy associations, occupational therapy boards, and others.

Program Description

Myofascial Release I is a twenty-hour, hands-on introductory course that includes instruction in Anatomy of Fascia and Related Structures, Whole-Body Inter-Relationships, Development of Palpation Skills, Myofascial Release Techniques, and

Craniosacral Therapy. This is a prerequisite for more advanced seminars.

The twenty-hour Cervical-Thoracic Myofascial/Osseous Release Seminar covers specific myofascial release, joint mobilization, and muscle energy techniques for the thoracic-lumbar region, sternum, rib cage, thoracic spine, and other areas.

The twenty-hour Fascial-Pelvis Myofascial/Osseous Release Seminar covers specific myofascial release, joint mobilization, and muscle energy techniques for the erector spinae, pelvic floor, lumbar area, sacroiliac joints, lower extremities, and other areas.

The twenty-hour Myofascial Unwinding Seminar teaches an effective movement facilitation technique utilized to decrease pain, increase range of motion, eliminate subconscious holding or bracing patterns, and more.

In the twenty-hour Myofascial Release II Seminar, students learn advanced myofascial release techniques and cranial procedures.

Twelve-hour introductory workshops include a Myofascial Mobilization Workshop that introduces myofascial release for upper and lower extremities, cervical, thoracic, and lumbar areas; and Pediatric Myofascial Release, in which myofascial release is presented for the evaluation and treatment of head injuries, cerebral palsy, birth trauma, scoliosis, pain, headaches, and more.

Admission Requirements

Applicants must be licensed to touch, i.e., as a physical therapist, physical therapy assistant, occupational therapist, occupational therapy assistant, massage therapist, athletic trainer, or speech and language therapist.

Tuition and Fees

Tuition for the Myofascial Release I, Fascial Pelvis Myofascial/Osseous Integration, Cervical Thoracic Myofascial/Osseous Integration, Myofascial Unwinding, and Myofascial Release II Seminars is $650 per seminar, $595 if registered two weeks prior to seminar date. Tuition for the Myofascial Mobilization Workshop and Pediatric Myofascial Release Workshop is $400 per seminar, $350 if registered two weeks prior to seminar date. Fees include workbook and materials.

New England School of Homeopathy

356 Middle Street
Amherst, Massachusetts 01002
PHONE: (413) 256-5949
FAX: (413) 256-6223
E-MAIL: herscu@nesh.com
WEBSITE: www.nesh.com

The New England School of Homeopathy (NESH) was founded in 1987 by Dr. Paul Herscu, N.D., D.H.A.N.P., and Dr. Amy Rothenberg, N.D., D.H.A.N.P. Most courses are held in the Northeast. There are four instructors, with an average of twenty-five to thirty students per class.

Accreditation and Approvals
Accreditation is pending.

Program Description
NESH has provided training in classical homeopathy for over 2,000 students in the United States and abroad. Courses are designed to educate the beginner and to enhance and broaden the practicing homeopath's knowledge so that consistent, favorable results are delivered.

A Post Graduate Course in Homeopathy is a two-year course designed for the licensed medical practitioner. The goal of the course is to enhance the practitioner's ability through an in-depth study of philosophy, case taking, case analysis, materia medica, and the repertory. Beginners to homeopathy will be required to complete Practical Applications: The Pivotal Points of Chronic Prescribing (a twenty-four-hour video class) or the equivalent prior to or concurrently with the Post Graduate class. The class will meet in western Massachusetts every third month for four days over a period of two years, beginning in February 1999. Videotaped lectures will be used for distance learning between sessions and all students will be required to be on-line for class discussions and support.

The Professional Homeopathy Course is a three-year class for those who wish to become professional homeopaths but do not currently have a medical degree. The emphasis is on using the Herscu method of understanding homeopathy through the study of the cycles each remedy presents and the segments that run through the cycle. Also included are case taking, case analysis, materia medica, and study of the repertory. The class began in September 1997 (students may join this class with permission of the instructors); a new section will begin in 2000.

An Introduction to Homeopathy is a comprehensive thirty-six-hour audiocassette series on introductory homeopathy. Topics covered include What Is Homeopathy?, Common Vocabulary, Introductory Philosophy, Repertory and Materia Medica, First Aid, and Acute Prescribing.

Admission Requirements
The NESH student body includes a wide range of health care practitioners, from medical, osteopathic, and naturopathic doctors to nurses, acupuncturists, chiropractors, psychologists, and nondoctor professional homeopaths. NESH also welcomes interested laypeople at every level, from beginners to experienced practitioners. Applicants must submit a completed application form.

Tuition and Fees
Tuition ranges from $500 to $3,800, depending on the length of the course.

Financial Assistance
A payment plan is available.

New Hampshire Institute for Therapeutic Arts

153 Lowell Road
Hudson, New Hampshire 03051
PHONE: (603) 882-3022
FAX: (603) 598-9101

MAINE LOCATION:
39 Main Street
Bridgton, Maine 04009
PHONE: (207) 647-3794

The New Hampshire Institute for Therapeutic Arts (NHITA) was founded in 1983. The institute in Hudson, New Hampshire, shares space and clinical facilities with the Merrimack Valley

Integral Health Center. The Bridgton, Maine, facility also serves as a clinic for massage therapy and natural therapeutics.

Accreditation and Approvals

The massage therapy program at NHITA is a candidate for accreditation with the Commission on Massage Training Accreditation (COMTA), and meets licensing requirements for the states of Maine and New Hampshire. Graduates are qualified to take the National Certification Examination for Therapeutic Massage and Bodywork (NCETMB). NHITA is approved by the National Certification Board for Therapeutic Massage and Bodywork (NCBTMB) as a continuing education provider.

Program Description

The nine-month, 750-hour massage therapy program includes courses in Embryology; First Aid, CPR, and Emergency Procedures; Anatomy and Physiology; Swedish Massage; Ethics and Professionalism; Reflexology; Reflex and Pressure Point Therapies; Public Health and Hygiene; Pathology; Hydrotherapy; Neuromuscular Technique; Human Sexuality; Nutrition; Neurology; Circulatory Massage; Lymphatic Drainage Massage; Eastern Techniques; Sports Massage; Polarity; and Health Service Management, as well as a research report, research presentation, and massage practicum.

Admission Requirements

Applicants must be at least 18 years of age, have a high school diploma or equivalent, and interview with an admissions representative.

Tuition and Fees

Tuition is $6,000. Additional expenses include a $35 application fee; books, approximately $300; massage table, approximately $500; and oils and linens, approximately $125.

Financial Assistance

A payment plan is available; NHITA is approved by the Canadian Department of Educaiton for financial aid.

Nurturing the Mother

8703 Rollingwood Road
Chapel Hill, North Carolina 27516

PHONE: (919) 929-4253 / (919) 933-5562
E-MAIL: wandasund@aol.com
            clairmar@bellsouth.net

Taught by Claire Marie Miller and Wanda Sundermann, Nurturing the Mother workshops were first offered in 1990. The teaching staff is expanding to six instructors, with an average of fourteen to twenty students per class. Workshops are held at various locations throughout the United States.

Accreditation and Approvals

Nurturing the Mother is approved by the National Certification Board for Therapeutic Massage and Bodywork (NCBTMB) as a continuing education provider (twenty-eight CEUs).

Program Description

The thirty-two-hour Nurturing the Mother certification workshop is a body/mind/spirit approach to pre- and perinatal massage. Workshops run Thursday evening through Sunday and cover Preconception Massage, Pregnancy Massage, Support for Labor and Delivery, Postpartum Massage, and Infant Massage.

Admission Requirements

The program is recommended for massage therapists, childbirth educators, labor assistants, midwives, labor and delivery nurses, and anyone who desires a deeper knowledge of birth and massage.

Tuition and Fees

Tuition varies with location, but is typically $535 to $600 including manual (meals and lodging additional at some locations).

Financial Assistance

Discount for advance registration and for sign-up with a friend; payment plans may be available to those with demonstrated need.

Ohashi Institute

12 West 27th Street
New York, New York 10001

PHONE: (800) 810-4190
FAX: (212) 447-5819
E-MAIL: ohashiinst@aol.com
WEBSITE: www.ohashi.com

The Ohashi Institute was founded in 1974 by Ohashi, a Japanese healer who created a program of bodywork, Ohashiatsu®, that incorporates Eastern healing philosophy, natural movement, and touch techniques to balance body, mind, and spirit. Ohashiatsu focuses on the giver's health, consciousness, and well-being, and maintains and improves the giver's posture and movement. The Ohashiatsu curriculum is taught in more than thirty locations around the world. There are an average of fourteen students per class.

Program Description
The 300-hour Ohashiatsu Program consists of nine required courses: Beginning Ohashiatsu I and II, Anatomy I and II for Ohashiatsu, Oriental Diagnosis, Intermediate Ohashiatsu I and II, and Advanced Ohashiatsu I and II. In addition, students are required to attend a minimum of twenty practice classes and receive ten private sessions from four or more Certified Ohashiatsu Instructors or Consultants.

Continuing Education
Postgraduate education is offered through the Instructor Training Program or the Consultant Program.

Instructor training takes twelve to eighteen months to complete and prepares the instructor to teach Beginning I and II levels. The course includes conducting practice classes, assisting Certified Ohashiatsu Instructors during four courses, and confirming teaching techniques through tutorials.

The Consultant Program allows graduates to continue their education and to use the Ohashiatsu trade name in developing their clientele. This entails continuing education, annual training, and tutorials.

Admission Requirements
Applicants need only have an open mind and a willingness to learn; there is no minimum age or educational requirement.

Tuition and Fees
Students proceed at their own pace and pay for each course individually.

The Beginning I course costs $395. Ohashi's Beginning I course taught by Ohashi costs $485. The Beginning II course costs $450. The Intermediate I course costs $525. The Intermediate II course costs $625. The Advanced I course costs $795. The Advanced II course costs $910. The Oriental Diagnosis course costs $395. The Anatomy I and II courses cost $340.

Additional expenses include: three tutorials, $65 each; Advanced II tutorial, $150; Advanced II practical exam fee, $150; private sessions, $65; certificate of completion, $30; and required texts.

Financial Assistance
A work-study program is available. A $30 discount is offered for early registration, and a $60 discount for same-semester registration.

Pacific College of Oriental Medicine

E-MAIL: jmiller@ormed.edu
WEBSITE: www.ormed.edu

SAN DIEGO CAMPUS:
7445 Mission Valley Road, Suite 105
San Diego, California 92108-4408
PHONE: (619) 574-6909 / (800) 729-0941
FAX: (619) 574-6641

NEW YORK CAMPUS:
915 Broadway, Third Floor
New York, New York 10010
PHONE: (212) 982-3456 / (800) 729-3468
FAX: (212) 982-6514

The Pacific College of Oriental Medicine was founded by Joseph Lazzaro, Ana de Vedia, Alex Tiberi, and Richard Gold. The Pacific College of Oriental Medicine, San Diego, was founded in 1986 and has fifty faculty members; the Pacific College of Oriental Medicine, New York, was founded in 1993 and has thirty faculty members. Class sizes at both campuses average about thirty-five students. The college has recently added a third branch in Chicago; call for details.

Accreditation and Approvals
The Master of Traditional Oriental Medicine degree (offered in San Diego), Master of Science in Oriental Medicine and the

Master of Science in Acupuncture (offered in New York) are accredited by the Accreditation Commission for Acupuncture and Oriental Medicine (ACAOM). Both campuses are approved by the California Acupuncture Committee, a division of the state medical board. Graduates of the Master of Traditional Oriental Medicine and Master of Science in Oriental Medicine Programs are eligible to take the State of California Acupuncture Licensing Examination. Graduates of all three programs are eligible to take the national certification exam given by the National Commission for the Certification of Acupuncturists (NCCA) and/or any acupuncture licensing exam required by New York.

Program Description

The 3,349-hour Master of Science in Traditional Medicine (San Diego and Chicago) and Master of Science in Oriental Medicine (New York) Programs may be completed in a 3.6-year track or in four years or longer. Course requirements include Oriental Medicine, Acupuncture Points, Herbology, Anatomy, Tui Na, Tai Chi Chuan, Clinical Techniques, Introduction to Orthopedic and Neurological Evaluation, Biophysics, CPR, Needle Techniques, Ethics/Philosophy, Pathophysiology, Biochemistry, Clinical Herbs, Clinical Science, Pharmacology, Biology, Diagnosis/ Evaluation, Physical Exam, Eastern Nutrition, Qigong, and others.

Students in the 2,586-hour Master of Science in Acupuncture Program (New York) may complete it in 3.3 years, depending on student ability and class availability. Courses include many of those required in the four-year programs.

The San Diego campus also offers several programs of instruction in massage.

The 133-hour Massage Technician Program includes classes Circulatory Massage, Public Safety and Hygiene, Business Management and Ethics, Anatomy, and Tui Na Hand Techniques. An accelerated program may be completed in three weeks.

The 500-hour Massage Therapist Certificate Program includes those classes listed under the Massage Technician Program plus Oriental Medicine, Acupuncture Points, East-West Deep Tissue, Tui Na Structural Techniques, CPR/First Aid, Jin Shin, Qigong, Thai Massage, Shiatsu Massage, electives, and supervised massage practice. The program generally takes three trimesters to complete.

The 1,000-hour Holistic Health Practitioner Program includes those classes listed under the Massage Therapists Certificate Program plus Tai Chi Chuan, Clinical Tui Na, Seitai Shiatsu, Alexander Technique, Clinical Counseling, Pediatric Tui Na, Sports Tui Na, Eastern Nutrition, Western Nutrition, and supervised massage practice. The program generally takes five to six trimesters to complete; graduates may apply to the city of San Diego for licensing as a Holistic Health Practitioner.

Students may also take a combination of courses that lead to certificates in Tui Na, Chinese Health and Exercise, or an Oriental Body Therapist Certificate that meets the curriculum standards of the American Oriental Bodywork Therapy Association (AOBTA).

Admission Requirements

For the Master of Traditional Oriental Medicine, Master of Science in Oriental Medicine, and Master of Science in Acupuncture, applicants must have completed at least sixty semester units (two years) at the baccalaureate level or equivalent. Applicants must also submit a personal essay, interview with the admissions committee, and be able to communicate in English.

Tuition and Fees

There is a $50 application fee and a $20 registration fee for each trimester.

In California, tuition for the Master of Traditional Oriental Medicine Program is $31,520 plus fees, CPR, and supplies (estimated at $2,431). Tuition for the Massage Technician Program is $800, plus fees and supplies (estimated at $100). Tuition for the Massage Therapist Program is $4,480 plus fees, supplies (estimated at $175), CPR and First Aid. Tuition for the Holistic Health Practitioner Program is $10,300 plus fees, supplies (estimated at $350), CPR, and First Aid.

In New York, tuition for the Master of Science in Oriental Medicine Program is $36,445 plus fees, CPR, and supplies (estimated at $2,628). Tuition for the Master of Science in Acupuncture Program is $37,500 plus fees, CPR, and supplies (estimated at $1,681).

Financial Assistance

Federal grants and loans are available to eligible acupuncture/traditional Oriental medicine students who are enrolled on at least a half-time basis.

Pacific Institute of Aromatherapy

P.O. Box 6723
San Rafael, California 94903
PHONE: (415) 479-9121
FAX: (415) 479-0119

In addition to their correspondence program (see page 469), Pacific Institute of Aromatherapy offers certification seminars in a variety of locations including New York, Chicago, Los Angeles, San Francisco, Toronto, and others.

Program Description
The three-day Progress in Aromatherapy Seminar is taught by Kurt Schnaubelt and Carole Addison. Topics covered include How and Why Oils Work, Essential Oils, Chemistry and Pharmacology, Self Medication with Essential Oils, Essential Oils for the Skin, and The Psychology of Fragrance.

Tuition and Fees
Tuition is $495.

Phoenix Rising Yoga Therapy

P.O. Box 819
402 Park Street, 2nd Floor
Housatonic, Massachusetts 01236
PHONE: (413) 274-3515 / (800) 288-9642
FAX: (413) 274-6166
E-MAIL: moreinfo@pryt.com
WEBSITE: www.pryt.com

Phoenix Rising Yoga Therapy was founded in 1986 by Michael Lee, who holds a master's degree in holistic education and has directed programs at the Kripalu Center for Yoga and Health. The school currently holds training in Lenox, Massachusetts; Santa Barbara, California; Columbia, Maryland; Gainsville, Florida; and Canada, and has offered programs in Canada, Pennsylvania, Oregon, Georgia, Arizona, the state of Washington, and Washington, D.C. There are three instructors, with an average of twenty-five students per class.

Accreditation and Approvals
Phoenix Rising Yoga Therapy is an approved provider with the National Board of Certified Counselors (NBCC). CEU credits are available for some nursing associations.

Program Description
Professional Certification Training courses are offered at three levels.

Level 1 consists of thirty-two hours of instruction focusing on the principles and practice of Phoenix Rising Yoga Therapy. Students learn techniques for assisting clients in yoga therapy postures, precautions, physical benefits, counterpostures, how to guide clients in a body scan to determine areas of tension, and general outlines for yoga therapy sessions.

Level 2 consists of forty-two hours and focuses on therapeutic dialogue techniques, including listening, following, questioning, and responding techniques, as well as how to use the yoga therapy session as part of a transformational life process.

Level 3 takes the form of an internship/practicum. It requires forty-eight practice sessions, attendance at two week-long residentials focusing on refinement of skills, a presentation of the student's work, selected readings, exchange sessions with peers, and attendance at practice days in the student's area. Work is spread over six months (600 hours).

Admission Requirements
Level 1 is open to those who have been practicing any traditional style of yoga regularly for at least three months, or who have been engaged in another body-oriented discipline. Level 1 is a prerequisite for Level 2, and Level 2 is a prerequisite for Level 3.

Tuition and Fees
Tuition for Level 1 is $545; for Level 2, $680; and for Level 3, $2,850.

Financial Assistance
Payment plans are available.

Polarity Realization Institute

126 High Street
Ipswich, Massachusetts 01938-1248
PHONE: (978) 356-0980 (Ipswich) / (508) 747-4333 (Plymouth) / (207) 828-8622 (Portland)
WEBSITE: www.polarity-therapy.com

The Polarity Realization Institute, founded in 1980, supports and promotes higher levels of self-healing and self-realization through honoring the life force with love, respect, and integrity. Programs are currently offered in Ipswich and Plymouth, Massachusetts, and Portland, Maine.

Accreditation and Approvals

Programs at the Polarity Realization Institute are accredited by the Integrative Massage and Somatic Therapies Accreditation Council (IMSTAC) and approved by the American Polarity Therapy Association (APTA). The massage trainings of 600 hours or more qualify students to take the National Certification Examination for Therapeutic Massage and Bodywork (NCETMB). The 880-hour Holistic Massage and Bodywork Program meets the New Hampshire licensing exam eligibility requirements. The institute is licensed by the Commonwealth of Massachusetts Department of Education and by the State of Maine Department of Education.

Program Description

The 650-hour Polarity Realization Certification Program is divided into two levels: a 160-hour Level 1 training and an additional 490-hour Level 2 training. The levels may be taken together or individually, and may be completed in eighteen months or longer.

Level 1 prepares students to receive the Associate Polarity Practitioner (A.P.P.) level of recognition from APTA. Students are guided toward an understanding of healing energies and polarity principles and assisted with personal healing and professional needs, with an emphasis on reaching higher levels of clarity, harmony, and inner peace. Additional requirements include thirty documented student practice sessions, five sessions received from professional polarity practitioners, and five additional outside study hours.

Level 2 prepares students to receive Registered Polarity Practitioner (R.P.P.) registration from APTA. There are nine components to this training: Polarity Systems Work (176 hours); Polarity Yoga and Nutrition (forty-eight hours); Anatomy and Physiology (forty-eight hours); Business Skills (thirty-two hours); Raising Your Sublime Energies (fifteen hours); Lifestyle Commitment; Outside Work (100 sessions given, ten sessions received, and First Aid/CPR); Internship (forty hours); and Clinical Supervision (twenty-four hours).

Holistic Massage and Bodywork Programs are offered in lengths of 180, 600, and 880 hours. The 180-hour Therapeutic Massage Program requires Module 1—Therapeutic Massage and Basic Anatomy and Physiology. The 600-hour Holistic Massage and Bodywork program requires Modules 1, 2A or 2B, 190 hours in Module 3, and Modules 4 and 5. The 880-hour Holistic Massage and Bodywork Program requires Modules 1, 2A, 438 hours in Module 3, and Modules 4 and 5.

Module 1—Therapeutic Massage consists of 180 hours: 96 hours of therapeutic massage, forty-eight hours of anatomy and physiology, thirty documented sessions (thirty hours), and six professional sessions received (six hours). Module 1 may be taken without continuing with other modules.

Module 2A—Polarity Realization Associate Certification consists of 160 hours: polarity realization therapy theory and bodywork (120 hours), thirty documented sessions given (thirty hours), five professional sessions received (five hours), and additional outside study (five hours).

Module 2B—Intermediate Therapeutic Massage consists of 160 hours: massage theory and bodywork (120 hours), thirty documented sessions given (thirty hours), five professional sessions received (five hours), and additional outside study (five hours).

Module 3 consists of 190 to 460 hours in advanced bodywork and massage electives that include clinics, hydrotherapy, business skills, and other topics.

Module 4 consists of fifty-six hours in advanced anatomy and physiology.

Module 5 consists of twenty-four hours in advanced Integration and evaluation.

RYSE (Realizing Your Sublime Energies) is the most advanced level training offered at the institute. Developed by Nancy Risley, R.P.P., this training teaches professionals how to be aware and in control of clearing their energies. The initial training consists of sixteen hours, with RYSE Practitioner Trainings of 120 hours for Level 1, 124 hours for Level 2, and 124 hours for Level 3. The RYSE Practitioner Training includes audio CDs of teaching supported by a crystal bowl sound track that clears the energies. Sessions may be done individually or in groups.

Programs may be taken on a full- or part-time basis.

Admission Requirements

Applicants must be at least 18 years of age, have a high school diploma or equivalent, and have a personal interview. Level 1 is a prerequisite for Level 2.

Tuition and Fees

Tuition for Polarity Level 1 is $1,425. Additional expenses include a $50 registration fee; five required sessions, $200 to $300; books and supplies, $80; and a massage table, $300 to $600.

Tuition for Level 2 is $4,560. Additional expenses include a $50 registration fee (waived for students going directly from Level 1 to Level 2); ten required sessions, $400 to $600; books and supplies, $80; and First Aid/CPR, $60.

Tuition for the 180-hour massage program is $1,710; for the 600-hour program, $5,985; and for the 880-hour program, $8,930. Additional costs include books and supplies, $110 to $160, and a massage table, $350 to $550. Outside sessions are additional. Modules and classes may be taken individually.

Tuition for RYSE is $400; for Practitioner Training Level 1, $1,535; Level 2, $2,200; and Level 3, $2,200.

Financial Assistance

Student loans and interest-free payment plans are available.

R. J. Buckle Associates, LLC

P.O. Box 868
Hunter, New York 12442
PHONE: (518) 263-4402
FAX: (518) 263-4031
E-MAIL: janebuckle001@aol.com
WEBSITE: www.rjbuckle.com

The Aromatherapy for Health Professionals Program was founded in 1995 by Jane Buckle, who then founded R. J. Buckle Associates, LLC. Classes are held throughout the United States. A home study program is also offered; see page 467.

Accreditation and Approvals

Each module earns sixteen CEUs through either the American Association of Critical Care Nurses AACN or the National Certification Board for Therapeutic Massage and Bodywork (NCBTMB).

Program Description

Aromatherapy for Health Professionals is a five-module clinically-based program in the use of essential oils developed for licensed health professionals. Topics covered include the composition and clinical use of thirty-three essential oils with reference to research, and the 'm' technique®, a registered method of touching patients where standard massage may be inappropriate. Certification follows successful completion of the written, oral, and practical exams.

Tuition and Fees

Tuition for each module and exam is $250 for AHNA (American Holistic Nurses Association) members, $275 for nonmembers.

The Rubenfeld Synergy Center

115 Waverly Place
New York, New York 10011
PHONE: (212) 254-5100
FAX: (212) 254-1174
E-MAIL: rubenfeld@aol.com

The Rubenfeld Synergy Center teaches a professional certification program in the Rubenfeld Synergy Method. Developed over thirty-five years ago by Ilana Rubenfeld, the Rubenfeld Synergy Method is a dynamic system for the integration of body, mind, emotions, and spirit that combines elements of bodymind teachers F. M. Alexander and Moshe Feldenkrais, the Perls' gestalt theory, and Erickson's hypnotherapy. This method uses verbal expression, movement, breathing, body posture and hands-on techniques to develop a "listening touch." There are over 300 certified Rubenfeld Synergists worldwide. The Training Program takes place in a variety of locations in the United States and Canada.

Program Description

The four-year, 1,660-hour professional Rubenfeld Synergy Training Certification Program meets for three seven-day modules over four years. The curriculum includes Rubenfeld Synergy Bodymind Exercises; Somatic Skill Building; Use of Touch and Movement; Somatic Skill Practicum; Theory, Technique and Art of a Rubenfeld Synergy Session; Rubenfeld Synergy Practicum; Principles of Humanistic Psychology; Ethics, Values and Professional Practice; Personal Rubenfeld Synergy Sessions; Practice and Model Clients; Regional Supervision; and Advisor/Advisee Contact. Certification hinges on evaluation by faculty and staff. Two days are added in the fourth year for certification.

Admission Requirements

Applicants must submit an application and two written references and participate in a workshop conducted by Ilana Rubenfeld.

Tuition and Fees

Tuition is $3,600 per year; additional expenses include a $50 application fee and a $275 charge in the fourth year for the two additional days.

Sage Femme Midwifery School

P.O. Box 91
O'Brien, Oregon 97534
PHONE: (800) BIRTHCARE
FAX: (541) 596-2543
E-MAIL: wisearth@cdsnet.net
WEBSITE: sagefemme.net

Sage Femme was founded in 1985 and has graduated more than 100 students. The school has one administrative office in O'Brien, Oregon, and several learning sites in different states; all sites offer the same curriculum. There are eight faculty members, with an average of seven students (maximum twelve) per class.

Accreditation and Approvals

Sage Femme has achieved pre-accreditation status with the Midwifery Education Accreditation Council (MEAC). Students may receive continuing education credits through the Oregon State Licensing Board, California Association of Midwives, and other selected institutions.

Program Description

The Midwifery curriculum consists of academics and clinical training; students may choose to take only the academics and acquire an apprenticeship separately.

First Year courses (26.3 credits) include Foundations, Natural Health and Nutrition, Alternative Care, Intuitive Development, Normal Pregnancy Care, Diagnostics and Lab, Complications of Pregnancy: Level One, Case Review, HIV/Public Health, Scientific Method, Medical Interface, Normal Labor and Birth, Assisting Skills, Complications of Labor and Birth: Level One, Postpartum, Current Issues, Field Trip, Normal Newborn, Lactation, Complications of Postpartum, Newborn Complications, Natural Care Alternatives, Research and Testing, Community Service, and Clinical Work Introduction.

Second Year courses (twenty-eight credits) include Skills, Biology/Chemistry, Intuitive Development, NARM Preparation, Well Woman Gynecology, Immunology, Epidemiology, Natural Nutrition, Counseling, Communication, Advanced Course Work, Professionalism, Case Review, New Mothers Practicum, Community Service, and Research Seminar.

Clinical Training in the first through third years includes prenatals observed and birth attendance, assist/observe at prenatals, primary prenatal management, assist/observe at births, primary birth management, primary postpartum management, and primary newborn exams.

Graduation requirements include completion of all course work; an evaluation in good standing by clinical preceptors; participating in fifty births, twenty-five as primary caregiver; and participating in one hundred prenatals and forty postpartum visits.

Admission Requirements

Applicants must have a high school diploma or equivalent and may be asked to submit an example of writing skills; reentry students or transfer students may be asked to take an entrance exam. Prospective applicants are encouraged to have attended at least three births as an observer or in some other capacity prior to admission.

Tuition and Fees

Tuition is $187 per credit hour. Additional expenses include a $25 application fee and materials fees of $100 the first year, $200 the second year.

Financial Assistance

Payment plans are available on an individual basis.

The School for Body-Mind Centering®

189 Pondview Drive
Amherst, Massachusetts 01002-3230
PHONE: (413) 256-8615
FAX: (413) 256-8239
E-MAIL: bmcschool@aol.com

Body-Mind Centering® is a system of movement reeducation and hands-on repatterning developed by Bonnie Bainbridge Cohen. It is an experiential study based on the embodiment and application of anatomical, physiological, and developmental principles, utilizing movement, breath, touch, voice, and awareness. There are twelve core faculty members; classes may be as large as seventy-five students, but occasionally break into supervision groups of ten students or less. Certification classes are taught in Amherst, Massachusetts, and Berkeley, California; shorter workshops are also offered in additional locations.

Program Description

The Body-Mind Centering Certification Programs are divided into two phases. In Phase 1, the emphasis is on the foundations and fundamentals of Body-Mind Centering. The courses and modules in this phase may be taken individually on a noncertification basis. Phase 2 is the certification phase and the focus is on a deeper personal understanding and embodiment through integration and application of the material. This phase is open only to students who have successfully completed Phase 1.

Material is presented in a modular format, with each module lasting approximately three weeks. Two courses are usually offered in each module. There are two modules per year in each program, and the whole certification program takes approximately three to three and one half years to complete.

Admission Requirements

The certification program is designed for those with some experience in the fields of movement, dance, bodywork, body-related psychotherapy, or other body-mind disciplines.

Tuition and Fees

The cost for Phase 1 is $2,395 per module and included five modules. The total cost for Phase 2 is $7,485 and includes three modules. Books and supplies are additional. Tuition varies for individual courses.

Financial Assistance

A $100 per module discount is given for early registration; a $250 per module discount is given for certification students in good standing.

School for Self-Healing

2218 48th Avenue
San Francisco, California 94116
PHONE: (415) 665-9574
FAX: (415) 665-1318
E-MAIL: school@self-healing.org
WEBSITE: www.self-healing.org

The School for Self-Healing, founded in 1984, offers training in San Francisco, throughout the United States, and in England, Brazil, and Israel; courses in the self-healing method are also sponsored by other organizations. Founder Meir Schneider, Ph.D., L.M.T., is the author of *Self-Healing: My Life and Vision* and coauthor of *The Handbook of Self-Healing: Your Personal Program for Better Health and Increased Vitality*. Though blind at birth, Schneider used his unique self-healing method to restore his vision. There are two instructors, with an average of twelve students per class.

Accreditation and Approvals

The School for Self-Healing is licensed by the State of California and is approved to offer continuing education credits to nurses. A Massage Practitioner Certificate is awarded upon successful completion of Segment B; this satisfies the requirements for a license in San Francisco.

Program Description

The Meir Schneider Self-Healing Method combines massage, movement, and other tools into powerful therapies that can strengthen vulnerable organ systems and reverse degenerative conditions.

The Self-Healing Practitioner/Educator training consists of Level One (Segments A and B), Level Two, and an apprenticeship. Segment A (Supporting Breathing, Circulation, Digestion, and the Spine and Joints) consists of eighty hours in eight consecutive days of beginning massage and movement. Segment B (Supporting Muscles, the Nervous System, and the Visual System) consists of eighty-four hours in eight and a half consecutive days of intermediate massage and movement and beginning vision improvement exercises. In Level Two: Professional Training (one hundred hours), students perform about forty hands-on sessions with clients and participate in evaluating many more; topics include advanced client evaluation and assessment, client-related pathology, exercise selection and invention, advanced discussion of self-healing principles, beginning client education, and more. In the apprenticeship, students spend 500 hours working directly under the supervision of Meir Schneider or another instructor, and self-healing principles and techniques are integrated into full practice.

Admission Requirements
Segment A applicants must have a high school diploma or equivalent and be able, in the opinion of the instructor, to complete the course work with the accommodations that the school is able to offer.

Tuition and Fees
Tuition for Segment A is $1,200, plus $99 for books and materials; tuition for Segment B is $1,100, plus $74 for books and materials; tuition for Level Two is $1,900; and tuition for the apprenticeship is $1,900. There is a $100 registration fee for each course; the total cost of the program is $6,673.

Financial Assistance
Payment plans are available; some discounts apply.

Southeastern School of Neuromuscular and Massage Therapy

WEBSITE: www.se-massage.com

JACKSONVILLE CAMPUS:
9088 Golfside Drive
Jacksonville, Florida 32256

PHONE: (904) 448-9499
FAX: (904) 448-9270

CHARLOTTE CAMPUS:
4 Woodlawn Green, Suite 200
Charlotte, North Carolina 28217
PHONE: (704) 527-4979
FAX: (704) 527-3104

CHARLESTON CAMPUS:
7410 Northside Drive, Suite 105
North Charleston, South Carolina 29420
PHONE: (803) 569-7444
FAX: (803) 569-7446

COLUMBIA CAMPUS:
3007 Broad River Road
Columbia, South Carolina 29210
PHONE: (803) 798-8800
FAX: (803) 798-0003

GREENVILLE CAMPUS:
850 South Pleasantberg Drive, Suite 105
Greenville, South Carolina 29607
PHONE: (864) 421-9481
FAX: (864) 421-9483

SPARTANBURG CAMPUS:
1000 North Pine Street
Suite 2B Pinewood Mall
Spartanburg, South Carolina 29303
PHONE: (864) 591-1134
FAX: (864) 582-7805
E-MAIL: Sesptg@aol.com

The Southeastern School of Neuromuscular and Massage Therapy was founded in 1992. President and director Kyle C. Wright also founded the Wright Center of Neuromuscular Therapy. There are twenty-five to thirty students per class and eight faculty members.

Accreditation and Approvals
The school is licensed by the Florida State Board of Independent Postsecondary Vocational, Technical, Trade, and Business Schools, Florida Department of Education. The curriculum is

approved by the Florida Department of Business and Professional Regulation Board of Massage. Graduates are qualified to take the National Certification Examination for Therapeutic Massage and Bodywork (NCETMB).

Program Description

The Master Program curriculum of over 500 hours includes Anatomy and Physiology I and II, Swedish Massage, Neuromuscular Therapy, Advanced Neuromuscular Therapy, Theory and Practice of Hydrotherapy, Practice Parameters, Allied Modalities (ninety-seven hours that may include Sports Massage, Craniosacral Therapy, Myofascial Release, Oriental Philosophy and Technique, Shiatsu, Flexibility/Movement/Therapy, Dynamic Structural Learning/Teaching, Corporate Chair Massage, Prenatal and Postpartum Massage, Health and Hygiene, Business Practices and Development, Reiki, Clinical Documentation, and Insurance Reimbursement), HIV/AIDS, and a Practical Internship in which students perform and document a minimum of fifty full-body sessions. Day and evening classes are available.

Admission Requirements

Applicants must be at least 18 years of age, have a high school diploma or equivalent, be of good moral character and appearance, submit three personal references (including one from a licensed health professional), and interview with one of the directors.

Tuition and Fees

Tuition is $5,300 for the Master Program, which includes a $100 application fee and $200 for books and supplies.

Financial Assistance

Payment plans, student loans, and veterans' benefits are available.

Southwest Acupuncture College

SANTA FE CAMPUS
2960 Rodeo Park Drive West
Santa Fe, New Mexico 87505
PHONE: (505) 438-8884

FAX: (505) 438-8883
E-MAIL: 105315.3010@compuserve.com
WEBSITE: www.swacupuncture.com

ALBUQUERQUE CAMPUS
4308 Carlisle NE, Suite 205
Albuquerque, New Mexico 87107
PHONE: (505) 888-8898
FAX: (505) 888-1380

BOULDER CAMPUS
6658 Gunpark Drive
Boulder, Colorado 80301
PHONE: (303) 581-9955
FAX: (303) 581-9944

Southwest Acupuncture College was founded in 1980. An Albuquerque branch was opened in 1993 and a Boulder, Colorado, branch was opened in 1997. There are a total of fifty-five instructors, with an average class size of thirty students.

Accreditation and Approvals

The college's professional master's degree program is accredited by the Accreditation Commission for Acupuncture and Oriental Medicine (ACAOM) and approved by the New Mexico Board of Acupuncture and Oriental Medicine and the Colorado Acupuncture Association. The school is also a member of the Council of Colleges of Acupuncture and Oriental Medicine (CCAOM).

Program Description

The college is a classical school of Oriental medicine and offers a professional program leading to a Master of Science degree in Oriental medicine. The 2,800-hour program is the equivalent of four academic years, and may be taken on a full-time, part-time, or accelerated basis (with completion in three calendar years).

The master's degree program consists of training in the five branches of traditional Oriental medicine: acupuncture, herbal medicine, physical therapy, nutrition, and exercise/breathing therapy, with the greatest number of hours devoted to acupuncture and herbal medicine. Courses include Botany, Chinese Medical Theory, Chinese Nutrition, Point Energetics, Point Location, Clinical Observation, Oriental Physical Therapy, Personal Energetics/Tai Chi or Qigong, Techniques of

Acupuncture and Moxibustion, Introduction to Diagnosis, Chinese Herbal Materia Medica, Human Anatomy and Physiology, CPR, Tui Na, Needle Technique Practicum, Chinese Herbal Patent Medicines, Chinese Medical Theory/Zang Fu, Western Pathology and Diagnosis, Clinical Herbal Prescribing, and more. Over 1,000 hours are clinical.

Admission Requirements

Applicants must be twenty years of age or older, have completed at least two years of general education at the college level, submit two letters of recommendation, and have a personal interview.

Tuition and Fees

The total tuition is $30,888; books and supplies are additional.

Financial Assistance

Federal loans, scholarships, and a payment plan are available.

Stens Corporation

6451 Oakwood Drive
Oakland, California 94611-1350
PHONE: (510) 339-9053 / (800) 257-8367
FAX: (510) 339-2222
E-MAIL: sales@stens-biofeedback.com
WEBSITE: www.stens-biofeedback.com

The Stens Corporation offers professional biofeedback training at locations throughout the country, and is a national leader in sales of biofeedback equipment. There are two instructors, and a maximum class size of twenty students.

Accreditation and Approvals

The Professional Biofeedback Certificate Program is accredited by the Biofeedback Certification Institute of America (BCIA). The program provides most of the hours required to take BCIA's national examination, with the exception of the required thirty hours of clinical supervision and ninety hours of direct treatment with patients. Stens Corporation can help with finding an appropriate supervisor for clinical supervision. Direct treatment can be done with clients in your own office or in another therapist's office; supervision is not required.

Program Description

The Professional Biofeedback Certificate Program consists of two parts:

Part One: Didactic Education and Clinical Biofeedback Training is a four-day, thirty-six-hour program held Saturday through Tuesday. The program covers Introduction to Biofeedback and Clinical Applications (Fight/Flight Response, Selye's General Adaptation Syndrome, Behavioral Medicine, Progressive Relaxation, Diaphragmatic Breathing, and more), Instrumentation (Environmental Noise, Terms and Concepts, EMG, EEG, GSR and TEMP, Respiration, Panel Controls, and more), and Hands-On Training (including EMG Lab, TEMP Lab, GSR Lab, Computer Experience, Patient Demonstration, and Role-Playing).

Part Two: Clinical Applications and Case Conference is a five-day, forty-four-hour program held Wednesday through Sunday. The program covers Stress-Related Disorders and Procedures: Clinical History and Evaluation (Structure of the Autonomic Nervous System, Treatment Planning, Migraine Headaches, Asthma, Dental Disorders, Anxiety, EMG Scanning, Current Research, and more), Business and Financial Issues (Forms and Records, Insurance Reimbursement, Referral Sources, and more), and Adjunctive Techniques (including Learning Theory, Visualization, Placebo, Nutrition, Medications, Autogenic Training, Guided Imagery, and Hypnosis).

The Stens Corporation also offers a computer software program, Self-Assessment in Biofeedback, that is based on the BCIA test blueprint.

Community and Continuing Education

The first two days of Surface EMG for Chronic Pain Management (a four-day seminar) and Clinical Applications of EEG Biofeedback (a four-day seminar) are combined with the last two days of Part II in the same location.

Admission Requirements

There are no minimum age or educational requirements.

Tuition and Fees

Tuition for Part One of the Professional Biofeedback Certificate Program is, $995; Part Two is also $995. Tuition for the Surface EMG for Chronic Pain Management Seminar is $995; the Clinical Applications of EEG Biofeedback Seminar is also $995.

Financial Assistance

Financial Assistance may be arranged on a case-by-case basis.

3HO International Kundalini Yoga Teachers Association

Route 2 Box 4 Shady Lane
Espanola, New Mexico 87532
PHONE: (505) 753-0423
FAX: (505) 753-5982
E-MAIL: ikyta@3ho.org
WEBSITE: www.kundaliniyoga.com

3HO, founded in 1969, offers KRI Kundalini Yoga Teacher Certification in Kundalini Yoga as taught by Yogi Bhajan, Ph.D., Master of Kundalini Yoga. Certification programs are offered in several cities throughout the United States and worldwide, and each summer in Espanola, New Mexico.

Program Description

The 200-hour Level 1 Kundalini Yoga Teacher Training Certification Program covers The Eight Limbs of Yoga and the Patanjali Sutras; History and Philosophy of Kundalini Yoga; Kundalini Yoga Kriyas, Fundamentals of Posture and Alignment, Mudras, Asanas, Mantras, Pranayam and Meditations; Yogic and Western Anatomy; Humanology; 3HO Lifestyle including Sadhana for the Aquarian Age and the Science of Hydrotherapy; and Practicums in class presentation.

Level 2 Teacher Training Certification consists of four modules (Modules 3 through 6) and provides advanced yogic challenges and presents more in-depth study of the yogic arts and sciences. Module 3 consists of Approaches to Healing; Yogic Diet; Yogic Cooking; Herbs and Healing; and Yogic Healing Practices. Topics in Module 4 include Tour of the Body; Advanced Study of Kundalini Yoga; Posture and the Spine; Inner Dynamics of the Human Body; and Sat Nam Rasayan. Module 5 covers Communication: Power of the Word; Naad; Inner Communication; Effective Communication; Chakras; Divine Communication; and Prayer. Module 6 includes Humanology; Teachings for Men; Teachings for Women; Death; Addiction; Child Development; and Personality Assessment.

The KRI Young Adults Certification Program is the same as the Level 1 program except that it is taught in two parts over two summers. Module 1 includes Kundalini Yoga Basics: Yoga for Daily Life, History of Yoga in the East, Kundalini Yoga in the West, The Art of being a Student of Yoga, Golden Chain of the Teacher; Breath; Meditation; Kriyas; Mantras; Mudras Asanas; and Bandhas. Module 2 covers Gunas; Tattwas; Reincarnation; Dharma and Karma; Spiritual Teacher; Yogic Anatomy; Ten Bodies; Western Anatomy; Basic Humanology; and Yogic Lifestyle.

Admission Requirements

Applicants must be between 13 and 21 years of age for the Young Adults Teacher Training Program; over 17 years of age for all other Teacher Training Programs.

Tuition and Fees

Tuition (estimated) is $1,500; $1800 for the summer intensive program; $450 for Module 1 summer Young Adults Program. Both summer programs include camping and meals.

Financial Assistance

A discount is given for prepayment.

Touch For Health Kinesiology Association

P.O. Box 392
New Carlisle, Ohio 45344-0392
PHONE: (937) 845-3404
FAX: (937) 845-3909
E-MAIL: Tch4Hlth@aol.com
WEBSITE: www.tfh.org

The Touch for Health Kinesiology Association (TFHKA) supervises and does referrals for the 500+ Touch For Health Instructors located throughout the United States. Although there is not a central school, Touch For Health has been taught to both laypeople and alternative health practitioners since the 1970s. Touch For Health is a safe and practical touch-healing process of balancing the body's natural energies to ease common aches, pains, and stress. (See page 456 for membership information.)

Accreditation and Approvals

TFHKA courses are recognized by the Associated Bodywork and Massage Professionals (ABMP), the American Massage

Therapy Association (AMTA), and the National Certification Board for Therapeutic Massage and Bodywork (NCBTMB) for continuing education units.

Program Description

The Touch For Health Certification Process is divided into five parts: Introductory (four hours), TFH 1 (sixteen hours), TFH 2 (sixteen hours), TFH 3 (sixteen hours) and TFH 4 (eight hours).

Introductory courses include Maximum Athletic Performance System; Self-Help for Stress and Pain; Tibetan Energy and Vitality; Stress Release Made Easy; Enhanced Learning; and the Top Ten Series.

The Touch For Health Introductory Workshop (TFH 1) provides practical skills to manage stress, reduce physical and mental pain, and increase energy. Also included are specific tests, exercises, and movements for enhancing learning, improving coordination, and finding food allergies, and techniques of applied kinesiology and acupressure massage.

TFH 2, 3, and 4 are designed to provide expansion of understanding and ability as a touch healer. Topics covered include basic human anatomy and muscle movements, causes of pain, ways to improve personal health, the basics of the Oriental health system (five elements), and comprehensive training in massage and applied kinesiology.

Continuing Education

Several courses are open to those who have completed the certification process above.

The sixty-hour Instructor Training Workshop prepares the student to become a Touch For Health Instructor. Training covers Marketing (enrollment skills, giving effective demos, presentation skills, networking), Logistics and Management (site selection, record keeping, project management, handout materials), and Teaching (mastering the TFH techniques, structuring hands-on practice, how to use TFH texts, communication skills, presentation strategies). Graduates are certified by the International Kinesiology College (IKC) and the Touch for Health Association (TFHA).

Professional Kinesiology Practitioner (PKP) Training is available at three levels: the forty-hour Level I Certification Training, the fifty-hour Level II Certification Training, and the fifty-hour Level III Certification Training. Students will become proficient at properly clearing emotions to avoid the sabotage of corrections; expand their repertoire of energy-balancing methods; work more effectively with athletes, dancers, and people in the workplace; know which technique to use when; and experience the power of these procedures first-hand during practice sessions. Graduates are certified by the IKC and TFHA.

Admission Requirements

Touch For Health Certification is designed for massage therapists, nutritionists, nurses, shiatsu and acupressure therapists, and other health practitioners. Courses may be taken for personal growth or professional use.

Tuition and Fees

Tuition will vary with instructor.

The Trager Institute

21 Locust
Mill Valley, California 94941-2806
PHONE: (415) 388-2688
FAX: (415) 388-2710
E-MAIL: admin@trager.com

The Trager® approach is a system of movement education created and developed by Milton Trager, M.D. The approach uses gentle movements to help release deep-seated physical and mental patterns and facilitate deep relaxation, increased physical mobility, and mental clarity. The positive results are reinforced by Mentastics®, simple movements that the client can do on his or her own. There are fourteen instructors. Trainings are held throughout the country.

Accreditation and Approvals

The Trager Institute is approved by the National Certification Board for Therapeutic Massage and Bodywork (NCBTMB), by the California Board of Registered Nursing, and by the State of California as a continuing education provider; the institute is also approved by the Florida Department of Professional Regulation to provide continuing education credits for Florida state massage therapists. In the State of California, the Trager Certification program is approved by the Bureau for Private Postsecondary and Vocational Education.

Program Description

The Trager Institute's professional certification program takes a minimum of six months to complete. The program consists of a six-day Beginning training, a five-day Intermediate training, and a six-day Anatomy and Physiology training, with a period of fieldwork and evaluations after the Beginning and Intermediate trainings. The fieldwork consists of giving at least sixty Trager sessions without charge and receiving at least twenty sessions, as well as completing at least five tutorials (private lessons).

Exemption from the anatomy and physiology training is given to those with medical or paramedical licensure, or those who are graduates of massage certification programs of 500 hours or more.

Expansion of certification requirements is under consideration.

Continuing Education

A certified Trager practitioner is required to take at least one three-day practitioner training per year for the first three years; after that time, one training is required every three years. In addition, one tutorial is required for each year of practice, along with receiving four sessions from certified practitioners.

Admission Requirements

Student license status in the Trager Institute is a prerequisite for beginning the program. Applicants must receive at least two sessions from a certified Trager practitioner, or receive one session and attend either an introductory workshop or six hours of Mentastics classes.

Tuition and Fees

Student status fees are $85 per year. Tuition for the Beginning training is $750; for the Intermediate training, $665; and for Trager anatomy and physiology, $750. One-day introductory workshops range from $65 to $85. Public Mentastics classes range from $5 to $8 per hour. Sessions with certified practitioners range from $35 to $75. Tutorials range from $30 to $50 per hour and usually last two hours. The total certification program is approximately 270 hours and costs approximately $3,000 plus student license fees.

Utah College of Massage Therapy

TOLL FREE: (800) 617-3302
E-MAIL: info@ucmt.com
WEBSITE: www.ucmt.com

SALT LAKE CITY CAMPUS
25 South 300 East
Salt Lake City, Utah 84111
PHONE: (801) 521-3330
FAX: (801) 521-3339

UTAH VALLEY CAMPUS
135 South State Street, Suite 12
Lindon, Utah 84042
PHONE: (801) 796-0300

LAYTON, UTAH AUXILIARY CLASSROOM
1992 West Antelope Drive, Suite 3D
Layton, Utah 84041
PHONE: (801) 779-0300
FAX: (801) 779-0330

LAS VEGAS, NEVADA CAMPUS
Nevada School of Massage Therapy
2381 East Windmill Lane, Suite 14
Las Vegas, Nevada 89123
PHONE: (702) 456-4325/ (800) 750-HEAL
FAX: (801) 456-9910

The Utah College of Massage Therapy (UCMT) was founded by Norman Cohn in 1986. There are over 100 instructors, with approximately fifty students per class. Programs are offered Salt Lake City, Lindon, and Layton, Utah, and in Las Vegas, Nevada.

Accreditation and Approvals

The Utah College of Massage Therapy is accredited by the Commission on Massage Training Accreditation (COMTA) and by the Accrediting Council for Continuing Education and Training (ACCET). Graduates are qualified to take the National Certification Examination for Therapeutic Massage and Bodywork (NCETMB).

Program Description

There are five Massage Therapy Programs offered at UCMT.

The 815.5-hour Professional Massage Therapy Program (offered over six months of full-time day study or twelve months of evening study) consists of instruction in Acupressure, AIDS Awareness, CPR/First Aid, Anatomy/Physiology, Movement for Massage Therapists, Reflexology, Massage Therapy, Professional Development, Seated Massage, Cranio Sacral Therapy, Infant Massage, Sports Massage, Student Clinical Internship, Touch for Health, Deep Tissue Bodywork, Advanced Deep Tissue Bodywork, Injury Massage, Facilitated Stretching, Shiatsu, and Trigger Point Therapy.

The ten-month, 1,175-hour Clinical Career Track Program (offered days) includes all of the coursework in the Professional Massage Therapy Program with additional classes in Cranio-Sacral Therapy, Advanced Eastern Paradigm, Advanced Structural Bodywork, Medical Terminology, Neurology, Pathology, Kinesiology, Hydrotherapy, Health Related Topics, Neuromuscular Therapy, and Advanced Clinical Internship.

The twelve-month, 1290.5-hour Sports Massage Career Track Program (offered days) includes all of the coursework in the Professional Massage Therapy Program plus Advanced Sports Massage courses that include Common Injuries, Post-Event Massage, Advanced Russian Massage, Pre-Event Massage, Protocols for Partial Massage, Specific Sports Massage, Sports Biochemistry, Sports Nutrition, Sports Pathology, Sports Physiology, Sports Psychology, Taping, Training Massage, and Sports Externship.

The ten-month, 1179.5-hour Structural Integration Career Track Program (offered days) includes all of the coursework in the Professional Massage Therapy Program plus advanced Structural Integration bodywork courses that include Advanced Structural Bodywork, Advanced Structural/Functional Anatomy, and the Ten Session System of Structural Integration.

Community and Continuing Education

UCMT offers an eighteen-hour introductory course in massage therapy several times per year. This course is not required for enrollment, but is designed to give the prospective student an experience of the quality of education at UCMT. It is open to the public, individuals, or couples.

Admission Requirements

Applicants must have a high school diploma or equivalent or pass an ability to benefit test; international students must demonstrate proficiency in English during the interview and by written documentation, and must have completed the equivalent of a high school education in the United States.

Tuition and Fees

Tuition and fees are as follows: for the Professional Massage Therapy day and evening program, $8,595; for the Clinical Career Track Program, $11,994; for the Sports Massage Career Track Program, $13,098; and for the Structural Integration Career Track Program, $12,538.

Figures include tuition, registration fee, books and manuals, lab fees, massage table/bolster, Feldenkrais table (if applicable), clinic shirt, and one gallon of massage cream.

Financial Assistance

Federal grants, loans, and veterans' benefits are available.

Wellness Institute

P.O. Box 251
Nathrop, Colorado 81236
PHONE: (719) 395-6290

Wellness Institute was founded in 1990 by Roger Gilchrist. Formerly located in Taos, New Mexico, the institute recently moved near the Mt. Princeton Hot Springs in Colorado; ongoing training programs are also offered in Washington, D.C., and New York City. There are six instructors, with an average class size of twelve students.

Accreditation and Approvals

The Associate Polarity Practitioner (A.P.P.) and Registered Polarity Practitioner (R.P.P.) Programs are approved by the American Polarity Therapy Association (APTA). The institute is approved by the APTA, the American Massage Therapy Association (AMTA), and the National Certification Board for Therapeutic Massage and Bodywork (NCBTMB) as a continuing education provider.

Program Description

The three-week Polarity Therapy Professional Certification Training, when combined with follow-up supervision, qualifies the student to become an Associate Polarity Practitioner (A.P.P.). Topics covered include theory and research on the Human Energy System, principles of energy movement, practical techniques for balancing life energy, emotional qualities inherent in specific areas of the body, anatomical adjustment through energy balancing, craniosacral balancing, and clinical supervision of thirty sessions.

The twelve-week Comprehensive Polarity Therapy Training allows students to complete all necessary studies for the R.P.P. credential in a single continuous program. The program begins with a three-week certification intensive and continues with eight R.P.P. modular classes. The eight modules are Cranio-Sacral Therapy and the Energetic Body, Process Oriented Bodywork, Energetic and Structural Assessment, Deepening Polarity Therapy, Trauma Resolution in the Healing Arts, The Healing Process, Business in the Healing Arts, and Clinical Supervision.

The Core Process Cranio-Sacral Therapy Program emphasizes the original principles of the work, based in osteopathic medicine. The program consists of two year-long trainings composed of five-day classes three times per year. Courses include Cranio-Sacral Therapy and the Energetic Body; Body Architecture and the Cranio-Sacral System; Cranial Base Patterns and Whole Body Dynamics; and The Spine, Dura, Ventricles, and Spaces.

Tuition and Fees

Tuition for the Polarity Therapy Professional Certification Training is $2,100. Tuition for the Comprehensive Polarity Therapy Training is $6,375. Figures for these two programs include lodging; tuition-only prices without lodging are also available. There is a $35 application fee.

Advanced modules and five day courses are $435 (lodging not included; lodging is available for $150 per week).

The Wellness Institute

3716 274th Avenue SE
Issaquah, Washington 98029
PHONE: (425) 391-9716 / (800) 326-4418
FAX: (425) 391-9737
E-MAIL: heartcenter@wellness-institute.org
WEBSITE: www.wellness-institute.org

The Wellness Institute was founded by Diane Zimberoff in 1985. Six-day certification seminars are offered in various locations throughout the country, including Chicago, New York, Houston, Syracuse, Boston, Seattle, and Atlanta, and around the world. There are eight instructors, with an average of thirty students per class.

Accreditation and Approvals

The six-day certification in hypnotherapy is approved for continuing education units for MSWs, Ph.D.s, MFCCs, and others by many national associations and state licensing boards.

Program Description

The Wellness Institute offers a six-day Certification in Hypnotherapy. Training combines traditional hypnosis, Ericksonian techniques, and NLP with Gestalt and Transactional Analysis into a therapeutic approach called Heart-Centered Hypnotherapy that addresses mind, body, and spirit. Topics include Introduction to Hypnosis, How to Induce and Deepen Hypnotic Trance, Self-Hypnosis, Treating the Dysfunctional Family with Hypnotherapy, the Mind/Body Connection, Sexual Abuse, Multiple Personality, NLP and Ericksonian Techniques, Hypnosis with Children, Eating Disorders, Birth Trauma, and others.

Continuing Education

Advanced training is available.

Admission Requirements

Certification is open to Ph.D. and master's-level therapists or the equivalent in practice.

Tuition and Fees

Tuition is $895.

Financial Assistance

A discount is given for early registration.

Wyrick Institute for European Manual Lymph Drainage

P.O. Box 99745
San Diego, California 92169
PHONE: (619) 273-9764

Wyrick Institute was founded in 1984 by Dana Wyrick, who has been practicing manual lymph drainage since 1982. Classes are held in San Diego and elsewhere in the United States.

Program Description

The institute offers Basic and Advanced courses in manual lymph drainage.

In the five-day Basic Body Course, students receive an introduction to manual lymph drainage theory, learn the five basic movements, and use these movements in routines effective on all parts of the body. Students receive a certificate of completion.

In the five-day Advanced Body Course, students perfect the basic techniques and learn therapeutic movements for the head, abdomen, and joints. An examination is given and a diploma awarded.

Admission Requirements

Applicants must have a health license or local minimal massage license.

Tuition and Fees

Tuition is $500 to $600 per course.

Canada

Canadian College of Massage and Hydrotherapy / West Coast College of Massage Therapy

PHONE: (877) 748-7800
FAX: (877) 748-7801
E-MAIL: DMahedyjr@aol.com
WEBSITE: www.collegeofmassage.com

HEAD OFFICE AND NEWMARKET CAMPUS:
Canadian College of Massage and Hydrotherapy
543 Timothy Street
Newmarket, Ontario L3Y 1R1
Canada

HEAD OFFICE AND VANCOUVER CAMPUS:
West Coast College of Massage Therapy
555 West Hastings Street, 6th Floor
Vancouver, British Columbia V6B 4N4
Canada

KITCHENER CAMPUS:
59 Frederick Street
Kitchener, Ontario N2H 2L3
Canada

TORONTO CAMPUS:
Canadian College of Massage and Hydrotherapy
5160 Yonge Street, Suite 505
North York, Ontario M2N 6L9
Canada

VICTORIA CAMPUS:
637 Bay Street, Suite 101
Victoria, British Columbia V8T 5L2
Canada

WINDSOR CAMPUS:
2970 College Avenue
Windsor, Ontario N9C 1S5
Canada

Established in 1946 in Ontario and in 1983 in British Columbia, the Canadian College of Massage and Hydrotherapy founded therapeutic massage in Canada. There are approximately fifty instructors, with an average of fifty students per class.

Accreditation and Approvals

Graduates of the Naturopathic Medicine program will be eligible for licensure as Doctors of Naturopathic Medicine in the province of British Columbia, other Canadian provinces, and certain American states.

Program Description

Offered in British Columbia, the three-year, 3,150-hour Massage Therapy Program includes 560 hours of clinical practicum training. The curriculum includes General Anatomy and Physiology, Musculoskeletal Anatomy, Principles of Practice, Manual Skills, Personal Awareness and Development, Neurology, Communication Skills, General Pathology, Hydrotherapy, Actinotherapy and Physical Agents, Fascial Release, Therapeutic Exercise, Professionalism: Ethics and Conduct, Orthopedic Pathology, Medicine and Surgery, Manual Lymph Drainage, Joint Mobilization, Systemic Dysfunction Treatment, Clinical Management and Assessment, General Orthopedic Treatment,

Professional Practice, Clinical Practicum, Nutrition, Neurological Treatment, Sports Massage and Athletic Treatment, Cranio-Sacral Mobilization, Pain and Stress Management, Spinal Orthopedic Treatment/Intro to Muscle-Energy Techniques, Selected Topics in Professional Practice (group projects), Research and Statistics, Regional Orthopedic Treatment, Business and Practice Management, Anatomy, Physiology and Pathology Review, Musculoskeletal Anatomy and Kinesiology Review, Clinical Science Treatment Synthesis and Integration Review, Clinical Case Presentation, and Jurisprudence.

Offered in Ontario, the two-year, 2,200-hour Massage Therapy Program includes 150 hours of clinical practicum training. The curriculum includes Anatomy and Physiology, Client/Therapist Relationship (Professional Development), Massage Theory and Techniques, Palpation Lab, Regional Anatomy, Study Skills, Assessments, Clinical Practicum, Neurology, Pathology, Principles of Treatment, Regional and Visceral Anatomy, Hydrotherapy, Law and Ethics, Pathological Treatments, Remedial Exercise, Business, Kinesiology, Microbiology/Infection Control, and Nutrition.

The four-year, 4,670-hour Naturopathic Medicine Program includes 1,400 hours of clinical practicum. Year One courses include Human Gross Anatomy; General Anatomy and Physiology; Biochemistry; Naturopathic History, Philosophy, and Principles of Practice; Personal Awareness, Development, and Health; Neuroscience; Pathology; Pharmacology; Communication Skills; Botanical Medicine; and Human Dissection Lab. Year Two courses include Pathology, Botanical Medicine, Clinical/Physical Diagnosis, Public Health and Epidemiology, Pharmacology, Nutrition, Laboratory Diagnosis, Diagnostic Imaging, and Emergency Procedures/CPR; students take the NPLEX Basic Science Exams at the end of Year Two. Year Three courses include Nutrition, Manual Therapy, Hydrotherapy, Chinese Medicine, Counseling Skills and Techniques, Diagnostic Imaging, Environmental Medicine, Clinical Education, Research Methodology and Statistics, Preventive and Therapeutic Exercise, Homeopathy, Medical Procedures, Psychological Assessment, Neurology, Dermatology, Clinical Ecology, Addictions and Disorders, Medical Jurisprudence and Ethics, Gastroenterology, Cardiology and Pulmonology, Gynecology, Obstetrics, Pediatrics, and Endocrinology. Year Four courses include Urology/Proctology, EENT, Geriatrics, Oncology, Family Medicine, Minor Surgery, Clinical Education, Orthopedics

and Sports Medicine, Rheumatology, Practice Management, Clinical Case Review, Clinical Case Presentation, and Advanced Naturopathic Principles of Practice.

Admission Requirements

Three-year Massage Therapy applicants must have completed one year at university, biology, grade 12 chemistry, and have a high school diploma. Two-year Massage Therapy applicants must have a high school diploma and two OAC Science courses. Naturopathic Medicine applicants must have completed three years or fifteen program-appropriate credits at a university level.

Tuition and Fees

There is a $100 application fee.

Tuition for the three-year Massage Therapy Program is $24,900 plus $1,500 for books and supplies.

Tuition for the two-year Massage Therapy Program is $12,950 plus $700 for books and supplies.

Tuition for the Naturopathic Medicine Program is $52,800 plus $2,500 for books and supplies.

Financial Assistance

Payment plans and student loans are available.

Canadian Holistic Therapist Training School/Mississauga School of Aromatherapy

2155 Leanne Boulevard
200A Sheridan Corporate Centre
Mississauga, Ontario L5K 2K8
Canada
PHONE: (905) 822-5094 / (800) 326-9491
FAX: (905) 822-0856
E-MAIL: Aromanet@sprint.ca
WEBSITE: www.Aroma.net

Canadian Holistic Therapist Training School and Mississauga School of Aromatherapy were founded in the early 1990s by Lynn Bosman, who remains the primary instructor. Courses are taught across Canada in Toronto, Mississauga, London, Ontario, Windsor, Vancouver, Victoria and Kelowna, and through correspondence. Correspondence programs are described on pages 467-68.

Program Description

The two-week Aromatherapy Certification Program consists of twenty-one lessons: Aromatherapy Explained; Aromatherapy History; Essential Oil Production/Extraction/Quality; Essential Oils/Therapeutic/References/Detailed Study; Pregnancy/ Childcare/Breastfeeding; Varied Applications; Skin Care; Aromatherapy in Application; The Holistic Approach; Aromatherapy Aiding Different Conditions; Skeletal System; Muscular System; Cardiovascular System; Nervous System; Digestive System; Respiratory System; Genito-Urinary System; Endocrine System; Skin; and Massage Techniques and Case Study Assignments.

The Aromatherapy Advanced Diploma Program may be taken in class or by correspondence. The twenty-four lessons cover Aromatherapy in This Current Era; Botanical Classification; Obscure and Dangerous Oils; Botanical Families; Terpeneless Oils; Chemistry; Actions of Chemical Groups; Chemical Classifications; Major Chemical Compositions of Essential Oils; Essential Oils From Various Species and Countries; Glossary of Terms; Basic Chemical Composition of Essential Oils; Chemical Compositions; Immune Response; Clinical Reference Chart; Pregnancy and Essential Oils; Cancer; Oils; Menopause; Aromatherapy and Meditation/Herbs and Bach Flowers; Anatomy, Physiology, Arteries and Veins; Cells; The Nervous System; and Joints and Bones.

The three-day Aromatherapy Natural Beauty Spa Course is a natural skin care program offered twice per year. Students learn how to combine oils in a spa setting and how to safely incorporate the benefits of plants in effective body and face treatments.

The forty-hour Iridology course covers History and Analysis of the Iris and includes use of an Iriscope, slide presentation, and case studies.

The Reflexology course consists of thirty hours of class time and sixty hours of practical and case studies covering principles of reflexology.

Admission Requirements

Applicants must have completed grade 12 or have mature student status.

Tuition and Fees

Tuition for the Aromatherapy Certification Program is $1,250 plus a $50 exam fee. Tuition for the Aromatherapy Advanced Diploma is $1,300 plus a $50 exam fee. Tuition for the Aromatherapy Natural Beauty Spa Course is $500. Tuition for the Iridology Course is $700. Tuition for the Reflexology Course is $545.

Dr. Vodder School—North America

P.O. Box 5701
Victoria, British Columbia V8R 6S8
Canada
PHONE: (250) 598-9862
FAX: (250) 598-9841
E-MAIL: drvodderna@vodderschool.com
WEBSITE: www.vodderschool.com

The Dr. Vodder School—North America was founded in 1994, although the Dr. Vodder method of manual lymph drainage was started by Emil and Estrid Vodder in France in the 1930s and has been taught in North America since the 1970s. Current Director Robert Harris has been teaching the technique since 1987. There are ten instructors, with an average of twelve students per class.

Accreditation and Approvals

The Dr. Vodder School—North America is approved by the National Certification Board for Therapeutic Massage and Bodywork (NCBTMB) as a continuing education provider. Courses may be eligible for continuing education credit from various local and national licensing bodies.

Program Description

The school offers postgraduate training in manual lymph drainage and combined decongestive therapy. The program is supervised by a physician specializing in lymphatic disorders who also teaches the pathology part of the program.

Manual Lymph Drainage and Combined Decongestive Therapy Training is offered in four consecutive parts (Basic and Therapy I, II, and III), each of which lasts five days, for a total of 160 hours of classroom education. The first two courses are offered independently at various locations throughout North America.

The forty-hour Basic Program covers anatomy and physiology of the lymph vessel system, connective tissue, effects of

MLD, contraindications, and MLD treatment of the full body, including all basic strokes. The forty-hour Therapy I covers special techniques for the joints, the head, and deep abdominal work, introducing the student to therapeutic applications; advanced theory and current research is discussed. Therapy II and III, taught consecutively for eighty classroom hours, cover various pathologies with an emphasis on lymphedema treatment in the context of combined decongestive therapy; bandaging, exercise therapy, skin care, and specific MLD treatments are taught. Students who successfully complete the oral, written, and practical exams at the end of the course may describe themselves as Vodder-Certified MLD Therapists.

Continuing Education

An annual twenty-five-hour review course is available to therapists to update and review their skills. Certified therapists must attend a review at least every two years to maintain their certification.

Admission Requirements

Enrollment is open to licensed or certified health care practitioners, including massage therapists who have completed a minimum of 500 hours at a massage therapy school, or who have successfully completed the national certification exam.

Tuition and Fees

Tuition is approximately $550 to $650 per five-day course.

Sivananda Ashram Yoga Camp

673 Eighth Avenue
Val Morin, Quebec J0T 2R0
Canada
PHONE: (819) 322-3226 / (800) 263-YOGA
FAX: (819) 322-5876
E-MAIL: HQ@sivananda.org
WEBSITE: www.sivananda.org

In 1968, Swami Vishnu-devananda developed the first Yoga Teacher's Training course in the West. Since then, more than 9,000 teachers have been trained in accordance with his program. Teacher's Training courses are taught in Quebec, California, New York, Europe, the Bahamas, and India. There are ten to fifteen instructors per course, with an average of twenty (maximum forty) students per class.

Program Description

Four-week Yoga Teacher's Training courses are taught by senior disciples personally trained by Swami Vishnu-devananda. The full daily schedule reflects the ancient yogic Gurukula system of training, in which the student's daily life itself was his or her yoga practice. The curriculum includes Asanas (to increase flexibility, strength, and concentration and receive training in teaching techniques); Pranayama (daily practice of breathing exercises); Meditation; Mantras and Japa yoga (science of the spiritual power of sound vibrations); Vedanta and Philosophy (study of the wisdom of India's sages); Bhagavad Gita (study of the classical paths of yoga); Chanting; Karma yoga (the yoga of selfless service); Yogic Diet (the principles behind vegetarianism); and Kriyas (purification techniques). No meat, fish, eggs, alcohol, tobacco, or nonprescription drugs are allowed, and participation in all classes is mandatory.

Admission Requirements

A basic knowledge of yoga postures is helpful but not essential.

Tuition and Fees

Teacher's Training courses in Canada and the United States cost $1,450 (U.S.) for tent or shared rooms, and $1,700 to $2,050 (U.S.) for dormitory lodging; books are additional.

Financial Assistance

Scholarships are occasionally available in exceptional circumstances.

Appendices

Accrediting Agencies and Councils on Education

Before you commit to a program, be sure you've compared schools, are aware of which accreditations and approvals are the norm in your field, and are acutely aware of the licensing requirements in the city and state in which you intend to practice. The agencies listed here can verify the accreditation status of a particular school or answer other questions you may have about accreditation.

GENERAL

Accrediting Commission of Career Schools and Colleges of Technology (ACCSCT)

2101 Wilson Boulevard, Suite 302
Arlington, Virginia 22201
PHONE: (703) 247-4212
FAX: (703) 247-4533
E-MAIL: info@accsct.org
WEBSITE: www.accsct.org

ACCSCT is an accrediting agency for private colleges and schools offering occupational, trade, and technical education. In order to become accredited, institutions must be open to the public, have been in operation for at least two years, have graduated at least one class of students from its longest program, and conduct a self-assessment that evaluates how well the school meets accreditation standards. Schools must submit documentation of compliance with standards in the areas of admission policies, advertising and promotion, enrollment agreement, faculty, financial stability, instructional materials, placement, student complaints, student progress, student recruitment, and tuition and refund policies. The commission conducts on-site reviews to verify information in the self-assessment.

Accrediting Council for Continuing Education and Training (ACCET)

1722 N Street NW
Washington, DC 20036
PHONE: (202) 955-1113
FAX: (202) 955-1118
WEBSITE: www.accet.org

ACCET is a voluntary group of educational organizations affiliated for the purpose of improving continuing education and training. Through its support of an independent accrediting commission, ACCET promulgates and sustains the standards for accreditation, along with policies and procedures that measure and ensure educational standards of quality. ACCET is recognized for this purpose by the U.S. Secretary of Education and, accordingly, is listed by the U.S. Department of Education as a nationally recognized accrediting agency. ACCET is also certified as an ISO9001 Quality Management System.

In order to become accredited by ACCET, schools must have been in operation for at least two years, must document financial and administrative capability, and must document their educational mission within prescribed guidelines. School representatives must attend a pre-accreditation workshop and document compliance with standards, after which the council conducts an on-site review.

ACUPUNCTURE AND ORIENTAL MEDICINE

Accreditation Commission for Acupuncture and Oriental Medicine (ACAOM)

1010 Wayne Avenue, Suite 1270
Silver Spring, Maryland 20910

PHONE: (301) 608-9680
FAX: (301) 608-9576
E-MAIL: acaom1@compuserve.com

ACAOM was established in June 1982 by the Council of Colleges of Acupuncture and Oriental Medicine (CCAOM) as a means of fostering excellence in acupuncture and Oriental medicine education. The commission acts independently to evaluate professional master's degree and master's-level certificate and diploma programs in acupuncture and Oriental medicine, with a concentration in both acupuncture and herbal therapies. The commission establishes accreditation criteria, arranges site visits, evaluates programs, and publicly designates those that meet the criteria. The commission is the sole agency recognized by the U.S. Department of Education and the Commission on Higher Education Accreditation to accredit professional programs in this field.

To be eligible for accreditation, a program must comply with fourteen essential requirements that provide minimum guidelines for assessment of broad areas of institutional structure. These include purpose, legal organization, governance, administration, records, admissions, evaluation, program of study, faculty, student services and activities, library and learning resources, physical facilities and equipment, financial resources, and publications and advertising.

To meet the requirements of ACAOM, a professional program in acupuncture must be a resident program of at least three academic years in length; must demonstrate attainment of professional competence; must have both adequate clinical and biomedical clinical sciences components; and must include the minimum core curriculum as outlined in the *Accreditation Handbook*.

A professional program in Oriental medicine must be a resident program of at least four academic years in length; must demonstrate attainment of professional competence; must have both adequate clinical and biomedical clinical sciences components; and must include the minimum core curriculum as outlined in the Accreditation Handbook.

As of 1999, twenty-nine programs had achieved ACAOM accreditation and eleven had achieved candidacy status.

AROMATHERAPY
National Association for Holistic Aromatherapy (NAHA)

2000 2nd Avenue, Suite 206
Seattle, Washington 98121
PHONE: (206) 256-0741 / (888) ASK-NAHA
E-MAIL: Info@NAHA.org
WEBSITE: NAHA.org

The National Association for Holistic Aromatherapy (NAHA) is a nonprofit educational organization whose mission is to promote and maintain high standards of education in the field of Aromatherapy. NAHA also establishes professional and ethical standards and provides public education of the practice of Aromatherapy.

NAHA has established core curriculum requirements in Professional Aromatherapy education (Level Two). Over twenty schools and independent educators have chosen to voluntarily comply with NAHA standards. NAHA has also set a national exam to certify practitioners in the field of Aromatherapy.

Schools wishing to comply with NAHA's approved standards for professional aromatherapy education for Level Two: Professional Aromatherapy Certification must provide a minimum of 200 hours of training and practical instruction in the fields of aromatherapy, essential oil studies, and anatomy and physiology. The aromatherapy and essential oil studies should include the following core curriculum requirements: history and modern development; basics of botany; properties of essential oils within a holistic and clinical framework; methods of extraction; organic chemistry; carrier oils; blending techniques; methods of application; safety and aromatherapy; consultation and treatment program design; basics of business development; and legal and ethical issues. Anatomy and physiology requirements include the teaching of specific body systems and common ailments. Student graduation requires a research paper, a minimum of ten case histories, and passing an examination given by the school. For information on certification, see page 436; for NAHA membership, see page 448.

BIOFEEDBACK

Biofeedback Certification Institute of America (BCIA)

10200 West 44th Avenue, Suite 310
Wheat Ridge, Colorado 80033-2840
PHONE: (303) 420-2902

BCIA was established in 1981 to create and maintain standards for biofeedback practitioners, and to certify those who meet these standards (see page 437). The BCIA Didactic Education Accreditation program was established in 1990 to recognize quality providers of didactic education in biofeedback training.

The didactic hours required for educational programs to be eligible for BCIA accreditation include: Introduction to Biofeedback (three hours); Preparing for Clinical Intervention (six hours); Neuromuscular Intervention: General (six hours); Neuromuscular Intervention: Specific (three hours); Central Nervous System Interventions: General (two hours); Autonomic Nervous System Interventions: General (seven hours); Autonomic Nervous System Interventions: Specific (eight hours); Biofeedback and Distress (four hours); Instrumentation (eleven hours); Adjunctive Techniques and Cognitive Interventions (seven hours); and Professional Conduct (three hours).

Educational institutions, private training programs, state chapters, clinics, and individuals may all be accredited through this program.

CHIROPRACTIC

Council on Chiropractic Education (CCE)

7975 North Hayden Road, Suite A210
Scottsdale, Arizona 85258-3246
PHONE: (602) 443-8877
FAX: (602) 483-7333
E-MAIL: CCE@adata.com
WEBSITE: cce-usa (domain name)

The Council on Chiropractic Education (CCE), incorporated in 1971, is the agency recognized by the U.S. Secretary of Education for accreditation of programs and institutions offering the doctor of chiropractic degree.

The CCE criteria for accreditation address the areas of mission, assessment and planning, organization, support services, and curriculum. Criteria requirements include a minimum of 4,200 hours that must address at least twenty-five required subject areas including anatomy; biochemistry; physiology; microbiology; pathology; public health; physical, clinical and laboratory diagnosis; gynecology; obstetrics; pediatrics; geriatrics; dermatology; otolaryngology; diagnostic imaging procedures; psychology; nutrition/dietetics; biomechanics; orthopedics; first aid and emergency procedures; spinal analysis; principles and practice of chiropractic; adjustive techniques; research methods and procedures; and professional practice ethics.

There are currently sixteen chiropractic programs and institutions in the United States, all accredited by CCE.

HERBOLOGY

American Herbalists Guild

P.O. Box 70
Roosevelt, Utah 84066
PHONE: (435) 722-8434
FAX: (435) 722-8452
E-MAIL: ahgoffice@earthlink.net
WEBSITE: www.healthy.net/herbalists

There is currently no agency that accredits, approves, or regulates schools of herbology. However, the Education Committee of the American Herbalists Guild (AHG) is presently occupied with a number of projects mandated by the governing council. These include the development of educational guidelines for professional herbalists as a means of providing general direction to students to further their study of herbal medicines; the development of guidelines for clinical training; development of a mentorship program, in which a newer member would be teamed up with an experienced herbalist through the first one or two years of professional membership; and the establishment of a council of schools that is intended to be a forum for the discussion and development of appropriate methods of ensuring that adequate standards are adhered to in the training of clinicians of herbal medicine.

The AHG recommendations for training in the Western biomedical model include a total of 640 hours in Western sciences (including anatomy, pathology, botany, toxicology, and related disciplines), 730 hours in the herbal and therapeutic areas (including materia medica, therapeutics applications, ethnobotany, herbal pharmacy, formulating and prescribing, and dispensing), ninety hours in the area of therapeutic orientation (covering Western constitutional and clinical approaches, history and philosophy of Western medicine, and ethics in clinical practice), ninety hours in additional modalities (such as psychology, counseling, nutrition, and CPR and First Aid), and 400 hours of clinical practicum. Other recommended topics include political and legislative issues, developing teaching skills, stress management, and growing herbs.

The AHG *Directory of Herbal Education* is available for $10. For membership information, see page 450.

HOMEOPATHY
Council on Homeopathic Education (CHE)

801 North Fairfax Street, Suite 306
Alexandria, Virginia 22314
PHONE: (518) 392-7975
E-MAIL: ched@igc.org
WEBSITE: www.chedu.org

The Council on Homeopathic Education (CHE) was founded in 1982 as an independent agency to assess homeopathic training in the United States and Canada. Its goals are to establish, maintain, ensure, and improve the quality of education within the discipline of homeopathy; to serve as a resource center, providing information about the content and format of lectures, seminars, academic programs, and institutions dealing with the art and science of homeopathy; and to establish standards for such presentations, and to evaluate presentations and institutions for endorsement or certification.

The council has been active in the evaluation of homeopathic training since 1982. The board consists of representatives from member organizations, endorsed schools, and the public at large. Participating organizations include the American Homeopathic Pharmacist Organization, the American Institute of Homeopathy, the Council on Homeopathic Certification, the Homeopathic Academy of Naturopathic Physicians,

the National Center for Homeopathy, and the North American Society of Homeopaths.

Beginning and advanced programs are evaluated at the graduate and postgraduate level. Episodic programs for continuing education units (CEU) are endorsed as well.

Ontario Homeopathic Association (OHA)

P.O. Box 258
Station P
Toronto, Ontario M5S 2S7
Canada
PHONE: (416) 488-9685
E-MAIL: root@ontariohomeopath.com
WEBSITE: ontariohomeopath.com

According to the Ontario Homeopathic Association, homeopathy is currently unregulated in Canada and anyone can claim to be a homeopath or homeopathic doctor. But in 1859, homeopathy was regulated in Ontario; a homeopathic doctor required three years of training, including medical sciences, plus a clinical externship. OHA, founded in 1992, considers standards similar to these to be the minimum that should be implemented in Canada now, and accredits professional educational programs accordingly. For membership information, see page 453.

HYPNOTHERAPY
International Medical and Dental Hypnotherapy Association (IMDHA)

4110 Edgeland, Suite 800
Royal Oak, Michigan 48073-2285
PHONE: (248) 549-5594
FAX: (248) 549-5421
E-MAIL: aspencer@infinityinst.com
WEBSITE: www.infinityinst.com

While the International Medical and Dental Hypnotherapy Association (IMDHA) does not accredit hypnotherapy programs, it does provide a list of approved schools throughout the United States, Canada, Australia, Brazil, and the West Indies. The main function of the organization is to certify hypnotherapists through an examination process and continued education, and to maintain a directory of certified hypnotherapists. For information on certification, see page 440; for membership information, see page 454.

MASSAGE THERAPY AND BODYWORK

American Massage Therapy Association (AMTA)

AMTA Council of Schools
820 Davis Street, Suite 100
Evanston, Illinois 60201-4444
PHONE: (847) 864-0123
FAX: (847) 864-1178
E-MAIL: info@inet.amtamassage.org
WEBSITE: www.amtamassage.org

AMTA is the oldest and largest national organization representing the massage therapy profession, with over 37,000 members in thirty countries. AMTA played a major role in the development and launching of the Commission on Massage Therapy Accreditation (COMTA), which is now an independent body (see below).

The AMTA Council of Schools was founded in 1982 as a forum for massage therapy school owners, administrators, and faculty to explore common interests, make new contacts, gather information from the experience of others, and participate in the growth and development of the massage therapy profession. In order to become members in the AMTA Council of Schools, schools must offer a minimum 500-hour program of study for massage therapists and/or bodyworkers, and must meet all legal requirements for operation within its jurisdiction.

For specialty exam information, see page 440; for membership, see pages 454-55.

American Oriental Bodywork Therapy Association (AOBTA)

Laurel Oak Corporate Center, Suite 408
1010 Haddonfield-Berlin Road

Voorhees, New Jersey 08043
PHONE: (856) 782-1616
FAX: (856) 782-1653
E-MAIL: www.aobta.org

While AOBTA is not an accrediting agency, sixteen schools of Oriental bodywork are members of the AOBTA Council of Schools and Programs (COSP). In order to be accepted for membership, schools and programs must successfully meet certain criteria that include offering a program of at least 500 hours of study. Contact AOBTA for additional information. For membership information, see page 455.

Associated Bodywork and Massage Professionals (ABMP)/Integrative Massage and Somatic Therapies Accreditation Council (IMSTAC)

1271 Sugarbush Drive
Evergreen, Colorado 80439
PHONE: (800) 458-2267
FAX: (303) 674-0859
E-MAIL: expectmore@abmp.com
WEBSITE: www.abmp.com

In 1995, ABMP announced the inception of its program accreditation for schools of massage, bodywork, and somatic therapies. ABMP's Integrative Massage and Somatic Therapies Accreditation Council (IMSTAC) standards are based on academic climate, financial viability, logistical/operational function, accountability, and professionalism. In order for a program to be considered for accreditation, it must offer a minimum of 500 hours of education at an established school, with a minimum of one year in operation and a minimum of one graduating class. Currently, twenty-one schools have met IMSTAC accreditation standards; contact ABMP/IMSTAC for a complete listing.

In addition, ABMP reviews curricula of state-approved schools offering an education in massage and bodywork therapy. Graduates of curriculum reviewed schools are eligible for ABMP membership upon graduation. This is not a guarantee of training or employment; it is an indication that the educational program meets or exceeds professional membership standards.

For membership information, see page 455.

Commission on Massage Training Accreditation (COMTA)

820 Davis Street, Suite 100
Evanston, Illinois 60201-4444
PHONE: (847) 864-0123
FAX: (847) 864-1178
E-MAIL: costendo@inet.amtamassage.org
WEBSITE: www.comta.org

COMTA is the primary accrediting agency for schools and programs in the field of massage therapy. The American Massage Therapy Association (AMTA) played a major role in the development and launching of COMTA; however, in 1994 COMTA became an independent affiliate of AMTA, operating separately and under its own mission, policies, and procedures.

Currently, thirty-three schools at forty-three locations have met the requirements for accreditation; COMTA's Approved program for massage schools expired in March 1999.

Accreditation is a voluntary process that identifies and acknowledges educational programs and/or institutions for achieving and maintaining a level of quality, performance, and integrity that meets meaningful standards. The five-step accreditation process involves application; pre-accreditation workshop; self-study and a self-study report; an on-site visit; and deliberation and decision. Programs must offer at least 500 hours of faculty-supervised instruction that includes massage therapy theory and technique, anatomy, physiology, and business ethics; graduates must also complete First Aid and CPR training. Schools must demonstrate that they continue to meet COMTA standards by engaging in the self-study process at least every five years.

Feldenkrais Guild® of North America

3611 SW Hood Avenue, Suite 100
Portland, Oregon 97201
PHONE: (503) 221-6612/ (800) 775-2118
FAX: (503) 221-6616

E-MAIL: guild@feldenkrais.com
WEBSITE: www.feldenkrais.com

The Feldenkrais Guild® of North America is the professional organization of Guild Certified Feldenkrais Practitioners/ Teachers® and also maintains standards of practice, certification, training accreditation, and professional conduct. Accredited trainings offer a minimum of 800 class hours over a minimum of three years; most trainings meet over four years. See pages 455-56 for membership information.

International Myomassethics Federation (IMF)

IMF Home Office
1720 Willow Creek Circle, Suite 517
Eugene, Oregon 97402
PHONE: (800) 433-4463
FAX: (541) 485-7372
E-MAIL: myomasseth@aol.com

The International Myomassethics Federation (IMF), founded in 1971, is primarily a professional membership organization (see page 456), but also offers curriculum approval to schools of myomassology and related fields throughout the country. Contact IMF for additional information.

MIDWIFERY

Midwifery Education Accreditation Council (MEAC)

200 West Birch
Flagstaff, Arizona 86001
PHONE: (520) 214-0997
FAX: (520) 773-9694
E-MAIL: meac@altavista.net
WEBSITE: www.mana.org/meac

MEAC was formed in 1991 by the National Coalition of Midwifery Educators as a not-for-profit corporation. The purpose of the council is to accredit direct-entry midwifery educational programs and institutions under the rules of the Department of Education. MEAC has applied for recognition as a federally recognized accrediting agency by the Department of Education.

MEAC's standards for accreditation were developed by expert midwifery educators from a variety of direct-entry educational programs in the United States. Institutions and programs accredited by MEAC provide the student with the requirements necessary to qualify for the North American Registry of Midwives national examination leading to certification as a Certified Professional Midwife (CPM). To become accredited, each program or institution must make a self-evaluation study of its own operations; open its doors to a thorough inspection by an outside examining committee; submit its curriculum for review; and repeat the process every three to five years.

There are currently eight MEAC accredited or pre-accredited programs and institutions in the United States.

NATUROPATHY

Council on Naturopathic Medical Education (CNME)

c/o Robert B. Lofft, Executive Director
P.O. Box 11426
Eugene, Oregon 97440-3626
PHONE: (541) 484-6028
E-MAIL: dir@cnme.org
WEBSITE: www.cnme.org

CNME, founded in 1978, is recognized by the U.S. Secretary of Education as the national accrediting agency for educational programs leading to the Doctor of Naturopathy or Doctor of Naturopathic Medicine (N.D.) degrees. Accreditation or candidacy is a requirement for American colleges to participate in federal student loan programs.

CNME considers for accreditation only four-year, in-residence, doctoral-level programs that prepare students to become licensed naturopathic physicians in the eleven states, Puerto Rico, and five Canadian provinces that recognize the profession. Accredited programs must consist of at least 4,200 clock hours, including 1,200 clinic hours under the supervision of licensed physicians. The council does not accept accreditation applications from correspondence schools and does not provide information about them.

Currently, three schools are accredited (Bastyr University, National College of Naturopathic Medicine, and Southwest College of Naturopathic Medicine) and one is a candidate for accreditation (Canadian College of Naturopathic Medicine).

POLARITY THERAPY

American Polarity Therapy Association (APTA)

P.O. Box 19858
Boulder, Colorado 80308
PHONE: (303) 545-2080/ (800) 359-5620 (messages only)
FAX: (303) 545-2161
E-MAIL: satvaHQ@aol.com
WEBSITE: www.PolarityTherapy.org

APTA approves schools and training centers that develop course descriptions based on the APTA Standards for Practice, which defines competencies required for practitioners to be certified by APTA at two levels: an entry level (155 hours of training) called Associate Polarity Practitioner (A.P.P.), and an advanced level (615 hours of training) called Registered Polarity Practitioner (R.P.P.). Currently, forty schools offer A.P.P. training and seventeen offer R.P.P. training; contact APTA for an updated list.

As a nonprofit organization, APTA's primary mission is to advance the profession of polarity therapy. See pages 459–60 for membership information.

YOGA

American Yoga Association

P.O. Box 19986
Sarasota, Florida 34276
PHONE: (941) 927-4977
FAX: (941) 921-9844
E-MAIL: yogamerica@aol.com
WEBSITE: users.aol.com/amyogaassn

Currently there is no national certification of yoga instructors, nor any national agencies accrediting or approving schools of yoga. Some organizations may certify teachers after a week of instruction; others, after three or more years of study and practice.

The American Yoga Association recommends that prospective students ask the following questions: Does the teacher practice yoga exercise, breathing, and meditation daily? Does the teacher study regularly with a teacher of his or her own? Is the teacher a vegetarian? Does he or she smoke or use drugs? Is he or she nutritionally aware? Yoga should influence the teacher's entire lifestyle. Is the teacher knowledgeable in anatomy and physiology; in the effects of the exercises, breathing, and meditation; and in varying exercises for each person's capabilities?

For additional information, contact the American Yoga Association.

Licensing and Certification

Probably the most crucial thing to consider before committing to a program is whether or not it will provide you with adequate training to practice in your desired location. In some areas, licensing requirements are determined at the state level; in others, the individual county or city determines the level of education needed for a license.

This section gives a brief description of the laws and licensing requirements that are currently in place for a number of fields of alternative medicine, followed by agencies who can help you determine the current legal status of each field and whether the program you plan to attend will meet legal requirements.

Students are strongly urged to contact the appropriate licensing boards in the state in which they intend to practice before putting down a deposit on any educational program.

ACUPUNCTURE AND ORIENTAL MEDICINE

At the present time, acupuncture licensing is required in thirty-two states and the District of Columbia. In almost all of these jurisdictions, NCCAOM certification is a requirement to fulfill some or all of the licensure requirements; graduation from an ACAOM-accredited or candidate school is required for a large and increasing number of states for licensure eligibility. Students attending an unaccredited or noncandidate school may find upon graduation that they are unable to get a license in the state in which they'd hoped to practice.

The Accreditation Commission for Acupuncture and Oriental Medicine (ACAOM) has accredited twenty-nine schools in the United States; an additional eleven programs are candidates for accreditation.

For updated information on acupuncture laws by state, visit the website: www.acupuncture.com/StateLaws/statelaws.htm.

For information on NCCAOM certification, visit www.nccaom.org.

Contact these organizations for additional information:

American Academy of Medical Acupuncture (AAMA)

5820 Wilshire Boulevard, Suite 500
Los Angeles, California 90036
PHONE: (323) 937-5514
FAX: (323) 937-0959
E-MAIL: jdowden@prodigy.net
WEBSITE: www.medicalacupuncture.org

AAMA was founded in 1987 by a group of physicians who were graduates of the Medical Acupuncture for Physicians training programs sponsored by UCLA School of Medicine. AAMA serves as an educational, certifying, and professional (see pages 445-46) organization.

AAMA has created a proficiency examination for physicians who have incorporated acupuncture into their medical practice; the Board of Directors awards a Certificate of Proficiency in Medical Acupuncture to individuals who successfully pass this exam. The exam is the first step toward establishing a formal, recognized, board certification program. The examination is held at various locations throughout the United States, and the examination fee is $500. An optional review course is given on the two days prior to the exam; see pages 384-85.

National Certification Commission for Acupuncture and Oriental Medicine (NCCAOM)

11 Canal Center Plaza, Suite 300
Alexandria, Virginia 22314

PHONE: (703) 548-9004
FAX: (703) 548-9079
E-MAIL: info@nccaom.org
WEBSITE: www.nccaom.org

At the present time acupuncture licensing is required in thirty-six states and the District of Columbia (see website for a complete listing). In almost all of these jurisdictions, NCCAOM certification is a requirement to fulfill some or all of the licensure requirements. Since giving its first examination in 1985, the NCCAOM has certified over 7,000 acupuncturists, over 2,000 Chinese herbologists, and 200 Oriental bodywork therapists. NCCAOM is accredited by the National Commission for Certifying Agencies of the National Organization for Competency Assurance.

NCCAOM has three separate certification programs: Diplomate in Acupuncture, Diplomate in Chinese Herbology, and Diplomate in Oriental Bodywork Therapy. Earning the Diplomate designation demonstrates to patients and employers that the recipient has met national professional standards of skill and knowledge necessary for a safe and competent practice.

To meet the NCCAOM requirements in acupuncture, Chinese herbology, and Oriental bodywork therapy, practitioners must be at least 18 years old, qualify to take the examination through one of four defined routes of eligibility, subscribe to a national code of ethics, pass all portions of the NCCAOM examinations, and successfully complete a Clean Needle Technique Course.

The NCCAOM examination in acupuncture features a written exam and a point location exam. Certification fees are $900 for acupuncture ($400 application fee and $500 examination fee), $750 for Chinese herbology ($400 application fee and $350 examination fee), and $750 for Oriental bodywork therapy ($400 application fee and $350 examination fee).

AROMATHERAPY

The practice of aromatherapy is largely unregulated. Though aromatherapists can't legally diagnose and treat illnesses, they may teach others how to prepare blends, create aromatic bath oils, and use essential oils to treat themselves and their family members, and may produce and sell a variety of aromatic products. Aromatherapy used in conjunction with massage is covered under a massage therapy license.

There are as yet no legal standards for aromatherapy training or certification in the United States; however, the National Association for Holistic Aromatherapy (NAHA) has developed guidelines for aromatherapy education and certification; see below.

National Association for Holistic Aromatherapy (NAHA)

2000 2nd Avenue, Suite 206
Seattle, Washington 98121
PHONE: (206) 256-0741 / (888) ASK-NAHA
E-MAIL: Info@NAHA.org
WEBSITE: NAHA.org

The National Association for Holistic Aromatherapy (NAHA) is a nonprofit educational organization whose mission is to promote and maintain high standards of education in the field of aromatherapy. NAHA also establishes professional and ethical standards of the practice of aromatherapy and provides public education to enhance public knowledge of this holistic healing modality.

NAHA's education committee, the Council for Aromatherapy Schools and Educators, has passed core curriculum requirements for national aromatherapy education. NAHA has also released a national examination for its professional aromatherapist category of membership. NAHA maintains a member registry for professional aromatherapists with the United States.

For information on accreditation, see page 428; for NAHA membership, see page 448.

BIOFEEDBACK

Biofeedback practitioners are not required by law to be certified; in states that license psychologists, nurses, and other professionals, the state license is all that is required to practice biofeedback, and technicians may work under their employer's license. Practitioners may be certified by BCIA; see below.

Biofeedback Certification Institute of America (BCIA)

10200 West 44th Avenue, Suite 310
Wheat Ridge, Colorado 80033-2840
PHONE: (303) 420-2902

Biofeedback practitioners are not required by law to be certified. BCIA was established in 1981 to create and maintain standards for practitioners who use biofeedback, and to certify those who meet these standards.

The certification process involves a review of credentials, written and practical examinations, and recertification. All applicants for certification must hold a bachelor's degree or higher in an approved health care field from an accredited institution and have at least 200 hours of training that includes sixty hours of didactic education in biofeedback, including a course in human anatomy or physiology and a counseling course and practicum; personal experience with biofeedback; and 140 hours of supervised clinical biofeedback training.

Candidates must obtain their didactic biofeedback education from either a regionally accredited academic institution or a BCIA-accredited training program in the eleven Blueprint Areas, which are: Introduction to Biofeedback; Preparing for Clinical Intervention; Neuromuscular Intervention: General; Neuromuscular Intervention: Specific; Central Nervous System Interventions: General; Autonomic Nervous System Interventions: General; Autonomic Nervous System Interventions: Specific; Biofeedback and Distress; Instrumentation; Adjunctive Techniques and Cognitive Interventions; and Professional Conduct.

Candidates should be prepared to document that they are licensed in a BCIA-approved health care field or are supervised by an individual who meets BCIA's qualifications for supervisors.

Certification is granted for four years. Examinations are offered twice each year. Fees are $25 for the application packet and $375 for initial application fees. Recertification every four years requires continuing formal education and payment of applicable fees.

For information on BCIA accreditation, see page 429.

CHIROPRACTIC

All fifty states plus the District of Columbia, the U.S. Virgin Islands, and Puerto Rico license chiropractors as health care providers. In general, students must have completed two years (in some states, four years) of a preprofessional, college-level education prior to attending a four-year (at least 4,200-hour) chiropractic college. For a graduate to be eligible for licensure, the chiropractic college must be accredited by the Council on Chiropractic Education (CCE) and/or approved by the state board; national exams and some state assessment are also required.

Legally, chiropractors are permitted to do much more than align a spine. Like any doctor, a chiropractor will take a medical history and conduct a physical exam, and may order lab tests or X-rays in order to arrive at a diagnosis. Most chiropractors will also work with their patients to develop a plan for a healthier lifestyle through better nutrition, exercise, improved posture, and other changes.

State statutes set boundaries for chiropractors that often fall far short of what is permissible for physicians, however: currently no state allows chiropractors to prescribe drugs or perform major surgery. Some states, like Michigan, prohibit venipuncture for lab diagnosis or the dispensing of vitamin supplements; others, like Oregon, are more liberal, allowing chiropractors to perform minor surgery and pelvic and rectal exams, and to collect blood specimens for diagnosis. For specific information on licensure and legal scope of practice by state, visit the website www.ncschiropractic.com/ahcpr/part5.htm.

For additional information regarding licensure, contact:

Federation of Chiropractic Licensing Boards

901 54th Avenue, Suite 101
Greeley, Colorado 80634
PHONE: (970) 356-3500
FAX: (970) 356-3599

HOMEOPATHY

The legal status of the practice of homeopathy is somewhat muddled. In most states, homeopathic remedies can legally be prescribed by M.D.s, D.O.s, N.D.s, dentists, and veterinarians; in some states, chiropractors are also permitted to administer homeopathic remedies. The practice of homeopathy may also be legal if done under the supervision of a physician or other licensed practitioner.

Currently, eight states have laws protecting the physician's use of homeopathy and other alternative therapies; three states (Arizona, Connecticut, and Nevada) offer an additional homeopathic license to previously licensed physicians. Nevada also offers professional status for Advanced Practitioners of Homeopathy who work in collaboration with an M.D. or D.O. Homeopathy is currently unregulated in Canada.

For additional information on homeopathy and the law, contact the National Center for Homeopathy (see page 453 or visit www.homeopathic.org) or one of the agencies listed here:

American Board of Homeotherapeutics

801 North Fairfax Street, Suite 306
Alexandria, Virginia 22314
PHONE: (703) 548-7790

The American Board of Homeotherapeutics is a medical specialty board in homeopathic medicine. Candidates who successfully pass the written and oral examinations are awarded the Diplomate in Homeotherapeutics (D.Ht.), signifying the attainment of the requisite knowledge and experience necessary to engage in homeopathic medical practice. Only M.D.s and D.O.s may apply for the examination.

In order to be eligible for the examination, applicants must meet the following prerequisites: be eligible for American Institute of Homeopathy membership (currently licensed medical or osteopathic physicians in the United States); hold an M.D. or D.O. degree and be licensed to practice medicine in the state or province in which they reside; have practiced homeopathy for a minimum of three years; have accumulated at least 150 hours of approved homeopathic education credits and provide documentation of such; function under unquestionable moral and ethical standards, to which two members of ABHt have attested; present ten chronic treated cases, each of which must have been treated for at least one year; and apply to the office of the National Center for Homeopathy, which serves as the

central office of the American Board of Homeotherapeutics, at least two months prior to the examination.

Council for Homeopathic Certification (CHC)

P.O. Box 460190
San Francisco, California 94146
PHONE: (415) 789-7677
FAX: (415) 695-8220
E-MAIL: mail@homeopathy-council.org
WEBSITE: homeopathy-council.org

The Council for Homeopathic Certification (CHC) was created to provide recognition for homeopathic practitioners who have attained a high level of competence, and to assist the public in choosing appropriately qualified homeopaths from all professional backgrounds. The council's board is comprised of homeopaths from major health care professions as well as professional homeopaths, and cooperates with existing homeopathic educational and professional organizations to promote excellence in classical homeopathic practice.

In order to be eligible to take the certification exam, candidates must have a total of 500 hours of training in homeopathy from an established teaching institution, or a total of 500 hours from a formal institution and external seminars. For those who have taught themselves homeopathy or learned under the personal guidance of another practitioner, CHC has devised a point system so that practitioners may qualify for the exam in different ways. Candidates should have at least one year of practical experience in practicing homeopathy and must submit five cases with follow-up interviews over a six-month period.

The seven hour certification exam consists of a written exam covering both classical homeopathy and human sciences, and an oral exam given at a separate time (at present, conducted over the phone) that focuses on the candidate's clinical knowledge, case management, and other aspects of the candidate's professional practice. Exams are held in various locations throughout the country. The application fee of $300 consists of a $250 exam fee and a nonrefundable $50 application fee. Successful candidates will receive a certificate stating that they are

Certified in Classical Homeopathy and may use the designation "CCH."

Homeopathic Academy of Naturopathic Physicians (HANP)

Susan Wolfer, Executive Director
12132 SE Foster Place
Portland, Oregon 97266
PHONE: (503) 761-3298
FAX: (503) 762-1929
E-MAIL: hanp@igc.apc.org
WEBSITE: www.healthy.net/hanp

Naturopathic physicians may take the HANP Board Certification Examination (HBCE) in order to become board certified in homeopathy. In order to be eligible for board certification, physicians must be a graduate of an HANP-approved naturopathic college; be licensed to practice naturopathic medicine; have completed 250 hours of specialty training in homeopathy; submit five cured chronic cases with one year follow-up; pass the written and oral examinations; be in practice for at least one year prior to certification; and present two letters of recommendation.

National Board of Homeopathic Examiners (NBHE)

President: Dr. Marcia C. Sasso, D.C.
5663 NW 29th Street
Margate, Florida 33063
PHONE: (305) 974-3456
FAX: (954) 974-3568
E-MAIL: Msassodc@aol.com
WEBSITE: www.NBHE.com

The National Board of Homeopathic Examiners was incorporated in 1987 to create standardized interprofessional testing for the certification of homeopathic practitioners.

The board administers a comprehensive exam every six months that tests basic proficiency in homeopathic philosophy, materia medica, case taking, miasms, preparations and potencies, repertorization, Einsteinian quantum physics, Arndt Schultz law, all of Hahnemann's Aphorisms in the Organon, and the keynotes, essences, and indications for remedy prescription. The examination consists of closed- and open-book exams, plus a practical/oral examination in which the examinee is required to take a case history and make recommendations. Upon successful completion of all three parts, a candidate is granted status with the NBHE.

Eligibility for taking the exam for diplomate status requires that candidates have previously earned a Ph.D., D.C., M.D., D.O., A.P., N.D., O.M.D., or equivalent-level degree and have received training in homeopathy at a board certified institution. Certificate status is available to nondoctorate candidates. Annual renewal requirements include continuing education, service requirements, and an annual renewal fee.

Visit the NBHE website for detailed information regarding the board, examinations, and member profiles.

North American Society of Homeopaths (NASH)

1122 East Pike Street, Suite 1122
Seattle, Washington 98122
PHONE: (206) 720-7000
FAX: (206) 329-3445
E-MAIL: nashinfo@aol.com
WEBSITE: www.homeopathy.org

The North American Society of Homeopaths (NASH) is an organization of professional practitioners dedicated to developing and maintaining high standards of homeopathic practice. It is a professional membership organization (see page 453 for membership information) that also certifies and maintains a register of qualified homeopaths.

HYPNOTHERAPY

There are many organizations that offer certification upon successful completion of a training program and an exam; usually these organizations require a minimum of 120 to 150 hours of classroom-based training. However, it's not difficult for a school to itself become a certifying agency; "certification" may only mean that you've completed their course.

Certification, whatever it means, has little to do with licensing. Indiana is the only state that licenses hypnotherapists and offers a State Certification for hypnotherapists; applicants must be graduates of state-licensed schools. Otherwise, hypnotherapists may operate in any state with any amount of training.

International Medical and Dental Hypnotherapy Association (IMDHA)

4110 Edgeland, Suite 800
Royal Oak, Michigan 48073-2285
PHONE: (248) 549-5594
FAX: (248) 549-5421
E-MAIL: aspencer@infinityinst.com
WEBSITE: www.infinityinst.com

The purpose of the IMDHA is to provide the public with excellently trained certified hypnotherapists who work in harmony with health care professionals to assist those undergoing medical procedures or challenges. Hypnotherapy helps reduce stress and pain for patients, thereby promoting healing.

The association certifies hypnotherapists and provides referrals. To become certified, a hypnotherapist must have completed 120 hours of basic and advanced training from an approved school of hypnotherapy; pass oral and written certification exams; use hypnotherapy as a professional, full- or part-time; and agree to complete thirty CEUs annually for renewal of membership.

Certified member dues are $135 for new members and $75 for renewal; associate membership is $50 per year.

For information on course approvals, see pages 430-31. For membership, see page 454.

MASSAGE THERAPY AND BODYWORK

Currently, twenty-nine states plus the District of Columbia regulate the massage and bodywork profession. Although twenty-one of those twenty-nine states utilize the National Certification Exam for Therapeutic Massage and Bodywork (NCETMB) either by statute or in rule, not all states regulate the profession by licensure. Whether or not a given state administers massage practice laws, local or county laws may still apply; large cities and counties often utilize the NCETMB in their local ordinances. In states that govern massage, the potential practitioner should contact the Board of Massage (generally a function of the Department of Health) for requirements.

In 1992, the National Certification Board for Therapeutic Massage and Bodywork (NCBTMB) began administering the only nationally accredited certification examination for the therapeutic massage and bodywork profession. In order to become eligible to sit for the NCETMB, candidates must have graduated from a formal education training program of at least 500 hours, or its equivalent. This program must have included 100 hours of anatomy and physiology, 200 hours of massage/bodywork theory and application, and 200 hours of related education. For a copy of the current Candidate Handbook, contact the NCBTMB at (703) 610-0281, or visit their website at www.ncbtmb.com.

The American Massage Therapy Association (AMTA) chapter in any state will also be able to provide up-to-date information on massage laws; it might also be useful to contact a massage therapist currently practicing in the desired locality.

Visit the AMTA website for more information: www.amtamassage.org/about/lawstate.htm.

American Massage Therapy Association (AMTA)

820 Davis Street, Suite 100
Evanston, Illinois 60201-4444
PHONE: (847) 864-0123
FAX: (847) 864-1178
E-MAIL: info@inet.amtamassage.org
WEBSITE: www.amtamassage.org

The AMTA administers an Event Sports Massage specialty exam. The exam is open to all active AMTA members in good standing. For additional information, contact the AMTA education programming manager.

For information on the AMTA Council of Schools, see page 431; for membership information, see pages 454-55.

National Certification Board for Therapeutic Massage and Bodywork (NCBTMB)

8201 Greensboro Drive, Suite 300
McLean, Virginia 22102
PHONE: (703) 610-9015 / (800) 296-0664
FAX: (703) 610-9005
E-MAIL: mdownes@ncbtmb.com
WEBSITE: www.ncbtmb.com

NCBTMB is an independent, private, nonprofit organization that fosters high standards of ethical and professional practice through a recognized credentialing program that assures the competency of practitioners of therapeutic massage and bodywork.

Candidates may demonstrate eligibility to take the national certification examination either through traditional formal education/training or through the portfolio review process.

In the first method, candidates must have completed 500 clock hours of formal training at an established school of massage and/or bodywork (these hours must have been completed at a state-licensed training institute or the school must show exemption from licensing status), with at least 100 hours in anatomy and physiology; at least 200 clock hours in massage and/or bodywork theory and practice, including at least two clock hours of ethics; and the remainder of clock hours in related education. Candidates must show successful completion of their entire program (i.e., if a program is 700 hours in length, candidates must have successfully completed all 700 hours).

Candidates whose education does not meet the above requirements may be eligible through the portfolio review process. Course work requirements are 200 hours of formal education and training in massage therapy and/or bodywork, including at least two hours of ethics; 100 hours of anatomy and physiology; and 200 hours of adjunct/related education and/or professional experience.

The national certification examination application fee is $195; portfolio review candidates must submit an additional $75 review fee. Once a candidate is determined to be eligible to take the exam, the candidate will be sent a list of testing center locations. Exams are administered on a computerized testing system. The exam covers human anatomy, physiology, kinesiology, clinical pathology and recognition of various conditions, massage/bodywork theory, assessment and practice, adjunct techniques and methods, and business practices and professionalism. Contact NCBTMB for a complete application packet.

The Zero Balancing® Association

P.O. Box 1727
Capitola, California 95010
PHONE: (831) 476-0665
FAX: (831) 475-0525
E-MAIL: ZBAOffice@aol.com
WEBSITE: www.zerobalancing.com

The Zero Balancing® Association was founded in 1973 by Fritz Frederick Smith, M.D. The association offers a Certification Program in Zero Balancing (ZB), a hands-on bodywork system designed to align a person's energy body with their physical structure. The Certificate Program is an advanced studies program for the licensed health care professional; it does not provide a person with the legal base to handle another person.

Upon acceptance, the applicant embarks on an eighteen- to twenty-four-month self-paced course of study as a candidate for recognition as a Certified Zero Balancer. Applicants are connected with a faculty member or a candidate in the Teacher Training Program who will act as advisor, mentor, and coach.

Tuition for the Certification Program is $500, which covers processing of application, the cost of overseeing the program, reviewing written work, administration, and student membership in the Zero Balancing Association; it does not cover the cost of ZB classes, individual ZB sessions or tutorial sessions.

Training requirements include class study, correspondence study, and practical experience. Students must attend four or more ZB classes to total a minimum of 100 hours of class time. Required classes (fifty hours) are Core ZB Segment I and II with Practical Experience of three to six months between segments. The remaining fifty hours of course work may be completed in elective classes such as Alchemy of Touch, Geometry of Healing, ZB Master Class, Advanced ZB, or others. The correspondence study consists of performing and reporting on fifty pure ZB sessions, plus two creative essays. Personal ZB experience requirements include receiving a minimum of four ZB sessions and performing a minimum of four ZB sessions. A final examination follows.

Those interested in receiving ZB sessions may contact the association for a Practitioner Directory.

MIDWIFERY

To become licensed by the state or certified by the North American Registry of Midwives (NARM), a national certifying agency, a Direct-Entry midwife must demonstrate a certain level of skill and academic knowledge on the NARM or state exam, and must have participated as the primary midwife on a prescribed number of births and pre- and postnatal visits.

At this writing, direct-entry midwifery is legal and regulated, or legal and unregulated, in a total of twenty-nine states, including California, New York, and Texas; it is legally prohibited or effectively prohibited in a total of seventeen states, including Illinois, New Jersey, and Pennsylvania; and in five states, the legal status of direct-entry midwifery is unclear. Eleven states require national certification (NARM or ACNM) for direct-entry midwives.

For updated information on state midwifery laws, visit midwife.org/prof/direct.htm.

North American Registry of Midwives (NARM)

P.O. Box 41705
Nashville, Tennessee 37204
PHONE: (615) 964-3996

The North American Registry of Midwives (NARM) was launched in 1992 by MANA as a separately incorporated entity. NARM has since developed a competence-based certification process whereby a midwife who successfully passes the NARM Written Examination, documents a specified amount of clinical experience, and demonstrates competence in a broad range of skills, is granted the title Certified Professional Midwife (CPM).

NATUROPATHY

Several correspondence schools (none included in this book) offer programs leading to an N.D. degree; it is not illegal for them to do so, nor for their graduates to use the initials "N.D."

after their names. However, they may not legally represent themselves as physicians or engage in the practice of medicine unless they are otherwise licensed. The CNME does not consider graduates of such courses to be part of the naturopathic medical profession, and points out that the accrediting agencies listed by such schools are not recognized by the U.S. Secretary of Education or the Council for Higher Education Accreditation. For more information, visit the www.cnme.org.

Eleven states and four provinces have laws that specifically license or register naturopathic physicians, and N.D.s practice in virtually all of the remaining states and provinces under various legal provisions. Those states that license naturopathic physicians require graduation from an approved resident college program of 4,200 hours or more, and many require graduates to take the Naturopathic Physicians Licensing Exam (NPLEX), a national licensing examination, and/or another licensing exam.

The NPLEX includes basic science exams (Anatomy, Physiology, Pathology, Biochemistry, and Microbiology/Immunology) and clinical science exams (Clinical and Physical Diagnosis, Laboratory Diagnosis and Diagnostic Imaging, Botanical Medicine, Pharmacology, Nutrition, Physical Medicine, Homeopathy, Minor Surgery, Psychology and Lifestyle Counseling, and Emergency Medicine).

For information on licensing legislation in the United States and Canada contact:

American Association of Naturopathic Physicians (AANP)

601 Valley Street, Suite 105
Seattle, Washington 98109
PHONE: (206) 298-0126
Referral Line: (206) 298-0125
FAX: (206) 298-0129
WEBSITE: www.naturopathic.org

NUTRITION

In general, nutritional counselors are permitted to educate their clients about diet and nutrition, but are not permitted to diagnose or prescribe.

Macrobiotic Educators Association (MEA)

Kushi Institute
P.O. Box 7
Becket, Massachusetts 01223-0007
PHONE: (413) 623-5741 /(800) 975-8744
FAX: (413) 623-8827
E-MAIL: kushi@macrobiotics.org
WEBSITE: www.macrobiotics.org

MEA was created to establish and maintain qualifications for teachers of the Kushi approach to the macrobiotic way of life. The Kushi Institute (see pages 204-5) welcomes all experienced and knowledgeable macrobiotic educators to join the MEA by successfully completing a five-day residential testing program that is held twice yearly at the Kushi Institute. The program currently assesses membership qualifications in two fields of macrobiotic education—macrobiotic health care and macrobiotic cooking instructors—and includes a written exam, an oral presentation on either macrobiotic health care or macrobiotic cooking, a media-style interview, an original written composition, and demonstration of personal education sessions or cooking classes. Teachers may apply for one or both programs.

Requirements for admission into the five-day testing program are: previous certification by the Kushi Institute or prior Kushi Institute Review Board status; at least five years' macrobiotic teaching experience; or completion of the three levels of the former Kushi Institute Leadership Program or the current Macrobiotic Career Training Program (or their equivalent), and letters of recommendation from two macrobiotic teachers.

MEA members are included in a special referral directory, receive a 30 percent discount at most Kushi Institute USA programs, are recommended to media representatives requesting macrobiotic contacts, and are invited to attend an annual three-day MEA Continuing Education Conference for teacher development with Michio and Aveline Kushi.

Nutritional Consultants Organization of Canada (NCOC)

1201 Division Street
Kingston, Ontario K7K 6X4

Canada
PHONE: (613) 382-8161 / (800) 406-2703
FAX: (613) 382-8593
E-MAIL: ncoc@king.igs.net
WEBSITE: www.canlink.com/ncoc

NCOC was founded in 1983 as a voluntary, independent, non-profit organization that provides standards of practice for nutritional consultants. The organization awards two designations to those applicants who have been approved by the Board of Examiners: Registered Nutritional Consultant (R.N.C.) and Registered Nutritional Consulting Practitioner (R.N.C.P.).

The educational requirements for designation may be met by a bachelor's degree in holistic nutrition or equivalent. Proficiency must be demonstrated at the postsecondary level in clinical nutrition research, geriatric nutrition, digestion, therapeutic and clinical nutrition, biology, lipid metabolism, life cycle, sports nutrition, pathology, anatomy, chemistry, biochemistry, vitamins, minerals, allergies, preventive nutrition, environmental pollution, and several other areas.

Additional requirements for Level I: Registered Nutritional Consultant requires ten hours of upgrading each year. This level is appropriate for those involved in writing, publishing, offering seminars, teaching, etc., and who do not see clients on a regular basis and do not require malpractice insurance.

Level II: Registered Nutritional Consulting Practitioner requires forty hours of upgrading each year, and R.N.C.P.s must carry malpractice insurance. R.N.C.P. is the only level that can offer insurance receipts to clients who have coverage for alternative therapies

To receive either designation, applicants must also be active members of NCOC. The one-time registration fee of $294 for Level I, $348 for Level II, covers the application fee and a one-year membership; an annual fee of $107 is required to maintain RNC registration.

REFLEXOLOGY

There is no national licensure for reflexologists, though practitioners may choose to be certified by the American Reflexology Certification Board (ARCB; see below).

In some states, reflexologists are categorized as massage therapists; nine states and six large cities require that reflexologists hold a massage therapy license. In general, a reflexologist who is licensed for nursing, physical therapy, cosmetology, or barbering is probably not required to meet massage therapy standards. For detailed information on the increasingly mucky legal battle over the status of reflexology, visit the web pages prepared by Kevin and Barbara Kunz at www.foot-reflexologist.com.

American Reflexology Certification Board (ARCB)

P.O. Box 620607
Littleton, Colorado 80162
PHONE: (303) 933-6921
FAX: (303) 904-0460

ARCB is a nonprofit corporation whose primary goal is to certify the competency of reflexologists meeting certain basic standards. ARCB is an independent organization and its certification process does not interfere with or negate the certification programs offered by individual schools.

In order to take the certification exam, applicants must be eighteen years of age or older; have a high school diploma or equivalent; have completed a hands-on reflexology course of at least 110 hours; and submit documentation of ninety postgraduate sessions on ARCB forms. Effective January 1, 1999, it is required that the 110 hours of instruction include forty hours of reflexology instruction covering theory, history, and hands-on work; forty hours of anatomy and physiology correlated to reflexology; fifteen hours of anatomy and physiology specifically focused on the study of the lower leg and foot; five hours of business practice; and ten hours of practicum (supervised classroom or clinical work).

The examination has three parts: a written component that tests theoretical knowledge; a practical component that tests technique, pressure, and flow; and client documentations. The total testing fee is $250. Exams are conducted nationally on an ongoing basis.

Professional Associations and Membership Organizations

A great source of information about a particular school or field of study is a professional organization within that field. This section lists just a fraction of the hundreds of organizations that cater to the needs of practicing professionals, but that may also be open to students of the profession or interested individuals. These organizations usually offer a newsletter and/or magazine to their members, as well as discounts, referrals, and general information about the field.

ALTERNATIVE MEDICINE—GENERAL

American Holistic Health Association

P.O. Box 17400
Anaheim, California 92817-7400
PHONE: (714) 779-6152
E-MAIL: ahha@healthy.net
WEBSITE: ahha.org

A nonprofit organization incorporated in 1989, the American Holistic Health Association (AHHA) is the leading national resource connecting people with vital wellness solutions. AHHA supports personal involvement through source lists for practitioner referrals, treatment options, and wellness tools. Membership contributions allow AHHA to provide these materials at no charge. Special memberships offer networking opportunities for holistic health care practitioners, companies, organizations, and healing centers.

Membership contributions are $25 for General Membership, $50 for Practitioner Membership, and $100 for Organizational or Institutional Membership.

National Center for Complementary and Alternative Medicine (NCCAM)

NCCAM Clearinghouse
P.O. Box 8218
Silver Spring, Maryland 20907-8218
PHONE: (888) 644-6226
FAX: (301) 495-4957
E-MAIL: nccamc@altmedinfo.org
WEBSITE: nccam.nih.gov

The National Center for Complementary and Alternative Medicine (formerly the Office of Alternative Medicine) was created at the National Institutes of Health (NIH) by Congressional mandate in 1992 to facilitate the evaluation of alternative medical treatment modalities. The NCCAM sponsors research, provides technical support for preliminary studies of alternative medical practices and provides a public information clearinghouse. Materials currently available at no cost include a General Information Package, topical fact sheets, and a quarterly NCCAM newsletter, *Complementary and Alternative Medicine at the NIH*. The NCCAM website also includes this information.

ACUPUNCTURE AND ORIENTAL MEDICINE

American Academy of Medical Acupuncture (AAMA)

5820 Wilshire Boulevard, Suite 500
Los Angeles, California 90036
PHONE: (323) 937-5514
FAX: (323) 937-0959

E-MAIL: jdowden@prodigy.net
WEBSITE: www.medicalacupuncture.org

AAMA was founded in 1987 by a group of physicians who were graduates of the Medical Acupuncture for Physicians training programs sponsored by the UCLA School of Medicine. Their goal is to promote the integration of traditional and modern forms of acupuncture with Western medical training. AAMA creates and endorses courses in medical acupuncture (see pages 384-85); conducts an annual symposium; publishes a scientific journal, *Medical Acupuncture;* provides information about news in the field; and serves as a resource for practitioners. AAMA has also developed a proficiency exam that leads to a Certificate of Proficiency in Medical Acupuncture (see page 435).

Membership is limited to physicians (M.D., D.O., or equivalent) and full-time fellows, residents, and medical students with an interest in acupuncture. Annual dues range from $50 for students to $285 for a full membership.

American Association of Oriental Medicine (AAOM)

433 Front Street
Catasauqua, Pennsylvania 18032
PHONE: (610) 266-1433 / (888) 500-7999
FAX: (610) 264-2768
E-MAIL: AAOM1@aol.com
WEBSITE: aaom.org

AAOM was incorporated in 1983, and is the oldest and largest professional organization of its kind in the United States. The organization has become the nation's strongest advocate for national recognition of the Oriental medicine profession. Its goals are to have acupuncturists licensed in every state as independent health care providers; to have acupuncturists as covered providers under all insurance policies and Medicare; and to promote research, educate the public, and set high standards for the education of acupuncture practitioners. AAOM offers referrals to qualified practitioners through their toll-free number (above).

Membership benefits include a subscription to *The American Acupuncturist* newsletter, referral services, update bulletins covering association news and legislative reports, member discounts on seminars and supplies, and more. The association also maintains a library of articles on treatments for particular diseases.

Annual dues are $35 for students currently enrolled in a school of acupuncture, and $195 for joint or allied health professionals ($70 for a first-year practitioner, $100 for a second-year practitioner).

Canadian Medical Acupuncture Society

9904 106 Street
Edmonton, Alberta T5K 1C4
Canada
PHONE: (403) 426-2760
FAX: (403) 426-5650
E-MAIL: steven@hippocrates.family.med.ualberta.ca
WEBSITE: www.geocities.com/~skha/

CMAS was founded in 1994 to encourage a recognition of the essential therapeutic importance of medical acupuncture; to act as a liaison between members and national, provincial, or international medical organizations; to provide advice to licensing and other organizations; and to serve as a forum for the exchange of academic and clinical information and for ongoing professional development in medical acupuncture.

Membership is open to licensed professionals, medical students, residents or interns studying both medicine and medical acupuncture in Canada; associate membership is open to those licensed to practice medicine in any other country with acupuncture training approved by CMAS.

National Acupuncture and Oriental Medicine Alliance

14637 Starr Road SE
Olalla, Washington 98359
PHONE: (253) 851-6896
FAX: (253) 851-6883
WEBSITE: www.naoma.org

The National Acupuncture and Oriental Medicine Alliance was founded in 1994 as a member-driven organization committed to fostering open dialog within the profession and working to advance the field of acupuncture and Oriental medicine in the United States. Its membership is composed of individuals and organizations who use acupuncture and Oriental medicine principles in their work and lives. Its mission is to foster high quality health care, professional development and research; to expand public awareness of and access to acupuncture and Oriental medicine; and to work with consumers and other health care providers to develop standards of competency for those who practice acupuncture and Oriental medicine.

Membership is open to licensed/national board certified acupuncturists and Chinese herbal practitioners, acudetox specialists, other health care professionals, students, consumers, colleges, state associations, and vendors. Membership benefits include a subscription to the quarterly newsletter *The Forum;* a listing in the Acupuncture Alliance phone, fax and web referral service for professional members; discounts on professional liability insurance and telephone services; and discounts on books, publications, seminars and the annual conference.

Annual dues start at $20 for consumers and acudetox specialists, $25 for students, $50 for other health care providers, and $50 to $170 for professional members, depending on the number of years of practice.

APPLIED KINESIOLOGY

International College of Applied Kinesiology®—U.S.A.

6405 Metcalf Avenue, Suite 503
Shawnee Mission, Kansas 66202-3929
PHONE: (913) 384-5336
FAX: (913) 384-5112
E-MAIL: icakusa@usa.net
WEBSITE: www.icakusa.com

The International College of Applied Kinesiology®—U.S.A. (ICAK), founded in 1975, is a professional association that promotes the science of applied kinesiology through research programs, training seminars, and regional and annual meetings.

Membership is open to licensed physicians, including chiropractors, dentists, and M.D.s, and students enrolled in pro-

grams leading to such licensing. Annual dues are $400 for professionals and $25 for students. Membership benefits include quarterly and semiannual newsletters, annual publications, annual meetings, patient referrals, and more.

Introductory courses offered by the International College of Applied Kinesiology are part of the Essentials of Applied Kinesiology—The One-Hundred-Hour Certified Course, which is divided into eight individual sessions. These two-day sessions are offered throughout the United States and the world. Other courses that have been offered beyond the Essentials courses include Common Sense in Nutrition from Pediatrics to Geriatrics, Hands-On Pain Relief, the Definitive Disc Seminar, Relieving Fatigue, Chiropractic and Pain Control, and others. Fees for courses vary, depending on the instructor. Interested physicians should contact ICAK for a course schedule.

AROMATHERAPY AND FLOWER ESSENCE THERAPY

American Alliance of Aromatherapy

P.O. Box 309
Depoe Bay, Oregon 97341
PHONE: (800) 809-9850
FAX: (800) 809-9808
E-MAIL: aaoa@wcn.net
WEBSITE: www.aaoa.org

The American Alliance of Aromatherapy is a nonprofit organization established as a resource center and voice for aromatherapy in North America.

Membership benefits for Individuals ($40) include a subscription to *AAoA News Quarterly,* a complementary issue of *The International Journal of Aromatherapy,* and a listing in the AAoA Resource Database. Professional memberships ($55) also include a listing in the AAoA Resource Guide and an additional issue of the journal. Business ($75) and Business Sponsor ($125) memberships confer additional benefits.

The International Journal of Aromatherapy is also available without membership; see page 469.

Flower Essence Society

P.O. Box 459
Nevada City, California 95959
PHONE: (530) 265-9163 / (800) 736-9222
FAX: (530) 265-0584
E-mail: fes@floweressence.com / info@flowersociety.org
WEBSITE: www.floweressence.com / www.flowersociety.org

The Flower Essence Society is a nonprofit, international network of flower essence practitioners, researchers, educators, and others dedicated to the advancement of flower essence therapy (see also pages 87 and 466). Membership benefits include a members' newsletter and access to their interactive website. Membership dues start at $25.

National Association for Holistic Aromatherapy (NAHA)

2000 2nd Avenue, Suite 206
Seattle, Washington 98121
PHONE: (206) 256-0741 / (888) ASK-NAHA
E-MAIL: Info@NAHA.org
WEBSITE: NAHA.org

NAHA is a nonprofit educational aromatherapy organization founded in 1988 and run entirely by volunteer members. The mission of NAHA is to promote and maintain high educational standards in the field of aromatherapy. NAHA also establishes professional and ethical guidelines for the practice of aromatherapy and provides public education to enhance the awareness and credibility of this field.

Membership benefits include a subscription to *Scentsitivity*, a quarterly journal featuring essential oil research, case studies, product reviews, information on aromatherapy education and the business aspects of running a practice, and a schedule of educational events. Members also receive a Source and Practitioner Directory listing reliable sources for aromatherapy products, schools, practitioners, and publications. Professional, Business, and Donor members are entitled to a listing in the NAHA Source and Practitioner Directory.

Membership dues are as follows: Friends, $45 per year U.S./$55 per year international; Professional and Business,

$100/$110; Professional Aromatherapist, $125; and Donor, $250 minimum.

For information on accreditation, see page 428; for certification, see page 436.

AYURVEDA
The Ayurvedic Institute

11311 Menaul NE
Albuquerque, New Mexico 87112
PHONE: (505) 291-9698
FAX: (505) 294-7572
E-MAIL: registrar@ayurveda.com
WEBSITE: www.ayurveda.com

In addition to classroom (see pages 242–43) and distance learning (see page 470) programs, the Ayurvedic Institute has a membership organization whose purpose is to promote the knowledge of Ayurveda. Membership benefits include the Ayurvedic Online Research Center, an encyclopedic collection of searchable hyperlinked Ayurvedic research; the quarterly journal *Ayurveda Today;* and a discount on seminars and products. Membership dues start at $25 for regular membership, $75 for membership with a one-year subscription to the Online Research Center.

BIOFEEDBACK
The Association for Applied Psychophysiology and Biofeedback (AAPB)

10200 West 44th Avenue, Suite 304
Wheat Ridge, Colorado 80033-2840
PHONE: (303) 422-8436 / (800) 477-8892
FAX: (303) 422-8894
E-MAIL: aapb@resourcenter.com
WEBSITE: www.aapb.org

Founded in 1969, AAPB is the foremost international association for the study of biofeedback and applied psychophysiology, with over 1,900 active members and forty-four state chapters. The organization encourages scientific research, seeks to integrate biofeedback with other self-regulatory methods, promotes high standards of professional practice, and disseminates information to the public.

Membership is open to both professionals and students. Benefits include reduced registration fees for the annual meeting and workshops; a subscription to the quarterly journal *Applied Psychophysiology and Biofeedback,* and the quarterly newsmagazine *Biofeedback;* discounts on AAPB publications; and a membership directory. Optional membership sections include Allied Professionals, Applied Respiratory Psychophysiology, Education, EEG, International, Optimal Functioning, Primary Care, Pediatric Care, and sEMG/ SESNA. Dues are $30 for students, $85 for regular or associate individual, and $275 for associate corporate; section memberships range from $5 to $150.

CHIROPRACTIC

American Chiropractic Association (ACA)

1701 Clarendon Boulevard
Arlington, Virginia 22209
PHONE: (703) 276-8800 / (800) 986-4636
FAX: (703) 243-2593
E-MAIL: memberinfo@amerchiro.org
WEBSITE: www.amerchiro.org

ACA is chiropractic's largest organization, with over 18,000 members. The ACA monitors legislation, maintains daily contact with key members of Congress and the Administration, enhances the image of chiropractic through public relations, and advocates the highest ethical standards for its members.

Membership benefits include access to legislative and legal information, Medicare and insurance coding information, proactive legislative/regulatory efforts, proactive media and public relations, credentials verification service, affinity credit cards, credit card processing services, discounted office products and supplies, discounted professional literature services, toll-free "Find A Doctor of Chiropractic" listing that can also be accessed by the public on ACA's website, group insurance programs, hotel and rental car discounts, retirement planning, product and seminar discounts, subscriptions to the monthly newsletter *ACA Today* and the *Journal of the American Chiropractic Association (JACA).* (Partial *JACA* subscription is available for student members.) Membership dues range from a one-time fee of $30 for students to $600 annually for general membership.

For information on the ACA catalog of products, see page 471.

International Chiropractors Association (ICA)

1110 North Glebe Road, Suite 1000
Arlington, Virginia 22201
PHONE: (703) 528-5000 / (800) 423-4690
FAX: (703) 528-5023
E-MAIL: chiro@chiropractic.org
WEBSITE: www.chiropractic.org

Founded in 1926 by B. J. Palmer, ICA is the oldest national chiropractic organization in the world. Its goals are to preserve and advance the chiropractic profession, and to represent the interests of chiropractors and their patients through advocacy, research, and education. Volunteer members staff committees dealing with legislative affairs, postgraduate education, practice management and development, production research, public relations, membership services, definitions and policies, legal affairs, and insurance and managed care.

Membership benefits include competitive professional liability insurance, group health insurance, seminars at special member rates, the bimonthly magazine *The ICA Review* and the newsletter *ICA Today,* a listing in the annual Membership Referral Directory, marketing materials, and more. Membership dues for chiropractic students is a one-time fee of $30 until graduation.

ENVIRONMENTAL MEDICINE

American Academy of Environmental Medicine

American Financial Center
7701 East Kellogg, Suite 625
Wichita, Kansas 67207-1705
PHONE: (316) 684-5500
FAX: (316) 684-5709

E-MAIL: aaem@swbell.net
WEBSITE: www.healthy.net/pan/pa/NaturalTherapies/aaem/

The American Academy of Environmental Medicine was founded to study and treat people with illnesses or health problems caused by adverse, allergic or toxic reactions to a variey of environmental substances. AAEM is accredited by the Accreditation Council for Continuing Medical Education to sponsor continuing medical education for physicians; for information on instructional courses, see pages 383–84.

Over 400 physicians in the United States and around the world are members of AAEM. There are eight categories of membership, with membership dues as follows: Student, $60; Associate or Affiliate, $250; and Member, Fellow or Retired, $420. Membership is open to physicians, nonphysicians working in the area of Environmental Medicine or supportive of its principles and practice, and to organizations. Membership benefits include a directory of members and reduced rates for seminars, courses, and publications.

National Foundation for the Chemically Hypersensitive

4407 Swinson-Newman Road
Rhodes, Michigan 48652
PHONE: (517) 689-6369

The National Foundation for the Chemically Hypersensitive is a nonprofit volunteer organization dedicated to research, education, dissemination of information, patient-to-doctor referrals, patient-to-attorney referrals, Social Security, Disability, and Workers Compensation information, networking, housing assistance, and compilation of case histories and studies. Dues are $20 (includes newsletter) for general membership, $45 for doctors who treat the chemically injured, and $175 for corporations, government agencies, and attorneys.

HERBOLOGY

American Herb Association (AHA)

P.O. Box 1673
Nevada City, California 95959

PHONE: (530) 265-9552
WEBSITE: jps.net/ahaherb

AHA is an educational and research organization dedicated to increasing the public's knowledge about herbs, and increasing the use of herbs and herbal products.

Members receive *The AHA Quarterly,* a twenty-page newsletter that reports on the latest scientific studies, herb books and audiovisual materials, international herb news, legal and environmental issues, and more. Annual membership is $20 ($24 for Canadian/Mexican members and $28 for foreign members). AHA also has an *Herb Education Directory* ($3.50), *Herb Products Directory* ($4), and *Recommended Herb Book List* ($2.50).

American Herbalists Guild (AHG)

P.O. Box 70
Roosevelt, Utah 84066
PHONE: (435) 722-8434
FAX: (435) 722-8452
E-MAIL: ahgoffice@earthlink.net
WEBSITE: www.healthy.net/herbalists

AHG, founded in 1989, is the only professional, peer-review organization in the United States for herbalists specializing in the medicinal uses of plants. AHG offers educational guidelines for herbalists and students (see pages 429–30); serves as an information referral center; represents herbalists to the FDA, Congress, and other regulatory agencies; and promotes further research, education, and study of herbal medicine.

Members receive the quarterly newsletter *The Journal of the AHG,* discounts on herb publications and databases, an optional referral listing in the membership directory, and a discount on the annual symposium. Membership is offered at three levels: Student, $35; Associate, $50; and Professional, $85. AHG also provides a membership directory (free for members; $5 for nonmembers), a *Directory of Herbal Education* ($10), a recommended reading list ($2), and other materials.

Herb Growing and Marketing Network

The Herbal Connection
P.O. Box 245

Silver Spring, Pennsylvania 17575-0245

PHONE: (717) 393-3295

FAX: (717) 393-9261

E-MAIL: herbworld@aol.com

WEBSITE: www.herbnet.com

www.herbworld.com

Founded in 1990, the Herb Growing and Marketing Network is the largest trade association for the herb industry, with over 2,000 members. The Network is an information service, with a library of over 3,000 books and over 200 periodicals.

Membership benefits include the bimonthly trade journal *The Herbal Connection* ($48 without membership; $6 for sample issue); an annual resource guide, *Herbal Green Pages* ($45 without membership); a free business listing in both the online and print versions of the *Herbal Green Pages;* group rates on insurance, discounts on phone service, free classified ads, discounts at the annual conference and one-day business seminars, and more. Annual membership is $95.

In addition, the Network offers *Herbalpedia,* a monthly monograph series covering five in-depth profiles of various botanicals. The monographs range from two to eight pages in length and come double-sided with punch holes. Cost is $48 per year. A sample monograph of rosemary is available for a large SASE with $.55 postage.

Herb Research Foundation (HRF)

1007 Pearl Street, Suite 200

Boulder, Colorado 80302-5124

PHONE: (303) 449-2265

FAX: (303) 449-7849

E-MAIL: info@herbs.org

WEBSITE: www.herbs.org

HRF, a nonprofit organization, was founded in 1983 and is a noted source for scientific, historical, and cultural information on herbs. HRF is dedicated to promoting better world health through the responsible and informed use of herbs, and draws from a research library containing more than 200,000 scientific articles on thousands of herbs and a unique in-house database.

Members receive *HerbalGram* or *Herbs for Health,* plus a quarterly newsletter and discounts on all services. Annual membership starts at $35.

Herb Information Packets contain selected articles and/or discussions by experts on individual herbs, supplements, health topics, and special subjects. Each packet is $7 for nonmembers, $5 for members.

Resource Lists are available on such topics as Herb Farming and Marketing Resources, Herb Business Resources, Natural Product Laboratories, Herb Education Programs, Herb Seed Source List, Herb Sources, Internet Resources, and more; lists are $2 for nonmembers, $1 for members.

The Natural Healthcare Hotline provides fast answers by phone, utilizing the HRF's unique proprietary database, on the health benefits and safety of herbs. Hotline services are $1.50 per minute for nonmembers, $1.10 per minute or less for members, depending on level of membership.

HRF also provides a Botanical Literature Research Service and an Herb Abstract Service for serious researchers; call for details.

The Ontario Herbalists' Association

11 Winthrop Place

Stoney Creek, Ontario L8G 3M3

Canada

PHONE: (416) 536-1509

FAX: (905) 664-1567

WEBSITE: www.herbalists.on.ca

Founded in 1979, the Ontario Herbalists' Association offers members a subscription to the quarterly journal *The Canadian Journal of Herbalism;* lectures by professional herbalists; the Annual Herb Day, a members-only event presenting lectures and discussions by professional practitioners, herb walks, and a vegetarian lunch; a lending library; guided walks led by professional herbalists; and the Annual Herb Fair, Canada's largest herb show and sale, held in Toronto. Membership is $30 General, $100 Professional, plus GST.

United Plant Savers

P.O. Box 98

East Barre, Vermont 05649

PHONE: (802) 479-9825
FAX: (802) 476-3722
E-MAIL: info@plantsavers.org
WEBSITE: www.plantsavers.org

United Plant Savers (UpS) is a nonprofit, grassroots membership organization dedicated to the conservation and cultivation of at-risk native medicinal plants. Their activities include identifying the at-risk plants species, researching cultivation and propagation techniques, securing and operating botanical sanctuaries, replanting and restoring at-risk medicinal plants, consulting, raising public awareness, networking, and working with the natural products industry to bring awareness to all concerned. UpS also rents slide shows, develops programs for creating botanical sanctuaries, and hosts conferences.

Membership benefits include the *United Plant Savers Newsletter;* membership dues start at $35.

HOLISTIC DENTISTRY

Holistic Dental Association

P.O. Box 5007
Durango, Colorado 81301
PHONE: (970) 259-1091
FAX: (970) 259-1091
E-MAIL: hda@frontier.net
WEBSITE: www.holisticdental.org

Founded in 1978, the Holistic Dental Association was created to provide a forum for the development and sharing of interdisciplinary health-promoting therapies.

Membership benefits include a subscription to the *Holistic Dental Association Newsletter,* conference discounts, information on programs and seminars in the health care field, and a directory of member dentists and the treatment disciplines they offer.

Annual membership dues are $250 for dental practitioners, $50 for students, and $125 for all others.

HOLISTIC NURSING

American Holistic Nurses' Association (AHNA)

P.O. Box 2130
Flagstaff, Arizona 86003-2130
PHONE: (520) 526-2752 / (800) 278-AHNA
FAX: (520) 526-2752
E-MAIL: AHNA-Flag@Flaglink.com
WEBSITE: www.ahna.org

AHNA was founded in 1980 by Charlotte McGuire and a group of nurses dedicated to bringing the concepts of holism to nursing practice. AHNA has developed Standards of Holistic Nursing Practice, published the *Core Curriculum for Holistic Nursing,* and supported the development of a credentialing body to create certification in Holistic Nursing. AHNA also offers state and regional conferences, supports the formation of local networking groups, provides and approves educational programs, grants continuing education credit for nurses, and endorses certificate programs for nurses that present content in holistic nursing and/or complementary healing modalities.

Membership benefits include the *Journal of Holistic Nursing,* the AHNA newsletter *Beginnings,* a membership handbook and directory, networking list, reduced rates to AHNA conferences and endorsed programs, discounts on AHNA resources and publications, Charlotte McGuire scholarships, and research grant activities. Annual dues are $50 for Student Membership, $100 for Active/Voting Membership (for currently licensed R.N.s or L.V.N./L.P.N.s) and for Non-Voting Membership (open to anyone).

HOMEOPATHY

Homeopathic Academy of Naturopathic Physicians (HANP)

Susan Wolfer, Executive Director
12132 SE Foster Place
Portland, Oregon 97266
PHONE: (503) 761-3298
FAX: (503) 762-1929
E-MAIL: hanp@lgc.apc.org
WEBSITE: www.healthy.net/hanp

HANP is a specialty society within the profession of naturo-pathic medicine, and is affiliated with the American Association of Naturopathic Physicians. It offers board certification in classical homeopathy to qualified naturopathic physicians, encourages the development and improvement of homeopathic curricula at naturopathic colleges, and publishes the quarterly professional journal *Simillimum,* which includes 120 pages of cured cases, materia medica, news, philosophy, and discussion of practical applications of homeopathic concepts.

General membership ($47) is open to everyone with an interest in homeopathy.

National Center for Homeopathy (NCH)

801 North Fairfax Street, Suite 306
Alexandria, Virginia 22314
PHONE: (703) 548-7790
FAX: (703) 548-7792
E-MAIL: info@homeopathic.org
WEBSITE: www.homeopathic.org

NCH is a nonprofit membership organization and the largest homeopathic organization in the United States. In addition to offering seminars and training programs in homeopathy for consumers and health care professionals (see pages 330-31), the center provides information and literature to the public, the media, the government, and the health care industry, and publishes the monthly magazine *Homeopathy Today.* The center also compiles the annual *NCH Membership Directory and Homeopathic Resource Guide* and coordinates over 160 affiliated study groups across North America.

Membership is open to all. Annual membership is $40 ($55 outside the United States and Canada), and includes the membership directory, the magazine, and discounts on NCH books, products, and its annual conference and summer school.

North American Society of Homeopaths (NASH)

1122 East Pike Street, Suite 1122
Seattle, Washington 98122
PHONE: (206) 720-7000
FAX: (206) 329-3445

E-MAIL: nashinfo@aol.com
WEBSITE: www.homeopathy.org

NASH is an organization of professional practitioners dedicated to developing and maintaining high standards of homeopathic practice. The organization certifies and maintains a register of practitioners (see page 439), supports the development of training programs in classical homeopathy, supports research, and promotes public awareness of homeopathy.

Associate membership is open to everyone. Membership benefits include a copy of the annual journal *The American Homeopath* and a quarterly newsletter. Dues are $55 for students, $80 for associate, and $150 for Special Friend of NASH.

Ontario Homeopathic Association (OHA)

P.O. Box 258
Station P
Toronto, Ontario M5S 2S7
Canada
PHONE: (416) 488-9685
WEBSITE: homeopathy.on.ca

The objectives of the OHA are to promote the science, art, and philosophy of homeopathy; to encourage professional and educational activities among members of the association; to encourage the standardization of educational requirements for homeopathic practitioners; and to encourage continuing research and trials in homeopathy. Graduates of accredited homeopathic schools who meet OHA guidelines are invited to apply for professional membership. Benefits include a referral service, computer services to repertorize cases, notification of lectures and seminars, continuing education, discounts on homeopathic books, and liability insurance.

Professional membership dues are $275 per year. Other health practitioners, students, and interested individuals are also welcome to join OHA at reduced rates ($25 to $150). Benefits for these members include discounts on publications and notification of lectures and seminars.

For information on accreditation, see page 430.

HYPNOTHERAPY

International Medical and Dental Hypnotherapy Association (IMDHA)

4110 Edgeland, Suite 800
Royal Oak, Michigan 48073-2285
PHONE: (248) 549-5594
FAX: (248) 549-5421
E-MAIL: aspencer@infinityinst.com
WEBSITE: www.infinityinst.com

The International Medical and Dental Hypnotherapy Association (IMDHA) certifies hypnotherapists (see page 440) and provides referrals to certified hypnotherapists. It also makes available a list of IMDHA-approved schools in the United States, Canada, Australia, Brazil, and the West Indies, and publishes a bimonthly newsletter, *Subconsciously Speaking.* Certified member dues are $135 for new members and $75 for renewal; associate membership is $50 per year.

For information on approved schools, see pages 430–31; for certification, see page 440.

National Association of Transpersonal Hypnotherapists

Eastern Institute of Hypnotherapy
P.O. Box 249
Goshen, Virginia 24439
PHONE: (540) 997-0325 / (800) 296-MIND
FAX: (540) 997-0324
E-MAIL: HypTrainer@aol.com
WEBSITE: members.aol.com/EIHNATH

The National Association of Transpersonal Hypnotherapists sponsors an annual conference, sells a variety of books appropriate for self-help or continuing education, and publishes a triannual newsletter, *The Bridge,* that includes articles on existing and new transpersonal methodology, book reviews, continuing education opportunities, legislative changes, and more. Annual dues are $60 for certified membership.

MASSAGE THERAPY AND BODYWORK

American Massage Therapy Association (AMTA)

820 Davis Street, Suite 100
Evanston, Illinois 60201-4444
PHONE: (847) 864-0123
(888) THE-AMTA or (888) 843-2682 [Find a Massage Therapist National Locator Service]
FAX: (847) 864-1178
E-MAIL: info@inet.amtamassage.org
WEBSITE: www.amtamassage.org

AMTA is the oldest and largest national organization representing the massage therapy profession. Founded in 1943, it has over 41,000 members in thirty countries and chapters in all fifty states. AMTA strives to advance the practice of professional massage therapy through the promotion of national certification, school accreditation, continuing education, professional publications, legislative efforts, and public relations. In 1990, AMTA created a nonprofit foundation to fund massage therapy-related scholarships, research, and community outreach.

AMTA played a major role in the development and launching of the Commission on Massage Training Accreditation (COMTA), which is now an independent body (see page 432).

AMTA provides up-to-date information on COMTA-accredited schools and programs, addresses of state boards administering massage practice laws, and a list of chapter contacts for further information.

In recent years the organization has established AMTA's National Massage Therapy Awareness Week, which is instrumental in further educating the public about the efficacy of massage and the professional quality of AMTA massage therapists; AMTA's website, which is recognized as a primary resource for information about massage and the profession; and AMTA's Find A Massage Therapist locator service, a free service that helps consumers and medical personnel find qualified massage therapists anywhere in the United States. These developments not only assist the public but are significant benefits for Professional Members.

Membership benefits also include professional liability insurance, a products discount, continuing education, the *Massage Therapy Journal,* a *Hands On* newsletter, an annual convention and conferences, and more. Dues are $169 for associate membership and $235 for professional active membership; state chapter dues are up to $30 additional.

For information on the AMTA Council of Schools, see page 431; for specialty exam information, see page 440.

American Oriental Bodywork Therapy Association (AOBTA)

Laurel Oak Corporate Center, Suite 408
1010 Haddonfield-Berlin Road
Voorhees, New Jersey 08043
PHONE: (856) 782-1616
FAX: (856) 782-1653
E-MAIL: aobta@prodigy.net
WEBSITE: www.aobta.org

Founded in 1990, AOBTA is a not-for-profit professional membership association of Oriental bodywork practitioners. Currently, the organization serves well over 1,400 members throughout the United States and abroad.

Membership benefits include protection and representation of the interests, rights, and professional standards of Oriental bodywork therapy; high-quality educational opportunities; the *Pulse* quarterly newsletter and biannual *Journal of Oriental Bodywork Therapy* (members receive an advertising discount); optional liability, group health, and disability coverage; membership directory; and more.

Membership is offered at three levels: Student ($30 dues plus $10 application fee); Associate (eligible after 150 hours of instruction; $75 dues plus $30 application fee); and Certified Practitioner (eligible after 500 hours of instruction; $100 dues and $30 application fee).

For information on the AOBTA Council of Schools and Programs, see page 431.

Associated Bodywork and Massage Professionals (ABMP)

1271 Sugarbush Drive
Evergreen, Colorado 80439
PHONE: (800) 458-2267
FAX: (303) 674-0859

E-MAIL: expectmore@abmp.com
WEBSITE: www.abmp.com

ABMP is dedicated to promoting ethical practices and legitimate standards of training, protecting the rights of practitioners, and educating the public as to the benefits of massage, bodywork, somatic and esthetic practices. ABMP has a current active membership of over 25,000.

Membership benefits include liability insurance with the highest limits available in the field, *Massage and Bodywork* magazine with six issues annually, *The Successful Business Handbook, ABMP Yellow Pages* and the *Touch Training Directory* (a nationwide listing of all state-approved schools offering a massage therapy program). In addition, ABMP provides regulatory support, a nationwide referral service, a members-only credit card with no annual fee, and discounts on rental cars, hotels, legal services, travel, office products, and amusement parks. Optional benefits include disability, personal property, and health insurance.

Student membership is $39; Professional-level member fees are $199.

For information on IMSTAC (the accrediting arm of ABMP), see pages 431-32.

The Feldenkrais Guild® of North America

3611 SW Hood Avenue, Suite 100
Portland, Oregon 97201
PHONE: (503) 221-6612 / (800) 775-2118
FAX: (503) 221-6616
E-MAIL: guild@feldenkrais.com
WEBSITE: www.feldenkrais.com

The Feldenkrais Guild® of North America is the professional organization of Guild Certified Feldenkrais Practitioners/Teachers®. The guild maintains standards of practice, certification, training, accreditation, a code of professional conduct, and a grievance process; provides information regarding legislative and licensing issues; publishes a directory, journals, and newsletters; maintains the North American Amherst Training Video Library; promotes Feldenkrais through public relations activities; and maintains a central office for the sale of books, tapes, and more.

Membership is open to graduates and trainees of accredited training programs. Benefits include a listing in the international directory and on the Internet; an annual issue of the *Feldenkrais Journal;* a quarterly newsletter; discounts on books, tapes, and brochures; group insurance information; and more.

Annual dues are $60 for students, and $350 for practitioners. See page 432 for information on accreditation.

International Massage Association (IMA)

92 Main Street, P.O. Drawer 421
Warrenton, Virginia 21088-0421
PHONE: (540) 351-0800
FAX: (540) 351-0816
WEBSITE: www.imagroup.com

IMA was founded in 1994; membership exceeded 24,000 within its first four years. Its goals are to take massage into the mainstream through the unity of massage practitioners; to educate those who have never tried massage; to assist in the success of its member practitioners; and to provide liability insurance to its members. The IMA assists its members with setting up a credit card merchant account, advertising, financial advice, marketing videos, a free Internet referral service, and liability insurance. The IMA has added several new divisions, which include: Yoga, Movement, Aromatherapy, Reflexology, Feng Shui, Kinesiology, Colonic Educators, Massage and Movement Schools, Dance Teachers, and soon, cosmetology, day spas, and more. Practicing Membership is $129; Student Membership is $50.

International Myomassethics Federation (IMF)

IMF Home Office
1720 Willow Creek Circle, Suite 517
Eugene, Oregon 97402
PHONE: (800) 433-4463
FAX: (541) 485-7372
E-MAIL: myomasseth@aol.com

IMF was founded in 1971 to serve the myomassology/ bodywork community. "Myomassethics" is a three-part term: "myo"

refers to muscle, "mass" refers to massage, and "ethics" is a tribute to the high personal and professional standards members hold for themselves.

IMF is an organization of health-service myomassologists who individually practice various forms of therapeutic touch. IMF's purposes are to improve the image and quality of massage services, to provide resources enabling massage professionals to increase their knowledge and skills, and to educate the public about the benefits and variety of healthy touch alternatives.

Membership benefits include an annual educational convention; continuing education programs and resource information; affiliation with state organizations; and *The Myomassethics Forum,* a quarterly publication. For membership categories and dues, contact IMF.

For information on curriculum approval, see page 432.

Touch For Health Kinesiology Association (TFHKA)

P.O. Box 392
New Carlisle, Ohio 45344-0392
PHONE: (937) 845-3404
FAX: (937) 845-3909
E-MAIL: Tch4Hlth@aol.com
WEBSITE: www.tfh.org

Touch For Health Kinesiology Association is a professional membership organization that teaches the Touch For Health technique (see pages 415-16) and supervises and provides referrals for Touch For Health Instructors. Membership benefits include a subscription to the *Keeping in Touch* newsletter, the *TFHKA Annual Journal,* a copy of the membership directory, discounts on catalog products and at TFHKA meetings and events, discounts on liability insurance, and more. Membership dues are $25 for Associate Members, $50 for Basic Members, and $100 for Instructor/Professional Members.

MIDWIFERY

Midwives' Alliance of North America (MANA)

4805 Lawrenceville Highway, Suite 116-279
Lilburn, Georgia 30047
PHONE: (888) 923-MANA
E-MAIL: info@mana.org
WEBSITE: www.mana.org

Founded in 1982, MANA was established to honor diversity in midwifery educational background and practice styles while fostering unity among midwives. All midwives are welcome as members. In addition to supporting the work of NARM (see page 442) and MEAC (see pages 432–33), MANA has developed and makes available the following documents: Aspiring Midwife Packet ($15), Direct-Entry and ACNM Accredited Training Programs ($2), Direct Entry U.S. and Canadian Associations ($1), Educational Resource Packet ($7), Legal Status of Direct-Entry Midwifery by State ($1), and others.

MANA welcomes as members all practicing and student midwives, supportive health care providers in complementary professions, and consumers. Membership includes a subscription to the *MANA News* and discounts for national and regional conferences. Dues are $35 to $50 for students, $60 to $85 for midwives.

NATUROPATHY

American Association of Naturopathic Physicians (AANP)

601 Valley Street, Suite 105
Seattle, Washington 98109
PHONE: (206) 298-0126
REFERRAL LINE: (206) 298-0125
FAX: (206) 298-0129
WEBSITE: www.naturopathic.org

AANP was founded in 1986 to represent the interests of its members, composed of licensed naturopathic physicians and N.D. students. AANP sponsors medical conferences and an annual convention, and makes available information on naturopathic medicine.

NUTRITION AND ORTHOMOLECULAR MEDICINE

American Natural Hygiene Society, Inc. (ANHS)

P.O. Box 30630
Tampa, Florida 33630
PHONE: (813) 855-6607
E-MAIL: anhs@anhs.org
WEBSITE: www.anhs.org

ANHS, founded in 1948, is the oldest natural health organization in the United States. ANHS advocates a total-health approach that emphasizes all aspects of healthful living.

Members receive *Health Science* magazine, discounts on seminars and conferences, a quarterly book and tape catalog, and discounts on all books, pamphlets, and video- and audiotapes. Membership dues are $25 in the United States and Canada, and $45 elsewhere.

The American Vegan Society

56 Dinshah Lane
P.O. Box 369
Malaga, New Jersey 08328-0908
PHONE: (856) 694-2887
FAX: (856) 694-2288

The American Vegan Society is a nonprofit educational membership organization teaching a compassionate way of living that includes veganism—living on the products of the plant kingdom—and excludes the use of animal products such as meats, fish, poultry, eggs, dairy products, leather, wool, fur, silk, and animal oils.

Members receive the quarterly publication *Ahimsa*, which contains articles, recipes, and a listing of available books, videos, charts, audiocassettes, and more pertaining to veganism. Membership is open to vegans, vegetarians, and nonvegetarians. Dues are $18 per year.

Canadian Natural Health Association Founded On Natural Hygiene

439 Wellington Street West #5
Toronto, Ontario M5V 1E7
Canada
PHONE: (416) 977-CNHA /   (416) 280-6025
E-MAIL: cnha@greenplanet.org
WEBSITE: greenplanet.org/cnha

The Canadian Natural Health Association was founded in 1960 as a nonprofit, educational, charitable organization dedicated to teaching healthful living in accordance with natural hygiene principles. Natural hygiene is a way of life that recognizes the needs of the body for pure, raw, vegan foods; proper sleep; exercise; fresh air; water; and sunlight. Emphasis is placed on the superiority of raw fruits and vegetables, nuts, and seeds; the harmful effects of too much protein, drugs, food additives, pesticides, meat and dairy products, and vaccination; fasting as a means of regaining and maintaining vigorous health; and the importance of fresh air, sunshine, exercise, rest and sleep, and emotional poise.

Members receive a newsletter, *Living Naturally;* a directory of practitioners offering discounts to members; discounts on books, charts, videos, and audiotapes; access to an extensive library of books and tapes; and reduced admission to CNHA-sponsored events. Membership dues start at $20 for seniors and students, and $40 for individuals (Canadian members must add GST).

International Society for Orthomolecular Medicine

UNITED STATES
Society for Orthomolecular Health Medicine (OHM)
President: Richard Kunin, M.D.
2698 Pacific Avenue
San Francisco, California 94115
PHONE: (415) 922-6462
FAX: (415) 346-4991

CANADA
Canadian Society for Orthomolecular Medicine (CSOM)
Secretary: Steven Carter
16 Florence Avenue
Toronto, Ontario M2N 1E9
Canada
PHONE: (416) 733-2117
FAX: (416) 733-2352
E-MAIL: centre@orthomed.org
WEBSITE: www.orthomed.org

Orthomolecular Medicine describes the practice of using nutrients, including vitamins and minerals, in therapeutic amounts to establish optimum health. The purpose of the International Society for Orthomolecular Medicine is to further the advancement and raise awareness of orthomolecular medicine throughout the world, and to unite the various groups already operating in the field.

Membership benefits include a subscription to the quarterly *Journal of Orthomolecular Medicine* and to the biannual *ISOM Newsletter,* and a listing in the international referral database. Dues are $195 per year.

North American Vegetarian Society

P.O. Box 72
Dolgeville, New York 13329
PHONE: (518) 568-7970
FAX: (518) 568-7979
E-MAIL: navs@telenet.net

The North American Vegetarian Society, founded in 1974, is a nonprofit educational organization dedicated to promoting vegetarianism and to providing support to new and longtime vegetarians.

Membership benefits include four issues of the NAVS newsmagazine, *Vegetarian Voice,* which features in-depth articles, recipes, reports on activism, book reviews, and local vegetarian group listings; discounted conference registration; and books and merchandise. Dues are $22 for U.S. and $25 for Canadian or foreign individuals; $28 for U.S. and $31 for Canadian or foreign families.

One Peaceful World (OPW)

Box 10, 308 Leland Road
Becket, Massachusetts 01223
PHONE: (413) 623-2322
FAX: (413) 623-6042
E-MAIL: opw@macrobiotics.org

One Peaceful World is an international macrobiotic information network and membership society founded by Michio and Aveline Kushi. There are national OPW offices in over twenty-six countries.

Membership benefits include a subscription to the *One Peaceful World* newsletter, featuring articles by Michio and Aveline Kushi, scientific-medical updates, recipes, menus, and news about macrobiotic activities around the world; a free book and discounts on selected books from One Peaceful World Press and other publishers of macrobiotic books and study materials; the latest information regarding macrobiotic, environmental, and holistic activities throughout the world; and the opportunity to take part in tours, seminars, and special programs.

Annual dues are $30 for individuals (one free book), $50 for families (two free books), and $100 for supporting members (three free books).

Triangle Macrobiotics Association

P.O. Box 2755
Durham, North Carolina 27715
PHONE: (919) 383-4265
FAX: (919) 383-7098
E-MAIL: ceilber@compuserve.com

Members of Triangle Macrobiotics Association, (TMA) receive a bimonthly newsletter that includes a calendar of North Carolina macrobiotic events, recipes, resources, and more, and may borrow audio- and videotapes on macrobiotic subjects free of charge. The *TMA Cookbook* of macrobiotic recipes is available for $5 plus $1.25 for postage; it is free to new members. Membership dues are $10 for students, $15 for individuals, and $20 for couples.

The Vegetarian Resource Group

P.O. Box 1463
Baltimore, Maryland 21203
PHONE: (410) 366-VEGE
FAX: (410) 366-8804
E-MAIL: vrg@vrg.org
WEBSITE: www.vrg.org

The Vegetarian Resource Group is a nonprofit organization working with businesses and individuals to bring about healthy changes in the school, workplace, and community. Physicians and registered dietitians aid in the development of nutrition-related publications and answer questions about the vegetarian diet. The group also develops and sells books, newsletters, and other resource materials; gives presentations at annual meetings of nutrition-related organizations; provides information to the media; sponsors gatherings and one-day conferences; and aids in the creation of local vegetarian groups.

Members receive *Vegetarian Journal*, a thirty-six-page, bimonthly publication covering such topics as vegetarian meal planning, nutrition, natural food product reviews, and more. Membership dues are $20 per year ($10 additional in Canada and Mexico, $22 additional in other foreign countries).

POLARITY THERAPY
American Polarity Therapy Association (APTA)

2888 Bluff Street, #149
Boulder, Colorado 80301
PHONE: (303) 545-2080
FAX: (303) 545-2161
E-MAIL: satvaHQ@aol.com
WEBSITE: www.PolarityTherapy.org

APTA is a nonprofit organization dedicated to the advancement of the profession of polarity therapy. In addition to approving educational programs (see page 433), APTA provides services that include practitioner certification, educational conferences, the quarterly newsletter *ENERGY,* a mail-order bookstore containing all polarity titles and related works, and referrals to trainings and practitioners.

Membership is open to all. Annual membership dues are $125 for R.P.P.s (Registered Polarity Practitioners), $85 for A.P.P.s (Associate Polarity Practitioners), $60 General, $40 for students, and $125 Institutional.

QIGONG
American Qigong Association

450 Sutter Street, Suite 2104
San Francisco, California 94108
PHONE: (415) 788-2227
FAX: (415) 788-2242
E-MAIL: eastwestqi@aol.com
WEBSITE: www.eastwestqi.com

The American Qigong Association is a chapter of the World Qigong Federation and a subsidiary of the East West Academy of Healing Arts (see page 393).

The association seeks to bring together scientists, professionals, institutions, and laypeople to promote research and education in the area of qigong; to establish standards of excellence and ethics in practice; to act as an information clearinghouse for qigong; to establish a resource library including print, audio, and video; to publish a directory of qigong professionals and institutions; and to promote an international coalition. Membership benefits include the *Qigong Newsletter,* free or reduced admission to designated monthly professional lectures on qigong, a discount on videos and publications, and international conferences.

Membership dues are $150 per year for individuals, $100 for full-time students and seniors.

REFLEXOLOGY
International Council of Reflexologists (ICR)

P.O. Box 30513
Richmond Hill, Ontario L4C 0C7
Canada
FAX: (905) 884-0294   E-MAIL: icr.samek@sympatico.ca

ICR was established in 1990 to meet the needs of the profession by providing an international forum for the exchange of ideas, promoting international conferences, and supporting the development of local, regional, and national associations.

Membership is $50 per year ($80 for two years). Benefits include the *ICR Newsletter,* discounts on conference fees, and printed research studies.

VETERINARY HOMEOPATHY
Academy of Veterinary Homeopathy

Larry A. Bernstein, V.M.D.
751 NE 168th Street
North Miami Beach, Florida 33162-2427
PHONE: (305) 652-1590
FAX: (305) 653-7244
E-MAIL: avhcs@TheAVH.org
WEBSITE: www.theavh.org

The Academy of Veterinary Homeopathy (AVH) was founded as a means to train other veterinarians in the practice of homeopathy for animals. The academy has been instrumental in providing basic and advanced training to veterinarians all over the world, and provides an essential link between veterinarians and persons seeking homeopathic treatment for their animal companions.

The academy provides guidelines and standards for the practice of veterinary homeopathy; training in veterinary homeopathy at introductory, basic, and advanced levels; certification for veterinarians completing specific course and practice requirements; an annual Case Conference; a quarterly newsletter; a referral network; general information for the public and media; and a Memorial Fund to honor the memory of departed animal companions and support the advancement of veterinary homeopathy.

Full membership is available to academy-certified veterinarians; affiliate membership is available to all veterinarians by application.

YOGA

B.K.S. Iyengar Association of Northern California

2404 27th Avenue
San Francisco, California 94116
PHONE: (415) 753-0909
FAX: (415) 753-0913
E-MAIL: iyisf@sirius.com
WEBSITE: www.iyoga.com/iyisf

The B.K.S. Iyengar Association of Northern California is a membership organization which owns and operates the Iyengar Yoga Institute of San Francisco (see pages 95 and 494). The mission of the organization is to promote the study, practice, and teaching of yoga as inspired by B.K.S. Iyengar and to foster a flourishing yoga community.

Membership benefits include a subscription to the *Iyengar Yoga Institute Review,* reduced prices for workshops and intensives, and automatic membership in the Iyengar Yoga National Association of the United States.

SELF-STUDY RESOURCES

This chapter provides a listing, arranged alphabetically by specialty, of distance-learning courses, periodicals, videos, catalogs, and other materials that offer basic instruction, serve as handy reference sources, offer a unique perspective, provide ongoing education, or otherwise serve to familiarize you with a field of study.

Although it may be tempting to forgo the expensive, time-consuming, and inconvenient classroom education in favor of a home-study course, you should think about how you want to apply your knowledge. Correspondence courses may be fine for learning how to treat yourself or your family, but if you are preparing for a career, classroom training is the only way to go: in fields that require licensing, classroom-based study is a requirement. As always, look into the licensing laws in the city and state in which you intend to practice prior to putting down money on any course, correspondence, or otherwise.

ALTERNATIVE MEDICINE—GENERAL

DISTANCE LEARNING

The Australasian College of Herbal Studies

P.O. Box 130
530 First Street, Suite A
Lake Oswego, Oregon 97034
PHONE: (503) 635-6652 / (800) 487-8839
FAX: (503) 636-0706
E-MAIL: achs@herbed.com
WEBSITE: www.herbed.com

Founded in New Zealand in 1978, the Australasian College of Herbal Studies, USA (ACHS), opened in 1991. ACHS is a State Licensed Private Career School offering CE credits to R.N.s, L.M.T.s, Veterinarians, and Pharmacists.

ACHS offers distance learning and residential certificate and diploma programs: The Basics of Herbalism; Certificate in Herbal Studies; Diploma in Herbal Studies; Introduction to Aromatherapy; Certificate in Aromatherapy; Diploma in Aromatherapy; Certificate in Nutrition, Bodycare and Herbalism; Certificate in Flower Essences; Certificate in Iridology; Certificate in Homeopathy; Certificate in Holistic Structure and Function of the Body; Certificate in Natural Therapies; Certificate in Homeobotanical Therapy; and Diploma in Homeobotanical Therapy. Lesson format includes virtual online library and real-time online classroom. Fees range from $300 to $3,500; sample lessons of all courses are available for $60 to $120. Payment plans and student loans are available.

For information on residential modules in aromatherapy, see pages 285–86.

The Michener Institute for Applied Health Sciences

222 St. Patrick Street
Toronto, Ontario M5T 1V4
Canada
PHONE: (416) 596-3177 / (800) 387-9066
FAX: (416) 596-3168
E-MAIL: info@michener.on.ca
WEBSITE: www.michener.on.ca

In addition to their diploma program in acupuncture (see pages 374–75), The Michener Institute offers print-based distance learning courses in Environmental Medicine, Principles of Herbology, Multicultural Medicine, Clinically Applied Nutrition, and Psychosomatic Medicine. Courses range from thirty to sixty instructional hours; course fees (including tuition and materials) range from $325 to $400.

Natural Healing Institute of Naturopathy

MAILING ADDRESS:

P.O. Box 230294

Encinitas, California 92023-0294

PHONE: (760) 943-8485 / (800) 559-4325

FAX: (760) 943-9477

E-MAIL: NHI@inetworld.net

CLASSROOM LOCATION:

2146 Encinitas Boulevard, Suite 105

Encinitas, California

The Natural Healing Institute (NHI), founded in 1997, is licensed and certified to operate by the Bureau for Private Post-secondary and Vocational Education and the Department of Consumer Affairs. NHI is approved by the California Board of Registered Nurses for continuing education credit hours (CEUs).

NOTE: Graduation from any of these programs does not qualify the graduate as a licensed primary health care provider, i.e., a medical doctor, nor to diagnose, prescribe, or treat symptom, defect, injury or disease pursuant to California Business and Professional Code 2052.

Distance-learning and self-directed training programs are offered in five areas: Clinical Herbology, Clinical Nutrition, Holistic Health Practitioner (HHP), Naturopathic Physician, and Massage Technician.

The Clinical Herbology program includes instruction in identifying and collecting wild medicinal herbs; how to purchase quality herbs; proper storage and methods of preparation. Over 300 Eastern and Western herbs are presented. Courses included are Introductory Herbology, Preparing Herbal Remedies, Eastern and Western Herbs Intermediate, and Advanced Herbology. Tuition and fees total $673. Students have the option of attending seven days of advanced training in Encinitas.

The Clinical Nutrition program includes Introduction to Nutrition, Major Dietary Systems, Vitamins and Minerals, Nutrient-Dense Super Foods, Antioxidants, Specialty Programs, and Environmental Nutrition and Detoxification. Tuition and fees total $796. Students have the option of attending seven days of advanced training in Encinitas.

The Holistic Health Practitioner program is a combination of the Clinical Herbology and Clinical Nutrition programs. Tuition and fees total $1,497.

The Naturopathic Physician Program consists of the Holistic Health Practitioner Program with additional training in such areas as health analysis, anatomy and physiology, therapeutic uses of amino acids, enzymes, dietary philosophies, homeopathy, fasting, and more. Tuition and fees total $2,376.

The 100-hour Professional Massage Technician Program combines home study with a required seven-day concentrated training. Tuition and fees total $796.

School of Natural Medicine

P.O. Box 7369

Boulder, Colorado 80306-7369

PHONE: (888) 593-6173

FAX: (888) 593-6733

E-MAIL: snm@purehealth.com

WEBSITE: www.purehealth.com

The School of Natural Medicine (SNM) offers natural physician training.

SNM home study courses are also offered separately. Iridology and the Foundation of Natural Medicine consists of fourteen lessons covering Philosophy of Natural Medicine; Symbolic Language of the Interior World; Iris Texture, Density, Constitution and Structure; Iris Signs; Iridian Psychology; The Rayid Model; Bach Flower Remedies; and the various body systems; tuition is $300.

Herbal Medicine covers History and Philosophy, Chemistry, Nutrition, Herbal Formulas, Materia Medica: Holotrophic Herbalism, Body Systems, Botany, Herbal Pharmacy/ Dispensary, and Subtle Healing in twelve lessons; tuition is $250.

The Naturopathy course covers History and Philosophy; Acute Disease; Chronic Disease; Earth, Water, Fire, Air and Ether Elemental Energetics; Heredity, Sexuality, Reproduction and Regeneration; Life Habits and Personal Hygiene; Purification, Regeneration and Transformation; and Naturopathic Sanitariums in twelve lessons; tuition is $250.

The Natural Physician program combines all three home study courses for $700.

For all programs, books, marking, diploma, seminar, summer school, and/or individual mentoring sessions are charged separately.

SNM also offers a clinic, an herbal pharmacy, and a publications department with books, audio- and videotapes, and equipment.

PERIODICALS

Alternative Medicine Magazine

Future Medicine Publishing
1640 Tiburon Boulevard, #2
Tiburon, California 94920
PHONE: (800) 333-HEAL
FAX: (415) 435-9448

Alternative Medicine is published bimonthly. It serves as a digest of journals, research, conferences, and newsletters in alternative medicine and includes feature articles, columns, and departments such as Prescribing—For Yourself, The Holistic Physician, Natural Pharmacy, The Politics of Medicine, and Alternative Medicine Reviews. Subscriptions are $20 for six issues or $35 for 12; back issues are available for $6 each.

Alternative Therapies in Health and Medicine

InnoVision Communications
P.O. Box 627
Holmes, Pennsylvania 19043-9650
PHONE: (800) 345-8112
FAX: (610) 532-9001
E-MAIL: alttherapy@aol.com
WEBSITE: www.healthonline.com/altther.htm

Alternative Therapies in Health and Medicine is a bimonthly peer-reviewed, research-based journal that deals with nonconventional medical practices; Larry Dossey, M.D., is executive editor. The journal includes research abstracts, news, features, conference calendar, and more. Subscription rates for individuals are $59 per year (six issues) U.S., $78 foreign; for institutions, $140 U.S., $160 foreign.

Dr. Andrew Weil's Self Healing

P.O. Box 2057
Marion, Ohio 43305-2057
PHONE: (800) 523-3296
WEBSITE: www.drweilselfhealing.com

Dr. Andrew Weil, probably our best-known holistic practitioner, is the author of several best-selling books, including *Natural Health, Natural Medicine,* and *Spontaneous Healing.* Dr. Weil publishes a monthly, eight-page newsletter that includes feature articles, tips on healthy living, self-healing recipes, health in the news, and Q & A. Subscriptions are $29 per year (twelve issues) in the U.S., $36 in Canada. Visit the website for a free issue and a first-year subscription rate of $16 U.S., $23 Canada.

New Age Journal

42 Pleasant Street
Watertown, Massachusetts 02172
PHONE: (617) 926-0200
WEBSITE: www.newage.com/journal

New Age Journal is published bimonthly with additional special issues published each fall and winter. It covers a broad range of body/mind and alternative health care practices, and includes features, special reports, and such departments as Tools for Living, Food, Natural Health Adviser, Mind/Body, and Arts and Media. It is widely available at newsstands or by subscription. Visit the website for subscription rates of $12 per year (six issues) in the United States, $15 in Canada.

ACUPRESSURE

CATALOGS AND PRODUCTS

Acupressure Institute

1533 Shattuck Avenue
Berkeley, California 94709
PHONE: (510) 845-1059 /(800) 442-2232
FAX: (510) 845-1496
WEBSITE: www.acupressure.com

In addition to their educational programs in acupressure (see pages 62–63), the Acupressure Institute offers a full-color *Hands-On Health Care* catalog of products, which includes healing books, instructional videos, charts, acupressure point flash cards, audio tapes, massage aids, workbooks and charts for equine and canine acupressure, and more.

DISTANCE LEARNING

The G-Jo Institute

P.O. Box 1460
Columbus, North Carolina 28722
PHONE: (828) 863-4660
FAX: (828) 863-4575
E-MAIL: office@g-jo.com
WEBSITE: www.g-jo.com

The G-Jo Institute, founded in 1976, offers a distance-learning program, the Master of G-Jo Acupressure Home Study certification program. The course includes a Basic G-Jo training manual, video, audiocassette, Advanced G-Jo manual, Master of G-Jo Acupressure Certification Test, wall chart, eye improvement program, and Inner Organ Balancing and "Tune-Up" program for $197, plus $5 for shipping and handling. Those successfully completing the course may become an Instructor of G-Jo Acupressure; contact the institute for details.

ACUPUNCTURE AND ORIENTAL MEDICINE

CATALOGS AND PRODUCTS

Insight Publishing

P.O. Box 18476
Anaheim Hills, California 92817
PHONE: (800) 787-2600 / (714) 779-1796
FAX: (714) 779-1798
WEBSITE: www.qi-journal.com

The publisher of *Qi: The Journal of Traditional Eastern Health and Fitness* (see below) also offers a catalog of over 1,700 products including books, CDs and cassettes, videos, wall charts, and models relating to Acupuncture, Bodywork/Tui Na, Qigong,

Philosophy, Herbs and Nutrition, Feng Shui, Tai Chi, Chinese Culture, and more.

PERIODICALS

The American Acupuncturist

Joining the American Association of Oriental Medicine entitles the member to receive the newsletter *The American Acupuncturist*. See page 446 for membership information.

Medical Acupuncture

Joining the American Academy of Medical Acupuncture entitles the member to receive the scientific journal *Medical Acupuncture*. See pages 445–46 for membership information.

Qi: The Journal of Traditional Eastern Health and Fitness

Insight Publishing
P.O. Box 18476
Anaheim Hills, California 92817
PHONE: (800) 787-2600 / (714) 779-1796
FAX: (714) 779-1798
WEBSITE: www.qi-journal.com

Qi Journal is a quarterly journal specializing in traditional Eastern health care practices. Topics include Acupuncture, Acupressure, TCM, Herbology, Qigong, Tai Chi, Shiatsu and Therapeutic Massage, Meditation, Taoism, Buddhism, Zen, and more. Subscription rates are $18.95 per year (four issues) U.S., $24.95 Canada.

AROMATHERAPY AND FLOWER ESSENCE THERAPY

CATALOGS AND PRODUCTS

Flower Essence Society

P.O. Box 459
Nevada City, California 95959
PHONE: (530) 265-9163 / (800) 736-9222
FAX: (530) 265-0584

E-MAIL: fes@floweressence.com / info@flowersociety.org
WEBSITE: www.floweressence.com / www.flowersociety.org

In addition to their weekend classes and week-long intensive (see page 87; see also page 448 for membership information), the Flower Essence Society offers a catalog of books, audiocassettes, flower essences, herbal flower oils, aroma lamps, and more. Shipping is additional. Practitioner discounts are available.

Les Herbes, Ltd.

9 Gerry Lane
Huntington, New York 11743
Phone/ FAX: (516) 271-4246
E-MAIL: info@aromatherapyinst.com
WEBSITE: www.aromatherapyinst.com

In addition to classroom and correspondence courses (see pages 253-54) offered through her school, the American Institute for Aromatherapy and Herbal Studies, Mynou de Mey has a catalog of aromatherapy products including essential oils, base oils, essential oil collections, vegan soaps, aromatherapy books, and more.

The Michael Scholes School for Aromatic Studies

4218 Glencoe Avenue #4
Marina Del Ray, California 90292
PHONE: (310) 827-7737 / (800) 677-2368
FAX: (310) 827-6068
E-MAIL: mhscholes@aol.com

In addition to their classroom and home study courses (see pages 401-2 and 468), The Michael Scholes School for Aromatic Studies offers a comprehensive line of books, essential oils, and other aromatherapy supplies, as well as three books: *The Most Commonly Asked Questions on Aromatherapy* and *A Pocket Guide to Aromatherapy* by Michael Scholes, and *A Pocket Guide to Aromatherapy and Pet Care* by Joan Clark. Send for a free catalog.

DISTANCE LEARNING

The American Institute for Aromatherapy and Herbal Studies

9 Gerry Lane
Huntington, New York 11743
PHONE/ FAX: (516) 271-4246
E-MAIL: info@aromatherapyinst.com
WEBSITE: www.aromatherapyinst.com

The American Institute for Aromatherapy and Herbal Studies offers a correspondence program in aromatherapy that offers the same training as their classroom-based course; see pages 253-54 for a description.

Aromaflex Centre of Healing Arts

511-2055 Carling Avenue
Ottawa, Ontario K2A 1G6
Canada
PHONE: (613) 725-9226
FAX: (613) 725-3402
E-MAIL: aromaflx@home.com
WEBSITE: www.comsearch-can.com/aromaflx.htm

In addition to classroom-based programs, Aromaflex offers a four-module Aromatology Correspondence Course, which includes samples of all oils and hydrosols discussed. Tuition is $950.

Atlantic Institute of Aromatherapy

16018 Saddlestring Drive
Tampa, Florida 33612
PHONE/FAX: (813) 265-2222
E-MAIL: Sylla@AtlanticInstitute.com
WEBSITE: AtlanticInstitute.com

In addition to classroom training (see pages 154-55), the Atlantic Institute of Aromatherapy offers self-study courses on the application of plant essential oils in health and well-being.

The Aromatherapy Practitioner Course is designed to be taken over six to twelve months. Though geared toward the health professional, the course is also open to beginning students or laypersons. Topics covered include what aromatherapy really is, types practices, history of aromatics, available essential oils, buying guidelines, basic essential oil chemistry, effect on human physiology, treatment methods and applications, research on skin absorption, dispelling the myths, contraindications, safety data and toxicity studies, and detailed study of fifty-seven essential oils. The course may be taken by massage therapists for continuing education credits. Cost of the course is $895; $1,070 with two recommended texts.

The Chemistry of Essential Oils and Principles of Perfumery is an advanced course covering such topics in both chemistry and perfumery. Chemistry topics include alkanes, alcohols and ethers, functional groups, alkenes and alkynes, physical properties, phenols, esters, diversity of nature, synthetic vs. natural, myths about essential oil chemistry, distillation, tips on detecting adulteration, and more; Perfumery topics include origins of perfumery, the fragrant art, the perfume types, fragrance user groups, fragrance families, personal fragrances using essential oils, essential oils and carrier oils, odor properties of essential oils, quality control of essential oils, chromatograms of essential oils, and isolated and synthetic fragrance materials. The course may be taken by massage therapists for continuing education credits. Cost of the course is $495.

R.J. Buckle Associates, LLC

P.O. Box 868
Hunter, New York 12442
PHONE: (518) 263-4402
FAX: (518) 263-4031
E-MAIL: janebuckle001@aol.com
WEBSITE: www.rjbuckle.com

In addition to classroom-based courses (see page 409), R. J. Buckle Associates offers a self-directed home study course, Foundations in Clinical Aromatherapy. The clinically based program includes 150 pages of referenced material, audiocassettes, and essential oils, and is approved for continuing education credit for nurses (AACN), massage therapists (NCBTMB), and physicians. Tuition is $500 for nurses/massage therapists, $750 for physicians.

An instructional video of the "m" technique and teaching booklet is $95; CEUs available for nurses and massage therapists.

Canadian Holistic Therapist Training School/Mississauga School of Aromatherapy

2155 Leanne Boulevard
200A Sheridan Corporate Centre
Mississauga, Ontario L5K 2K8
Canada
PHONE: (905) 822-5094 / (800) 326-9491
FAX: (905) 822-0856
E-MAIL: Aromanet@sprint.ca
WEBSITE: www.Aroma.net

Canadian Holistic Therapist Training School/Mississauga School of Aromatherapy offers both classroom-based (see pages 421–22) and distance learning courses in aromatherapy.

The Aromatherapy Certification Correspondence Program covers much of the same material as the classroom-based Certification course and is typically completed within three to six months. Topics include Aromatherapy History; Essential Oil Production/Extraction/Quality; Essential Oils/Therapeutic/References/Detailed Study; Pregnancy/Childcare/Breastfeeding; Skin Care; Aromatherapy in Application; The Holistic Approach; Aromatherapy Aiding Different Conditions; Skeletal System; Muscular System; Cardiovascular; Nervous System; Digestive System; Respiratory System; Genito-Urinary System; Endocrine System; Skin; and more. Locations are set for exam purposes; hands-on practical massage is offered to those who wish to incorporate bodywork. A week is set aside for the hands-on practical (covering ten essential oil blends for therapeutic uses), client assessment, and blending of oils. Students are required to write the final exam upon completion of twenty-five case studies. Tuition is $1,100 plus a $50 exam fee.

The Aromatherapy Advanced Diploma Program may be taken in class or by correspondence. The twenty-four lessons cover Aromatherapy in This Current Era; Botanical Classification; Obscure and Dangerous Oils; Botanical Families; Terpeneless Oils; Chemistry; Actions of Chemical Groups; Chemical Classifications; Major Chemical Compositions of Essential Oils; Essential Oils From Various Species and Countries; Glossary of Terms; Basic Chemical Composition of Essential Oils; Chemical Compositions; Immune Response; Clinical Reference Chart; Pregnancy and Essential Oils; Cancer; Oils; Menopause; Aromatherapy and Meditation/Herbs and Bach Flowers; Anatomy, Physiology, Arteries and Veins; Cells; The Nervous System; and Joints and Bones. Tuition is $1,300 plus a $50 exam fee.

Institute of Aromatherapy

3108 Route 10 West
Denville, New Jersey 07834
PHONE: (973) 989-1999
FAX: (973) 989-0770
E-MAIL: essence@aromatherapy4u.com
WEBSITE: www.aromatherapy4u.com

In addition to classroom-based programs, the Institute of Aromatherapy offers an Internet-based Aromatherapy Consultant program. The curriculum is similar to that of the classroom-based course, covering such topics as Aromatherapy: History and Modern Day Practices; The Sense of Smell; Essential Oils; Methods of Essential Oil Extraction and Yields; Essential Oil Adulteration, Qualtiy and Testing; Toxicity and Contraindications, Methods of Application, Dilutions and Dosages, Hydrosols, Carriers for Essential Oils, Essential Oils in Relation to the Body Systems, Aromatic Materia Medica, Aromachemistry, Botanical Families, Consultation Guidelines and Procedures, Business Practices and Ethics, and Tests and Quizzes. Additional requirements include case studies and a research paper. Applicants must be at least 18 years of age, comprehend English (reading and writing). and have access to a computer. Tuition is $2,995. Visit the website for more information and registration.

Jeanne Rose Aromatherapy

219 Carl Street
San Francisco, California 94117-3804
PHONE: (415) 564-6785
FAX: (415) 564-6799
E-MAIL: hydrosol@excite.com
WEBSITE: www.aromaticplantproject.com/jeannerose/

Jeanne Rose Aromatherapy offers correspondence courses in both aromatherapy and herbal studies (see page 475 for the Herbal Studies Course); the two courses may be combined for $870.

The two-volume, fifteen-chapter Aromatherapy Studies Course ($425) includes History of Aromatherapy, Blending, Guide to 375 Essential Oils and Hydrosols, Methods of Extraction, Aromatic Chemistry, How Herbalism and Aromatherapy Can Work Together, Skin Care, First Aid, and Massage.

The Michael Scholes School for Aromatic Studies

4218 Glencoe Avenue #4
Marina Del Ray, California 90292
PHONE: (310) 827-7737 / (800) 677-2368
FAX: (310) 827-6068
E-MAIL: mhscholes@aol.com

In addition to classroom instruction and a catalog of products (see pages 401–2 and 466), The Michael Scholes School for Aromatic Studies offers two home study courses designed to complement one another.

Beyond Scents, a twenty-hour course, consists of four ninety-minute audiocassettes, one ninety-five-minute video, a home study workbook, twenty-three essential oil samples, and additional supplies. The cost is $250.

The Aromatherapy Series, a 35-hour course, consists of five ninety-minute audiocassettes, fifty-five essential oil samples, a home study workbook, ten carrier oil samples, and several blending bottles, vials, and pipettes. The cost is $275.

Students may register for both courses for $450. Either course meets the prerequisite for attending the five-day certification course described on pages 401–2.

Pacific Institute of Aromatherapy

P.O. Box 6723
San Rafael, California 94903
PHONE: (415) 479-9121
FAX: (415) 479-0119

In addition to conferences and certification seminars offered in various locations (see page 407), Pacific Institute of Aro-

matherapy offers a six-part certification course in aromatherapy via correspondence. The course is usually completed
within 12 to 14 weeks and covers Essential Oils (including production methods, basics of distillation, purity and adulteration, and synthetic vs. natural), Structure and Energy
(essential oil chemistry and research on the effects of essential
oils on the body), Treatment of Disease (medical applications
of essential oils and aromatic hydrosols), Cosmetology (including typical applications of essential oils and hydrosols in skin
care, clays, natural creams, cleansers, and facial mask compositions), Psychology of Fragrance (effects of fragrance materials), and Toxicology (the safe use of essential oils). The course
costs $365, including essential oil samples.

PERIODICALS

The Aromatic Thymes

1804 Dundee Road, Suite 200
Barrington, Illinois 60010
PHONE: (847) 304-0975
FAX: (847) 304-0989
E-MAIL: editor@AromaticThymes.com
WEBSITE: www.AromaticThymes.com

The Aromatic Thymes is a quarterly magazine devoted to the
art and science of aromatherapy, covering such topics as essential oil recipes and uses, treatments, conferences, and more. Annual subscriptions (four issues) are $21.95 (Canada and
Mexico, $35 U.S.; foreign, $40 U.S.).

The International Journal of Aromatherapy

American Alliance of Aromatherapy
P.O. Box 309
Depoe Bay, Oregon 97341
PHONE: (800) 809-9850
FAX: (800) 809-9808
E-MAIL: aaoa@wcn.net
WEBSITE: www.aaoa.org

The American Alliance of Aromatherapy is a nonprofit membership organization (see page 447) that distributes *The International Journal of Aromatherapy,* a peer-reviewed journal that

includes research reports, essential oil profiles, clinical practices, case studies, book reviews, international news, conference reports and more. Members receive one or two free issues,
depending on level of membership. Nonmembers may purchase individual issues at $10 each or $60 for eight issues.

Scentsitivity Quarterly

Joining the National Association for Holistic Aromatherapy
(NAHA) entitles the member to receive their quarterly journal,
Scentsitivity Quarterly. See page 448 for membership informa-
tion.

AYURVEDA

CATALOGS AND PRODUCTS

American Institute of Vedic Studies

P.O. Box 8357
Santa Fe, New Mexico 87504-8357
PHONE: (505) 983-9385
FAX: (505) 982-5807
E-MAIL: vedicinst@aol.com
WEBSITE: www.vedanet.com

The American Institute of Vedic Studies offers a selection of
books, tapes, and distance-learning courses (below) in
Ayurveda, tantra, yoga, Vedic astrology, Vedas, and Hinduism.

DISTANCE LEARNING

American Institute of Vedic Studies

P.O. Box 8357
Santa Fe, New Mexico 87504-8357
PHONE: (505) 983-9385
FAX: (505) 982-5807
E-MAIL: vedicinst@aol.com
WEBSITE: www.vedanet.com

The American Institute of Vedic Studies was founded in 1988 by
David Frawley (Vamadeva Shastri), a Vedic teacher, Oriental
medical doctor, and professional herbalist.

The institute's comprehensive correspondence course is designed for both health care professionals and serious students; no medical background is required. The 250-hour course consists of four parts. Part I: Principles of Ayurveda 1 covers History of Ayurveda, Sankhya and Yoga Philosophy, Ayurvedic Anatomy and Physiology, The Biological Humors (doshas and subdoshas), Prana, Tejas and Ojas, Summary of Medical Systems, and more. Part II: Principles of Ayurveda 2 includes Constitutional Analysis, Mental Nature, The Disease Process, Humors and Tissues in the Disease Process, Differential Diagnosis of Disease Syndromes, Ayurvedic Psychology, and The System of Yoga. Part III: Ayurvedic Treatment Methods covers such topics as The Six Tastes, Dietary Treatment and Therapeutic Food List, Ayurvedic Herbalism, and Ayurvedic Therapeutic Measures. Part IV: Advanced Treatment Methods includes Subtle Healing Modalities of Aromas, Color, Gems and Mantras; Yoga Psychology Therapies and Ayurvedic Counseling; Herbal Treatment of the Channel Systems; Marma Points and Ayurvedic Massage; and more.

Course fee is $325; books and shipping are additional.

Ayurveda Holistic Center

82A Bayville Avenue
Bayville, New York 11709
PHONE: (516) 628-8200
E-MAIL: mail@ayurvedahc.com [Distance learning]
       lotusfair@aol.com [Classroom-based program]
WEBSITE: ayurvedahc.com/aycertif.htm

The Ayurveda Holistic Center offers a two-year certification program in Ayurveda in both classroom-based courses and through correspondence. (See page 255 for program description.)

The Ayurvedic Institute

11311 Menaul NE
Albuquerque, New Mexico 87112
PHONE: (505) 291-9698
FAX: (505) 294-7572
E-MAIL: registrar@ayurveda.com
WEBSITE: www.ayurveda.com

MAILING ADDRESS:
P.O. Box 23445
Albuquerque, New Mexico 87192-1445

In addition to classroom instruction (see pages 242-43) and a membership organization (see page 448), The Ayurvedic Institute offers an Ayurvedic Correspondence Course by Dr. Robert Svoboda. The course is an introduction to Ayurvedic principles and philosophy as well as a new way of thinking about health and disease. The course consists of twelve individual lessons: History and Philosophy; The Three Doshas; The Human Constitution; Doshas, Dhatus and Malas; Pathology; Diagnosis; Therapeutic Theory; Therapeutics of Indigestion; Food; Medicinals; Lifestyle and Routine; Rejuvenation and Virilization. Tuition is $270. The student is allowed one year to complete the course. The course is also available in Spanish.

Institute for Wholistic Education

33719 116th Street
Twin Lakes, Wisconsin 53181
PHONE: (414) 877-9396
FAX: (414) 889-8591

The Institute for Wholistic Education offers a four-part Ayurvedic home study course covering the fundamental principles of Ayurveda. This first-year program covers such topics as Basic Foundations and Principles of Ayurveda; Anatomy and Physiology from an Ayurvedic Perspective; Ayurvedic Etiology, Symptomatology, and Therapeutics; Ayurvedic Nutrition; Ayurvedic Herbology; Stress Management; and Health, Longevity, and the Disease Process. The cost is $250, including books.

A second-year program is offered to those who have completed the first-year program, and includes such topics as the Disease of Lightness and Nourishing Therapy, the Disease of Heaviness and Lightening Therapy, the Disease of Dryness and Oleation Therapy, the Multiple Attribute Diseases, and others. The cost is $250, including books.

Other courses include Hidden Science Behind Hatha Yoga ($250), Psycho-Bio-Cosmosis ($350), and Spiritual Path of Knowledge ($195).

The institute also sells a wide variety of books, body care products, bulk herbs and spices, herbal formulas, essential oils, and more.

PERIODICALS

Ayurveda Today

Joining the Ayurvedic Institute entitles the member to receive their quarterly journal, *Ayurveda Today.* See page 448 for membership information.

BIOFEEDBACK

DISTANCE LEARNING

Biofeedback Institute of Los Angeles

3710 South Robertson Boulevard, Suite 216
Culver City, California 90232-2351
PHONE: (310) 841-4970 / (800) 246-3526
FAX: (310) 841-0923

Biofeedback Institute of Los Angeles has conducted professional biofeedback training programs under the direction of Marjorie K. Toomim, Ph.D., since 1973. In addition to classroom-based programs (see pages 68-69), the institute offers a Home Study Course that includes the text materials used in the classroom program plus one hour of telephone consultation with Dr. Toomim. Topics covered include biofeedback history and theory; the basic psychophysiology of the stress response and stress-related disorders; a variety of relaxation, imagery, and suggestion techniques; biofeedback instrumentation; clinical applications; and ethical principles. Tuition is $425 plus shipping.

PERIODICALS

Biofeedback / Applied Psychophysiology and Biofeedback

Joining the Association for Applied Psychophysiology and Biofeedback (AAPB) entitles the member to receive their quarterly newsmagazine, *Biofeedback,* and their quarterly journal, *Applied Psychophysiology and Biofeedback.* See pages 448-49 for membership information.

CHIROPRACTIC

CATALOGS AND PRODUCTS

American Chiropractic Association (ACA)

1701 Clarendon Boulevard
Arlington, Virginia 22209
PHONE: (703) 276-8800 / (800) 986-4636
FAX: (703) 243-2593
E-MAIL: memberinfo@amerchiro.org
WEBSITE: www.amerchiro.org

The ACA has a catalog of software packages, audiotapes, videotapes, slides, and books for the practitioner or student. For professionals, the catalog includes chiropractic billing and nutrition software, chiropractic exercise videos, new patient orientation slides, and more. The catalog is available in print or online at the ACA website.

PERIODICALS

ACA Today/Journal of the American Chiropractic Association (JACA)

Joining the American Chiropractic Association (ACA) entitles the member to receive their monthly newsletter, *ACA Today,* and the *Journal of the American Chiropractic Association* (student members receive a partial subscription to *JACA*). See page 449 for membership information.

The ICA Review / ICA Today

Joining the International Chiropractors Association (ICA) entitles the member to receive the bimonthly magazine *The ICA Review* and the newsletter *ICA Today.* See page 449 for membership information.

ENVIRONMENTAL MEDICINE

PERIODICALS

Our Toxic Times

Chemical Injury Information Network (CIIN)
P.O. Box 301

White Sulphur Springs, Montana 59645
PHONE: (406) 547-2255

The Chemical Injury Information Network, a nonprofit organization, publishes a monthly newsletter, *Our Toxic Times,* by, for and about those suffering from chemically-related health problems. Topics recently covered include carpet testing, Gulf War Syndrome, chemical hazards, state news, and workplace air quality. A minimum contribution of $15 per year is encouraged.

GUIDED IMAGERY

DISTANCE LEARNING

Academy for Guided Imagery

P.O. Box 2070
Mill Valley, California 94942
PHONE: (415) 389-9324 / (800) 726-2070
FAX: (415) 389-9342
E-MAIL: agi1996@aol.com
WEBSITE: www.interactiveimagery.com

Martin Rossman, M.D., and David E. Bresler, Ph.D., founded the Academy for Guided Imagery in 1989 to provide instruction for health professionals in the imagery process. (See pages 59-60 for their 150-hour certification program.)

Interactive Guided Imagery(SM), the first module in the certification program, is available as an accredited, self-paced study program that includes four video and/or nine audio instructional tapes, two experiential audiotapes, a companion notebook with lecture outlines, and a 500+-page manual of articles, research, scripts, and patient handouts. This thirteen-hour program teaches fundamental skills to help clients work successfully with imagery. The cost is $195 (plus $9 shipping).

The academy also offers the *Healing Yourself* program, which includes nine highly effective imagery techniques in a comprehensive program for home use. The complete program, including book and six cassette tapes containing prerecorded imagery scripts, is $69.95 (plus $7 shipping); the book is available separately for $14.95 (plus $4 shipping), the tape series for $59.95 (plus $7 shipping).

HERBOLOGY

CATALOGS AND PRODUCTS

American Botanical Council

P.O. Box 144345
Austin, Texas 78714-4345
PHONE: (512) 926-4900
FAX: (512) 926-2345
E-MAIL: abc@herbalgram.org
WEBSITE: www.herbalgram.org

In addition to publishing *HerbalGram* (see page 479), the American Botanical Council has a catalog of hard-to-find books on general herbals, specific herbs, women's topics, field guides, general botany, history, ethnobotany, food and nutrition, technical works, psychoactive plants, essential oils, pharmacognosy, and many other topics. The catalog also includes *HerbalGram* back issues, botanical booklets, special reports, software, audio- and videotapes, CD-ROMs, monographs, and more. Gift certificates are available.

Ellen Evert Hopman

P.O. Box 219
Amherst, Massachusetts 01004
E-MAIL: saille333@mindspring.com
WEBSITE: www.neopagan.net/WillowsGrove/

Ellen Evert Hopman, M.Ed., is a psychotherapist, master herbalist, lay homeopath, and international coordinator of Keltria, the International Druid Fellowship. In addition to offering classes in herbal healing (see page 202), Ms. Hopman has written three herbals (*Tree Medicine, Tree Magic, A Druid's Herbal,* and *The Children's Herbal*—each is $12.95 plus $3 postage) and produced a seventy-minute video, *Gifts From the Healing Earth.* In it, she demonstrates the preparation of an herbal salve, birch beer, heart wine, lavender wine, dandelion salad, an Arabic powder for the gums, vegetable tonic, a comfrey poultice, and a cedar and sage smudgestick; $39.95 plus $3 postage.

Susun S. Weed

Ash Tree Publishing
P.O. Box 64
Woodstock, New York 12498
PHONE/FAX: (914) 246-8081
E-MAIL: [checked infrequently] weedwise@webjogger.net or ashtree@webjogger.net

Susun S. Weed, green witch and author of the Wise Woman Herbals, offers videos and books in addition to her programs at the Wise Woman Center (see page 271) and correspondence courses (see page 477).

Susun offers the one-hour videos, *Menopause Metamorphosis* and *Weeds to the Wise;* $29.95 each. *Menopausal Years: The Wise Woman Way* is available as a book ($9.95) or two audiotapes ($15.95). Other books include *Breast Cancer? Breast Health!* ($14.95), *Healing Wise: The Second Wise Woman Herbal* ($12.95), and *Wise Woman Herbal for the Childbearing Year* ($9.95). Add $3 shipping per order. Order toll-free (800) 356-9315 or through amazon.com.

DISTANCE LEARNING

The American Herbal Institute

3056 Lancaster Drive NE
Salem, Oregon 97305
PHONE: (503) 364-7242
E-MAIL: raw2103@aol.com

The American Herbal Institute offers classroom instruction in herbal studies (see pages 283–84) as well as a Modern Herbal Studies correspondence course. This course consists of six sections: Herbology I and II, Nutrition, Anatomy and Physiology, Herbal Remedies Lab (twenty-three projects/lessons), and How to Practice Medicine Without a License (legal issues involved in the practice of herbal medicine). The $600 tuition includes all books, videos, and instructional materials.

Artemisia Institute

P.O. Box 190
Jackson's Point, Ontario L0E 1L0
Canada

PHONE: (905) 722-1074
FAX: (905) 722-8617
E-MAIL: artemis@ils.net

Artemisia Institute was founded in 1972 by Christine DeVai, founder and former president of the Ontario Herbalists Association. The institute offers an Herbal Correspondence Course that covers Nutritional Aspects, including cleansing herbs, detoxification, vitamins and minerals, fasting and repairing, and kitchen herbs; Medicinal Aspects, such as Bach flowers, poultices, fomentations, tinctures, ointments, internal and external use of herbs, Chinese, Tibetan, and Ayurvedic herbs; and other topics such as homeopathy, ceremonial use of herbs, aromatherapy, gardening with herbs, wildcrafting, and more. The course includes two cassette tapes, four books, and reprints. There is no time limit for completion. Tuition is $440 (CDN), paid in advanced or four installments of $125 (CDN).

California School of Traditional Hispanic Herbalism

Charles Garcia
2810 Lincoln Avenue
Richmond, California 94804
PHONE: (510) 233-5837
E-MAIL: cgarcia@dnai.com
clh_2554@hotmail.com

In addition to classroom-based instruction (see page 75), the California School of Traditional Hispanic Herbalism offers online classes. Lectures are sent to students weekly via e-mail; questions and comments are expected within four days for inclusion in the following lecture. Occasionally a question-and-answer session is scheduled through a chat forum.

Classes currently offered are Introduction to Hispanic Herbalism (four classes covering history of California Hispanic herbalism, herbs for minor ailments, poultices, teas, decoctions, folklore; $45); Traditional Hispanic Herbalism and Magic (seven classes covering the hierarchy of lay healers, teas, wines, vinegars, magic, poisons as used in healing, treatment of serious ailments; $75); Hispanic Materia Medica (eight classes covering native and European herbs; $100); and Hispanic Ritual and Magic (two classes covering history, ritual, witchcraft, psychoactive plants, and more; $50). Additional courses are planned on Herbal Sweat Therapies, HIV Issues, Long Term Survival Herbalism, Local Herb Walks, and Magic, Folklore and Legend: Aspects of Native Healing.

Center for Herbal Studies

86437 Lorane Highway
Eugene, Oregon 97405
PHONE: (541) 484-6708
E-MAIL: chs@cpplus1.com
WEBSITE: www.cpplus1.com/~chs

The Center for Herbal Studies, founded in 1993 by Cherie Capps, offers on-site classes (pages 288–89) which are nearly identical to the correspondence program, which is comprised of two courses: the Herbal Studies Diploma and the Clinical Herbology Diploma.

The Herbal Studies Diploma program consists of two units. Unit I covers Basic Herbal Concepts, Harvesting and Preserving, Historical Perspectives, Legal Issues, Herbal Studies, and Herbal Preparations; tuition is $120. Unit II covers Herbal Actions, Botany, Herbal Constituents, Herb Study/ Walks, and Course Review; tuition is $180.

The Clinical Herbology Diploma consists of two units. Unit I covers Healthy Herbs and Foods, Monitoring the Healing Process, Tissue Cleansing, Nutrition: Vitamins and Minerals, Hydrotherapy, Body Cells and Tissues, and Pharmocokinetics; tuition is $120. Unit II consists of eighteen lessons covering the nine major body systems, the immune system, cancer, and treatments using natural therapies; tuition is $540.

Manuals and a video or cassette tape are included with each lesson; recommended texts are additional.

Dominion Herbal College

7527 Kingsway
Burnaby, British Columbia V3N 3C1
Canada
PHONE: (604) 521-5822
FAX: (604) 526-1561
E-MAIL: herbal@uniserve.com
WEBSITE: www.dominionherbal.com

Dominion Herbal College (DHC) was founded by Dr. Herbert Nowell, a naturopathic physician, in 1926. DHC offers Clinical Herbal Therapist, Clinical Aromatherapy, and Marketing Herbs for Industry classroom programs in Vancouver and Toronto (see pages 361–62), as well as several self-paced home study programs covering various aspects of herbal medicine.

The four-year Clinical Phytotherapy Tutorial course is a certified vocational course in the science and art of Herbal Therapeutics. The program includes approximately twenty to thirty hours of home study per week, annual week-long summer seminars (held in Vancouver), a minimum of 500 hours of clinical training under the supervision of a qualified practitioner, and a clinical exam at the end of the fourth year. Students must have completed high school-level chemistry and biology courses or high school chemistry and the Chartered Herbalist Program (below). The curriculum in Year One covers Anatomy and Physiology, Biochemistry, Biology, Botany, Herbal Materia Medica, History and Practice of Herbal Medicine, and First Year Seminar. Year Two includes Pathology, Anatomy, Physiology, Herbal Materia Medica, Clinical Assessment, Second Year Seminar, and Examinations. Year Three covers Nutrition and Dietetics, Pharmacology, General Medicine, Clinical Assessment, Differential Assessment, Third Year Seminar and Examinations. Year Four consists of Gynecology, Obstetrics and Pediatrics, Pharmacy, Medical Laboratory Science, General Medicine, Dermatology, Geriatrics, Psychiatry, Ethics and Medical Jurisprudence, Fourth Year Seminar, Examinations, and Clinical Examination. Tuition is $411 per quarter plus a $75 registration fee; books, seminars, written exams, equipment, and clinical training are not included in tuition.

The Chartered Herbalist diploma program consists of sixty lessons in three parts, and is usually completed in six to twelve months. Topics include Anatomy and Physiology of the Human Body, Pathology and Etiology of Disease, History of Herbalism, herbal remedies and their preparation, selected herbal formulas for various ailments, properties and conditions for use of over 200 herbs, environmental pollution, tonics for babies and small children, animal health care, and more. The cost is $1,000.

Upon successful completion of the Chartered Herbalist Program, students are eligible to apply to the six-month Master Herbalist Program, which includes research and a 10,000-word thesis on an aspect of herbalism; the cost is $500.

The Specially Structured Clinical Phytotherapy course is offered to health care professionals at the physician's level who are interested in developing a working knowledge of botanical medicine. The course is divided into four modules, each taking three to six months to complete. First Module covers Herbal Materia Medica and Philosophy and Practice of Herbal Medicine. Second Module covers Herbal Materia Medica, Pharmacology, Gynecology, Obstetrics, and Pediatrics, and Nutrition and Dietetics. Third Module consists of Pharmacology, Gynecology, Obstetrics, and Pediatrics, Herbal Pharmacy, and Dermatology. Fourth Module covers Dermatology, Pharmacy, Nutrition and Dietetics, Medical Ethics and Jurisprudence, Fourth Year Seminar, Written Examinations, and Clinical Examination. Tuition is $454 per module plus a $75 registration fee; books, seminars, equipment, clinical training, and clinical examination costs are additional.

Payment plans are available.

East West School of Herbology

Box 275
Ben Lomond, California 95005
PHONE: (800) 717-5010
FAX: (831) 336-4548
E-MAIL: herbcourse@planetherbs.com
WEBSITE: planetherbs.com

The East West School of Herbology was founded by Michael Tierra, L.Ac. OMD, who maintains an herb and acupuncture clinic in Santa Cruz, has created a line of herbal products, teaches, and writes about the uses of herbs. A week-long seminar is offered in each year in the mountains near Santa Cruz; see pages 82–83.

The school is approved by the California Board of Registered Nursing to offer continuing education credit for 400 contact hours.

Introduction to East West Herbalism is designed for the beginning herbal student; it includes seven lessons in the basic principles of herbal home health care, including remedies for particular conditions, herbal therapeutics, the use of food and herbs in health and healing, and the foundations of planetary herbal theory. The course costs $100. There are no tests in this introductory course.

A home study course in herbal medicine includes twelve lessons presented with Michael Tierra's book *The Way of Herbs.* Topics include the History of Herbology, A Balanced Diet: The Key to Health, Herbs as Special Foods, Ayurveda Tridosha Theory, Chinese Theory: Yin and Yang, the Chinese Theory of Five Elements, Chinese Differential Diagnosis, the Nature of Medicinal Herbs, Herbal Formulary, Herbal Remedies, and Herbal Therapeutics. The course costs $225.

The Professional Herbalist correspondence course includes the twelve lessons covered in the herbal medicine course above, followed by an additional twenty-four lessons covering over 500 herbs in the Materia Medica, Advanced Oriental Diagnosis, the Six Stages of Disease, Empty-Full Analysis and Water, Blood and Chi Diseases, the Four Radicals and Symptom-Sign Diagnosis, Specific Diseases and Their Treatments, and the Art of Simpling. The course costs $575, or each of the three twelve-lesson sections may be purchased individually for $225.

Jeanne Rose Aromatherapy

219 Carl Street
San Francisco, California 94117-3804
PHONE: (415) 564-6785
FAX: (415) 564-6799
E-MAIL: hydrosol@excite.com
WEBSITE: www.aromaticplantproject.com/jeannerose/

Jeanne Rose Aromatherapy offers correspondence courses in both Herbal Studies and Aromatherapy (see page 468 for the Aromatherapy course description); the courses may be combined for $870.

The 1,200-page, thirty-six-lesson Herbal Studies Course ($550) includes Seasonal Herbal (twelve lessons covering Folklore and Symbolism, Herbs and Diet, Internal Care, External Care, Gardening, Aromatherapy and Color Therapy, Astrology, and more); Medicinal Herbal/Therapeutics (twelve lessons covering herbal remedies for each of the organ systems); and Herbal Practice (twelve lessons covering Herbs in History, Materia Medica, Ancient Herbalism, Moonlore, Herbal Foods, Ritual, and more).

Sage Mountain Herbal Retreat Center

P.O. Box 420
East Barre, Vermont 05649

Rosemary Gladstar is the founder of United Plant Savers (see page 451) and of the California School of Herbal Studies, and cofounder of Sage Mountain Herbs. She teaches workshops in Vermont and around the world (see pages 322–23), and offers a correspondence course.

The ten-lesson course, *The Science and Art of Herbology*, covers such topics as Wild Plant Identification, Herbal Preparation, Medicinal Terminology, Herbal First Aid, Herbal Therapeutics, Hay Fever and Allergies, Traditions of Herbalism, Herbs for Children, Herbal Stimulants, Kitchen Medicine, Herbs for Women's Health, Herbs for Winter Health, Herbs for Men's Health, Herb Gardening, Treatment of Infections and Infestations, Preventive Health Care, Sources of Nutrition in Herbs, Guide for Skin Care and Hydrotherapy, Legal Herbalism, Understanding Flower Essences, Aromatherapy for the Herbalist, the Immune System, and more.

The entire program costs $350; Lesson One may be purchased for $20 to sample the course, and the payment may be applied to the remainder of the tuition.

The School of Natural Healing

P.O. Box 412
Springville, Utah 84663
PHONE: (801) 489-4254 / (800) 372-8255
FAX: (801) 489-8341
E-MAIL: snh@avpro.com
WEBSITE: www.schoolofnaturalhealing.com

The School of Natural Healing, founded by John R. Christopher, N.D., in 1953, offers correspondence courses in herbology and iridology.

The five-level Nutritional Herbologist Program enables the student to understand the basic principles of natural healing. Course levels 100 through 500 focus on preventative methods of avoiding illness, cleansing the internal body, and nourishing the body overall. Tuition is $560.

The Herbalist Program consists of course levels 600 through 1300, focusing on building an herbal foundation, understanding the body's inherent power to heal, and naturally removing the cause of disease. Tuition is $1,000.

The Advanced Herbalist Program consists of course levels 1400 through 2200. The program gives students the skills to become a qualified teacher of herbology. Tuition is $1,275.

To receive the Master Herbalist designation, after completing the correspondence study, students must attend a six-day certification seminar at the school's health retreat in the Wasatch Mountains and take the Master Herbalist exam. Tuition for the seminar is an additional $795 and includes meals.

Herbology courses may also be taken individually.

The Iridology Program consists of two levels of home study and a seminar, all by Dr. David J. Pesek. Level One: Basic Iridology includes twelve hours of home study instruction in the history of iridology, reading a live eye, how to develop a health program using iridology, understanding nutritional requirements through analysis of the eye, and more. Included is Health 100: Be Your Own Doctor. Tuition is $595.

Level Two: Intermediate Iridology offers 15.6 hours of home study instruction in constitutional typing, brain flares of iridology, treatment of conditions and accumulations, extensive training in reading a live eye, understanding the iris and zone map, and more. Tuition is $595. Levels One and Two may be purchased together for $990.

Level Three: Advanced Iridology is a 4-day seminar in Utah open to students who have completed Levels One and Two. Topics covered include training and protocols for reading a live eye and the use of iris photography, lighting techniques, iris topography, sclera indicators, and techniques for building an iridology practice. Tuition is $595 and includes meals.

To receive the Certified Iridologist designation, students must complete an advanced-level oral and written exam, given after the four-day seminar or with Dr. Pesek at the International Institute of Iridology in North Carolina by appointment. The certification exam is $150.

Tuition for correspondence programs includes all required books and materials.

Spirit of the Earth Centre for Herbal Education and Earth Awareness

5871 Bells Road
London, Ontario N6P 1P3
Canada
PHONE: (519) 652-0230
FAX: (519) 652-9190
E-MAIL: shantree@hotmail.com

Spirit of the Earth Centre for Herbal Education and Earth Awareness, formerly known as Balance Life Gardens, offers two home study courses in addition to classroom instruction (see pages 378–79).

Herbal Home Study Course is a systematic, in-depth study of herbs that encourages hands-on learning as students are active in herbal preparation, research, formulation, plant identification, and herb projects; the cost is $695 for ten lessons.

The Therapeutic Herbalism Correspondence Course uses a clinically oriented approach to the use of Western herbal medicine and lays a foundation for the skilled use of herbal medicines with a holistic practice. The course is intended for both the professional health care practitioner and the student of holistic medicine; the cost is $695 for ten lessons.

Susun S. Weed

Wise Woman Center
P.O. Box 64
Woodstock, New York 12498
PHONE/FAX: (914) 246-8081
E-MAIL: [checked infrequently] weedwise@webjogger.net or ashtree@webjogger.net

Susun S. Weed, green witch and author of the Wise Woman Herbals, offers three correspondence courses in addition to her books and videos (see page 473) and her programs at the Wise Woman Center (see page 271).

The *Green Witch* course focuses on developing personal and spiritual connections: to plants, to the earth, and to oneself. Students learn to create rituals, prepare an herbal first-aid kit, and develop Wise Woman ways of living and healing.

The *Spirit and Practice of the Wise Woman Tradition* course examines the three traditions of healing (Wise Woman, Heroic, and Scientific) and the Six Steps of Healing. Students learn to use all modalities of medicine: homeopathic to allopathic and beyond.

The *Green Allies* course explores herbal medicine through direct experiences with plants, plant spirits, and plant medicines. Students spend a full year with one plant of their choice.

Each course is $350 and includes a booklet of twenty-six projects and experiments, video- and audiotapes, the student's choice of books, erratic mailings, three hours of phone time with Susun, and a 50 percent discount at her classes. Payment may be made in four installments.

Wild Rose College of Natural Healing

#400, 1228 Kensington Road, NW
Calgary, Alberta T2N 4P9
Canada
PHONE: (403) 270-0936 / (888) WLD-ROSE
FAX: (403) 283-0799
E-MAIL: coordinators@wrc.net
WEBSITE: wildrosecollege.com

The Wild Rose College of Natural Healing, founded in 1975, offers two correspondence programs: Master Herbalist and Wholistic Therapist. Correspondence courses may be taken individually or as part of a program; prices range from $95 to $500. Some evening and weekend classes are offered in Calgary.

The 560-credit Master Herbalist Program may be completed in nine months to two years. Mandatory courses include Human Biology, Physiology, Herbology, Pharmacognosy, Iridology, Counseling Options, and a thesis. Students are also required to complete forty credits in hands-on therapies such as reflexology, acupressure, Touch for Health, or massage. Cost of the mandatory courses is $1,495; a 20 percent discount is given if the full package is purchased at once.

The 925-credit Wholistic Therapist diploma program is the minimum training recognized by the Canadian Association of Herbal Practitioners for alternative practice in Canada. Mandatory courses include Human Biology, Physiology, Herbology, Pharmacognosy, Nutrition, Vitamins and Minerals, Iridology, Counseling Options, and a thesis. Students are also required to complete one hundred general interest credits and 105 credits in hands-on therapies such as reflexology, acupressure, Touch for Health, or massage. Cost of the mandatory courses is $1,885; a 20 percent discount is given if the full package is purchased at once.

Wild Rose offers a Building Health Holistically Correspondence Course that fulfills the requirement for one hundred general interest credits. This eighteen-lesson course teaches the science of building health and stimulating the natural healing process through nutritional and herbal therapies. The cost of this course is $175.

The college also offers several correspondence courses that fulfill the requirement for sixty credits of Counseling Options. Students may complete the Counseling Option by enrolling in a classroom course or workshop or Wild Rose College or at another institute, or by taking any three Wild Rose Counseling Workshop Options correspondence courses chosen from Arthritis and You, Candida and Immune System, Chronic Fatigue Syndrome, Low Blood Sugar, Spring Cleanse, or Premenstrual Syndrome. These options are $50 each.

Wilderness Leadership International

24414 University # 34
Loma Linda, California 92354-2611
PHONE: (909) 796-8501 / (800) 500-7342
FAX: (909) 799-7122
E-MAIL: outdoorsurvival@yahoo.com

Wilderness Leadership International offers several correspondence courses of interest to the beginning herbalist. Wild Plants to Eat covers the identification, edible parts, habitat, preparation, and nutritive value of over one hundred edible wild plants found in North America. The cost is $50 plus $16.90 for books.

Natural Remedies covers hydrotherapy, massage, uses of charcoal, diseases and their home remedies, medicinal herbs, and more. The cost is $50 plus $15.45 for books.

In Introduction to Herbal Usage, students learn about the uses of common herbs, herbal formulas, herbs for health problems, herbal aid for emergencies, nutritional value/toxicity, herbal preparations, and cleansing. The cost is $50 plus $6.95 for books.

Herbs For Health covers single herbs and their uses, herbal combinations, herbal remedies for more than one hundred ailments, gathering and preserving of herbs, first aid with herbs, and more. The cost is $65 plus $21.90 for books.

Dining on the Wilds is a six-hour set of videos with two reference manuals covering the identification, habitat, season, edible parts, preparation, herbal usage, and nutritive value of 280 wild edible plants. The cost is $149.95 plus $10 for shipping.

PERIODICALS

The AHA Quarterly

Joining the American Herb Association (AHA) entitles the member to receive the twenty-page newsletter *The AHA Quarterly*. See page 450 for membership information.

The Business of Herbs

Northwind Publications
439 Ponderosa Way
Jemez Springs, New Mexico 87025-8036
PHONE: (505) 829-3448
FAX: (505) 829-3449
E-MAIL: HerbBiz@aol.com

The Business of Herbs is a bimonthly, international publication for the herb businessperson and the serious herb enthusiast. Regular features include in-depth articles by herb experts, interviews, marketing and advertising ideas, regional resources, herb book reviews, science and business notes, trends, calendar of events, sources of wholesale supplies, and more. Subscription rates are $24 per year (six issues) U.S., $30 Canadian, $36 international; sample issue $4.75.

The Canadian Journal of Herbalism

Joining the Ontario Herbalists' Association entitles the member to receive the quarterly journal *The Canadian Journal of Herbalism*. See page 451 for membership information.

The Herb Companion

Box 7713
Red Oak, Iowa 51591-2713
PHONE: (800) 456-5835
WEBSITE: www.Interweave.com

Published by Interweave Press, *The Herb Companion* is a bi-monthly magazine that covers herb gardening; using herbs in vinegars, beauty products and crafts; herbal remedies; cooking with herbs; book reviews; and more. Subscription rates are $24 per year (six issues) U.S., $34 Canadian.

The Herbal Connection

Joining the Herb Growing and Marketing Network entitles the member to receive the bimonthly trade journal *The Herbal Connection*. See pages 450–51 for additional literature and membership information.

HerbalGram

American Botanical Council
P.O. Box 144345
Austin, Texas 78714-4345
PHONE: (512) 926-4900
FAX: (512) 926-2345
E-MAIL: abc@herbalgram.org
WEBSITE: www.herbalgram.org

In addition to offering a catalog of items relating to herbal medicine (see page 472), the American Botanical Council, in conjunction with the Herb Research Foundation, publishes *HerbalGram*. This quarterly magazine includes feature-length articles, research reviews, conference reports, and book reviews. Annual subscription rates are $29 U.S., $36 Canadian, $44 foreign.

HerbalGram/Herbs for Health

Joining the Herb Research Foundation entitles the member to receive a subscription to either *HerbalGram* or *Herbs for Health*. See page 451 for additional literature and membership information.

The Journal of the AHG

Joining the American Herbalists Guild entitles the member to receive the quarterly newsletter *The Journal of the AHG*. See page 450 for membership information.

Herbs for Health

Box 7707
Red Oak, Iowa 51591-2707
PHONE: (800) 456-6018
WEBSITE: www.Interweave.com

Herbs for Health is a bimonthly magazine that includes features, Q & A, book reviews, news breaks in herb research, a calendar of events, and more. Subscription rates are $19.95 per year (six issues) U.S., $29.95 Canadian.

Medical Herbalism

P.O. Box 20512
Boulder, Colorado 80308
PHONE: (303) 541-9552 / (888) 237-4637
E-MAIL: bergner@concentric.net
WEBSITE: medherb.com

Medical Herbalism: A Journal for the Clinical Practitioner is published four times a year by Paul Bergner, Director of Clinical Education at the Rocky Mountain Center for Botanical Studies. Features include clinical case studies with commentary, materia medica reviews, international literature reviews, side effects and drug-herb interactions, clinical tips and practitioner reports, TCM, Ayurveda, educational resources, and book, video, and software reviews. One-year subscriptions are $36 U.S. ($25 for students and first-time subscribers), $39 Canadian; back issues are available at $8 each.

United Plant Savers Newsletter

Joining the United Plant Savers entitles the member to receive the *United Plant Savers Newsletter*. See pages 451–52 for membership information.

HOLISTIC DENTISTRY

Holistic Dental Association Newsletter

Joining the Holistic Dental Association entitles the member to receive the *Holistic Dental Association Newsletter*. See page 452 for membership information.

HOLISTIC NURSING

Journal of Holistic Nursing / Beginnings

Joining the American Holistic Nurses' Association entitles the member to receive the *Journal of Holistic Nursing* and the newsletter *Beginnings*. See page 452 for membership information.

HOMEOPATHY

CATALOGS AND PRODUCTS

Homeopathic Educational Services

2124 Kittredge Street
Berkeley, California 94704
PHONE: (510) 649-0294 / (800) 359-9051 (orders only)
FAX: (510) 649-1955
E-MAIL: mail@homeopathic.com
WEBSITE: www.homeopathic.com

Under the direction of Dana Ullman, M.P.H., Homeopathic Educational Services provides health professionals and the general public with homeopathic information, education, and products. Their catalog contains an exhaustive collection of books, directories, research, remedies, audio- and videotapes, kits, external applications, software, veterinary homeopathy products, and introductory-, intermediate-, and advanced-level courses on tape. See pages 483–84 for homeopathic correspondence study courses.

DISTANCE LEARNING

The American Academy of Clinical Homeopathy

612 Upland Trail
Conyers, Georgia 30012

PHONE: (770) 922-2644 / (800) 448-7256
FAX: (770) 388-7768
WEBSITE: www.newtonlabs.nat/academy.htm

The American Academy of Clinical Homeopathy offers a two-part correspondence course in clinical homeopathy. The course was developed by Luc Chaltin, president of Newton Laboratories (a producer of homeopathic remedies) and a practicing homeopathic physician for over thirty years.

Part I: Theory covers such topics as the theory of homeopathy, the Hahnemanian concepts, the origin and evolution of diseases, homeopathic constitutional typology, the miasms and their influence on health, the typology of Dr. Henri Bernard, and more. The cost is $300 plus $5 for shipping.

Part II: Practice offers instruction in the diagnosing and homeopathic treatment of acute and chronic diseases, clinical materia medica, clinical repertory listing the remedies used with chronic diseases, and more. The cost is $300 plus $5 for shipping.

An introductory section serves as a primer and prerequisite to the correspondence course and explains the principles of homeopathic diagnosing and prescribing; the registration fee and introductory section cost $10 plus $5 for shipping.

Ashwins Publications

P.O. Box 1686
Ojai, California 93024
PHONE: (805) 646-6622
E-MAIL: ashwins@aol.com

Ashwins Publications' home study course, *Homeopathic Medicine in the Home,* is designed for parents, health professionals, and others interested in receiving a practical introduction to homeopathy. Topics covered include Women's Health, Homeopathy for Children and Newborns, Immunizations, Psychological Homeopathy, Homeopathy Principles and Philosophy, Homeopathic Materia Medica: Remedy Pictures, Homeopathy for Accidents and Injuries, Homeopathic Pet Care, and more. The twelve lessons, consisting of reading and written assignments, each require about seven hours' work; the average course completion time is six months. The complete course fee of $355 includes three required texts. This course is commended by the Council on Homeopathic Education.

Homeopathic Medicine in the Home is also available without individualized tutoring; the program contains an answer and case analysis key, enabling the self-motivated student to do the entire course independently. The cost of the course books with answer key is $93.

The British Institute of Homoeopathy

520 Washington Boulevard, # 423
Marina Del Rey, California 90292
PHONE: (310) 577-2235 / (800) 494-9790
FAX: (310) 577-0296
E-MAIL: BIHUS@thegrid.net

The British Institute, founded in London in 1987, offers home study courses in homeopathy, human sciences, nutrition and herbology, and homeopathic pharmacy.

The Diploma Course in homeopathy consists of twenty-nine lessons, covering History of Homeopathy, Sources of Remedies, Homeopathic Pharmacy, Homeopathic Materia Medica, Constitutional Prescribing, Combination Remedies, Case Histories, Computerized Homeopathy, and more. The cost is $1,595.

The Postgraduate Course is available to graduates of the Diploma Course or those with at least 300 classroom hours and experience in homeopathy; it includes twenty-six lessons and takes one to two years to complete. Topics include Advanced Homeopathic Pharmacy, Current Research in Homeopathy, New Remedies, Advanced Bach Remedies, Establishment and Management of a Homeopathic Practice, Setting Up a Research Program, and more. The cost is $1,995.

The Veterinary Basic Course consists of ten lessons covering veterinary homeopathy, animal first aid, and acute care. The cost is $650.

The Veterinary Diploma Course is designed for licensed veterinarians and includes twenty-nine lessons covering the homeopathic treatment of dogs, cats, horses, cattle, sheep, poultry, and small animals, constitutional prescribing, animal case histories, animal nutrition, and more. The cost is $1,750.

The Nutrition and Herbology Program consists of ten lessons covering Herbal Medicine, Common Medicinal Herbs, Nutritional Therapy, Vitamins—Sources, Minerals, Trace Elements, Amino Acids, Protein, Phytochemicals, Enzymes, and more. The cost is $450.

The Bach Flower Practitioner's Course includes fourteen lessons covering the history, theory, and practice of Bach Flower Therapy, materia medica of the Bach Flower Remedies, and application of Bach Flower Therapy in special conditions. The cost is $975.

Other courses include Women's Health: Pregnancy-Childbirth ($500), Case Taking and Repertorization ($1,150), Establishing and Managing a Practice ($350), Anatomy and Physiology ($450), and Pathology and The Nature of Disease ($450).

Programs may be combined for a discount. Books are available at additional cost.

The British Institute of Homoeopathy Canada

1445 St. Joseph Boulevard
Gloucester, Ontario K1C 7K9
Canada
PHONE: (613) 830-4759 / (800) 579-HEAL
FAX: (613) 830-9174
E-MAIL: bihcanada@sprint.ca
WEBSITE: www.homeopathy.com

The British Institute of Homoeopathy (BIH) Canada works closely with the British Institute of Homoeopathy in London, which was founded in 1987 and has been active in Canada since 1988. Courses are offered in the departments of Homeopathy, Homeopathic Pharmacy, Veterinary Homeopathy, Sciences, General Studies, and Continuing Education. Courses are offered primarily via distance learning, though some classes are also available in a classroom setting or by independent study in a clinical setting.

The Department of Homeopathy distance learning courses include Homeopathy 001: Introduction to Homeopathy/First Aid (seven to nine hours; $85); Homeopathy 200: Principles/Materia Medica/Acute Case-Taking (500 hours; $1,500); Homeopathy 302: Repertorization/Case-Taking Skills (350 hours; $1,150); Homeopathy 400: Advanced Homeopathic Principles and Topics (500 hours; $1,800).

Distance-learning courses offered by the Department of Homeopathic Pharmacy include Pharmacy 100: Introduction to Homeopathic Pharmacy (150 hours; $600), and Pharmacy 200: Advanced Homeopathic Pharmacy and Principles (500 hours; $1,650).

Department of Veterinary Homeopathy courses include Veterinary 100: Introduction to Veterinary Homeopathy (150 hours; $650), and Veterinary 200: Veterinary Homeopathy (500 hours; $1,650).

Department of Sciences distance-learning courses include Human Sciences 100: Anatomy and Physiology (150 hours; $400), and Human Sciences 200: Pathology and Nature of Disease (150 hours; $400).

Department of General Studies distance-learning courses include Nutrition 100: Nutrition and Herbal Medicine (100 hours; $450); Business 100: Establishing a Successful Complementary Practice (25 hours; $350); and Flower Essence 200: Bach Flower Practitioner Diploma (200 hours; $975).

BIH offers an online study group; new courses are in development and are listed on the website.

Caduceus Institute of Classical Homeopathy

516 Caledonia Street
Santa Cruz, California 95062
PHONE: (800) 396-9778
FAX: (831) 466-3516
E-MAIL: HomeoUSA@aol.com
WEBSITE: www.homeopathyhome.com/caduceus

Caduceus Institute of Classical Homeopathy was founded in 1997 by Willa Esterson Keizer and is a candidate for accreditation with the Council on Homeopathic Education (CHE). The Caduceus Distance Learning Program is designed for health professionals and serious students of homeopathy. The program consists of six modules; each module includes videotaped sessions, exercises, reading, quizzes, and mentoring by correspondence.

Module One is a complete course in acute homeopathy. It may be taken on its own, or serve as the foundation for further modules. In each session of Module One, a different therapeutic topic is covered, such as gastrointestinal conditions or ear, nose, and throat, and the entire acute case-taking process is taught, including repertorization. This module takes about six months to complete based on twenty hours of study per month.

Modules Two through Six are a complete course in constitutional or chronic homeopathy. Homeopathic philosophy, case taking, case analyses, case management, materia medica, and potency selection are covered in these modules as well as other advanced topics such as miasms, client-practitioner relationship, and use of nosodes. These five modules take about two and one half years to three years to complete.

Tuition is $600 per module; required texts are additional. Payment in two or three installments may be arranged.

A summer clinical intensive is offered in Santa Cruz, California, to students who have completed Module One or equivalent training. It consists of five days of observing and participating in a live case-taking situation, as well as studying cases on video. Tuition is $375 for the intensive.

Canadian Academy of Homeopathy

1173 Boul de Mont-Royal
Outremont, Quebec H2V 2H6
Canada
PHONE: (514) 279-6629
FAX: (514) 279-0111

The Canadian Academy of Homeopathy was founded in 1986 by a group of naturopathic physicians. The program is open to primary contact health care professionals trained in pathology and diagnosis (N.D., M.D., D.O., D.C., D.D.S., nurse practitioners, physician's assistants, midwives, D.V.M., pharmacists, nurses, and psychologists), or to students enrolled in such a program.

The Homeopathic Program is offered in videotape format in four successive parts totaling 728 hours of instruction. Part I (70 hours) consists of Introduction to Homeopathy, Homeopathic First Aid, and Principles and Practice of Acute Prescribing. Part II is an Introduction to Chronic Prescribing (154 hours). Part III: Advanced Chronic Prescribing (504 hours) is the most comprehensive segment of the program, covering such topics as History, Philosophy, the Basis of Medicine, Homeopathy: The Science of Therapeutics, Practice (including case taking, case analysis, repertorization, the prescription, the follow-up visit, the second prescription, difficult cases, homeopathy and prophylaxis, diet regimen and supportive measures during homeopathic treatment, and the use of the computer in homeopathy), Materia Medica, Study of the Repertory, Clinics, and 152 hours of practice. Students may study to become a Fellow of the Canadian Academy of Homeopathy (FCAH).

Tuition for the entire program is $9,450 (plus shipping and handling); a 10 percent discount is offered for payment in full by check. The program may also be purchased in six segments of eighty-four hours each over three years, or individual topics may be purchased separately.

Hahnemann College of Homeopathy

80 Nicholl Avenue
Pt. Richmond, California 94801
PHONE: (510) 232-2079
FAX: (510) 412-9044
E-MAIL: hahnemann@igc.apc.org
WEBSITE: www.hahnemanncollege.com

In summer 2000, Hahnemann College of Homeopathy plans to add a home study program to their curriculum; visit the website for updated information. (See pages 87–88 for classroom-based programs.)

Health Academy of North America

P.O. Box 3024
Pagosa Springs, Colorado 81147
PHONE: (970) 731-9681
WEBSITE: alchemilla.com

The Health Academy of North America (HANA) offers a homeopathic home study course that includes 600 hours of taped seminars and 3,000 pages of written materials. The forty-five tape sets and four books cost $3,400. The course includes Emergency and Acute Care, Children's and Women's Health, and Psychological and Chronic Diseases. Studies in Repertory and Materia Medica, Alchemy, Spagyrics, and Medical Astrology are available. Portions of the course may be purchased separately; there is a 20 percent discount when the entire course is purchased.

The School of Homeopathy

Homeopathic Educational Services
2124 Kittredge Street
Berkeley, California 94704
PHONE: (510) 649-0294 / (800) 359-9051 (orders only)
FAX: (510) 649-1955
E-MAIL: mail@homeopathic.com
WEBSITE: www.homeopathic.com

Under the direction of Dana Ullman, M.P.H., the Homeopathic Educational Services' School of Homeopathy offers a three-year Flexible Learning Program in Homeopathy that combines 2,000 hours of correspondence course study with compulsory attendance at study days and seminars. Students have the flexibility of taking longer than three years to complete the program if they wish, or to stop at any point along the way. The program includes over eighty hours of taped classroom lectures and clinic case-takings with comprehensive supporting study notes. Essay assignments are marked by experienced practicing U.K. homeopaths who provide individual support; e-mail tutors are available. The material used in the correspondence program is the same as that used in the school's U.K. course, which is recognized by the U.K. Society of Homeopaths. All parts of the program count towards the North American Society of Homeopaths (NASH) registration requirements.

Students receive a Foundation Certificate upon completion of Study Units 1–10, a Study Day and three-day Seminar; an Advanced Diploma upon completion of Study Units 11–18, Anatomy and Physiology, a Study Day and three-day Seminar; a Clinical Certificate upon completion of the Advanced Diploma plus a three-day Seminar and twelve- to fourteen-day Clinical Workshops and Assessments; and a Practitioner Diploma upon completion of the Clinical Certificate plus Pathology and Disease and Case Supervision (ten cases).

There is a $100 registration fee for new students. Tuition for Units 1–7 is $1,695; for Units 8–14, $1,695; for Units 15–18, $1,165. Students may pay for Years 1–3 together for $3,895, or pay $635 for two or three units at a time.

See page 480 for a catalog of homeopathic products.

Toronto School of Homeopathic Medicine

17 Yorkville Avenue, Suite 200
Toronto, Ontario M4W 1L1
Canada
PHONE: (416) 966-2350 / (800) 572-6001
FAX: (416) 966-1724
E-MAIL: info@homeopathycanada.com
WEBSITE: www.homeopathycanada.com

Toronto School of Homeopathic Medicine offers a Professional Home-Study Certification Program, which is based on their accredited classroom-based lecture program; see pages 380-81 for description.

PERIODICALS

The American Homeopath

Joining the North American Society of Homeopaths entitles the member to receive the annual journal *The American Homeopath,* and a quarterly newsletter. See page 453 for membership information.

Homeopathy Today

Joining the National Center for Homeopathy entitles the member to receive the monthly magazine *Homeopathy Today.* See page 453 for membership information.

New England Journal of Homeopathy

New England School of Homeopathy
356 Middle Street
Amherst, Massachusetts 01002
PHONE: (413) 256-5949
FAX: (413) 256-6223
E-MAIL: herscu@nesh.com
WEBSITE: www.nesh.com

The New England School of Homeopathy publishes the *New England Journal of Homeopathy,* a journal published twice each year that includes cases, materia medica, book reviews, and more. A one-year subscription (two issues) costs $45.

Simillimum

Joining the Homeopathic Academy of Naturopathic Physicians (general membership is open to everyone with an interest in homeopathy) entitles the member to receive the quarterly professional journal *Simillimum.* See pages 452-53 for membership information.

HYPNOTHERAPY

CATALOGS AND PRODUCTS

Hypnotism Training Institute of Los Angeles

Westwood Publishing Company
700 South Central Avenue
Glendale, California 91204
PHONE: (818) 242-1159
FAX: (818) 247-9379
WEBSITE: www.GilBoyne.com

Westwood Publishing Company offers a catalog of hypnotism, hypnotherapy, mind power, and self-improvement products, including books, training videos, book and audiocassette sets, and self-hypnosis motivation cassettes. Classroom instruction (see pages 91-92) and a home study course (see page 485) are also available.

DISTANCE LEARNING

Hypnosis Motivation Institute

18607 Ventura Boulevard, Suite 310
Tarzana, California 91356
PHONE: (818) 758-2747 /   (818) 344-4464, ext. 747
WEBSITE: www.hypnosismotivation.com

The Hypnosis Motivation Institute offers over 100 hours of hypnotherapy instruction on a nine-volume video series, Foundations In Hypnotherapy. Topics include many of those covered in the classroom-based program (see page 90), such as Hypnotic Modalities, NLP, Ericksonian Hypnosis, Kappasinian Hypnosis, Hypnotic Regression, Dream Therapy, Hypno-Diagnostic Tools, Hypnodrama, Advanced Child Hypnosis, Medical Hypnosis, Fears and Phobias, Defense Mechanisms,

Emotional and Physical Sexuality, Systems Theory, Adult Children of Dysfunctional Families, Sexual Dysfunction, Low Blood Sugar, Eating Disorders, Substance Abuse, Crisis Intervention, Counseling and Interviewing, Habit Control, Law and Ethics, Advertising and Promotion, First Consultation, Mental Bank Seminar, and others. In addition, tutors are available for one hour per volume for questions and the sharing of practical experiences. Those who complete the program are eligible for Master Hypnotist certification with the Hypnotists' Union.

The Foundations in Hypnotherapy program is open to applicants at least 18 years of age. The cost of the entire program is $4,455; each of the nine volumes may be purchased separately in any order for $495 per volume.

Hypnotism Training Institute of Los Angeles

700 South Central Avenue
Glendale, California 91204
PHONE: (818) 242-1159
FAX: (818) 247-9379
WEBSITE: www.GilBoyne.com

In addition to classroom-based instruction (see pages 91-92), the Hypnotism Training Institute of Los Angeles also offers a Home Study Hypnotherapy Training Program. The program includes six videos, fourteen books, nineteen audiocassettes, two manuals, and a transcript of the #501 Training video. The cost of the program is $750. After completing the home study course, students may attend the Professional Hypnotism Training Program for an additional $200 tuition (regular tuition is $750).

Midwest Training Institute of Hypnosis

2121 Engle Road, Suite 3A
Fort Wayne, Indiana 46809
PHONE: (219) 747-6774
FAX: (219) 747-6774

In addition to classroom-based instruction, Midwest Training Institute of Hypnosis offers two of its programs as correspondence courses. See page 187 for a complete description.

Wesland Institute

3367 North Country Club Road
Tucson, Arizona 85716
PHONE/FAX: (520) 881-1530
E-MAIL: ninoc@primenet.com

Wesland Institute offers a 100-hour, classroom-based hypnotherapy certification program that is also available as a home study program on videotape for $1,200. Included with the videotapes are classroom handouts and a blank audio tape for student questions. Topics covered are the same as those in the classroom-based program (see page 58).

Home study audiotapes are offered in English and Spanish; please visit the website for more information.

PERIODICALS

The Bridge

Joining the National Association of Transpersonal Hypnotherapists entitles the member to receive the triannual newsletter *The Bridge*. See page 454 for membership information.

Subconsciously Speaking

Joining the International Medical and Dental Hypnotherapy Association entitles the member to receive the bimonthly newsletter *Subconsciously Speaking*. See page 454 for membership information.

MASSAGE AND BODYWORK

CATALOGS AND PRODUCTS

BioSomatics

P.O. Box 206
Grand Junction, Colorado 81502
PHONE: (800) 321-6032
FAX: (970) 241-5653
E-MAIL: biosomatics@gj.net
WEBSITE: www.biosomatic.com

In addition to the seminars offered throughout the United States and Canada (see pages 387-88), BioSomatics offers two instructional videos. *Reflexes 101* (seventy-six minutes) covers an overview of sensory motor amnesia, how it can be overcome by movement reeducation, and the three pathological processes by which it occurs. *Spine and Joints 102* (forty minutes) is based on movement patterns for the well-being of the spine, the long muscles of the back, and the small muscles joining the vertebrae. Each video is $39.95 plus $4 shipping.

The Day-Break Geriatric Massage Project

P.O. Box 1815
Sebastopol, California 95473-1815
PHONE: (707) 829-2798
FAX: (707) 829-2799
E-MAIL: daybreak@monitor.net
WEBSITE: www.daybreak-massage.com

In addition to their Certification Program in Geriatric Massage (see pages 390–91), Day-Break offers a selection of videos on both geriatric and general massage, as well as books and supplies. Videos on geriatric massage include *The A-B-C of Geriatric Massage* (two parts; $99.95), *Massaging the Alzheimer's Patient* ($39.95), and *Massaging the Elderly* ($49.95). Shipping additional; discounts available for GMP members.

Dr. Vodder School—North America

P.O. Box 5701
Victoria, British Columbia V8R 6S8
Canada
PHONE: (250) 598-9862
FAX: (250) 598-9841
E-MAIL: drvodderna@vodderschool.com
WEBSITE: www.vodderschool.com

In addition to classroom instruction (see pages 422–423), Dr. Vodder School—North America offers an informational videotape, *The Dr. Vodder Method of Manual Lymph Drainage and the Treatment of Lymphedema.* The nineteen-minute video reviews the basic course material covering effects and indications of MLD and the anatomy of the lymph system; lymphedema is discussed, and a synopsis of the treatment and bandaging of an edema patient is shown. The cost is $25 U.S., $30 Canadian (includes GST, postage, and handling).

The Feldenkrais® Guild® of North America

3611 SW Hood Avenue, Suite 100
Portland, Oregon 97201
PHONE: (503) 221-6612 / (800) 775-2118
FAX: (503) 221-6616
E-MAIL: guild@feldenkrais.com
WEBSITE: www.feldenkrais.com

The Feldenkrais Guild® of North America, the professional organization of Guild Certified Feldenkrais Practitioners and Teachers®, has a catalog of materials that includes books, articles, a directory of practitioners and teachers, merchandise, and audio- and videotapes. Of particular interest are *The Feldenkrais Method: Awareness Through Movement,* in which Stephen Rosenholtz, Ph.D., discusses posture, breathing, and using the imagination to increase smooth functioning and effective movement in two series of eight lessons ($39.95 for each of four videotapes or $125 for the complete set); *Workstation Workout,* a set of two videos demonstrating various movement methods (including Feldenkrais) designed for use in the workspace ($49 per set); and *Excerpts from Workstation Workout,* which features two fifteen-minute sections from the original *Workstation Workout* ($19.95). A twelve-minute video that gives an overview of the Feldenkrais method and its founder, Moshe Feldenkrais, is available for $20. Shipping and handling are additional.

See page 455 for additional information.

Feldenkrais® Resources

830 Bancroft Way, Suite 112
Berkeley, California 94710
PHONE: (800) 765-1907 / (510) 540-7600
FAX: (510) 540-7683
E-MAIL: feldenres@aol.com
WEBSITE: www.feldenkrais-resources.com

Feldenkrais® Resources is the exclusive producer of Dr. Feldenkrais's audio and video programs. Exercise sets available include *Relaxercise,* the *San Francisco Evening Class Volumes 1–3,* and *The Work of Moshe Feldenkrais.* Also available are books covering such topics as cognitive science, somatic philosophy, anatomy and physiology, and development. For information on Feldenkrais Professional Training Programs, see page 393-94.

International Alliance of Health Care Educators®

11211 Prosperity Farms Road, Suite D-325
Palm Beach Gardens, Florida 33410-3487
PHONE: (561) 622-4334 /   (800) 311-9204
FAX: (561) 622-4771
E-MAIL: iahe@iahe.com
WEBSITE: www.iahe.com

In addition to their classes and workshops (see pages 396-97), the International Alliance of Healthcare Educators (IAHE) offers a line of instructional videos, charts, audiotapes, posters, and slides dealing with Upledger Craniosacral Therapy®, Visceral Manipulation, Mechanical Link, Zero Balancing®, Process Acupressure, Neuromuscular Therapy, and Lymph Drainage Therapy, among other modalities. Contact IAHE for current prices.

McKinnon Institute

2940 Webster Street
Oakland, California 94609-3407
PHONE: (510) 465-3488
E-MAIL: mckinnon@aol.com

The McKinnon Institute sells the video, *Full Body Massage: The McKinnon Touch,* for $40 plus tax and $4 shipping.

Phillips School of Massage

101 Broad Street
P.O. Box 1999
Nevada City, California 95959
PHONE: (530) 265-4645
FAX: (530) 265-9485

E-MAIL: psm@jps.net
WEBSITE: www.jps.net/psm/

Judy Phillips, founder of the Phillips School of Massage, has produced a video, *Massage and Meditation,* that offers instruction in massage techniques; the body-mind connection and how massage influences the body, emotions, memories, and thoughts; and relaxation through a guided visualization. The cost is $29.95 plus $3 for postage and handling.

RxUB Corps

P.O. Box 14198
Columbus, Ohio 43214
PHONE: (614) 329-1245 / (500) 674-6635

RxUB Corps, founded in 1990 by Al Rimmel, offers a series of continuing education instructional video correspondence courses; certification and CEUs are available. Courses currently offered include *Hot Herbal Bodywraps/Lipolysis Massage; Mud Bath/Thalassotherapy; Paraffin Bath;* and *Pore Manipulation and Exfoliation.* Each of these courses range in price from $50 to $80 and include manuals, all materials, and most equipment necessary; shipping, handling, and Ohio sales tax are additional. Equipment and materials are also available separately. Other courses under development include *How to Determine Percent Body Fat Using Calipers; Posture Analysis; Manual Muscle Testing; Stretching; Proprioceptive Neuromuscular Facilitation; Reflexes, Myotomes, and Dermatomes; Post (Caesarian) Partum Low Back Pain; Soft Tissue Injuries by Symptom;* and *Soft Tissue Injuries by Region.* Call or write for details.

Shiatsu Massage School of California

2309 Main Street
Santa Monica, California 90405
PHONE: (310) 396-4877 / (310) 396-2130
FAX: (310) 396-4502
E-MAIL: shiatsanma@aol.com
WEBSITE: home.earthlink.net/~shiatsuanma

In addition to classroom instruction (see pages 117-18), the Shiatsu Massage School of California (SMSC) offers shiatsu/anma therapy instruction on video. Level I: Long Form shows amma meridian massage (one hour; $35); Level I (Short Form) addresses acupressure therapy (thirty minutes; $20); Level II: Intermediate Level covers shiatsu/ anma massage therapy (one hour; $35). Textbooks are available, including *DoAnn's Long Form and Short Form* ($27.50) and *DoAnn's Do-In* ($25.50). A discount is given on multiple titles; postage is $1.50 per video.

Shiatsu School of Canada

547 College Street
Toronto, Ontario M6G 1A9
Canada
PHONE: (416) 323-1818 / (800) 263-1703
FAX: (416) 323-1681
E-MAIL: info@shiatsucanada.com
WEBSITE: www.shiatsucanada.com

The Shiatsu School of Canada (see pages 377–78) offers two videos by director and founder Kaz Kamiya. *Meridian Shiatsu!* demonstrates a full-body, free-form meridian shiatsu treatment, with each position explained and supported with detailed charts. In *Shiatsu Stretching,* over sixty different stretches are demonstrated and include both examination and treatment methods. The cost for each video in the U.S. $30 plus $6 S/H, or $54 for both videos plus $9 S/H; in Canada, each video is $40 plus GST plus $7 S/H, or $72 plus GST plus $7 S/H. Allow four to six weeks for delivery.

DISTANCE LEARNING

Bev Johnson

Whole Resources
12303 East Prince of Peace Drive
Eagle River, Alaska 99577
PHONE: (907) 696-6009

Bev Johnson has been a massage practitioner since 1979 and is approved by the National Certification Board for Therapeutic Massage and Bodywork (NCBTMB) as a continuing education provider under Category A. Home study courses currently offered that meet recertification requirements include Profes-

sional Ethics (three credits), Intuitive Massage and Bodywork (three credits), Complementary Healing (six credits), and Independent Study (twenty credits), an interactive course that is partially designed by the student. Tuition is $10 per credit and includes shipping.

The Day-Break Geriatric Massage Project

P.O. Box 1815
Sebastopol, California 95473-1815
PHONE: (707) 829-2798
FAX: (707) 829-2799
E-MAIL: daybreak@monitor.net
WEBSITE: www.daybreak-massage.com

Day-Break offers a correspondence course as part of their modular Certification Program in Geriatric Massage; see pages 390–91.

PERIODICALS

Feldenkrais® Journal

Joining the Feldenkrais Guild® of North America entitles the member to receive the annual *Feldenkrais Journal* and a quarterly newsletter. See page 455 for membership information.

Journal of Oriental Bodywork Therapy / Pulse

Joining the American Oriental Bodywork Therapy Association entitles the member to receive the biannual *Journal of Oriental Bodywork Therapy* and the quarterly newsletter, *Pulse*. See page 455 for membership information.

Keeping in Touch / TFHKA Annual Journal

Joining the Touch for Health Kinesiology Association entitles the member to receive the *Keeping in Touch* newsletter and the *TFHKA Annual Journal*. See page 456 for membership information.

Massage and Bodywork Magazine

Joining the Associated Bodywork and Massage Professionals entitles the member to receive the bimonthly *Massage and Bodywork Magazine*. See page 455 for membership information.

Massage Magazine

1315 West Mallon Avenue
Spokane, Washington 99201-2038
PHONE: (800) 533-4263 / (509) 326-3955
WEBSITE: www.massagemag.com

Massage is the only independent news source for the massage and bodywork field. The magazine features articles on technique, business, related modalities, profiles of therapists, book and video reviews, resources, and more. Subscription rates for students are $20 per year (six issues) U.S., $24 Canadian.

Massage Therapy Journal

Subscription Department
820 Davis Street, Suite 100
Evanston, Illinois 60201-4444
FAX: (847) 864-1178
WEBSITE: www.amtamassage.com

Joining the American Massage Therapy Association entitles the member to receive *Massage Therapy Journal,* a quarterly magazine that features articles on such subjects as technique, massage for special populations, research, and more, along with book reviews, events, and more. See pages 454-55 for membership information.

Nonmembers may subscribe for $25 per year (four issues) U.S. and Canadian. Visit the website for a special introductory subscription price of $15 per year.

The Myomassethics Forum

Joining the International Myomassethics Federation entitles the member to receive the quarterly publication *The Myomassethics Forum*. See page 456 for membership information.

MIDWIFERY

DISTANCE LEARNING

Utah College of Midwifery

230 West 170 North
Orem, Utah 84057
PHONE: (801) 764-9068 / (888) 489-1238
E-MAIL: midwife@uswest.net

The core courses for Utah College of Midwifery's midwifery programs are offered through correspondence as well as classroom-based training. See pages 321-22 for a description.

PERIODICALS

MANA News

Joining the Midwives' Alliance of North America entitles the member to receive a subscription to the *MANA News*. See page 457 for additional literature and membership information.

NUTRITION

CATALOGS AND PRODUCTS

Kushi Institute

P.O. Box 7
Becket, Massachusetts 01223-0007
PHONE: (413) 623-5741/ (800) 975-8744
FAX: (413) 623-8827
E-MAIL: kushi@macrobiotics.org
WEBSITE: www.macrobiotics.org

In addition to their programs and seminars in macrobiotics and natural health (see pages 204-5), the Kushi Institute has a catalog of books, videotapes, audiotapes, kitchenware, cookware, and hard-to-find macrobiotic staples such as sea vegetables, dried foods, beverages, and more. A Macrobiotic Starter Kit features two books (*The Cancer Prevention Diet Book* and *The Macrobiotic Cancer Prevention Cookbook)*, a macrobiotic cooking video, and a selection of macrobiotic staple foods for $125 plus shipping.

DISTANCE LEARNING

American Academy of Nutrition

College of Nutrition
1212 Kenesaw
Knoxville, Tennessee 37919-7736
PHONE: (423) 524-8079 / (800) 290-4226
E-MAIL: aantn@aol.com
WEBSITE: www.nutritioneducation.com

The American Academy of Nutrition is accredited by the Accrediting Commission of the Distance Education and Training Council, the only U.S. Department of Education agency accrediting independent study schools. Courses at the academy have been approved for continuing education credits by numerous organizations including the American Dietetic Association. The Comprehensive Nutrition Program is a nondegree program designed for health and nutrition professionals or those who wish to help family and friends on an informal basis. The program includes six courses: Understanding Nutrition I and II, Environmental Challenges and Solutions, Vegetarian Nutrition, Anatomy and Physiology, and Nutritional Counseling Skills. Tuition is $1,790. Students are allowed fifteen months to complete the program.

To earn an Associate of Science degree in applied nutrition, students must complete sixty credit hours of study. Courses include Understanding Nutrition I and II, Vegetarian Nutrition, English: Reading Enhancement, Anatomy and Physiology, Environmental Challenges and Solutions, Human Biology, General Chemistry, Eating Disorders and Weight Management, Organic Chemistry and Biochemistry, Nutrition Counseling Skills, Business Mathematics, Clinical Nutrition, and both general and nutrition electives chosen from Direct Marketing, Psychology, Managing a Small Business, Public Speaking, Child Development, Sports Nutrition, Community Nutrition, Women's Special Health Concerns, Medicinal Herbs and Other Alternative Therapies, and Pregnancy, Pediatric, and Adolescent Nutrition. Tuition is $1,485 per segment; each segment consists of five courses. Students are allowed twelve months to complete each of the four segments.

Any course may also be taken individually for $345 per course, including study guide; books and videos are purchased separately. Students are allowed four months to complete each course.

The academy participates in the American Council on Education program for the transfer of college credits. Students wishing to transfer credits to another college or university must take a proctored exam upon completion of each course. There is a $20 fee for each exam.

Applicants must have a high school diploma or equivalent.

American Health Science University/The National Institute of Nutritional Education

1010 South Joliet, #107
Aurora, Colorado 80012
PHONE: (303) 340-2054 / (800) 530-8079
FAX: (303) 367-2577
E-MAIL: healthynine@earthlink.net
WEBSITE: www.ahsu.com

American Health Science University (AHSU) offers distance-education programs in the field of Nutrition Science. Students who complete the university's six-course certificate program in Nutrition Science and pass a national board examination receive the designation C.N. (Certified Nutritionist).

AHSU is an accredited member of the Distance Education and Training Council (DETC). The accrediting commission of DETC is a member of the Commission on Recognition of Postsecondary Accreditation and is listed by the U.S. Department of Education as a nationally recognized accrediting agency. AHSU is approved and regulated by the Colorado Department of Higher Education, Division of Private Occupational Schools. AHSU's six-course certificate program in Nutrition Science has been validated for college credits by the American Council on Education.

Each of the six courses in the Nutrition Science certificate program consists of twelve to eighteen modules. Students take self-grading quizzes at the end of each section (a section has three to five modules) as well as proctored midterm and final exams. Class titles include Health and Wellness Survey, Anatomy and Physiology, Normal Nutrition, Contemporary Clinical Nutrition, Professional Aspects of Counseling, and Nutrition Assessment.

In order to receive the C.N. designation, the student must complete the six courses with a cumulative average above a C (2.0), satisfy all financial obligations to AHSU, pass the national board examination, and agree to abide by the CN Professional Code of Ethics. The program takes about eighteen to twenty-four months for the average student to complete.

Applicants must have a baccalaureate degree from a four-year accredited college or university. Applicants who do not have such a degree but feel they should be eligible to enroll because of a combination of education and work experience are invited to take the course Anatomy and Physiology; entry requirements will be waived for those who receive a grade of C (2.0) or better. Applicants must submit an enrollment agreement, a résumé and goals statement, two letters of recommendation and official transcripts.

Tuition, registration, and administration fees are $2,920 for the six-course program (tuition may be paid on a per course basis); books are an additional $420.

The institute promotes professional continuing education courses for C.N.s interested in maintaining their certification. For more information on this program, contact the Continuing Education Department.

Canadian School of Natural Nutrition

10720 Yonge Street, Suite 220
Richmond Hill, Ontario L4C 3C9
Canada
PHONE: (905) 737-0284 / (800) 569-9938
FAX: (905) 737-7830
E-MAIL: info@csnn.ca
WEBSITE: www.csnn.ca

CORRESPONDENCE COURSE DIVISION:
PHONE: (905) 852-9660 / (800) 328-0743 / (888) 837-0337 (en français)
FAX: (905) 852-4616

The four-module correspondence course in natural nutrition qualifies graduates for the same R.N.C. designation as the classroom program and consists of the same curriculum (see pages 368-69 for course description). The correspondence program takes approximately 500 study hours to complete; a final

exam is required. Tuition is $2,055 (plus GST), including books; there is an extra charge for foreign students. Tuition may be paid in four installments of $524 (plus GST), due prior to receipt of each of the four modules.

Vegedine

3835 Route 414
Burdett, New York 14818
PHONE/ FAX: (607) 546-4091

The Association of Vegetarian Dietitians and Nutrition Educators (VEGEDINE) offers a correspondence course in basic nutrition for vegetarians/vegans under the instruction of George Eisman, R.D. Mr. Eisman has been a Registered Dietitian since 1978 and has taught nutrition at the college level since 1980.

The correspondence course covers the basic elements of human nutrition, vegetarian (vegan) sources of nutrients, vegetarian food analysis, and the chronic disease risk implication of dietary change toward vegetarianism. The eighteen study units cover Carbohydrates, Fiber, Fats, Protein Quality and Quantity, Digestion and Absorption, Weight Control, Fat-Soluble Vitamins, Major Minerals, Trace Minerals, Vegetarian Foods, Diet-Related Chronic Disease, Life Cycle and Vegetarianism, and Risks and Benefits of Vegetarian Diets. The course fee is $118, payable as a $10 application/processing fee and three installments of $36 each.

This course is also available in book form for those who prefer to teach themselves; the cost is $21.95 postpaid.

Mr. Eisman's first book, *The Most Noble Diet,* is available for $9.95 postpaid.

PERIODICALS

Ahimsa

Joining the American Vegan Society entitles the member to receive the quarterly publication *Ahimsa.* See page 457 for membership information.

Health Science

Joining the American Natural Hygiene Society entitles the

member to receive the bimonthly magazine *Health Science*. See page 457 for membership information.

Journal of Orthomolecular Medicine / ISOM Newsletter

Joining the International Society for Orthomolecular Medicine entitles the member to receive the quarterly *Journal of Orthomolecular Medicine* and the biannual *ISOM Newsletter*. See page 458 for membership information.

Living Naturally

Joining the Canadian Natural Health Association Founded on Natural Hygiene entitles the member to receive the bimonthly newsletter *Living Naturally*. See page 458 for membership information.

One Peaceful World

Joining One Peaceful World entitles the member to receive the newsletter *One Peaceful World*. See page 459 for membership information.

TMA Cookbook / Newsletter

Joining the Triangle Macrobiotics Association entitles the member to receive the *TMA Cookbook* of macrobiotic recipes and a bimonthly newsletter. See page 459 for membership information.

Vegetarian Journal

Joining the Vegetarian Resource Group entitles the member to receive the bimonthly *Vegetarian Journal*. See page 459 for membership information.

Vegetarian Times

P.O. Box 420235
Palm Coast, Florida 32142-0235
PHONE: (800) 829-3340 / (904) 446-6914
WEBSITE: www.vegetariantimes.com

Vegetarian Times, published monthly, includes features and departments such as In the Kitchen, Monthly Fare, Close to Home, and Mind/Body. It is widely available at newsstands or by subscription for $24 per year (twelve issues) U.S., $27 Canadian.

Vegetarian Voice

Joining the North American Vegetarian Society entitles the member to receive the newsmagazine *Vegetarian Voice*. See page 458 for membership information.

Veggie Life

308 East Hitt Street
P.O. Box 440
Mt. Morris, Illinois 61054-7659
WEBSITE: www.veggielife.com

Veggie Life is a ninety-two-page bimonthly magazine emphasizing gardening, diet, health, nutrition, and natural remedies. It is widely available at newsstands or by subscription for $17.97 per year (six issues) U.S., $23.97 Canadian.

POLARITY THERAPY

PERIODICALS

ENERGY

Joining the American Polarity Therapy Association entitles the member to receive the quarterly newsletter *ENERGY*. See pages 459–60 for membership information.

QIGONG

CATALOGS AND PRODUCTS

The Qigong and Human Life Research Foundation

Eastern Healing Arts International Training Center
Tian Enterprises, Inc.
2188 Vernon Road
Cleveland, Ohio 44118

PHONE: (800) 859-4343
FAX: (216) 932-2968
E-MAIL: te@modex.com
WEBSITE: www.qi-healing.com

The Qigong and Human Life Research Foundation offers classroom and correspondence training (see page 281 and below) as well as courses on video.

The five videos available include the basic contents of the elective courses Qigong I and II offered by the Foundation at Case Western Reserve University School of Medicine. Their titles are *Qigong Meditation Relaxation, Qigong and Standing Form Self-Healing Practice, Special Shao-Lin Sticks, Tai-Chi Qigong 17,* and *Acupressure Self-Massage 40 Forms.*

Contact Tian Enterprises for descriptions, prices, and selection recommendations for particular needs.

DISTANCE LEARNING

The Qigong and Human Life Research Foundation

Eastern Healing Arts International Training Center
Tian Enterprises, Inc.
2188 Vernon Road
Cleveland, Ohio 44118
PHONE: (800) 859-4343
FAX: (216) 932-2968
E-MAIL: te@modex.com
WEBSITE: www.qi-healing.com

Programs offered at the Qigong and Human Life Research Foundation are a combination of classroom and correspondence study; see page 282 for a complete description. For videos, see above.

PERIODICALS

Qigong Newsletter

Joining the American Qigong Association entitles the member to receive the *Qigong Newsletter.* See page 460 for membership information.

REFLEXOLOGY

PERIODICALS

ICR Newsletter

Joining the International Council of Reflexologists entitles the member to receive the quarterly *ICR Newsletter.* See page 460 for membership information.

REIKI

CATALOGS AND PRODUCTS

International Center for Reiki Training

21421 Hilltop Street, # 28
Southfield, Michigan 48034
PHONE: (248) 948-8112 / (800) 332-8112
FAX: (248) 948-9534
E-MAIL: center@reiki.org
WEBSITE: www.reiki.org

In addition to their professional level Reiki training programs (see pages 212–13), the International Center for Reiki Training offers a catalog of Reiki-related products including Reiki tables, books and tapes, Reiki clothing, tools, gift items, and other products.

DISTANCE LEARNING

Reiki Plus® Institute

707 Barcelona Road
Key Largo, Florida 33037
PHONE: (305) 451-9881
FAX: (305) 451-9841
E-MAIL: reikiplu@bellsouth.net
WEBSITE: www.reikiplus.com

In addition to classroom instruction (see page 166), Reiki Plus Institute (RPI) offers the following home study courses: Reiki Plus First Degree ($100; review tapes $50); Reiki Plus Second Degree ($300; review tapes $100); Psycho-Therapeutic Reiki Plus ($300; review class $75); Advanced Psycho-Therapeutic Reiki Plus ($200); Intuitive Evaluation of Client Consciousness ($100; review tapes $50); Astro-Physiology and Anatomy (in three segments: $90, $75, and $75); Applied Esoteric Psychology ($100; review tapes $50); Esoteric Anatomy ($100; review tapes $50); Breath of Light ($20); Spiritual Discernment Review Tapes ($50); and New Format PSEB Level 1 Review Tapes ($50). Contact RPI for course descriptions.

VETERINARY MASSAGE

CATALOGS AND PRODUCTS

Equissage

P.O. Box 447
Round Hill, Virginia 22141
PHONE: (540) 338-1917 / (800) 843-0224
FAX: (540) 338-5569
E-MAIL: equissage@webtv.net
WEBSITE: www.equissage.com

In addition to classroom training (see pages 329–30), Equissage offers two videos, *Sports Massage for the Equine Athlete* (fifty-five minutes, $49.95) and *Therapeutic Massage for Dogs* (forty-seven minutes, $39.95), plus a book, *The (How To) Manual of Sports Massage for the Equine Athlete* ($32.99).

Integrated Touch Therapy for Animals, Inc.

7041 Zane Trail Road
Circleville, Ohio 43113
PHONE: (740) 474-6436 / (800) 251-0007
FAX: (740) 474-2625
E-MAIL: wshaw1@bright.net

In addition to courses in equine, canine, and feline massage (see pages 277–78), Integrated Touch Therapy for Animals (ITTA) offers videos on Equine Massage and Canine Massage ($39.95 each) and companion books ($29.95 each); add $5 for shipping. The videos cover techniques of massage, application, and a choreography of a full body massage.

YOGA

CATALOGS AND PRODUCTS

Iyengar Yoga Institute of San Francisco

2404 27th Avenue
San Francisco, California 94116
PHONE: (415) 753-0909
FAX: (415) 753-0913
E-MAIL: iyisf@sirius.com
WEBSITE: www.iyoga.com/iyisf

In addition to offering public classes and a teacher training program (see page 95), the Iyengar Yoga Institute of San Francisco (IYISF) has a mail order catalog of books and periodicals, yoga clip art, videos, and audiocassettes for beginners to advanced students. (IYISF is owned and operated by the B.K.S. Iyengar Association of Northern California; see page 461.)

Nada Productions

2216 NW 8th Terrace
Ft. Lauderdale, Florida 33311
PHONE: (800) 964-2553
E-MAIL: yogihari@aol.com
WEBSITE: www.yogihari.com

In addition to the Yoga Teacher Certification course offered at Yogi Hari's Ashram (see page 168), Nada Productions sells a wide variety of books, audio- and videotapes in basic and advanced yoga, most of which are produced by Yogi Hari; see catalog or website for details.

The *Yoga At Home with Yogi Hari* video series offers beginners, two levels of intermediate, and advanced instruction in yoga, each with precise instructions and soothing background music. The Beginners Level costs $19.95; the Intermediate Level I and II, $24.95 each; and the Advanced Level, $29.95. Shipping is $4 for the first video, 50 cents for each additional video.

United States Yoga Association

2159 Filbert Street
San Francisco, California 94123
PHONE: (415) 931-YOGA
FAX: (415) 921-6676
E-MAIL: tony@usyoga.org
WEBSITE: www.usyoga.org

In addition to the teacher training program described on page 124, the United States Yoga Association offers the video *Yoga Challenge I,* which shows a one-hour Tony Sanchez hatha yoga class with easy-to-follow voice-over instructions. Included are modified exercises for common limitations and advanced positions for the experienced practitioner. The video is $24.95; the audio version is $10.95, and the poster recommended for use with the audio is $14.98 (audio and poster together are $21.95); shipping is $4.50 per item.

PERIODICALS

Iyengar Yoga Institute Review

Joining the B.K.S. Iyengar Yoga Association of Northern California entitles the member to receive the *Iyengar Yoga Institute Review.* See page 461 for membership information.

Yoga Journal

P.O. Box 469088
Escondido, California 92046-9088
PHONE: (800) 600-9642

Yoga Journal is a bimonthly publication of the California Yoga Teachers Association, a nonprofit California educational corporation. Departments include Food, Practice, Well-Being, Asana, World of Yoga, Self-Care for Beginners, Profile, and others. *Yoga Journal* is widely available at newsstands or by subscription for $21.95 per year (six issues) in the United States, $27.95 in Canada.

Conventional and Osteopathic Medical Schools Offering Courses in Alternative Medicine

Increasingly, conventional medical schools and schools of osteopathic medicine are finding the need to address in some way the ever-growing role of alternative medicine in the lives of their patients—either because they are sympathetic to the cause and want to know how to incorporate alternative therapies into their practices, or because patients are discussing with their physicians alternative practitioners they have consulted, remedies they have tried, or supplements that they're taking. What follows is a list of alternative and osteopathic medical schools that offer some instruction, however brief, in alternative medicine. This list was compiled independently by the author; any omissions are due to a failure of the schools to respond to requests for information. Please contact the individual medical schools for additional information.

CONVENTIONAL MEDICAL SCHOOLS— UNITED STATES

ARIZONA

University of Arizona College of Medicine Program in Integrative Medicine

P.O. Box 245153
Tucson, Arizona 85724-5153
PHONE: (520) 626-7222
FAX: (520) 626-6484

The Program in Integrative Medicine at the University of Arizona College of Medicine is a new approach to medical education. The program consists of a fellowship, a teaching clinic, a professional development/continuing education program for individuals in practice, and a research program. See page 52 for a complete description.

CALIFORNIA

University of California—Los Angeles UCLA School of Medicine

Center for Educational Development and Research
Los Angeles, California 90095
PHONE: (310) 794-7016
FAX: (310) 794-7465

Course titles:
"Introduction to Complementary Medicine"
"Alternative/ Complementary Medicine"

DISTRICT OF COLUMBIA

Georgetown University School of Medicine and Health Sciences

2300 Eye Street NW
Washington, D.C. 20037
PHONE: (202) 994-8749

A week-long intensive is offered by the Center for Mind-Body Medicine:
"Mind-Body-Spirit Medicine: A Professional Training Program"

FLORIDA

Nova Southeastern University

Health Professions Division
3200 South University Drive
Fort Lauderdale, Florida 33328
PHONE: (954) 262-1100 / (800) 356-0026

Second-year course:
"Alternative Medicine"

University of Miami School of Medicine

P.O. Box 016159
Miami, Florida 33101
PHONE: (305) 243-6791
FAX: (305) 243-6548

Courses offered for continuing medical education (CME) credits:
"The Art and Science of Acupuncture, Part I: The Basic Course" (100 CME hours)
"The Art and Science of Acupuncture, Part II: The Advanced Course" (150 CME hours)

GEORGIA

Emory University School of Medicine

3107 Rollins Research Center
1510 Clifton Road
Atlanta, Georgia 30322
PHONE: (404) 727-5948
FAX: (404) 727-0293

An informal series (not for credit; brown bag lunch format) called "Whole Person Health" covers alternative medicine and mind/body/spirit topics.

ILLINOIS

Chicago Medical School
Finch University of Health Sciences

3333 Green Bay Road
North Chicago, Illinois 60064
PHONE: (847) 578-3206
FAX: (847) 578-3284

Sophomore required course:
"Preventive Medicine" (includes environmental medicine)
Sophomore elective course:
"Overview of Alternative/Complementary Medicine"
Sophomore elective offered outside the medical school:
"Health Promotion and Complementary Medicine" (offered by Nutrition and Clinical Dietetics Department)
Senior elective course:

"Contemporary Clinical Nutrition" (includes intense nutritional support and nutritional assessments)

Southern Illinois University School of Medicine

P.O. Box 19230
Springfield, Illinois 62794
PHONE: (217) 782-2860
FAX: (217) 785-5538

Courses to be offered in the 1999–2000 school year:
"Complementary Medicine: A Critical Review (Carbondale)"
"Alternative Systems of Healing"
"Complementary Medicine (Springfield)"
"Lakota Culture: A Perspective of Healing"

KANSAS

University of Kansas School of Medicine

3901 Rainbow Boulevard
Kansas City, Kansas 66160
PHONE: (913) 588-5283
FAX: (913) 588-5259

Four-week elective course:
"Alternative Medicine"
An Alternative/Integrative Medicine Interest Group also sponsors presentations by guest lecturers.

KENTUCKY

University of Kentucky College of Medicine

800 Rose Street
Lexington, Kentucky 40536
PHONE: (606) 323-5261
FAX: (606) 323-2076

Sixteen-week first- or second-year elective:
"Integrative Medicine (Mind-Body-Spirit-Environment)"

University of Louisville School of Medicine

Health Sciences Center
Louisville, Kentucky 40292
PHONE: (502) 852-5193

Course title:
"A Scientific Look at Alternative Medicine"

LOUISIANA

Tulane University School of Medicine

1430 Tulane Avenue
New Orleans, Louisiana 70112
PHONE: (504) 588-5187
FAX: (504) 585-6462

Freshman-year elective:
"Alternative Medicine"

MARYLAND

Johns Hopkins University School of Medicine

720 Rutland Avenue
Baltimore, Maryland 21205
PHONE: (410) 955-3182

Clinical elective (three-week intensive) offered to third- and fourth-year medical students:
"The Philosophy and Practice of Healing"

University of Maryland at Baltimore School of Medicine

655 West Baltimore Street
Baltimore, Maryland 21201-1559
PHONE: (410) 706-7476
FAX: (410) 706-8311

Four-week senior elective course offered by the Department of Family Medicine:
Complementary Medicine Program at Kernan Hospital:
"Introduction to Complementary and Alternative Medicine (CAM)"

MASSACHUSETTS

Boston University School of Medicine

80 East Concord Street
Boston, Massachusetts 02118
PHONE: (617) 638-4510

"Public Health Perspectives on Alternative Health Care"

Harvard Medical School

25 Shattuck Street
Boston, Massachusetts 02115
PHONE: (617) 432-1550

Core course for second-year students:
"Preventive Medicine and Nutrition"
Elective courses:
"Alternative Medicine: Implications for Clinical Practice and Research"
"Human Health and Global Environmental Change"
"Clinical Experience in Occupational and Environmental Medicine"
"Spirituality and Healing in Medicine"

MICHIGAN

Wayne State University School of Medicine

540 East Canfield Avenue
Detroit, Michigan 48201
PHONE: (313) 577-1466
FAX: (313) 577-1330

A one-month course offered to fourth-year medical students:
"Introduction to Complementary/ Alternative Medicine"

MINNESOTA

University of Minnesota— Duluth School of Medicine

10 University Drive
109 Medical Building

Duluth, Minnesota 55812
PHONE: (218) 726-8511
FAX: (218) 726-6235

Lectures on alternative medicine topics are included in the first-year course, "Family Medicine I."

University of Minnesota Medical School—Minneapolis

420 Delaware Street SE
Minneapolis, Minnesota 55455
PHONE: (612) 624-8601
FAX: (612) 626-4200

A three-week Clinical Rotation is offered in "An Introduction to Complementary and Alternative Therapies." Students witness complementary care providers in action, participate in weekly seminars, and complete a special project.

MISSOURI

St. Louis University School of Medicine

1402 South Grand Boulevard, LRC 101
St. Louis, Missouri 63104
PHONE: (314) 577-8622
FAX: (314) 771-9316

First-year elective:
"Alternative Medicine: Unconventional Healing Practices"

NEVADA

University of Nevada School of Medicine

Reno, Nevada 89557
PHONE: (702) 784-6063
FAX: (702) 784-6194

Elective course offered to fourth-year medical students:
"Alternative/ Complementary Medicine"
Jeffrey Millman, M.D.

NEW JERSEY

New Jersey Medical School University of Medicine and Dentistry of New Jersey

185 South Orange Avenue
Newark, New Jersey 07103-2714
PHONE: (973) 972-4631

Courses offered by the Department of Preventive Medicine and Community Health include:
"General Preventive Medicine and International Health" (includes the role of environmental pollutants in major diseases)
"Nutrition and Aging" (studies of vitamin supplementation and free radicals are underway)

NEW MEXICO

University of New Mexico School of Medicine

Albuquerque, New Mexico 87131
PHONE: (505) 277-4766

Four-week senior elective course offered by the Department of Pediatrics:
"Alternative and Complementary Medicine"

NEW YORK

Columbia University College of Physicians and Surgeons

630 West 168th Street
New York, New York 10032
PHONE: (212) 305-3595

Course title:
"Survey in Alternative/ Complementary Medicine"

State University of New York—Buffalo School of Medicine and Biomedical Sciences

Biomedical Education Building
Bailey Avenue

Buffalo, New York 14214
PHONE: (716) 829-2802
FAX: (716) 829-2798

One-week elective for third-year students:
"Alternative Healing Modalities"
Four-week preceptorship for fourth-year students in the office with Dr. Sanford Levy:
"Preceptorship in Integrative Medicine"

State University of New York—Syracuse Health Science Center at Syracuse

155 Elizabeth Blackwell Street
Syracuse, New York 13210
PHONE: (315) 464-4570
FAX: (315) 464-8867

Individualized study featuring readings, conferences, and precepting with providers.
"Integrative Medicine"

NORTH CAROLINA

Wake Forest University School of Medicine

Winston-Salem, North Carolina 27157
PHONE: (910) 716-4264
FAX: (910) 716-5807

A Complementary Medicine Symposium (usually a one- to two-hour presentation) is offered each year to all students and faculty, and is required for first- and second-year medical students as part of the course "Medicine as a Profession."

Students have also organized lunchtime seminar sessions on alternative and complementary medicine topics, inviting acupuncturists, herbologists, and others to speak and demonstrate.

OHIO

Case Western Reserve University School of Medicine

10900 Euclid Avenue
Cleveland, Ohio 44106

PHONE: (216) 368-3450
FAX: (216) 368-4621

Students may take an Alternative Medicine Area of Concentration in which they learn basic techniques in healing touch, reiki, osteopathic manipulation, meditation, and acupuncture, and may learn homeopathic principles in the office of a homeopath. Students may choose a minimum of four electives from Alternative Medicine I, II and III; Diet, Nutrition, Cancer and Toxicity; Healing: An Inquiry; Faith, Religion and Medicine; Finding Balance: Stress and Wellness; Caring for the Soul; Introduction to Tibetan Medicine; Chinese Qigong I and II; Japanese Medicine: Acupuncture; and Medical Hypnosis/Biofeedback. Students also choose a minimum of one elective from either Clinical Alternative Medicine or Independent Study in Alternative Medicine.

Ohio State University College of Medicine

370 West Ninth Avenue
Columbus, Ohio 43210
PHONE: (614) 292-7137
FAX: (614) 292-1544

Course title:
"Maharishi Ayur-Veda"

University of Cincinnati College of Medicine

P.O. Box 670552
Cincinnati, Ohio 45267
PHONE: (513) 558-7314
FAX: (513) 558-1165

Fourth-year elective course:
"Complementary Medicine: Non-Allopathic Approaches"

TEXAS

Baylor College of Medicine

One Baylor Plaza, Room M301
Houston, Texas 77030-3498
PHONE: (713) 798-7760

In the required third-year course, "Longitudinal Ambulatory Clinical Experiences (LACE)," students may choose a module on alternative/complementary medicine, which includes information and experiences in homeopathy, acupuncture, naturopathy, herbalism, and martial arts.

Texas Tech University School of Medicine

Lubbock, Texas 79430
PHONE: (806) 743-2297

Two-week senior elective:
"Lifelong Learning: Complementary/Alternative Medicine" (includes pain control, hypnotism, Hispanic folk medicine, osteopathy and chiropractic, spiritual healing, tai chi and yoga)

VIRGINIA

University of Virginia School of Medicine

Charlottesville, Virginia 22908
PHONE: (804) 924-5579
FAX: (804) 982-4073

Elective course for medical students from LCME-approved schools:
"Integrative Medicine: Complementary Therapies for Health"

WASHINGTON

University of Washington School of Medicine

Box 357120
Seattle, Washington 98195-7120
PHONE: (206) 543-5145
FAX: (206) 685-7515

Course title:
"Alternative Approaches to Healing"

WISCONSIN

University of Wisconsin Medical School

1300 University Avenue
Madison, Wisconsin 53706

PHONE: (608) 263-4721
FAX: (608) 262-2327

Course title:
"Complementary Medicine"

CONVENTIONAL MEDICAL SCHOOLS—CANADA

Memorial University of Newfoundland Faculty of Medicine

Prince Philip Drive
St. John's, Newfoundland A1B 3V6
Canada
PHONE: (709) 737-6669
FAX: (709) 737-5190

Elective course with an emphasis on holistic medicine, teaching basic concepts in energetic medicine, homeopathy, acupuncture, and auricular acupuncture:
"Urban General Practice"

University of Saskatchewan College of Medicine

Saskatoon, Saskatchewan S7N 0W0
Canada
PHONE: (306) 966-8554

The M.D. curriculum includes six hours of instruction in complementary medicine in Year One and six hours in Year Three, for a total of twelve hours. These hours are part of other required courses covering a variety of topics, including chiropractic, traditional Chinese medicine, acupuncture, and Native traditional healing.

OSTEOPATHIC MEDICAL SCHOOLS— UNITED STATES

CALIFORNIA

Western University of Health Sciences

309 East Second Street
College Plaza
Pomona, California 91766-1854
PHONE: (909) 623-6116

Invited lecturers and occasional seminars in various areas of alternative or complementary medicine; no formal courses at this time.

IOWA

University of Osteopathic Medicine and Health Sciences

3200 Grand Avenue
Des Moines, Iowa 50312-4198
PHONE: (515) 271-1400
FAX: (515) 271-1545

"Nutrition" (includes prevention of disease and therapeutic diets)

MISSOURI

Kirksville College of Osteopathic Medicine

800 West Jefferson
Kirksville, Missouri 63501
PHONE: (816) 626-2354

Brief discussions of Herbal Medicine are included in the Pharmacology and Nutrition courses.

Bibliography

ALTERNATIVE HEALTH CARE—GENERAL

Cornellia Aihara and Herman Aihara with Carl Ferré. *Natural Healing from Head to Toe.* Garden City Park, NY: Avery Publishing Group, 1994. 264 pp. ISBN 0895294966.

The Aiharas' self-help guide to over 200 common disorders takes a macrobiotic view of treatment using whole foods and medicinal preparations. The book also contains an explanation of the healing concepts of macrobiotics and over 200 recipes.

Steven Bratman. *The Alternative Medicine Sourcebook: A Realistic Evaluation of Alternative Healing Methods.* Los Angeles: Lowell House, 1997. 254 pp. ISBN 1565658558.

Dr. Bratman combines his clinical experience with the medical literature to evaluate the scientific approaches to healing, such as naturopathy, herbal medicine, and diet, and the healing arts, including Chinese medicine, acupuncture, bodywork, chiropractic, and others. Also included are Bratman's recommendations for a variety of common illnesses.

The Burton Goldberg Group. *Alternative Medicine: The Definitive Guide.* Tiburon, California: Future Medicine Publishing, 1998. 1,100 pp. ISBN 1887299335.

A weighty tome, this book explains scores of alternative therapies from acupuncture to yoga, with descriptions of typical treatment sessions, conditions benefited, and where to find a practitioner, plus alternative treatment options for specific health conditions.

Essential for the home library.

Larry P. Credit, Sharon G. Hartunian, and Margaret J. Nowak. *Your Guide to Complementary Medicine.* Garden City Park, New York: Avery, 1998. 200 pp. ISBN 0895298317.

This quick reference, no-nonsense guide to alternative therapies covers what it is, how it works, and what to expect for each of thirty-seven therapies.

Teresa Hale. *The Hale Clinic Guide to Good Health: How to Choose the Right Complementary Therapy.* New York: The Overlook Press, 1996. 256 pp. ISBN 0879518057.

Founder of the Hale Clinic in London, Hale has produced a colorful, informative guide to alternative treatments for a variety of common health problems.

Mark Kastner and Hugh Burroughs. *Alternative Healing: A Complete A–Z Guide to More Than 150 Alternative Therapies.* La Mesa, CA: Halcyon Publishing, 1996. ISBN 0805046704.

This is a concise encyclopedia of alternative health care modalities that covers both the common (acupuncture, herbal medicine, and naturopathic medicine) and the not-so-common (Hoffman quadrinity process, radix, and urine therapy).

James E. Marti. *The Alternative Health and Medicine Encyclopedia.* New York: Gale, 1998. 462 pp. ISBN 0787600733.

Marti gives us a handy reference guide to alternative therapies and their applications, with chapters on Diet and Nutrition, Vitamins, Minerals and Trace Elements, Botanical Medicines, Exercise, Strengthening the Immune System, Holistic Pregnancy and Childbirth, Dental Care, Mental Health Disorders, and much more.

Michael Murray and Joseph Pizzorno. *Encyclopedia of Natural Medicine* 2nd ed. Rocklin, CA: Prima Publishing, 1997. 960 pp. ISBN 0761511571.

Another must-have for the home library, this book provides an explanation of the basic principles of health and an extensive discussion of nutritional, botanical, lifestyle, and other treatments for over seventy problems, from acne to varicose veins.

Gary Null. *The Clinician's Handbook of Natural Healing.* New York: Kensington Books, 1997. 870 pp. ISBN 1575662841.

Ten years of examination of scientific literature resulted in this comprehensive guide to peer-review studies of nutrients, herbs, amino acids, and phytochemicals. Useful for clinicians, researchers, writers, and the public.

Gary Null. *The Complete Encyclopedia of Natural Healing.* New York: Kensington Books, 1998. 612 pp. ISBN 1575662582.

Null has written an authoritative, useful, and complete A-to-Z guide to common conditions and their proven natural treatments. All of Null's books are keepers—this one especially so.

Louise Tenney. *The Encyclopedia of Natural Remedies.* Pleasant Grove, UT: Woodland Publishing, 1995. 400 pp. ISBN 0913923982.

A comprehensive guide that covers prevention, health maintenance, cleansing diets, children and health, nutritional supplements, and more, plus causes, herbal formulas, and nutritional therapy for over 100 ailments.

Andrew Weil. *Natural Health, Natural Medicine: A Comprehensive Manual for Wellness and Self-Care.* Boston: Houghton Mifflin, 1998. 370 pp. ISBN 0395911559.

Weil's first best-seller is a general guide to preventive health care using basic natural treatments. The book includes home remedies, such as nutritional supplements, herbs, dietary changes, exercise, and stress reduction, for common disorders.

ACUPRESSURE

Cathryn Bauer. *Pocket Guide to Acupressure Points for Women.* Freedom, CA: The Crossing Press, 1997. ISBN 0895948796.

The homework that the author, an acupressure practitioner, gave to clients became the basis for this book. Bauer simply and clearly explains the Five Elements Theory, and line drawings illustrate the various acupressure points. Nutrition and biological influences are also discussed.

ACUPUNCTURE AND ORIENTAL MEDICINE

Harriet Beinfield and Efrem Korngold. *Between Heaven and Earth: A Guide to Chinese Medicine.* New York: Ballantine Books, 1992. 432 pp. ISBN 0345379748.

Required reading at several schools of TCM, this book is a comprehensive guide for the serious student. Topics include eastern and western philosophy, yin and yang, diagnosis, the five-phase theory and archetypes, acupuncture, Chinese herbs, and culinary alchemy.

Sheila McNamara. *Traditional Chinese Medicine.* New York: Basic-Books, 1996. 288 pp. ISBN 0465006299.

This book provides an introduction to the history, philosophy, and principles of TCM, with an A-to-Z guide to conditions and their remedies. Addresses the use of herbs, acupuncture, qigong, and diet.

Gail Reichstein. *Wood Becomes Water: Chinese Medicine in Everyday Life.* New York: Kodansha, 1998. 215 pp. ISBN 1568362099.

The five elements—wood, fire, earth, metal, and water—are examined in the human life cycle and in the body, and treatments from acupuncture, dietary therapy, qi gong, and feng shui are discussed as corrective measures for out-of-balance conditions.

Robert Svoboda and Arnie Lade. *Tao and Dharma: Chinese Medicine and Ayurveda.* Twin Lakes, WI: Lotus Press, 1995. 155 pp. ISBN 0914955217.

Svoboda provides an introduction to and comparison of the theories and practices of traditional Chinese medicine and Ayurveda.

AROMATHERAPY

Kathi Keville and Mindy Green. *Aromatherapy: A Complete Guide to the Healing Art.* Freedom, CA: The Crossing Press, 1995. 158 pp. ISBN 0895946920.

This is a thorough guide to aromatherapy from its history and theories to therapeutic uses, instructions for creating skin care products, techniques for home distillation and blending, and a materia medica listing uses of common essential oils.

Roberta Wilson. *Aromatherapy for Vibrant Health and Beauty.* Garden City Park, NY: Avery Publishing Group, 1995. 244 pp. ISBN 0895296276.

Wilson provides an introduction to thirty-six essential oils that includes folklore and herbal heritage, medicinal uses, beauty benefits, emotional effects, primary actions, and cautions where appropriate, and lists common conditions that can be treated with aromatherapy.

AYURVEDA

David Frawley and Vasant Lad. *The Yoga of Herbs: An Ayurvedic Guide to Herbal Medicine.* Twin Lakes, WI: Lotus Press, 1986. 251 pp. ISBN 0941524248.

This book discusses the basics of Ayurvedic medicine and provides an explanation of herbal energetics and management of individual doshas. Detailed explanations of the uses of eighty-eight therapeutic herbs are given, plus how to prepare herbs according to Ayurvedic principles.

Angela Hope-Murray and Tony Pickup. *Discover Ayurveda: A First-Step Handbook to Better Health.* Berkeley, California: Ulysses Press, 1998. 112 pp. ISBN 1569750815.

One of a series of beginner health guides, this book introduces the novice to the basics of Ayurveda: the history and philosophy of Ayurveda, a personal step-by-step guide, and treatment with Ayurveda.

Vasant Lad. *Ayurveda: The Science of Self-Healing.* Wilmot, WI: Lotus Press, 1984. 175 pp. ISBN 0914955004.

Lad offers a simple, practical explanation of the principles and practical applications of Ayurveda. Topics covered include the five elements, the human constitution, disease process, attributes, diagnosis, lifestyle, medicinals, and more.

Light Miller and Bryan Miller. *Ayurveda and Aromatherapy: The Earth Essential Guide to Ancient Wisdom and Modern Healing.* Twin Lakes, WI: Lotus Books, 1995. 368 pp. ISBN 0914955209.

This book discusses the basics of Ayurveda and the use of aromatherapy for the correction of dosha imbalance. Applications of essential oils include Ayurvedic blending, personal care, cooking, health enhancement, Indian massage, and more.

Amadea Morningstar with Urmila Desai. *The Ayurvedic Cookbook: A Personalized Guide to Good Nutrition and Health.* Wilmot, WI: Lotus Press, 1990. 351 pp. ISBN 0914955063.

What's for dinner?

This book provides over 250 recipes specifically designed to balance each Ayurvedic constitution, but created with the Western diner in mind. General background on Ayurveda and the attributes and nutritional needs of each constitution are included.

CHIROPRACTIC

Daniel Kamen. *The Well-Adjusted Dog: Canine Chiropractic Methods You Can Do.* Cambridge, Massachusetts: Brookline Books, 1996. 165 pp. ISBN 1571290303.

Most states don't allow chiropractors to work on animals, and few vets know anything about chiropractic—so Dr. Kamen shows pet owners how, when, and why to adjust our own dogs.

Terry A. Rondberg. *Chiropractic First: The Fastest Growing Healthcare Choice Before Drugs or Surgery.* The Chiropractic Journal, 1996. ISBN 0964716828.

This is a very readable, easy-to-understand introduction to the history, philosophy, and practice of chiropractic.

ENVIRONMENTAL ILLNESS

Stephen Edelson. *Living with Environmental Illness: A Practical Guide to Multiple Chemical Sensitivity.* Dallas: Taylor Publishing, 1998. 226 pp. ISBN 087833968X.

Edelson examines the definition and causes of multiple chemical sensitivity, explores possible treatments, and tells the stories of some of the people affected. Especially helpful is the Resources chapter, which lists sources of nontoxic products for the home and family.

Robert Sampson and Patricia Hughes. *Breaking Out of Environmental Illness: Essential Reading for People with Chronic Fatigue Syndrome, Allergies, and Chemical Sensitivities.* Santa Fe: Bear and Company, 1997. 258 pp. ISBN 187918141X.

Sampson and Hughes give us a personal account of their battle with and recovery from environmental illness.

FLOWER ESSENCES

Lila Devi. *The Essential Flower Essence Handbook.* Carlsbad, California: Hay House, 1996. 347 pp. ISBN 156170511X.

While flower essence therapy is often taught in conjunction with herbal remedies or aromatherapy, it is a therapy that one can learn to use for self-help—Devi's book is a thorough introduction to the field. Covered in the book are the origins of flower essences and how they work, and detailed descriptions and applications of 20 essences.

GUIDED IMAGERY

Belleruth Naparstek. *Staying Well with Guided Imagery.* New York: Warner Books, 1994. 228 pp. ISBN 0446518212.

Written by a psychotherapist who also produces an audio tape series, this introduction to guided imagery explains what it is, how it works, and how to use it for personal growth. The book includes 20 scripts to aid the immune response and cardiovascular system and for common complaints such as headaches, allergies, and more.

HERBOLOGY

Michael Castleman. *The Healing Herbs: The Ultimate Guide to the Curative Power of Nature's Medicines.* Emmaus, PA: Rodale Press, 1991. ISBN 0878579346.

This book delineates the history, healing powers, dosages, and contraindications for one hundred healing herbs. It also includes a history of herbal healing and tips on storing, preparing, and obtaining herbs.

Logan Chamberlain. *A Consumer Guide to Herbal Supplements: What the Labels Won't Tell You.* Loveland, CO: Interweave Press, 1998. 120 pp. ISBN 1883010497.

Chamberlain's guide helps clear some of the confusion surrounding herbal remedies, covering such topics as decoding the labels, how supplements are manufactured, cautions about using herbs, deciding which herbal form to use, recommended herbal supplements for women and men, and up-and-coming herbs.

Steven Foster. *An Illustrated Guide to 101 Medicinal Herbs.* Loveland, CO: Interweave Press, 1998. 240 pp. ISBN 1883010519.

This handy guide offers sources, traditional and current uses, typical dosages, preparations, cautions, and full-color photographs of 101 medicinal herbs.

Mrs. M. Grieve. *A Modern Herbal in Two Volumes.* New York: Dover Publications, 1982. 902 pp. ISBN 0486227987 (volume I); 0486227995 (Volume II).

These volumes are unabridged republications of the original work first published in 1931. The serious herbologist's bible, Mrs. Grieve's books describe the properties, cultivation, folklore, and medicinal uses of herbs and other plants.

Christopher Hobbs. *Handmade Medicines: Simple Recipes for Herbal Health.* Loveland, CO: Interweave Press, 1998. 120 pp. ISBN 1883010500.

Hobbs has created a guide for both novice and experienced herbalists to finding and preparing herbs in teas, tinctures, compresses, and syrups.

Michael T. Murray. *The Healing Power of Herbs: The Enlightened Person's Guide to the Wonders of Medicinal Plants* / 2nd ed. Rocklin, CA: Prima Publishing, 1995. 410 pp. ISBN 1559587008.

This guide to thirty-seven herbs includes a general description, terminology, chemical composition, history and folk use, pharmacology, clinical applications, dosage, and toxicity for each, followed by recommended herbs for specific health conditions.

Louise Tenney. *Today's Herbal Health,* 3rd edition. Pleasant Grove, UT: Woodland Books, 1997. 384 pp. ISBN 1885670060.

This is a comprehensive guide to both single herbs and their combinations. For each herb, a description is given of the parts used, how it acts in the body, the vitamins and minerals it contains, and ailments for which it is commonly used.

Lesley Tierra. *The Herbs of Life: Health and Healing Using Western and Chinese Techniques.* Freedom, CA: The Crossing Press, 1992. 274 pp. ISBN 0895944987.

This is a comprehensive book for the beginning or intermediate student of herbology. The author clearly explains the concepts of heating and cooling energies of both herbs and illnesses, discusses the properties and indications of Western and Chinese herbs in turn, and provides step-by-step instructions in making poultices, plasters, tinctures, and more.

Gregory L. Tilford. *From Earth to Herbalist: An Earth-Conscious Guide to Medicinal Plants.* Missoula, MT: Mountain Press, 1998. 248 pp. ISBN 0878423729.

Tilford presents guidelines for the ethical harvesting of wild plants; the basics of herbal preparations; and a full-color field guide to medicinal plants, listing for each herb other names, parts used, actions, description, habitat and range, applications, care after gathering, warnings, and more.

Joyce A. Wardwell. *The Herbal Home Remedy Book: Simple Recipes for Tinctures, Teas, Salves, Tonics, and Syrups.* Pownal, VT: Storey Communications, 1998. 169 pp. ISBN 1580170161.

A practical how-to-do-it guide to gathering, drying, storing, and blending twenty-five common herbs and making your own herbal medicine cabinet of tinctures, syrups, lozenges, and more.

HOMEOPATHY

Wayne B. Jonas and Jennifer Jacobs. *Healing with Homeopathy: The Complete Guide.* New York: Warner Books, 1996. ISBN 0446518697.

Jonas and Jacobs offer a comprehensive yet readable guide to homeopathy that covers its origins, cycles, theory, and research, plus a guide to home treatment with chapters on injuries and first aid, babies, children's illnesses, women's health, and other common problems.

R. Donald Papon. *Homeopathy Made Simple: A Quick Reference Guide.* Charlottesville, VA: Hampton Roads, 1999. 262 pp. ISBN 1-57174-110-0.

Finding a homeopathic remedy for everyday problems couldn't be simpler than with the Five-Minute Prescriber in this book. Profiles of common remedies follow, with homeopathic solutions to candida overgrowth, hypoglycemia, depression, and other common problems.

Barry Rode and Christina Scott-Moncrieff. *Homeopathy for Women.* North Pomfret, VT: Trafalgar Square, 1998. 176 pp. ISBN 1850283923.

This useful do-it-yourself reference tool explains which homeopathic remedy to use for common problems of the breasts, reproductive system, pregnancy, menopause, and various systems of the body, plus treatments for metabolic and emotional problems.

HYPNOSIS

C. Roy Hunter. *The Art of Hypnotherapy.* Dubuque, IA: Kendall/Hunt Publishing, 1995. 314 pp. ISBN 078724287X.

Hunter gives the serious student of hypnotherapy a comprehensive guide to the field, covering the pre-induction interview, scripts for progressions, anchoring and triggers, hypnotic uncovering techniques, regression therapy, phobias, past-life regressions, common potential applications of hypnotherapy, and much more.

Ursula Markham. *Hypnotherapy: A Guide to Improving Health and Well-Being with Hypnosis.* North Pomfret, VT: Trafalgar Square, 1997. 127pp. ISBN 0091815193.

An easy-to-read introduction to field of hypnotherapy, this book covers the history of hypnosis, relaxation and visualization, smoking and obesity, phobias, common uses of hypnosis, and pain and illness.

John M. Yates and Elizabeth S. Wallace. *The Complete Book of Self-Hypnosis.* Chicago: Nelson-Hall, 1990. ISBN 0804104093.

This book is a primer in the use of self-hypnosis for the control of weight, pain, addictions, and more. It includes steps to self-hypnosis and hypnotic techniques.

IRIDOLOGY

Bernard Jensen and Donald V. Bodeen. *Visions of Health: Understanding Iridology.* Garden City Park, NY: Avery Publishing Group, 1992. 176 pp. ISBN 0895294338.

One of America's pioneering iridologists has written this detailed look at the art and science of iridology, with dozens of color photos, illustrations, and charts.

MASSAGE AND BODYWORK

Thomas Claire. *Bodywork: What Type of Massage to Get—and How to Make the Most of It.* New York: William Morrow, 1996. ISBN 0688149529.

This book explains in detail the practices and philosophies of various styles of massage including Swedish, myofascial release, shiatsu, reflexology, Reiki, therapeutic touch, craniosacral therapy, polarity therapy, and more, plus a glossary and resources.

Saul Goodman. *The Book of Shiatsu: The Healing Art of Finger Pressure,* 2nd ed. Garden City Park, NY: Avery Publishing Group, 1990. ISBN 0895294540.

This book takes an in-depth look at shiatsu, from how shiatsu works to step-by-step instructions for whole-body shiatsu, including acupressure points for specific symptoms and diagnostic techniques.

Shizuko Yamamoto and Patrick McCarty. *Barefoot Shiatsu.* New York: Avery Publishing Group, 1998. 160 pp. ISBN 0895298570.

Yamamoto, one of the world's leading authorities on shiatsu, shows us the unique attitude and techniques of barefoot shiatsu, correcting exercises, and how to perform self-diagnosis.

MIDWIFERY

Elizabeth Davis. *Heart and Hands: A Midwife's Guide to Pregnancy and Birth,* 3rd ed. Berkeley, CA: Celestial Arts, 1997. 287 pp. ISBN 0890878382.

This practical guide is an informative yet intimate introduction to midwifery for prospective midwives. Comprehensive and easy to read, the books explores prenatal care, problems in pregnancy, assisting at birth, complications in labor, postpartum care, becoming a midwife, and the midwife's practice.

Judith Pence Rooks. *Midwifery and Childbirth in America.* Philadelphia: Temple University Press, 1997. 548 pp. ISBN 1566395658.

Rooks offers an in-depth study of the history of midwifery, American midwifery from the first nurse-midwives to the development of direct-entry midwifery, the effectiveness of midwifery as practiced in the US, midwifery around the world, and recommendations for the future.

NUTRITION

James F. Balch and Phyllis A. Balch. *Prescription for Nutritional Healing,* 2nd ed. Garden City Park, NY: Avery Publishing Group, 1997. 600 pp. ISBN 0895297272.

This is a handy guide that lists important nutrients, including vitamins, minerals, enzymes, herbs, and amino acids, for use in the treatment of ailments from abscesses to yeast infections.

Robert Buist. *Food Chemical Sensitivity: What It Is and How to Cope with It.* Garden City Park, NY: Avery Publishing Group, 1986. ISBN 0895293994.

Readers will learn how the consumption of food additives can contribute to asthma, hyperactivity, skin disorders, migraines, and other ailments, and how to identify and eliminate contaminants in our diet.

Jean Carper. *Food: Your Miracle Medicine.* New York: HarperCollins, 1993. 528 pp. ISBN 0061013307.

Carper gives practical advice on using foods to feel better and smarter, prevent cancer and heart disease, and fight common infections and illnesses.

Carl Ferré. *Pocket Guide to Macrobiotics.* Freedom, CA: The Crossing Press, 1997. 126 pp. ISBN 0895948486.

A small book packed with lots of information, Ferré's guide covers the definition of macrobiotics, a macrobiotic approach to diet, macrobiotic yin and yang, and macrobiotic healing, all in a clear and concise format.

Elson M. Haas. *Staying Healthy with Nutrition: The Complete Guide to Diet and Nutritional Medicine.* Berkeley, CA: Celestial Arts, 1992. ISBN 0890874816.

Haas presents a comprehensive guide to diet and nutrition, featuring a detailed analysis of the various types of nutrients, an evaluation of foods and diets (including vegetarianism, macrobi-

otics, fasting, and more), how to build a healthy diet, and special diets and supplement programs for specific needs.

Carolyn Heidenry. *An Introduction to Macrobiotics: A Beginner's Guide to the Natural Way of Health.* Garden City Park, NY: Avery Publishing Group, 1992. 102 pp. ISBN 0895294648.

This book discusses the basic principles and practical application of the macrobiotic diet: disease as imbalance, nature's designs, recommended foods and foods to avoid, yin and yang, and more.

Bernard Jensen. *Foods That Heal.* Garden City Park, NY: Avery Publishing Group, 1993. ISBN 0895295636.

Jensen presents a history of use, therapeutic benefits, and nutrient information for dozens of fruits and vegetables, plus over 100 natural foods recipes.

Gayla J. Kirschmann and John D. Kirschmann. *Nutrition Almanac,* 4th ed. New York: McGraw-Hill, 1996. ISBN 007349223.

This book contains an in-depth look at the absorption and storage, dosages and toxicity, beneficial effects, deficiency effects, and human and animal tests conducted on vitamins, minerals, and other nutrients. Includes beneficial nutrients for dozens of ailments, a table of food composition, and a section on herbs.

Shari Lieberman and Nancy Bruning. *The Real Vitamin and Mineral Book,* 2nd ed. Garden City Park, NY: Avery Publishing Group, 1997. ISBN 0-89529-769-8.

This guide to nutritional supplements covers the RDAs, ODAs (Optimum Daily Allowance), adverse effects, and how to design your own supplement program, plus abstracts of scientific studies on vitamins, minerals, and other nutrients.

Gary Null. *The Complete Guide to Sensible Eating.* New York: Seven Stories, 1998. ISBN 188363614.

More a complete guide to sensible living, this book offers an introduction to various nutrients, detoxification, food allergies, vegetarianism, weight management, and a rotation diet, plus the basics of herbs, exercise, environmental medicine, candida, selecting a health practitioner, and much more.

Gary Null. *No More Allergies: Identifying and Eliminating Allergies and Sensitivity Reactions to Everything in Your Environment.* New York: Villard Books, 1992. 421 pp. ISBN 0679743103.

This book discusses how environmental toxins and food allergies can affect physical and mental functioning. It covers allergies and the immune system, chemical poisoning, childhood allergies, indoor pollutants, and much more.

George Ohsawa. *Essential Ohsawa: From Food to Health, Happiness to Freedom.* Garden City Park, NY: Avery Publishing Group, 1994. 238 pp. ISBN 0895296160.

The father of macrobiotics discusses the principles of macrobiotics and the philosophy that governed his productive life; includes photos and anecdotes from those who knew him best.

John Robbins. *Diet for a New America.* Tiburon, CA: H.J. Kramer, 1987. 423 pp. ISBN 0915811812.

In this compelling classic, Robbins gives Americans a wake-up call regarding the effects of an animal-based diet on our health, our consciousness, and our environment. A must for everyone considering a vegetarian diet (and their meat-eating friends).

Art Ulene. *The NutriBase Nutrition Facts Desk Reference.* Garden City Park, NY: Avery Publishing Group, 1995. 789 pp. ISBN 0895296233.

Here's where you'll find nutritional information for over 40,000 foods that includes calories, protein, carbohydrates, fat, saturated fat, sodium, cholesterol, fiber, vitamins, and minerals, plus information for fast food items by restaurant.

POLARITY THERAPY

Maruti Seidman. *Guide to Polarity Therapy: The Gentle Art of Hand-on Healing.* Elan Press, 1991. ISBN 0962870900.

Seidman offers an introduction to the theory and techniques of polarity therapy.

REFLEXOLOGY

Mildred Carter and Tammy Weber. *Healing Yourself with Foot Reflexology.* Englewood Cliffs, NJ: Prentice Hall, 1997. 288 pp. ISBN 0132441209.

This is a step-by-step guide to improving your life and that of others with reflexology. This book explains how reflexology works, complete with benefits, charts, and techniques.

Beryl Crane. *Reflexology: The Definitive Practitioner's Manual.* Rockport, MA: Element, 1997. 442 pp. ISBN 1862041253.

Both novice and professional reflexologists will appreciate this comprehensive guide to the history and concepts of reflexology; the zones, divisions, and meridians associated with the feet; reflexology of the hand, ear, face and head; and advice on setting up a practice, consultation procedures, and taking case histories.

Inge Douglas. *The Complete Illustrated Guide to Reflexology.* Rockport, MA: Element, 1996. ISBN 1852309105.

The basics of reflexology are explained and illustrated with color photos. The book covers reflexology and relaxation, understanding energy, foot anatomy, mapping of foot reflexes, techniques, case studies, and detailed treatment sequences.

Pauline Wills. *The Reflexology Manual.* Rochester, VT: Healing Arts Press, 1995. ISBN: 0892815477.

Wills covers the history of reflexology, pressure point and massage techniques, and step-by-step directions on giving treatments. The book also contains clear color photographs accompanied by arrows showing the direction of massage, making techniques easy to understand and perform.

REIKI

Tanmaya Honervogt. *The Power of Reiki: An Ancient Hands-on Healing Technique.* New York: Henry Holt, 1998. 143 pp. ISBN 0805055592.

A Reiki Master-Teacher gives us a clear and helpful introduction to Reiki, including its history and meaning, Reiki degrees and treatments, and Reiki in daily life.

Paula Horan. *Empowerment Through Reiki: The Path to Personal and Global Transformation.* Wilmot, WI: Lotus Light, 1998. ISBN 0941524841.

An experienced Reiki master describes how Reiki energy works, how it can be used, and the effects that may be achieved.

Sandi Leir Shuffrey. *Reiki: A Beginner's Guide.* North Pomfret, VT: Trafalgar Square, 1998. 90 pp. ISBN 0340720816.

Shuffrey explains in beginner's terms the origins and nature of Reiki, Reiki in practice and in combination with other therapies, and experiences with Reiki.

Diane Stein. *Essential Reiki: A Complete Guide to an Ancient Healing Art.* Freedom, CA: The Crossing Press, 1995. 156 pp. ISBN 0-89594-736-6.

This book provides an explanation of the ancient system of

"laying on of hands" that includes the first, second, and third degree. Covers the basic principles of Reiki, the Reiki symbols, distance healing, opening the Kundalini, passing attunements, teaching Reiki, and more.

VETERINARY CARE

George MacLeod. *Cats: Homoeopathic Remedies.* Santa Rosa, CA: Atrium Publishers Group, 1990. ISBN 0852071906.

Written for cat lovers interested in an alternative approach to the treatment of illnesses, this book uses only the common remedies. For each disorder, the author describes clinical signs and a number of suggested homeopathic treatments.

George MacLeod. *Dogs: Homoeopathic Remedies.* Santa Rosa, CA: Atrium Publishers Group, 1992. ISBN 085207218X.

This book is written in the same style and format as *Cats,* above. It is useful to any dog owner who wants to try homeopathic remedies for specific disorders.

Diane Stein. *The Natural Remedy Book for Dogs and Cats.* Freedom, CA: The Crossing Press, 1994. 341 pp. ISBN 0895946866.

This is a guide to the use of naturopathy, vitamins and minerals, herbs, homeopathy, acupuncture and acupressure, flower essences, and gemstones for the treatment of common disorders in dogs and cats.

YOGA

Alice Christensen. *The American Yoga Association Wellness Book.* New York: Kensington Books, 1996. ISBN 1575660253.

A step-by-step guide for the beginner or seasoned practitioner, this book includes basic daily routines, individualized programs for the treatment of specific disorders, and advanced techniques.

Rammurti S. Mishra. *Fundamentals of Yoga: A Handbook of Theory, Practice, and Application.* New York: Harmony Books, 1987. 198 pp. ISBN 051756422X.

This book explains the science of yoga for the serious beginner. It includes lessons on using yoga to control mental and physical states, and illustrations of yoga postures.

Rachel Schaeffer. *Yoga For Your Spiritual Muscles.* Wheaton, IL: Quest Books, 1998. 194 pp. ISBN 0835607631.

This step-by-step yoga program explores ways to use yoga to strengthen inner qualities such as awareness, acceptance, focus, confidence, compassion, energy, playfulness, and others.

Notes

INTRODUCTION

1. Deanne Tenney. *Introduction to Natural Health* (Provo, UT: Woodland Books, 1992), 5.
2. Karen Baar. "The Real Options in Healthcare," *Natural Health*, November/December 1994, 95.
3. Dana Ullman. "Renegade Remedies?" *Utne Reader*, November/December 1993, 42.

ACUPUNCTURE AND ORIENTAL MEDICINE

1. The Burton Goldberg Group. *Alternative Medicine: The Definitive Guide* (Fife, WA: Future Medicine Publishing, 1994), 450.
2. Sheila McNamara. *Traditional Chinese Medicine* (New York: BasicBooks, 1996), xiii.
3. *Ibid.,* 28.
4. Manfred Porkett with Christian Ullman. *Chinese Medicine* (New York: William Morrow, 1982), 69.
5. McNamara. *Traditional Chinese Medicine,* 99.
6. Mark Kastner and Hugh Burroughs. *Alternative Healing: The Complete A–Z Guide to Over 160 Different Alternative Therapies* (La Mesa, CA: Halcyon Publishing, 1993), 108.
7. The Burton Goldberg Group. *Alternative Medicine,* 37–38.
8. *Ibid.,* 38.
9. *Ibid.,* 44.
10. Dort Bigg, Executive Director ACAOM. E-mail. March 31, 1999.

AROMATHERAPY

1. The Burton Goldberg Group. *Alternative Medicine: The Definitive Guide* (Fife, WA: Future Medicine Publishing, 1994), 55.
2. *Ibid.,* 57.
3. Kathi Keville and Mindy Green. *Aromatherapy: A Complete Guide to the Healing Art* (Freedom, CA: The Crossing Press, 1995), 15.
4. Roberta Wilson. *Aromatherapy For Vibrant Health and Beauty* (Garden City Park, NY: Avery Publishing Group, 1995), 3.
5. Robert Tisserand. *Aromatherapy: To Heal and Tend the Body* (Twin Lakes, WI: Lotus Press, 1988), 163.

AYURVEDA

1. Vasant Lad. *Ayurveda: The Science of Self-Healing* (Twin Lakes, WI: Lotus Press, 1984), 18.
2. The Burton Goldberg Group. *Alternative Medicine: The Definitive Guide* (Fife, WA: Future Medicine Publishing, 1994), 68.
3. *Ibid.,* 70.
4. David Frawley and Vasant Lad. *The Yoga of Herbs: An Ayurvedic Guide to Herbal Medicine* (Twin Lakes, WI: Lotus Press, 1986), 15.

BIOFEEDBACK

1. Mark Kastner and Hugh Burroughs. *Alternative Healing: The Complete A–Z Guide to Over 160 Different Alternative Therapies* (La Mesa, CA: Halcyon Publishing, 1993), 37.
2. Ernest Lawrence Rossi. *The Psychobiology of Mind-Body Heal-*

ing: New Concepts of Therapeutic Hypnosis (New York: W.W. Norton, 1986), 109-110.

CHIROPRACTIC

1. International Chiropractors Association. "Consumer Information," www.chiropractic.org/consumerinfo/consumerinfo.htm, April 1999.
2. Nathaniel Altman. *Everybody's Guide to Chiriopractic Health Care* (Los Angeles: Jeremy P. Tarcher, 1990), 10–11.
3. *Ibid.*, 16–19.
4. Council on Chiropractic Education. *Biennial Report: February 1994–January 1996* (Scottsdale, AZ: Council on Chiropractic Education, 1996), 23.
5. International Chiropractors Association. "Consumer Information."
6. Ruth Sandefur. "Chapter V: Licensure and Legal Scope of Practice," www.homepathic.com/intro/tenques.htm, April 1999.

ENVIRONMENTAL MEDICINE

1. The Burton Goldberg Group. *Alternative Medicine: The Definitive Guide* (Fife, WA: Future Medicine Publishing, 1994), 206.
2. *Ibid.*, 206–207.
3. Sherry Rogers. *Tired or Toxic? A Blueprint for Health* (Syracuse, NY: Prestige Publishing, 1990), 21.
4. The Burton Goldberg Group. *Alternative Medicine*, 207–208.
5. John Bower. *The Healthy House: How to Buy One, How to Build One, How to Cure a "Sick" One* (New York: Carol Publishing Group, 1993), 16.

GUIDED IMAGERY

1. Belleruth Naparstek. *Staying Well with Guided Imagery* (New York: Warner Books, 1994), 18, 22, 26.
2. The Burton Goldberg Group. *Alternative Medicine: The Definitive Guide* (Fife, WA: Future Medicine Publishing, 1994), 248–249.

HERBAL MEDICINE

1. Michael T. Murray. *The Healing Power of Herbs, 2nd edition* (Rocklin, CA: Prima Publishing, 1995), 1.
2. *Ibid.*
3. Jeanne Rattenbury. "The Other Health Care Reform," *Chicago,* January 1995, 62.

4. Murray. *The Healing Power of Herbs,* 97–100.
5. David Hoffman. *The Information Sourcebook of Herbal Medicine* (Freedom, CA: The Crossing Press, 1994), 7.
6. Alan Gathright. "More Patients Are Looking Beyond Western Medicine to Herbal Treatments," Knight-Ridder/ Tribune News Service, September 2, 1994, 0902K6214.
7. Michael Castleman. "Legalize It!" *Mother Jones,* November–December 1994, 43.
8. Caren Goldman and Deborah France. "Days in Lives: Natural Health 1994 Career Guide," Natural Health, May–June 1994, 92.
9. Michael Tierra. "East West Master Course in Herbology" (Santa Cruz, CA: East West School of Herbalism), 9.

HOMEOPATHY

1. Christopher Hammond. *The Complete Family Guide to Homeopathy: An Illustrated Encyclopedia of Safe and Effective Remedies* (New York: Penguin Studio, 1995), 19.
2. Dana Ullman. "Ten Most Frequently Asked Questions on Homeopathic Medicine," www.homeopathic.com/intro/tenques. htm, April 1999.
3. *Ibid.*
4. The Burton Goldberg Group. *Alternative Medicine: The Definitive Guide* (Fife, WA: Future Medicine Publishing, 1994), 272.
5. *Ibid.*

HYPNOTHERAPY

1. The Burton Goldberg Group. *Alternative Medicine: The Definitive Guide* (Fife, WA: Future Medicine Publishing, 1994), 306.
2. John M. Yates and Elizabeth S. Wallace. *The Complete Book of Self-Hypnosis* (Chicago: Nelson-Hill, 1984) , 1.
3. Lewis R. Wolberg. *Hypnosis: Is It For You?* (New York: Dembner Books, 1982), 22.
4. Yates and Wallace. *The Complete Book of Self-Hypnosis,* 30.
5. *Ibid.*, 4–6.

IRIDOLOGY

1. Mark Kastner and Hugh Burroughs. *Alternative Healing: The Complete A–Z Guide to Over 160 Different Alternative Therapies* (La Mesa, CA: Halcyon Publishing, 1993), 130.
2. Dr. Bernard Jensen and Dr. Donald V. Boden. Visions of Heatlh: Understanding Iridology (Garden City Park, NY: Avery Publishing Group, 1992), 74–83.
3. *Ibid.*

MASSAGE THERAPY AND BODYWORK

1. Mary Crews and Rick Rosen/American Massage Therapy Association. "A Guide to Massage Therapy in America," 1995, 9.
2. Gayle MacDonald. "A Review of Nursing Research: Massage for Cancer Patients," *Massage Therapy Journal,* Summer 1995, 54, citing Ferrell-Torry A. T. and Glick O. J. "The Use of Therapeutic Massage as a Nursing Intervention to Modify Anxiety and the Perception of Cancer Pain," Cancer Nursing, 1993, 16:93–101.
3. Jessica Cohen. "The Healing Touch," *The Natural Way,* February–March 1995, 61.
4. "Alternative Medicine: Expanding Medical Horizons: A Report to the National Institutes of Health on Alternative Medical Systems and Practices in the United States," prepared under the auspices of the Workshop on Alternative Medicine, Chantilly, VA, September 14–16, 1992, citing *The New England Journal of Medicine,* January 28, 1993.
5. *Ibid.,* 125.
6. *Ibid.,* 128.
7. Rosemary Feitis. *Ida Rolf Talks About Rolfing and Physical Reality* (New York: Harper and Row, 1978), 31.
8. "Alternative Medicine," 132.
9. American Massage Therapy Association. "Massage Therapy in the United States: Meeting the Growing Demand Among Consumers," www.amtamassage.org/publications/markettrends.htm, April 1999.
10. National Certification Board for Therapeutic Massage and Bodywork. "NCBTMB State Summary of Nationally Certified Practitioners," March 15, 1999.

NATUROPATHY

1. National College of Naturopathic Medicine Catalog 1995–1997 (Portland, OR: National College of Naturopathic Medicine, 1995), 1–2.

NUTRITION

1. Elson M. Haas. *Staying Healthy with Nutrition: The Complele Guide to Diet and Nutritional Medicine* (Berkeley, CA: Celestial Arts, 1992), 775.
2. *Ibid.,* 361.
3. George Ohsawa. Essential Ohsawa: From Food to Health, Happiness to Freedom (Garden City Park, NY: Avery Publishing Group, 1994), 18–26.
4. Lavon J. Dunne. Nutrition Almanac: Third Edition (New York: McGraw-Hill, 1990), 78, 192.

5. *Ibid.,* 117.
6. *Ibid.,* 82, 80.

POLARITY THERAPY

1. Dr. Randolph Stone. *Polarity Therapy Vol II,* 207, quoted in *Polarity Therapy* (brochure), (Boulder, CO: American Polarity Therapy Association).
2. Alan Siegel. *Polarity Therapy: The Power That Heals* (San Leandro, CA: Prism Press, 1987), 5.
3. Thomas Claire. *Bodywork: What Type of Massage to Get—and How to Make the Most of It* (New York: William Morrow, 1995), 329.

REFLEXOLOGY

1. The Burton Goldberg Group. *Alternative Medicine: The Definitive Guide* (Fife, WA: Future Medicine Publishing, 1994), 109.
2. Thomas Claire. *Bodywork: What Type of Massage to Get—and How to Make the Most of It* (New York: William Morrow, 1995), 222.
3. The Burton Goldberg Group. *Alternative Medicine,* 109.
4. *Ibid.*
5. Kevin Kunz and Barbara Kunz. "Consequences of the Massage Regulation of Reflexology," www.foot-reflexologist.com/massf.htm, April 1999.

VETERINARY MASSAGE

1. Mary Schreiber. "Healing Hands," *Practical Horseman,* July 1993, 55.
2. International Association of Equine Sports Massage Therapists. "Analysis/ Tabulation of 1995 National ESMT Survey," *Stable Talk,* Summer 1995.

YOGA

1. Clint Willis. "Fitness," *Lear's,* November 1993, 40.
2. *Ibid.*
3. The Burton Goldberg Group. *Alternative Medicine: The Definitive Guide* (Fife, WA: Future Medicine Publishing, 1994), 474.
4. *Ibid.,* 471.

Index

AAMA. *See* American Academy of Medical
Acupuncture
AANP. *See* American Association of Naturopathic
Physicians
AAoA News Quarterly 447
AAOM. *See* American Association of Oriental
Medicine
ABMP. *See* Associated Bodywork and Massage
Professionals
ACA. *See* American Chiropractic Association
Academy for Five Element Acupuncture 150–51
Academy for Guided Imagery 59–60, 472
Academy for Myofascial Trigger Point Therapy 295
Academy of Chinese Culture and Health Sciences
60–61
Academy of Chinese Healing Arts 151–52
Academy of Classical Oriental Sciences 359
Academy of Court Reporting 61
Academy of Healing Arts 152–53
Academy of Massage Therapy 230
Academy of Natural Healing 253
Academy of Natural Therapy 129
Academy of Oriental Medicine — Austin 309–10
Academy of Professional Careers 61–62
Academy of Somatic Healing Arts 168–69
Academy of Veterinary Homeopathy 460
ACAOM. *See* Accreditation Commission for
Acupuncture and Oriental Medicine
ACA Today 449, 471
ACCET. *See* Accrediting Council for Continuing
Education and Training
Accreditation Commission for Acupuncture and
Oriental Medicine xvii, 4, 427–28, 435
Accrediting Commission of Career Schools and
Colleges of Technology 427
Accrediting Council for Continuing Education and
Training 427
ACCSCT. *See* Accrediting Commission of Career
Schools and Colleges of Technology
ACNM. *See* American College of Nurse Midwifery
Acupressure 17, 34, 56–57, 62–63, 67, 70, 74, 96, 106,
120, 154, 253, 356, 360, 397, 464–65. *See also*

Shiatsu; Massage therapy and bodywork; Jin Shin
Do
Acupressure-Acupuncture Institute 153–54
Acupressure Institute 62–63, 464–65
Acupuncture xvii, 3–4, 34–35, 51, 87, 115–16, 119,
127–28, 151, 177, 183, 197–98, 206–7, 219–20,
259–60, 262–64, 268–71, 291, 336–38, 342–43,
358, 360–63, 375, 382, 384–85, 398–99, 406,
427–28, 435–36, 445–47, 465. *See also* Oriental
medicine; Traditional Chinese medicine;
Herbology
Acupuncture Center 350
Adinolfi, Melodie A. 295
Advanced Fuller School of Massage 325–26
AHA. See American Herb Association
AHA Quarterly 450, 478
AHG. *See* American Herbalists Guild
Ahimsa 457, 491
Aihara, Cornellia 125
Aihara, Herman 125
Aisen Shiatsu School 173–74
Alberta Institute of Massage 353
Alchemical hypnotherapy. *See* Hypnotherapy
Alchemy Institute of Healing Arts 63–64
Alexandar, Aliesha 334
Alexandar School of Natural Therapeutics 334
Alexander, F. Mathias 17
Alexander technique 17
Alexandria School of Scientific Therapeutics 186
Alive and Well! Institute of Conscious Bodywork
64–65
Alternative Conjunction Clinic and School of
Massage Therapy, The 295–96
Alternative Medicine Magazine 464
Alternative Therapies in Health and Medicine 464
Alves, Kate 73
Ambrose, Satya 291
American Academy of Clinical Homeopathy 480
American Academy of Environmental Medicine 9,
383–84, 449–50
American Academy of Medical Acupuncture
384–85, 435, 445–46, 465

American Academy of Nutrition 490
American Academy of Reflexology 27
American Acupuncturist, The 446, 465
American Alliance of Aromatherapy 447, 469
American Association of Naturopathic Physicians
442, 457
American Associaton of Oriental Medicine 446, 465
American Association of Poison Control Centers 11
American Board of Homeotherapeutics 438
American Botanical Council 472, 479
American Chiropractic Association 449, 471
American College of Acupuncture and Oriental
Medicine 310–11
American College of Nurse Midwifery 22, 442
American College of Traditional Chinese Medicine
65–66
American Health Science University 490–91
American Herbal Institute, The 283–84, 473
American Herbalists Guild 235, 429, 450, 479
American Herb Association 450, 478
American Holistic Health Association 445
American Holistic Nurses' Association 452, 480
American Homeopath, The 453, 484
American Institute for Aromatherapy and Herbal
Studies, The 253–54, 466
American Institute of Massage Therapy 66–67
American Institute of Vedic Studies 469–70
American Massage Therapy Association 17, 21, 431,
432, 440, 454–55, 489
American Medical Association 14, 25
American Natural Hygiene Society 457, 491
American Oriental Bodywork Therapy Association
xviii, 431, 455, 488
American Polarity Therapy Association xviii–xix,
26, 433, 459–60, 492
American Qigong Association 460, 493
American Reflexology Certification Board 27, 444
American School for Energy Therapies 198–99
American University of Complementary Medicine
67
American Vegan Society, The 457, 491
American Viniyoga Institute 385

American Yoga Association 385–86, 433–34
Amma 19, 178–79, 263–64
Amrita Aromatherapy 394
AMTA. *See* American Massage Therapy Association
Anderson, Jane 208
Andrusiak, Ken 363
Animal Natural Health Center 284
Ann Arbor Institute of Massage Therapy 208
Anton, Shannon 103
AOBTA. *See* American Oriental Bodywork Therapy Association
Apollo Herbs 304–5
Applied kinesiology 17–18, 447
Applied Kinesthetic Studies 326
Applied Psychophysiology and Biofeedback 449, 471
APTA. *See* American Polarity Therapy Association
ARCB. *See* American Reflexology Certification Board
Arizona School of Integrative Studies 49
Aromaflex Centre of Healing Arts 366, 466
Aromatherapy 4–5, 18, 35–36, 68, 78, 123, 130, 145, 154–55, 202, 236, 254, 265–66, 280–81, 285–86, 325–26, 335, 341, 356, 366, 373, 394–96, 401–2, 407, 409, 422, 428, 436, 447–48, 466–69. *See also* Flower essence therapy
Aromatherapy Center 326
Aromatherapy Institute and Research 68
Aromatic Thymes, The 469
AromaYoga™ 326–27
Artemisia Institute 473
Artemis Institute of Natural Therapies 129–30
Aschendorf, Marcia L. 278
Ashland Massage Institute 284–85
Ashmead College School of Massage 334–35
Ash Tree Publications 271, 473
Ashwins Publications 480–81
Associated Bodywork and Massage Professionals 431–32, 455, 489
Association for Applied Psychophysiology and Biofeedback, The 448–49
Association for Research and Enlightenment 327
Association of Vegetarian Dietitians and Nutrition Educators. *See* Vegedine
Asten, Paige 386
Asten Center of Natural Therapeutics 386
Aston, Judith 228
Aston-Patterning ® 228–29
Atlanta School of Massage 169–70
Atlantic Academy of Classical Homeopathy 254–55
Atlantic Institute of Aromatherapy 154–55, 466–67
Atlantic Institute of Oriental Medicine 155–56
Austin School of Massage Therapy 311–12
Australasian College of Herbal Studies, The 285–86, 462
Avena Botanicals 191–92
Avenoso, Michael 59
Avicenna 16
Ayurveda xvii, 5–7, 26, 36, 67, 71–72, 105, 141, 189–90, 202, 242–43, 253, 255, 397–98, 448, 469–71
Ayurveda Holistic Center 255, 470
Ayurveda Today 448, 471
Ayurvedic Institute, The 242–43, 448, 470, 471

Bach Flower Remedies 481. *See also* Flower essence therapy

Balance Life Gardens. *See* Spirit of the Earth Centre for Herbal Education and Earth Awareness
Ball, Barbara 104
Baltimore School of Massage 195–96
Bancroft School of Massage Therapy 199–200
Barber, T. X. 7
Barnes, John F. 402
Barnes, Randy 246
Barnes, Susan 246
Bashan, Barbera 178
Bastyr University 335–38
Baylor College of Medicine 500–1
BCIA. *See* Biofeedback Certification Institute of America
Beaulieu, John 257
Beebe, Walter 265
Beginnings 452, 480
Bellerue, Ilene 174
Bellerue, Thomas 174
Benham, Jan 373
Benjamin, Ben E. 205
Benjamin System 205
Bensky, Dan 343
Bergner, Paul 479
Bernstein, Larry A. 460
Bhajan, Yogi 415
Bio-Energetics 211
Biofeedback xvii, 7–8, 36, 68–69, 387, 414–15, 429, 436–37, 448–49, 471
Biofeedback 449, 471
Biofeedback Certification Institute of America xvii, 7–8, 429, 437
Biofeedback Institute of Los Angeles 68–69, 471
Biofeedback Instrument Corporation 387
BioSomatics 387–88, 485–86
Birthingway Midwifery School 286–87
Birthwise Midwifery School 192–93
Bisenius, Edward 188
B.K.S. Iyengar Yoga Association of Northern California 95, 461, 495
B.K.S. Iyengar Yoga Association of Southern California 69
Black, Cindy 255
Blazing Star Herbal School 200–201
Blue Cliff School of Therapeutic Massage 388–90
Blue Sky Educational Foundation 349
Boardwine, Teresa 328
Boca Raton Institute 156
Body Dynamics School of Massage Therapy 243–44
Body-Mind Centering® 411
Body-mind integrative therapies 107–8, 193
Body-mind transformational psychology 57–58
Body Therapy Center 69–71
Body Therapy Institute 272
Bodywork. *See* Massage therapy and bodywork
Bolesky, Karen 345
Bontrager, Winona 299
Bosman, Lynn 421
Boston Shiatsu School. *See* East West Institute of Alternative Medicine
Boston University School of Medicine 498
Bothwell, Jane 78
Boulder College of Massage Therapy 130–31
Bourdelais, Maryalice 126
Boyne, Gil 91
Breckenridge, Mary 22

Breema bodywork, 71. *See also* Massage therapy and bodywork
Breema Center, The 71
Brenneke, Heida F. 338
Brenneke School of Massage 338–39
Bresler, David E. 59, 472
Brian Utting School of Massage 339
Bridge, The 454, 485
Brighid's Academy of Healing Arts 287
British Institute of Homoeopathy, The 481
British Institute of Homoeopathy Canada, The 481–82
British Journal of Occupational Therapy 4
British Medical Journal 13
Brotman, Dr. 387
Brown, Walter Matthew 352
Buckle, Jane 409
Burman, Iris 157
Burmeister, Mary 400
Business of Herbs, The 478
Butje, Andrea 255
Byers, Dwight 27

Caduceus Institute of Classical Homeopathy 482
Cale, Charles 99
Cale, Linnie 99
California College of Ayurveda 71–72
California College of Physical Arts 72–73
California Institute of Integral Studies 73
California Institute of Massage and Spa Services 73–74
California School of Herbal Studies 74–75, 476
California School of Traditional Hispanic Herbalism 75, 473–74
California Yoga Teachers Association 495
Canadian Academy of Homeopathy 482–83
Canadian Acupressure Institute 359–60
Canadian College of Acupuncture and Oriental Medicine 360–61
Canadian College of Massage and Hydrotherapy 420–21
Canadian College of Naturopathic Medicine 366–67
Canadian Holistic Therapist Training School 421–22, 467–68
Canadian Journal of Herbalism, The 451, 478
Canadian Medical Acupuncture Society 446
Canadian Memorial Chiropractic College 367–68
Canadian Natural Health Association Founded on Natural Hygiene 458, 492
Canadian School of Natural Nutrition 368–69, 491
Capps, Cheri 288, 474
Capri College 188
Career Training Academy 296–97
Carey, Michael C. J. 155
Carlson, Ruth A. 188
Carlson College of Massage Therapy 188–89
Carolina School of Massage Therapy 272–73
Carpenter, Carol 106
Cascade Institute of Massage and Body Therapies 287–88
Case Western Reserve University School of Medicine 500
Cassel-Beckwith, Bonita 300
Caster, Paul 8
Cayce, Edgar 327
Cayce/Reilly School of Massotherapy 327–28

CCAOM. *See* Council of Colleges of Acupuncture and Oriental Medicine
CCE. *See* Council on Chiropractic Education
Cedar Mountain Center for Massage 340
Celsus 16
Centennial College 369–70
Center for a Balanced Life 217
Center for Herbal Studies 288–89, 474
Center for Hypnotherapy Certification 76
Central California School of Body Therapy 76–77
Central Ohio School of Massage 276
Centre of the Web 201
Cernie, Sally 124
Certified natural health practitioner 374
Chan, Grace 379
Charleston School of Massage 305
Chaudhuri, Haridas 73
CHC. *See* Council for Homeopathic Certification
CHE. *See* Council for Homeopathic Education
Checkley, Beth 354
Chelnick, Robert 350
Chemical Injury Information Network 472
Chi Kung. *See* Qigong
Chicago Medical School 497
Chicago National College of Naprapathy 179–80
Chicago School of Massage Therapy 180, 208
Chichon, Patricia 230
Chips, Allen S. 328
Chiropractic xvii, 8–9, 36–37, 77, 98–100, 110, 146–47, 171–73, 182–83, 190–91, 221–24, 260–61, 293–94, 306, 316–18, 367–68, 429, 437, 449, 471
Chiropractic assistant 37, 316–17
Chiropractic technician 172–73
Chom, Barbara Seideneck 131
Choudhury, Bikram 128
Chow, Effie Poy Yew 393
Christensen, Alice 385–86
Chrysalis Center, The 230–31
Churchill, Randal 90
Cicchetti, Jane 231
Clark, Jill 143
Clayton, Clydette 326
Cleveland, C. S. 77, 222
Cleveland, Ruth R. 77, 222
Cleveland Chiropractic College of Kansas City 77, 222
Cleveland Chiropractic College of Los Angeles 77, 222
CNME. *See* Council on Naturopathic Medical Education
Cohen, Bonnie Bainbridge 411
Colbin, Annemarie 260
College of the Botanical Healing Arts 78
Collins, Barbara 346
Colorado Institute for Classical Homeopathy 131–32
Colorado Institute of Massage Therapy 132–33
Colorado School of Healing Arts 133–34
Colorado School of Traditional Chinese Medicine 134–35, 137
Columbia University College of Physicians and Surgeons 499
Commission on Massage Training Accreditation xviii, 21, 432
Community Wholistic Health Center 272

Complementary care 370
COMTA. *See* Commission on Massage Training Accreditation
Connecticut Center for Massage Therapy 144–45
Connecticut Institute for Herbal Studies 145
Connecticut School for Hypnosis and NLP, The 146
Constitutional medicine 379
Conway, John 314
Cooksley, Valerie 396
Coppola, Gloria 232
CORE Institute 156–57
Cottonwood School of Massage Therapy 135–36
Council for Higher Education Accreditation 24, 442
Council for Homeopathic Certification 438
Council of Colleges of Acupuncture and Oriental Medicine 428
Council on Chiropractic Education xvii, 9, 429, 437
Council on Homeopathic Education xviii, 430
Council on Naturopathic Medical Education xviii, 24, 433, 442
Counseling Psychology 97
Craig, Karen E. 307
Crane, Adam 387
Craniosacral therapy 18, 101, 111–12, 133–34, 139, 397, 419, 487
Crawford, Amanda McQuade 247
Creativity Learning Institute 390
Crestone Healing Arts Center 136
Cronin, Kyle 54
Cronin, Michael 54
Crystal Mountain Apprenticeship in the Healing Arts 244
Cumberland Institute for Wellness Education 306–7
Curentur University. *See* American University of Complementary Medicine
Curtiss, Neha 88
Curtiss, Paula 88

Dail, Nancy 193
Dallas Institute of Acupuncture and Oriental Medicine 312–13
Dalphin, Ruth 239
Dandelion Herbal Center 78–79
D'Arcy Lane Institute School of Massage Therapy 370–71
Davis, Elizabeth 103
Day-Break Geriatric Massage Project, The 390–91, 486, 488
Day-Star Method of Yoga 136–37
Dean, Frank E. 260
de Busy, Kathy 359
Deckebach, John 249
Deep muscle therapy 18, 70, 80, 160–61, 169, 186, 298. *See also* Massage therapy and bodywork
Deep tissue massage. *See* Deep muscle therapy
de la Tour, Shatoiya 81
de May, Mynou 253, 466
Desai, Yogi Amrit 203
Desert Institute of the Healing Arts 49–50
Desert Resorts School of Somatherapy 79–80
DeVai, Christine 473
de Vedia, Ana 405
Diamond Lights School of Massage and Healing Arts 80
Dietetics 337–38
Dinsdale, Janice M. 323

Discovery Institute of Clinical Hypnotherapy 208–9
Dr. Andrew Weil's Self Healing 464
Dr. Vodder School — North America 422–23, 486
Dr. Welbe's College of Massage Therapy. *See* Gateway College of Massage Therapy
Do-In 18
Dominion Herbal College 361–62, 474–75
Dongguk Royal University 81
Dossey, Larry 464
DoveStar Institute 391–93
Downeast School of Massage 193
Dreamtime Center for Herbal Studies 328
Driggers, V. Wendell 326
Dry Creek Herb Farm and Learning Center 81–82
Dull, Harold 117
Dunbar, William 350
D'Urso, Margaret L. 149
DuVerger, Douglas H. 229

Earth-Spirit 87
Easterbrooks, Sandra K. 171
Eastern Healing Arts International Training Center 281, 493
Eastern Institute of Hypnotherapy 328–29, 454
East West Academy of Healing Arts/Qigong Institute 393, 460
East-West College of the Healing Arts 289
East West Herb Course 12
East West Institute of Alternative Medicine 201–2
East West Medical Society 360
East West School of Herbology 82, 475
East-West School of Massage Therapy 297
Edge, Raymond 380
Edmonton School of Swedish Relaxation Massage 353–54
Educating Hands School of Massage 157–58
Edwards, Victoria 68
Eisman, George 491
Eisner, Birgit Ball 104
Elias, Jack 340
Ellis, Craig 273
Emory University School of Medicine 497
Emperor's College of Traditional Oriental Medicine 83
Energetic healing 9, 37, 80–81, 209–10, 225, 253, 273–74
ENERGY 459, 492
Energy work 56–57, 324–25
Environmental medicine 9–10, 37, 384, 449–50, 471
Equine sports massage. *See* Massage, veterinary
Equissage ® 28, 329–30, 494
Esalen Institute 83–84
Esalen massage 18, 84, 101
Essential oils therapy. *See* Aromatherapy
EverGreen Herb Garden and School of Integrative Herbology 84–85
EverGreen Wholistic Ministry 84
Expanding Light, The 85
Ezraty, Maty 128

Fairweather, Douglas R. 363
Faulds, Richard 203
FDA. *See* Food and Drug Administration
Federation of Chiropractic Licensing Boards 437
Feldenkrais, Moshe 18
Feldenkrais Guild ® 382

Feldenkrais Guild ® of North America 432, 455–56, 486, 488
Feldenkrais ® Institute of Somatic Education 382
Feldenkrais ® Journal 488
Feldenkrais ® Method 18, 113–14, 393–94, 486–87
Feldenkrais ® Resources 393–94, 486–87
Feldman, Murray 364
Feuerstein, Alice 232
Fiegen, Charles 188
Field, Tiffany 16
Fillmore-Patrick, Heidi 192
Finch University of Health Sciences 497
Finger Lakes School of Massage 255–56
Fischer, Pam 108
Fischer, Warren 359
Fitzgerald, William 27
Five Branches Institute 85–86
Five Elements Center 231
Five Element Training Program 86–87
Flanders, Susan 136
Flocco, Bill 27
Florida Academy of Massage 158
Florida College of Natural Health 158–60
Florida Health Academy 160
Florida Institute of Psychophysical Integration 160–61
Florida Institute of Traditional Chinese Medicine 161
Florida School of Massage 161–63, 255, 348
Florida's Therapeutic Massage School 163
Flower Essence Society 87, 448, 466
Flower essence therapy 35–36, 87, 253, 447–48. *See also* Aromatherapy
Flynn, Arcus 256
Flynn's School of Herbology 256
Food and Drug Administration 14
Foothills College of Massage Therapy 354
Footloose 193–94
Ford, Michael 304
Foster, Jim 320
Foster, Shirley 320
Foundation for Aromatherapy Education and Research, The 394–95
Frawley, David 469
French, Ramona Moody 79
Fritz, Sandy 209
Frontier, Anne M. 352
Frontier School of Midwifery and Family Nursing 22
Future Medicine Publishing 464

Gabriel, Jim 168
Gach, Michael Reed 62
Galante, Lawrence 254
Galen 16
Garcia, Charles 75, 473
Garden State Center for Holistic Health Care 232
Gateway College of Massage Therapy 227
Gauthier, Irene 213
Georgetown University School of Medicine and Health Sciences 496
Georgia Institute of Therapeutic Massage 170–71
GEO Touch 156
Gilchrist, Roger 418
Gill, Carol 236

G-Jo Institute, The 465
Gladstar, Rosemary 74, 82, 108, 322, 476
Glickstein, Bob 198
Gold, Richard 405
Goldberg, Gloria 69
Goodheart, George 17
Gordon, Marilyn 76
Granger, Jocelyn 208
Grant, Ulysses S. 16
Grant MacEwan Community College 355
Gray, Ronald D. 158
Gregg, Constance 156
Griffin, Perl B. 77, 222
Grigore, Gabrielle 229
Groves, Robert L. 282
Guided imagery 10–11, 37, 59–60, 472
Gulliver's Institute for Integrative Nutrition 256–57

Hahnemann, Samuel 13–14, 24
Hahnemann College of Homeopathy 87–88, 483
Hall, Patricia 366
Halpern, Mark 71
Hammerli, Hanna 112
Han, Larry L. 165
Hands of Light 203
Hands On 454
Hands-On Therapy School of Massage 313
Hanna, Thomas 388
HANP. *See* Homeopathic Academy of Naturopathic Physicians
Hao, Tianyou 281
Hari, Sri Yogi 168
Harris, Robert 422
Harrison, Benjamin 16
Harrison, Lewis 253
Harvard Medical School 498
Hawaiian Islands School of Body Therapies 175
Hawai'i College of Traditional Oriental Medicine 174
Healing Hands Institute for Massage Therapy 232–33
Healing Hands School of Holistic Health 88
Healing Hands School of Massage 233–34
Healing Heart Herbals 276–77
Health Academy of North America 483
Health Care Associates 133
Health Choices 234
Health Enrichment Center 209–10
Health Options Institute 298
Health Science 457, 492
Heartwood Institute 88–89
Heiny, Dodie 118
Heller, Joseph 395
Hellerwork 395
Hellerwork International 395
Helm, Bill 120
Helma Institute of Massage Therapy 234–35
Hendler, Denise 305
Hendler, Mark 305
Herbal Connection, The 451, 479
Herbalgram 451, 472, 479
Herbal medicine. *See* Herbology
Herbalpedia 451
Herbal Therapeutics School of Botanical Medicine 235
Herb Companion, The 479
Herb Growing and Marketing Network 450–51, 479

Herbology xviii, 11–12, 37–38, 51, 57–58, 67, 74–75, 78–79, 82, 84–85, 107–9, 118–19, 130, 140–41, 145, 146, 154, 160, 173, 183–84, 191–92, 200–03, 226, 230–31, 235, 247–50, 253, 256, 262–66, 270–71, 273–74, 277, 280–81, 284, 287, 288–89, 302, 304–5, 322–24, 328, 336–38, 351–52, 361–62, 363, 378–79, 381–82, 429–30, 450–52, 472. *See also* Traditional Chinese medicine; Oriental medicine
Herb Research Foundation 451, 479
Herbs for Health 451, 479
Herscu, Paul 403
High Tide 335
Himalayan International Institute of Yoga Science and Philosophy, The 298–99
Hippocrates 16, 23, 24
Hnizdo, Mercedes 235
Hobbs, Herbert 186
Hobbs, Ruthann 186
Hoffman, Beth 284
Holistic counseling 12–13, 478
Holistic Dental Association 452, 480
Holistic Dental Association Newsletter 452, 480
Holistic dentistry 452, 480
Holistic health care 57–58, 67
Holistic health education 12–13, 38–39, 73, 97, 106, 203–4, 302
Holistic health practitioner 12–13, 38–39, 60–61, 72–73, 79–80, 88, 89, 102–3, 106, 107–8, 116–17, 247, 355, 374, 392–93, 406, 477–78
Holistic nursing 13, 39, 263–64, 452, 480
Holistic nutrition. *See* Nutrition
Holistic studies 97, 323
Holmes, Peter 129
Homeopathic Academy of Naturopathic Physicians 439, 452–53, 484
Homeopathic College of Canada 371–72
Homeopathic Educational Services 480, 483
Homeopathy xviii, 13–14, 39, 67, 87–88, 92, 109, 112–13, 125, 131–32, 153–54, 182–83, 211, 220–21, 231, 254–55, 267–70, 290–91, 330–31, 364–65, 371–72, 380–81, 403, 430, 437–39, 452–53, 480–84
Homeopathy, veterinary 284, 460, 481, 482
Homeopathy Today 453, 484
Honolulu School of Massage 175–76
Hopman, Ellen Evert 202, 472
Howell, Patricia Kyritsi 173
Hsiang, Master Chang Yi 176
Hua-Ching Ni 127
Hubbard, Stanley 160
Humanities Center Institute of Applied Health School of Massage, The 163–64
Humber College 371
Hungerford, Myk 66
Hunter, H. Katharine 326
Hydrotherapy 18, 49, 162, 163, 255–56, 383. *See also* Massage therapy and bodywork
Hypnosis. *See* Hypnotherapy
Hypnosis Career Institute 244–45
Hypnosis Motivation Institute 90, 484–85
Hypnotherapy xviii, 14–15, 39–40, 57–58, 63–64, 76, 80, 90, 91–92, 107–8, 116–17, 123, 124–25, 146, 181, 187, 194, 208–11, 236, 242, 245, 275, 279–81, 328–29, 340–41, 353, 390, 392–93, 419, 430–31, 439–40, 454, 484–85

Hypnotherapy Training Institute 90–91
Hypnotism Training Institute of Los Angeles 91–92, 484, 485

ICA. *See* International Chiropractors Association
ICA Review 449, 471
ICA Today 449, 471
ICR. *See* International Council of Reflexologists
ICR Newsletter 460, 493
ICT Kikkawa College 372
ICT Northumberland College 372–73
Idaho Institute of Wholistic Studies 178–79
IMDHA. *See* International Medical and Dental Hypnotherapy Association
IMF. *See* International Myomassethics Federation
IMSTAC. *See* Integrative Massage and Somatic Therapies Accreditation Council
Indei, Fumihiko 173
Independent study degree programs 40
Infant massage 18
Infinity Institute International 210–11
Ingham, Eunice 27, 398
InnoVision Communications 464
Inner Quest Awareness Center of California 187
Insight Publishing 465
Institute for Integrated Therapies 149
Institute for Therapeutic Learning 340–41
Institute for Wholistic Education 470–71
Institute of Aromatherapy, The (ON) 373–74
Institute of Aromatherapy (NJ) 235–36, 468
Institute of Classical Homoeopathy 92
Institute of Dynamic Aromatherapy 341
Institute of Integrative Aromatherapy 395–96
Institute of Materia Medica 3
Institute of Natural Healing Sciences, The 313–14
Institute of Natural Health Sciences 211
Institute of Natural Therapies 211–12
Institute of Psycho-Structural Balancing 92–93
Integrated Touch Therapy for Animals 277–78, 494
Integrative Massage and Somatic Therapies Accreditation Council xviii, 431–32
Integrative medicine 15, 40, 52–53, 267, 496
Integrative Yoga Therapy 396–97
Interactive Guided Imagery (SM) 59–60, 472
International Academy for Reflexology Studies 278
International Alliance of Healthcare Educators® 397, 487
International Ayurvedic Institute 397–98
International Center for Reiki Training 212–13, 493
International Chiropractors Association 449
International College of Applied Kinesiology ® — USA 447
International College of Homeopathy 112–13
International College of Traditional Chinese Medicine of Vancouver 362–63
International Council of Reflexologists 460, 493
International Institute of Reflexology 398
International Institute of Chinese Medicine 245–46, 310
International Institute of Reflexology 27
International Journal of Aromatherapy, The 447, 469
International Massage Association 456
International Medical and Dental Hypnotherapy Association xviii, 210, 430–31, 440, 454, 485
International Myomassethics Federation 432, 456, 489
International Professional School of Bodywork 93–94

International Society for Orthomolecular Medicine 458, 492
International Veterinary Acupuncture Society 398–99
International Woodstock Retreat Center 257–58
International Yoga Studies 399–400
Interweave Press 479
Iqbal, M. 124
Irene's Myomassology Institute 213
Iridology 15–16, 40, 279–81, 378–79, 422, 476–77
ISOM Newsletter 458, 492
Iuppo, Vincent 235
Iyengar, B. K. S. 69
Iyengar Yoga Institute of San Francisco 95, 461, 494
Iyengar Yoga Institute Review 461, 495

Jacobs, Terry S. 67
Janssen, Douglas 198
Jarrell, David G. 166
Jeanne Rose Aromatherapy 468, 475
Jensen, Bernard 16
Jin Shin Do 18, 70, 95–96, 360. *See also* Acupressure
Jin Shin Do Foundation for Bodymind Acupressure 95–96
Jin Shin Jyutsu ® 18, 56–57, 400
John F. Kennedy University 96–97
Johns Hopkins University School of Medicine 498
Johnson, Bev 488
Johnson, Joy K. 160
Jones, Elizabeth 78
Jones, Feather 139
Jones, Mary Jo 252
Jordan, Alan 308
Journal of Holistic Nursing 452, 480
Journal of Oriental Bodywork Therapy 455, 488
Journal of Orthomolecular Medicine 458, 492
Journal of the AHG, The 450, 479
Journal of the American Chiropractic Association 449, 471

Kacera, Walter 378
Kalamazoo Center for the Healing Arts 213–14
Kaley, Deborah 315
Kali Ray Tri Yoga ® 400
Kaltsas, Harrey 151
Kamiya, Kaz 377
Kamiya, Yasuko 377
Kaneko, DoAnn T. 118
Kappas, John G. 90
Karsten, Paul 343
Kasprzyk, David 264
Keeping in Touch 456, 488
Keizer, Willa Esterson 482
Khalsa, Rose Diana 331
Kinnaman, Togi 132
Kinney, Charles 208
Kirksville College of Osteopathic Medicine 502
Kirtland Community College 214–15
Kitchie, George 134
Kitts, Steve 144
Knight-Wind Method of Restorative Therapies 175
Knott, Donald 227
Knott, Joan 227
Koblin, Seymour 116
Kong, Lam 177
Kousaleos, George 156
Kousaleos, Patricia 156

Kozak, Sandra Summerfield 399
Kraftsow, Gary 385
Kreisberg, Joel 269
Kripalu Center for Yoga and Health 203–4
Ku, Su Liang 161
Kubicek, Olga 232
Kunin, Richard 458
Kunz, Barbara 27
Kunz, Kevin 27
Kushi, Aveline 25, 204, 459
Kushi, Michio 25, 204, 459
Kushi Institute 204–5, 443, 489
Kyle, Laraine 396
Kyung San University 97–98

Lad, Vasant 242
LaFleur, Henry 199
LaForce, Jane I. 201
Lake Lanier School of Massage 171
Lakeside School of Massage Therapy 350
Lancaster School of Massage 299
Lancet 13
Lansing Community College 215–16
Lauterstein, David 314
Lauterstein-Conway Massage School, The 314–15
Layden, Bob 353
Lazzaro, Joseph 405
Le Centre Psycho-Corporel 382–83
Lee, Michael 407
Leer, Kitty 234
Lehigh Valley Healing Arts Academy 300
Leidecker Institute 180–81
Les Herbes, Ltd. 466
Levin, Cecile Tovah 100
Lewis, Blair 349
Lewis, Karen 349
Lewis, Rose Marie 186
Lewis School and Clinic of Massage Therapy 186–87
Liang, Shen Ping 311
Life Chiropractic College West 98–99
LifePath School of Massage Therapy 181–82
Life University School of Chiropractic 171–73
Light Lines Wholistic Center 236
Liljequist, Nils 16
Linden Tree Center for Wholistic Health, The 258–59
Ling, Peter 20
Living Naturally 458, 492
Living With Herbs Institute 173
Lofft, Robert B. 433
Logan, Hugh B. 223
Logan College of Chiropractic 223–24
Longo, Angela 177
Loraine's Academy 164–65
Los Angeles College of Chiropractic 99–100
Los Angeles East West Center Institute for Macrobiotic Studies 100
Louise, Roxanne 241
Luka, Robert M. 275
Lust, Benedict 23

McCormick, Patti 279
McGarry, Gina 287
McGrath, Marilyn 297
McGuire, Charlotte 452
McKay School of Massage and Hydrotherapy 383

McKinnon, Judith 100
McKinnon Institute 100–101, 487
McLaughlin, Christine 138
McLaughlin, Craig 138
Macrobiotic Educators Association 204, 443
Macrobiotics 25, 100, 125–26, 204–5
Maharishi International University. *See* Maharishi University of Management
Maharishi Mahesh Yogi 27–28, 189
Maharishi University of Management 27–28, 189–90
Maier, Kathleen 328
MANA see Midwives Alliance of North America
MANA News 457, 489
Mangus-Rogers, Mary E. 348
Manton, Mark 131, 134, 137
Manual lymph drainage 19, 79–80, 397, 420, 423, 486. *See also* Massage therapy and bodywork
Maryland Institute of Traditional Chinese Medicine 196–97
Mascelli, Anne 301
Massage, Oriental 19, 57–58, 67, 101, 185–86, 195–96, 309–11, 389–90, 406. *See also* Amma
Massage, pregnancy 19. *See also* Massage therapy and bodywork
Massage, sports 20, 56–58, 66–67, 70, 101, 126–27, 133–34, 138, 162–63, 184–85, 193, 296–97, 304, 327, 335, 356, 418. *See also* Massage therapy and bodywork
Massage, Swedish 20, 66–67, 101, 193, 276, 296–97, 304, 327. *See also* Massage therapy and bodywork
Massage, Veterinary 28, 47–48, 56–57, 277–78, 330, 371, 494
Massage and Bodywork 455, 489
Massage Institute of Memphis, The 307–8
Massage Institute of New England 205
Massage Magazine 489
Massage therapy and bodywork xviii, 16–21, 40–44, 49, 50, 51–57, 59, 61–62, 64–65, 69–74, 76–77, 79–80, 84, 88, 89, 92–94, 100–8, 111, 114, 116–17, 120–23, 126–27, 129–38, 143–45, 150, 152–54, 156, 157–60, 161–66, 167–71, 175, 176, 178–89, 193, 195–96, 199–200, 203–4, 205–18, 220, 225–30, 232–35, 237–41, 243–44, 246–53, 255–56, 263–65, 268–69, 272–76, 282, 282–83, 283, 285, 288, 289, 292, 295–300, 301–5, 307–9, 311–15, 319–20, 324–26, 332–35, 338–40, 345–50, 352–58, 363–64, 369–71, 373, 376–77, 379, 382–83, 386, 389–93, 404, 406, 412, 413, 417, 418, 421, 431–32, 440–41, 454–56, 485–89. *See also* Deep muscle therapy; Shiatsu; Acupressure; Hydrotherapy; Massotherapy
Massage Therapy Institute of Colorado 137
Massage Therapy Journal 454, 489
Massage Therapy Training Institute LLC 224–25
Massotherapy 279, 327–28, 382–83
Mata, Leela 168
Maternidad La Luz 315–16
Matthews, Nancy 49
Matusow, Vajra 80
Maupin, Edward W. 93
Mauro, Stuart 312
May, Ellen 59
MEA. *See* Macrobiotic Educators Association
MEAC. *See* Midwifery Education Accreditation Council
Medical Acupuncture 446, 465
Medical Herbalism: A Journal for the Clinical Practitioner 479

Medicine Wheel, The — A School of Holistic Therapies 246–47
Meditation instructor 273–74
Meiji College of Oriental Medicine 101–2
Memorial University of Newfoundland Faculty of Medicine 501
Mendocino School of Holistic Massage and Advanced Healing Arts 102–3
Mercer, Tami 308
Mercy College 259–60
Meridian Shiatsu Institute 300–301
Mesmer, Franz Anton 14
Michael Scholes School for Aromatic Studies, The 401–2, 466, 468
Michigan School of Myomassology 216
Michner Institute for Applied Health Sciences, The 374–75, 462
Middle Tennessee Institute of Therapeutic Massage 308
Midwest College of Oriental Medicine 350–51
Midwest Training Institute of Hypnosis 187, 485
Midwifery xviii, 22, 44–45, 103–4, 192–93, 203, 286–87, 293, 315–16, 321–22, 344–45, 410–11, 432–33, 457, 489
Midwifery Education Accreditation Council xviii, 22, 432–33
Midwifery Institute of California 103–4
Midwives Alliance of North America 22, 457, 489
Miesler, Dietrich 390
Mignosa, Laura 145
Miller, Brian 55
Miller, Claire Marie 404
Miller, K. C. 52, 55
Mind-body medicine 67
Minneapolis School of Massage and Bodywork 217–18
Minnesota Center for Shiatsu Study, The 218–19
Minnesota Institute of Acupuncture and Herbal Studies 219–20
Miracchi, Lucia 69
Miscampbell, Danielle 368
Mississauga School of Aromatherapy 421–22, 467–68
Mongan, Dorothy 129
Monterey Institute of Touch 104
Moore, Diana 324
Moore, Marie 76
Moore, Michael 58
Morris Institute of Natural Therapeutics 236–37
Mountain State School of Massage 348–49
Mountainheart School of Bodywork and Transformational Therapy 138
Mount Madonna Center 104–5
Mt. Nittany Institute of Natural Health 301–2
Mount Royal College 355–56
Mueller, E. W. 105
Mueller College of Holistic Studies 105–6
Mulder, Marleen 90
Murai, Master Jiro 400
Muscular Therapy Institute 205–6
Myofascial massage 19, 295, 402
Myofascial Release Treatment Centers and Seminars 402
Myomassethics Forum, The 456, 489
Myomassology 213, 216. *See also* Massage therapy and bodywork

Myotherapy 19, 72–73
Myotherapy College of Utah 320

Nada Productions 494
NAHA. *See* National Association for Holistic Aromatherapy
Naile, Carolyn Scott 313
Naparstek, Belleruth 10
Naprapathy 23, 45, 179–80
NARM. *See* North American Registry of Midwives
NASH. *See* North American Society of Homeopaths
Nassen, Don 146
National Acupuncture and Oriental Medicine Alliance 446–47
National Association for Holistic Aromatherapy 5, 428, 436, 448, 469
National Association of Transpersonal Hypnotherapists 328, 454, 485
National Board of Homeopathic Examiners 439
National Center for Complementary and Alternative Medicine 445
National Center for Homeopathy 330–31, 438, 453, 484
National Certification Board for Therapeutic Massage and Bodywork 21, 440, 441
National Certification Commission for Acupuncture and Oriental Medicine 4, 435, 435–36
National Certification Examination for Therapeutic Massage and Bodywork xviii, 21, 440, 441
National College of Chiropractic 182–83
National College of Naturopathic Medicine 289–91
National College of Oriental Medicine 165–66
National College of Phytotherapy 247–48, 256
National Commission for the Certification of Acupuncturists 12
National Foundation for the Chemically Hypersensitive 450
National Holistic Institute 106–7
National Institute of Massotherapy 278–79
National Institute of Nutritional Education 490–91
National Institutes of Health 17, 204, 445
National Iridology Research Association 16
Natural Gourmet Cookery School, The 260
Natural Healing Institute of Naturopathy 107–8, 463
Naturopathic medicine. *See* Naturopathy
Naturopathic Physicians Licensing Exam 24, 442
Naturopathy xviii, 23–24, 45, 54–55, 148, 290–91, 336–38, 367, 421, 433, 442, 457
NBHE. *See* National Board of Homeopathic Examiners
NCBTMB. *See* National Certification Board for Therapeutic Massage and Bodywork
NCCAM. *See* National Center for Complementary and Alternative Medicine
NCCAOM. *See* National Certification Commission for Acupuncture and Oriental Medicine
NCETMB. *See* National Certification Examination for Therapeutic Massage and Bodywork
NCOC. *See* Nutritional Consultants Organization of Canada
Nealy, Harold 194
Nealy, Jane 194
Nedelec, Mireille 326
Neurolinguistic programming 280–81, 329, 340–41. *See also* Hypnotherapy
Neuromuscular therapy 19, 133–34, 345–46. *See also* Massage therapy and bodywork

New Age Journal 464
New England Center for Aromatherapy. *See* Institute of Dynamic Aromatherapy, The
New England Institute of Ayurvedic Medicine. *See* International Ayurvedic Institute
New England Journal of Homeopathy 484
New England Journal of Medicine xxii, 17
New England School of Acupuncture 206–7
New England School of Clinical Hypnotherapy 194–95
New England School of Homeopathy 403, 484
New Hampshire Institute for Therapeutic Arts 403–4
New Jersey Medical School 499
New Mexico Academy of Healing Arts 248–49
New Mexico College of Natural Healing 249–50
New Mexico Herb Center, The 250
New Mexico School of Natural Therapeutics 250–51
New York Chiropractic College 260–61
New York College for Wholistic Health Education and Research 261–64
New York Institute of Massage 264–65
New York Open Center 265–66
Ni, Hua-Ching 127
Niemiec, Catherine 51
NIRA. *See* National Iridology Research Association
NMT. *See* Neuromuscular therapy
Nolte, Marcia 345
North American Registry of Midwives 22, 442
North American Society of Homeopaths 439, 453, 484
North American Vegetarian Society 458, 492
North Carolina School of Natural Healing 273–74
North Eastern Institute of Whole Health 229–30
Northeast School of Botanical Medicine 266
Northern Lights School of Massage Therapy 220
Northern Prairie Center for Education and Healing Arts 183–84
Northwestern Academy of Homeopathy 220–21
Northwestern College of Chiropractic 221–22
Northwestern Connecticut Community-Technical College 146
Northwestern School of Massage 356–57
Northwest Institute of Acupuncture and Oriental Medicine 342
Northwind Publications 478
Norwich University 323
Nova Southeastern University 496
Novak, Renate 234
Nowell, Herbert 361, 474
NPLEX. *See* Naturopathic Physicians Licensing Exam
Nurturing the Mother 404
Nutrition 24–26, 45, 57–58, 89, 107–8, 116–17, 172, 257, 260, 280–81, 337–38, 369, 442–43, 457–59, 476, 481, 489–92
Nutritional Consultants Organization of Canada 443

Occupational science degree program 57–58
Odey, Jackie 135
O'Donnell, Cynthia 151
Ohanian, Valerie 221
Ohashi 405
Ohashiatsu 405
Ohashi Institute 404–5
Ohio Academy of Holistic Health 279–81
Ohio State University College of Medicine 500

Ohlone Center for Herbal Studies 108–9
Ohm, Ilan Kwang 97
Ohm, Kwee Ja 97
Ohsawa, George 25
Okanagan Valley College of Massage Therapy Ltd. 363–64
Oklahoma School of Natural Healing 282–83
Olivier, Jocelyn 64
Omaha School of Massage Therapy 227–28
Omega Institute 266–67
One Peaceful World 459, 492
One Peaceful World 459, 492
On-site massage 19
Ontario Herbalists' Association 451, 478
Ontario Homeopathic Association 430, 453
Optissage 277
Oregon College of Oriental Medicine 291
Oregon School of Massage 291–92
Oregon School of Midwifery 292–93
Oriental bodywork. *See* Massage, Oriental
Oriental healing arts 89
Oriental massage. *See* Massage, Oriental
Oriental medicine xvii, 3–4, 34–35, 51, 56–57, 81, 83, 97–98, 101–2, 114–16, 119, 150–54, 165–66, 174, 176–77, 219–20, 245–46, 259–60, 262–64, 268–69, 290–91, 291, 310, 311–13, 318–19, 336–38, 343, 350–51, 360–61, 405–6, 413–14, 427–28, 435–36, 446–47, 465. *See also* Traditional Chinese medicine; Acupuncture; Herbology
Orthobionomy 19
Orthomolecular medicine 457–59. *See also* Nutrition
Orthopaedic Massage Therapy Institute, The 356–57
Othmer, Siegfried 387
Othmer, Susan 387
Our Lady of Lourdes Institute of Wholistic Studies 237–39
Our Toxic Times 472
Owens, Sister Helen 238

Pacheco, Jo-Anne 304
Pacific Academy of Homeopathy 109
Pacific College of Oriental Medicine 405–6
Pacific Institute of Aromatherapy 407, 468–69
Packard, Candis Cantin 84
Packard, Lonnie 84
Palkhivala, Aadil 347
Palmer, Daniel David 8, 23, 190
Palmer College of Chiropractic 110, 190–91
Palmer College of Chiropractic West 110
Palmer School of Chiropractic 23
Paracelsus 13
Parker, Carolee 300
Parker, Cindy 277
Parker, James William 316
Parker College of Chiropractic 316–17
Peck, Darrell J. 227
Pelava, Cari Johnson 218
Pennsylvania Institute of Massage Therapy 303
Pennsylvania School of Muscle Therapy 303–4
Perkinson, Stephen 278
Phillips, Judy 110, 487
Phillips School of Massage 110–11, 487
Phoenix Institute of Herbal Medicine and Acupuncture 50–51
Phoenix Rising Yoga Therapy 407

Phoenix Therapeutic Massage College 51–52
Platt, Vicki N. 170
Polarity Center and Shamanic Studies, The 331–32
Polarity Center of Colorado 139
Polarity Healing Arts 111–12
Polarity Realization Institute 407–9
Polarity therapy xviii–xix, 19, 26–27, 45–46, 56–57, 89, 111–12, 139, 162–63, 198–99, 248–49, 253, 257–59, 265–66, 331, 375–76, 407–9, 418–19, 433, 459–60, 492
Polarity Therapy Center of Marin 112
Porter, Arnold 359
Posse, Nils 16
Posse Institute 16
Potomac Massage Training Institute 149–50
Practical Horseman 28
Praxis College of Health Arts and Sciences 283
Pregnancy massage. *See* Massage, pregnancy
Program in Integrative Medicine xv, 15, 52–53, 496
Pryor, Cissie 309
Pryor, David 309
Pulse 455

Qi: The Journal of Traditional Eastern Health and Fitness 465
Qigong 19–20, 46, 55–56, 120, 281, 310, 393, 460, 493
Qigong and Human Life Research Foundation, The 281, 493
Qigong Newsletter 460, 493
Quantum-Veritas International University Systems 112–13
Quigley, David 63
Qutab, Abbas 398

Radha, Swami Sivananda 365
RainStar College 53–54
Rajkowski, Sister M. Janine 217
Ramm, Clark 102
Ramm, Theresa 102
Rand, William L. 212
Randolph, Theron G. 9, 10
Ray, Kali 400
Ray-Reese, Donna 113
Reaching Your Potential 375–76
Rebirthing 102–3
Redfern Training Systems School of Massage 184–85
Redinger, Brandie 178
Reel, Joseph P. 244
Reese, Mark 113
Reese Movement Institute 113–14
Reflexology 20, 27, 46, 55–56, 132–33, 135–38, 149, 162–63, 184–85, 193–94, 238–40, 265–67, 278–80, 300, 302, 325–26, 356, 366, 373–74, 398, 422, 443–44, 460, 493
Reiki 20, 46–47, 80, 166, 212–13, 242, 258–59, 279–81, 329, 392–93, 493–94
Reiki Plus Institute ® 166, 493–94
Reilly, Harold 327
Renner, Kamala 391
Rerucha, Nancy Ashmead 335
Rerucha, Paul 335
re-Source 114
Retuta, Dan 136
Ribeiro, Cynthia 126
Richmond Academy of Massage 332

Rimmel, Al 487
Ritchie, J. Frederick 252
R. J. Buckle Associates, LLC 409, 467
Rocky Mountain Center for Botanical Studies
    139–41, 479
Rocky Mountain Herbal Institute 226–27
Rocky Mountain Institute of Yoga and Ayurveda 141
Rogers, Robert 348
Rogers, Sherry 9
Rolf, Ida P. 20, 141
Rolfing 20
Rolf Institute of Structural Integration 141–42
Rongo, Jamie 49
Rongo, Joseph 49
Rosen, Rick 272
Rosen-Pyros, Mary 166
Rosen-Pyros, Michael 166
Rossman, Martin 59, 472
Rothenberg, Amy 403
Rotko, Marilyn A. 216
Rowland, Theresa 241
Royal University of America. *See* Dongguk Royal
    University
Rubenfeld, Ilana 409
Rubenfeld Synergy Center, The 409–10
Rubenfeld Synergy Method 409–10
Rudnianin, Harold Roy 211
Russell, Jody 53
RxUB Corps 487

Sage Femme Midwifery School 410–11
Sage Mountain Herbal Retreat Center 322, 476
St. Charles School of Massage Therapy 225–26
St. John, Paul 168
St. Louis University School of Medicine 499
Saito, Kensen 377
Samra University of Oriental Medicine 114–15
Sanchez, Tony 495
Santa Barbara College of Oriental Medicine 115–16
Sarasota School of Massage Therapy 166–67
Sasso, Marcia C. 439
Satchidananda, Sri Swami 332
Satchidananda Ashram — Yogaville 332–33
Sault College of Applied Arts and Technology
    376–77
Scentsitivity 448, 469
Schechter, Steve 107
Scherer Institute of Natural Healing 251–52
Schmeeckle, Wayne 52
Schneider, Meir 411
Scholes, Michael 401–2, 466
School for Body-Mind Centering ®, The 411
School for Self-Healing 411–12
School of Asian Healing Arts 239–40
School of Healing Arts 116–17
School of Homeopathy, The (CA) 483
School of Homoeopathy, New York, The 267–68
School of Natural Healing, The 320–21, 476
School of Natural Medicine 463–64
School of Shiatsu and Massage at Harbin Hot
    Springs 117
Schreiber, John 71
Schreiber, Mary 28
Seattle Institute of Oriental Medicine 343
Seattle Massage School. *See* Ashmead College School
    of Massage
Seattle Midwifery School 343–45

Sechuck, Joanna 230
Self-healing 411–12
Seminar Network International 167–68
7 Song 266
Shambhava School of Yoga 142–43
Shannon, Betty Z. 155
Shattuck, Arthur D. 351, 352
Shaw, Kristina 233
SHEN therapy. *See* Therapeutic touch
Sheppard-Hanger, Sylla 154
Sherman College of Straight Chiropractic 306
Shew, Cheryl 275
Shi, Cheng 134
Shiatsu 20, 47, 49–50, 56, 62–63, 70, 74, 117, 118,
    133–36, 153–54, 173–74, 193, 195–96, 201–2,
    218–19, 230, 237–40, 296–98, 301–2, 360,
    369–70, 377–78, 405–6, 487–88. *See also*
    Acupressure; Massage therapy and bodywork
Shiatsu Academy of Tokyo 377
Shiatsu Massage School of California 117–18, 487–88
Shaitsu School of Canada 377–78, 488
SHI Integrative Medical Massage School 281–82
Shutes, Jade 341
Siegel, Gary 258
Siegel, Regina 258
Sierra Institute of Herbal Studies 118–19
Silver, Faeterri 324
Simillimum 453, 484
Singingtree, Daphne 292
Sino-American Medical Rehabilitation Association
    114
Sivananda Ashram Yoga Camp 423
Slawson, David 289
Smith, Carey 272
Smith, Fritz Frederick 441
Smith, Michael 359
Smith, Oakley 23
Smith, Sherry 375
So, James Tin Yau 206
Sohn, Robert 262
Sohn, Tina 262
Soma Institute 345–46
Somatic Arts Institute 357–58
Somatic therapy 357–58
Somerset School of Massage Therapy 240–41
Sommerman, Eric 221
Soule, Deb 191
South Baylo University 119
Southeastern School of Neuromuscular and
    Massage Therapy 412–13
Southern Illinois University School of Medicine 497
Southwest Acupuncture College 310, 413–14
Southwest College of Naturopathic Medicine and
    Health Sciences 54–55
Southwest Institute of Healing Arts 55–58
Southwest School of Botanical Medicine 58
South West School of Massage 143–44
Spanos, Tasso 295
Spa treatments 56–57, 74, 138, 169–70, 184–86, 335.
    See also Massage therapy and bodywork
Spectrum Center School of Massage 346
Spirit of the Earth Centre for Herbal Education and
    Earth Awareness 378–79, 477
Spirituality, health and medicine 47, 336–38
Sports massage. *See* Massage, sports
State University of New York — Buffalo School of
    Medicine and Biomedical Sciences 499–500

State University of New York — Syracuse Health
    Science Center at Syracuse 500
Staying Well with Guided Imagery 10
Stens Corporation 414–15
Stephens, Eric 291
Stetser, Janet E. 194
Stewart, Gail 114
Stillpoint Clinics 356
Stillpoint Program at Greenfield Community
    College, The 207–8
Stocks, Susan E. 76
Stockwell, Shelly 390
Stone, Darlene 243
Stone, J. N. 317
Stone, Randolph 26
Strauss, Gary B. 111
Streicher, Christoph 394
Structural integration 20, 348–49, 418
Studio Yoga 241
Subconsciously Speaking 454, 485
Sundermann, Wanda 404
Sutherland, Christine 379
Sutherland-Chan School and Teaching Clinic
    379–80
Svoboda, Robert 242, 470
Swedish Health Institute 16
Swedish Institute School of Massage Therapy
    268–69
Swedish massage. *See* Massage, Swedish

Tai chi teacher training 47, 167–68
Tai Hsuan Foundation College of Acupuncture and
    Herbal Medicine 176–77
Taoist Sanctuary of San Diego 120
Taos School of Massage 252
Taylor, Charles 16
Taylor, George 16
Teeguarden, Marsaa 95
Teleosis School of Homeopathy 269–70
Tennessee Institute of Healing Arts 308–9
Tennessee School of Massage 309
Texas Chiropractic College 317–18
Texas College of Traditional Chinese Medicine
    318–19
Texas Tech University School of Medicine 501
TFHKA. *See* Touch for Health Kinesiology
    Association
TFHKA Annual Journal 456
Therapeutic Massage Training Institute 274
Therapeutic touch 21
3HO International Kundalini Yoga Teachers
    Association 415
Tian Enterprises 281, 493
Tiberi, Alex 405
Tierra, Michael 12, 82, 475
Tirtha, Swami Sada Shiva 255
Toomim, Marjorie K. 68, 471
Toporovsky, Jerry 195, 333
Toronto School of Homeopathic Medicine 380–81,
    484
Toronto School of Traditional Chinese Medicine
    381–82
Tosh, Robert W. 303
Touch for Health 280–81, 415–16
Touch for Health Kinesiology Association 415–16,
    456, 488
Touching for Health Center 121–22

Touch Research Institute 16, 17
Touch Therapy Institute ®, The 120–21
Traditional Acupuncture Institute 197–98
Traditional Chinese Medical College of Hawaii 177–78
Traditional Chinese medicine 3–4, 60–61, 65–66, 85–86, 127–28, 134–35, 145, 153–56, 161, 196–97, 342–43, 359, 362–63, 381–82, 427–28, 435–36, 445–47, 465. *See also* Oriental medicine; Acupuncture; Herbology
Trager, Milton 21, 416
Trager Institute, The 416–17
Trager ® Method 21, 416–17
Triangle Macrobiotics Association 459, 492
Tri-City School of Massage 346–47
Trigger point therapy 21, 295
Trinity College 122
Tri-State College of Acupuncture 270–71
Tsuei, Wei 60
Tufts University School of Veterinary Medicine 28
Tui Na see Acupressure
Tulane University School of Medicine 498
Twin Lakes College of the Healing Arts 122–23

Ullman, Dana 480, 483
Ulrich, Gail 200
United Plant Savers 322, 451–52, 476, 479
United Plant Savers Newsletter 452, 479
United States Secretary of Education 24, 442
United States Yoga Association 124, 495
Universal Therapeutic Massage Institute 252–53
University of Alberta 358
University of Arizona xv, 15, 52–53, 496
University of Bridgeport 146–48
University of Bridgeport College of Chiropractic 146–47
University of Bridgeport College of Naturopathic Medicine 147–48
University of California — Los Angeles UCLA School of Medicine 496
University of Cincinnati College of Medicine 500
University of Kansas School of Medicine 497
University of Kentucky College of Medicine 497
University of Louisville School of Medicine 497–98
University of Maryland at Baltimore School of Medicine 498
University of Medicine and Dentistry of New Jersey 499
University of Miami 16
University of Miami School of Medicine 497
University of Minnesota Duluth School of Medicine 498–99
University of Minnesota Medical School — Minneapolis 499
University of Nevada School of Medicine 499
University of New Mexico School of Medicine 499
University of Osteopathic Medicine and Health Sciences 502
University of Saskatchewan College of Medicine 501
University of Virginia School of Medicine 501
University of Washington School of Medicine 501

University of Wisconsin Medical School 501
Unlimited Potential Institute 241–42
Unruh, Gwynne 249
Utah College of Massage Therapy 417–18
Utah College of Midwifery 321–22, 489
Utting, Brian 339
Utting School of Massage, Brian. *See* Brian Utting School of Massage

Valley Hypnosis Center 124–25
Vancouver Homeopathic Academy 364–65
VanDeGrift, Karen 178
Vaupel, Jeannette 183
Vaurigaud, Geraldine 163
Vedic medicine 27–28, 47, 189–90
Vedic psychology 27–28, 47, 189–90
Vega Institute 125–26
Vegedine 491–92
Vegetarianism 25, 458, 459, 491–92
Vegetarian Journal 459, 492
Vegetarian Resource Group, The 459, 492
Vegetarian Times 492
Vegetarian Voice 458, 492
Veggie Life 492
Vermont College of Norwich University 323
Vermont School of Herbal Studies 323
Vermont School of Professional Massage 324
Veterinary health care 47–48, 284, 329–30, 398–99, 460. *See also* Massage, Veterinary; Homeopathy, Veterinary
Veterinary massage. *See* Massage, Veterinary
Viniyoga 385
Virginia School of Massage 333–34
Vishnu-Devananda, Swami 423
Vitamin therapy 25
Vodder, Emil 422
Vodder, Estrid 422
Vodder School — North America, Dr. *See* Dr. Vodder School — North America
von Peczely, Ignatz 15, 16

Wake Forest University School of Medicine 500
Walford, Lisa 128
Walker, Constance 284
Walker, Richard 284
Washer, Rhonda 181
Watsu ® 117
Watts, Stuart 310
Wayne State University School of Medicine 498
Weed, Susun S. 271, 473, 477
Weil, Andrew 52, 464
Welch, Carol 387
Wellness and Massage Training Institute 185–86
Wellness College of Vermont 324–25
Wellness consultant 225
Wellness Institute (CO) 418–19
Wellness Institute, The (WA) 419
Wellness Training Center 275
Wellspring School of Therapeutic Bodywork 216–17
Wesland Institute 58–59, 485
Westbrook University 255, 398
West Coast College of Massage Therapy 420–21

Western Institute of Neuromuscular Therapy 126–27
Western States Chiropractic College 293–94
Western University of Health Sciences 502
Westwood Publishing 484
Whalen-Shaw, Patricia 277
White, Ralph 265
White River School of Massage 59
Whole You School of Massage and Bodywork, The 275–76
Wholistic Innerworks Foundation 246
Wicke, Roger 12, 226
Wilderness Leadership International 478
Wild Rose College of Natural Healing 477–78
Wilk, Chester A. 8
Williams, Ruth 346
Williams, Sid E. 172
Wind, Lynn 175
Windsor, James 327
Winston, David 235
Winters, Nancy 319
Winters School, The 319–20
Wisconsin Institute of Chinese Herbology 351–52
Wisconsin Institute of Natural Wellness 352
Wise, Ruth 287
Wise, Tracy 287
Wise Woman Center 271, 473, 477
WMB Hypnosis Training Center 352–53
Wolfer, Susan 439, 452
Wolski, Rhonda A. 184
Wood, Mathew 192
World Health Organization 3, 11
World Qigong Federation 460
Worldwide Aquatic Bodywork Association 117
Wright, Kyle C. 412
Wu, Mary X. 381
Wyrick, Dana 419
Wyrick Institute for European Manual Lymph Drainage 419–20

Yasodhara Ashram 365
Yellow Emperor of China 3
Yen, Johanna Chu 155
Yoga xix, 28–30, 461, 494–95
Yoga Biomedical Trust 29
Yoga Center, The 198
Yoga Centers 347
Yoga College of India 128
Yoga Journal 28–29, 495
Yoga teacher training 48, 57, 69, 85, 95, 105, 124, 128, 129, 136–37, 141, 143, 168, 198, 203–4, 238–41, 267, 299, 326–27, 332–33, 347, 365, 385–86, 392–93, 396, 399, 400–1, 407, 415, 423, 433–34, 461, 494–95
Yoga Works 128–29
Yogi Hari's Ashram 168, 494
Yo San University 127–28

Zeng, Michael 245
Zero Balancing ® 397, 441–42
Zero Balancing Association ®, The 441–42
Zimberoff, Diane 419
Zukausky, Gisella 187